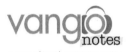

Hear it. Get It.

In partnership with Audible Education

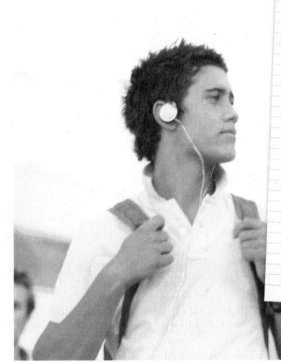

Pearson Nursing Reviews & Rationales

Medical-Surgical Nursing

Third Edition

SERIES EDITOR

MaryAnn Hogan, MSN, RN

Clinical Assistant Professor
School of Nursing
University of Massachusetts–Amherst
Amherst, Massachusetts

CONSULTING EDITORS

Nancy C. Dentlinger, RN, MS, EdD

Associate Professor
University of Central Oklahoma
Edmond, Oklahoma

Valeria Ramdin, PhD(c), MS, APRN-BC

Assistant Dean, Nursing
Northeastern University
Boston, Massachusetts

PEARSON

Boston   Columbus   Indianapolis   New York   San Francisco   Upper Saddle River
Amsterdam   Cape Town   Dubai   London   Madrid   Milan   Munich   Paris   Montréal   Toronto
Delhi   Mexico City   São Paulo   Sydney   Hong Kong   Seoul   Singapore   Taipei   Tokyo

Director of Readypoint™: Maura Connor
Executive Editor: Jennifer Farthing
Developmental Editor: Rachael Zipperlen
Editorial Assistant: Deirdre MacKnight
Director, Digital Product Development: Alex Marciante
Media Product Manager: Travis Moses-Westphal
Vice President, Director Sales & Marketing: David Gesell
Senior Marketing Manager: Phoenix Harvey
Marketing Coordinator: Michael Sirinides
Director of Media Production: Allyson Graesser
Media Project Manager: Rachel Collett

Managing Editor, Production: Patrick Walsh
Production Liaison: Maria Reyes
Production Editor: GEX Publishing Services
Manufacturing Manager: Lisa McDowell
Art Director/Cover Designer: Christopher Weigand
Cover Designer: Dina Curro
Cover image: Lisa F. Young/Shutterstock.com
Composition: GEX Publishing Services
Printer/Binder: Edwards Brothers Malloy
Cover Printer: Lehigh/Phoenix Color Hagerstown

Notice: Care has been taken to confirm the accuracy of the information presented in this book. The authors, editors, and the publisher, however, cannot accept any responsibility for errors or omissions or for the consequences for application of the information in this book and make no warranty, express or implied, with respect to its contents.

The authors and the publisher have exerted every effort to ensure that drug selections and dosages set forth in this text are in accord with current recommendations and practice at time of publication. However, in view of ongoing research, changes in government regulations, and the constant flow of information relating to drug therapy and drug reactions, the reader is urged to check the package inserts of all drugs for any change in indications of dosage and for added warnings and precautions. This is particularly important when the recommended agent is a new and/or infrequently employed drug.

The authors and publisher disclaim all responsibility for any liability, loss, injury, or damage incurred as a consequence, directly or indirectly, of the use and application of any of the contents of this volume.

Library of Congress Cataloging-in-Publication Data

Medical-surgical nursing. -- 3rd ed. / [edited by] MaryAnn Hogan ; consulting editors,
Nancy C. Dentlinger, Valeria Ramdin.
   p. ; cm. -- (Pearson nursing reviews & rationales)
 Includes bibliographical references and index.
 ISBN 978-0-13-308360-6 (pbk.)
 I. Hogan, Mary Ann, MSN. II. Dentlinger, Nancy C. III. Ramdin, Valeria. IV. Series:
Pearson nursing reviews & rationales series.
 [DNLM: 1. Nursing Process--Examination Questions. 2. Nursing
Process--Outlines. 3. Nursing Care--methods--Examination Questions. 4. Nursing
Care--methods--Outlines. 5. Perioperative Nursing--methods--Examination Questions.
6. Perioperative Nursing--methods--Outlines. WY 18.2]

 610.73--dc23
                        2012041769

10 9 8 7 6 5 4 3 2 1

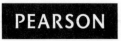

ISBN-13: 978-0-13-308360-6
ISBN-10: 0-13-308360-8

Contents

Welcome to the Pearson Nursing Reviews & Rationales Series!

This series has been specifically designed to provide a clear and concentrated review of important nursing knowledge in the following content areas:

- Anatomy & Physiology
- Nursing Fundamentals
- Nutrition & Diet Therapy
- Fluids, Electrolytes, & Acid–Base Balance
- Medical-Surgical Nursing
- Pathophysiology
- Pharmacology
- Maternal-Newborn Nursing
- Child Health Nursing
- Mental Health Nursing
- Health & Physical Assessment
- Leadership & Management

The books in this series are designed for use either by current nursing students as a study aid for nursing course work, for NCLEX-RN® exam preparation, or by practicing nurses seeking a comprehensive yet concise review of a nursing specialty or subject area.

This series is truly unique. One of its most special features is that it has been developed and reviewed by a large team of nurse educators from across the United States and Canada to ensure that each chapter is edited by a nurse expert in the content area under study. The series editor, MaryAnn Hogan, designed the overall series in collaboration with a core Pearson team to take full advantage of Pearson's cutting-edge technology. The consulting editors for each book, also experts in that specialty area, then reviewed all chapters and test questions submitted for comprehensiveness and accuracy. Finally, MaryAnn Hogan reviewed the chapters in each book for consistency, accuracy, and applicability to the NCLEX-RN® Test Plan.

All books in the series are identical in their overall design for your convenience. As an added value, each book comes with a comprehensive support package, including access to additional questions online, complete eText, and a tear-out *NursingNotes* card for clinical reference and quick review.

What's New to this Edition?

- Completely updated review material reflecting the 2013 NCLEX-RN® Test Plan
- Online access to NursingReviewsandRationales.com http://nursingreviewsandrationales.com/ where students can complete quizzes on the computer to practice for the NCLEX® experience
- Includes a fully searchable eText version of the book as well as valuable note-taking and highlighting tools
- 850 updated or brand-new NCLEX®-style practice test questions
- Features new alternate-item format questions
- The latest test prep advice from MaryAnn Hogan, trusted expert in what nursing students need to know

Study Tips

Use of this book should help simplify your review. To make the most of your valuable study time, also follow these simple but important suggestions:

1. Use a weekly calendar to schedule study sessions.
   - Outline the timeframes for all of your activities (home, school, appointments, etc.) on a weekly calendar.
   - Find the "holes" in your calendar, which are the times when you can plan to study. Add study sessions to the calendar at times when you can expect to be mentally alert and follow your plan!
2. Create the optimal study environment.
   - Eliminate external sources of distraction, such as television, telephone, etc.
   - Eliminate internal sources of distraction, such as hunger, thirst, or dwelling on items or problems that cannot be worked on at the moment.
   - Take a break for 10 minutes or so after each hour of concentrated study both as a reward and an incentive to keep studying.

3. Use pre-reading strategies to increase comprehension of chapter material.
   - Skim read the headings in the chapter (because they identify chapter content).
   - Read the definitions of key terms, which will help you learn new words to comprehend chapter information.
   - Review all graphic aids (figures, tables, boxes) because they are often used to explain important points in the chapter.
4. Read the chapter thoroughly but at a reasonable speed.
   - Comprehension and retention are actually enhanced by not reading too slowly.
   - Do take the time to reread any section that is unclear to you.
5. Summarize what you have learned.
   - Use the accompanying online resource, NursingReviewsandRationales.com, to test yourself with hundreds of NCLEX-RN®-style practice questions.
   - Review again any sections that correspond to questions you answered incorrectly or incompletely.

Test-Taking Strategies

Test-taking strategies accompany the rationales for every question in the series. These strategies will assist you to select the correct answer by breaking down the question, even if you do not know the correct response. Use the following strategies to increase your success on nursing tests or examinations:

- Get sufficient sleep and have something to eat before taking a test. Avoid concentrated sweets before a test, however, to prevent rapid upward and then downward surges in your blood glucose. Also avoid high-fat foods that will make you sleepy.
- Take deep breaths during the test as needed. Remember, the brain requires both oxygen and glucose as fuel.
- Read the question carefully, identifying the stem, all the options, and any critical words or phrases in either the stem or options.
  - Critical words in the stem such as "most important" indicate the need to set priorities, since more than one option is likely to contain a statement that is technically correct.
  - Remember that the presence of red flag words such as *never* or *only* in an answer option is more likely to make that option incorrect.

- Determine who is the client in the question; often this is the person with the health problem, but it may also be a significant other, relative, friend, or another nurse.
- Decide whether the stem is a true response stem or a false response stem. With a true response stem, the correct answer will be a true statement, and vice-versa.
- Determine what the question is really asking, sometimes referred to as the core issue of the question. Evaluate all answer options in relation to this issue, and not strictly to the "correctness" of the statement in each individual option.
- Eliminate options that are obviously incorrect, then go back and reread the stem. Evaluate those remaining options against the stem once more to make a final selection.
- If two answers seem similar and correct, try to decide whether one of them is more global or comprehensive. If one option includes the alternative option within it, it is likely that the more global option is the correct answer.

The NCLEX-RN® Licensing Examination

Upon graduation from a nursing program, successful completion of the NCLEX-RN® licensing examination is required to begin professional nursing practice. The NCLEX-RN® exam is a Computer Adaptive Test (CAT) that ranges in length from 75 to 265 individual (stand-alone) test items, depending on your performance during the examination. The blueprint for the exam is reviewed and revised every three years by the National Council of State Boards of Nursing using the results of a job analysis study of new graduate nurses practicing within the first six months after graduation. Each question on the exam is coded to a *Client Need Category* and an *Integrated Process*.

Client Need Categories. There are four categories of client needs, and each exam will contain a minimum and maximum percent of questions from each category. Each major category has subcategories within it. The *Client Needs* categories according to the NCLEX-RN® Test Plan effective April 2013 are as follows:

- Safe, Effective Care Environment
  - Management of Care (17–23%)
  - Safety and Infection Control (9–15%)
- Health Promotion and Maintenance (6–12%)
- Psychosocial Integrity (6–12%)
- Physiological Integrity
  - Basic Care and Comfort (6–12%)
  - Pharmacological and Parenteral Therapies (12–18%)

- Reduction of Risk Potential (9–15%)
- Physiological Adaptation (11–17%)

Integrated Processes. The integrated processes identified on the NCLEX-RN® Test Plan effective April 2013, with condensed definitions, are as follows:

- Nursing Process: a scientific problem-solving approach used in nursing practice; consisting of assessment, analysis, planning, implementation, and evaluation.
- Caring: client–nurse interaction(s) characterized by mutual respect and trust and that are directed toward achieving desired client outcomes.

- Communication and Documentation: verbal and/or nonverbal interactions between nurse and others (client, family, health care team); a written or electronic recording of activities or events that occur during client care.
- Teaching/Learning: facilitating client's acquisition of knowledge, skills, and attitudes that lead to behavior change.

More detailed information about this examination may be obtained by visiting the National Council of State Boards of Nursing website at http://www.ncsbn.org and viewing the *2013 NCLEX-RN® Test Plan.*[1]

---

[1]Reference: National Council of State Boards of Nursing, Inc. *2013 NCLEX-RN® Test Plan.* Effective April, 2013. Retrieved from https://www.ncsbn.org/2013_NCLEX_RN_Test_Plan.pdf.

HOW TO GET THE MOST OUT OF THIS BOOK

Each chapter has the following elements to guide you during review and study:

Chapter Objectives describe what you will be able to know or do after learning the material covered in the chapter.

Objectives

➤ Discuss the use of the nursing process as it applies to care of the adult client.
➤ Describe common physical assessment procedures used to examine the adult client.
➤ Identify laboratory tests commonly used to monitor the status of the adult client.
➤ Identify diagnostic tests commonly used to detect health problems in the adult client.

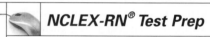

NCLEX-RN® Test Prep

Use the accompanying online resource, NursingReviewsandRationales, to test yourself with hundreds of NCLEX®-style practice questions.

Review at a Glance contains a glossary of key terms used in the chapter, with definitions provided up-front and available at your fingertips, to help you stay focused and make the best use of your study time.

Review at a Glance

afterload resistance that ventricles must overcome to eject blood into systemic circulation; directly related to arterial blood pressure

angina pectoris chest pain resulting from restricted blood flow to myocardium

bradycardia heart rate less than 60 beats per minute

cardiac cycle one complete heartbeat; includes 2 phases: systole (ventricular contraction) and diastole (ventricular relaxation and refilling)

cardiac output (CO) volume of blood in liters ejected by heart each minute; indicator of pump function of heart; normal adult CO is 4–8 L/min; $CO = HR \times SV$

Pretest provides a 10-question quiz as a sample overview of the material covered in the chapter and helps you decide in what areas you need the most—or the least—review.

PRETEST

1 A client with hypertension has a blood pressure of 158/90 after 6 months of intensive exercise and diet modifications. The nurse makes which appropriate statement to the client at this time?

1. "Continue the current treatment plan as your blood pressure is being adequately controlled."
2. "Your current treatment plan is ineffective and will be discontinued; medications will be required instead."
3. "Try to double your exercise time and maintain dietary modifications to continue to reduce your blood pressure."
4. "Medication therapy will likely need to be started along with continuing your exercise and diet program."

Practice to Pass questions are open-ended, stimulate critical thinking, and reinforce mastery of the chapter information.

Practice to Pass

A client newly admitted to a long-term care facility exhibits confusion. What client assessments would be necessary to determine whether the client is experiencing delirium (acute confusion) versus dementia (chronic confusion)?

NCLEX® Alert identifies concepts that are likely to be tested on the NCLEX-RN® examination. Be sure to learn the information highlighted wherever you see this icon.

Case Study, found at the end of the chapter, provides an opportunity for you to use your critical thinking and clinical reasoning skills to "put it all together." It describes a true-to-life client case situation and asks you open-ended questions about how you would provide care for that client and/or family.

Case Study

C. S., a 60-year-old truck driver, has been diabetic and has required insulin therapy for the past twenty years. Diabetic neuropathy has led to several complications, including end-stage renal disease, which he developed two years ago. He now receives hemodialysis three times a week and has an AV fistula in his left forearm. Yesterday, C. S. presented in the Emergency Department with a respiratory infection and was hospitalized with pneumonia, hypertension, and fluid overload. He will receive dialysis while on your nursing unit.

Posttest provides an additional 10-question quiz at the end of the chapter. It provides you with feedback about mastery of the chapter material following review and study. All pretest and posttest questions contain comprehensive rationales for the correct and incorrect answers and are coded according to cognitive level of difficulty, NCLEX-RN® Test Plan category of client need, and integrated process.

POSTTEST

1 A client presents with skin lesions that are raised, reddened, round, and covered with silvery white scales. The nurse concludes that the client most likely has which of the following conditions?

1. Eczema
2. Contact dermatitis
3. Psoriasis
4. Poison ivy

NCLEX-RN® Test Prep: NursingReviewsandRationales.com

For those who want to prepare for the NCLEX-RN®, practicing online will help you become more familiar with the computer-based testing experience, especially for the new alternate item formats such as media-enhanced, hot spot, and exhibit questions. With this new edition, use the code printed inside the front cover of the book to access Nursing Reviews and Rationales, which offers 850 practice questions using all NCLEX®-style formats. This includes the practice questions found in all chapters of the book as well as 30 additional questions per chapter. Nursing Reviews & Rationales allows you to choose two ways to prepare for the NCLEX-RN®. Both approaches personalize your practice experience according to what stage you are at in your NCLEX® preparation:

Nursing Reviews and Rationales includes the eText version *Pearson Medical-Surgical Nursing Reviews and Rationales*, Third Edition. This eText is fully searchable and includes features like note-taking, highlighting, and more. The eText allows you to take your review with you anywhere you have an internet connection to NursingReviewsandRationales.com.

NursingNotes Card

This tear-out card provides a reference for frequently used facts and information related to the subject matter of the book. These are designed to be useful in the clinical setting, when quick and easy access to information is so important!

About the Medical-Surgical Nursing Book

Chapters in this book cover "need-to-know" information about nursing management of a wide variety of health problems. The first chapter reviews nursing process and diagnostic and laboratory studies relevant to medical-surgical nursing. Chapters 2 through 16 explore health problems related to specific body systems. The final chapter discusses health problems commonly encountered in emergency and critical care settings. Mastery of the information in this book and effective use of the test-taking strategies described will help you be confident and successful in testing situations, including the NCLEX-RN®, and in actual clinical practice.

Acknowledgements

This book is a monumental effort of collaboration. Without the contributions of many individuals, this edition of *Medical-Surgical Nursing: Reviews and Rationales* would not have been possible. Thank you to all the contributors and reviewers who devoted their time and talents to the third edition. The contributors for this edition are Nancy Dentlinger, RN, MS, EdD, University of Central Oklahoma and Valeria Ramdin, PhD(c), MS, APRN-BC, Northeastern University. Additional contributors who reviewed and revised questions for this edition are Susan E. Lewis, MSN, RN, CNE, Delaware Technical Community College; Kathleen M. Reilly Dolin, DNP, RN, Northampton Community College; and Rosemary Timmerman, MSN, RN, CCRN-CSC-CMC, CCNS, Providence

Alaska Medical Center. The reviewers for this edition are Jamie L. Houchins, MSN, RN, Ivy Technical School of Nursing, Evansville, Indiana and Krystal Oliver-Green, MSN, RN, CNE, Georgia Southwestern State University, Americus, Georgia.

Thanks also to the contributors and reviewers who assisted with the previous editions of this book: Joan Davenport, RN, PhD, University of Maryland; Stacy Estridge, BSN, MN, Midlands Technical College; Dolores Zygmont, RN, PhD, Temple University; Julie A. Adkins, RN, MSN, FNP, Private Practice; Carol Wolfensperger Bashford, MS, RN, CS, Miami University; Jill C. Cash, RN-CS, MSN, FNP, Southern Illinois OB/GYN Associates; Joseann Helmes DeWitt, MSN, RN, C, CLNC, Alcorn State University, School of Nursing; Lynn L. Fletcher, MSN, FNP, RN-CS, West Palm Beach, Florida; Ann Marie John, MS, RN, Monroe Community College; Sammie L. Justesen; Susan Letvak, PhD, RN, University of North Carolina; Theresa Loan, PhD, RN, Eastern Kentucky University; Theresa Loan, PhD, RN, Eastern Kentucky University; Tomas M. Madayag, ARNP, MEd, MSN, EdD, Barry University; Eileen Reilly-Mitchell, MSN, RN, BC-APN, Family Nurse Practitioner; Joan Roche, PhD, APRN, MS, CCRN, University of Massachusetts; Deborah Jane Schwytzer, RN, MSN, CEN, University of Cincinnati; Debera Jane Thomas, DNS, FNP/ANP, RN-CS, School of Nursing, University of Connecticut; Daryle Wane, APRN, BC, MSN, BSN, Pasco-Hernando Community College; Mary L. Anthony, MSN, RN, MacMurray College; Sharon Chappy, RN, PhD, CNOR, University of Wisconsin; Martha Cobb, MS, RN, MEd, CWOCN, The University of Arizona; Deborah Conaway, RN, MSN, Samuel Merritt College/KaiserPermanente; Kelly Jo Cone, RN, PhD, St. Francis Medical Center, College of Nursing; Kathy Patton Hall, RN, MSN, OCN, Arkansas State University, Department of Nursing; Mary Beth Kuehn, RN, MSN, St. Olaf College; Mercy Popoola, RN, CNS, PhD, Georgia Southern University, School of Nursing; Vincent Salyers, EdD(c), RN, Palomar College; Marian Tabi, PhD, RN, Georgia Southern University. Their work will surely assist both students and practicing nurses alike to extend their knowledge in the area of medical-surgical nursing.

I owe a special debt of gratitude to the wonderful team at Pearson Nursing for their enthusiasm for this project, as well as their good humor, expertise, and encouragement as the series developed. Maura Connor, Director of Readypoint™, was unending in her creativity, support, encouragement, and belief in the need for this series. Jennifer Farthing, Executive Editor, Readypoint™, coordinated this revision with insight, talent, and zeal, and fostered a culture of true collaboration and team work. Rachael Zipperlen, Developmental Editor, devoted many long hours to coordinating different facets of this project, and tirelessly and cheerfully encouraged our efforts as well. Her high standards and attention to detail contributed greatly to the final "look" of this book. Editorial Assistant, Deirdre MacKnight, helped to keep the project moving forward on a day-to-day basis, and I am grateful for her efforts as well. A very special thank you goes to the designers of the book and the production team, led by Patrick Walsh, Managing Editor, Maria Reyes, Production Editor, and Christopher Weigand, Designer, who brought the ideas and manuscript into final form.

Thank you to the team at GEX Publishing Services, led by Project Coordinator Michelle Durgerian, for the detail-oriented work of creating this book. I greatly appreciate their hard work, attention to detail, and spirit of collaboration.

Finally, I would like to acknowledge and gratefully thank my children Michael Jr., Kathryn, Kristen, and William, who sacrificed precious hours of family time so this book could be revised. I would also like to thank my students, past and present, for continuing to inspire me with their quest for knowledge and passion for nursing. You are the future!

–MaryAnn Hogan

Nursing Process, Physical Assessment, and Common Laboratory and Diagnostic Tests

1

Chapter Outline

The Nursing Process
Assessment Phase
Diagnosis Phase
Planning Phase
Implementation Phase

Evaluation Phase
Documentation
History-Taking as Part of
   Physical Assessment

Physical Examination
   Techniques
Common Laboratory Tests
Common Diagnostic Tests

Objectives

➤ Discuss the use of the nursing process as it applies to care of the adult client.
➤ Describe common physical assessment procedures used to examine the adult client.
➤ Identify laboratory tests commonly used to monitor the status of the adult client.
➤ Identify diagnostic tests commonly used to detect health problems in the adult client.

 NCLEX-RN® Test Prep

Use the accompanying online resource, NursingReviewsandRationales, to test yourself with hundreds of NCLEX®-style practice questions.

Review at a Glance

assessment first step of nursing process that involves systematic gathering, sorting, and documentation of information collected

auscultation active listening to sounds within body to gather information about client's health status

database client-specific data collected through client health history, physical assessment, and diagnostic test findings

defining characteristics signs and symptoms that support a specific nursing diagnosis

diagnosis application of standardized nursing labels to identified health problems or needs identified during client assessment

etiology identifiable causes or contributing factors defining the presence of a client need or problem

evaluation analysis of data gathered about client's progress towards achievement of identified goals or outcomes

implementation operationalization of interventions assigned to achieve client-specific goals

inspection utilization of vision and smell to obtain information about a client's health status

nonverbal communication unspoken messages conveyed using body, facial expressions, or attitude

nursing process a systematic problem-solving approach to collaboratively identify client health

needs and provide nursing care to effectively meet those needs

objective data any observable information that can be corroborated with assessment and diagnostic testing

outcomes measurable achievement of goals of treatment

palpation touching of a client in a therapeutic manner to gain specific information pertinent to health status

percussion striking of one object against another to produce characteristic vibration sounds

PES format method for creating a client-specific nursing diagnostic statement by combining client's identified problem (need), etiology, and signs or symptoms that label the need

planning identification of achievable client goals and outcomes with assignment of appropriate interventions to achieve these goals

subjective data data obtained from a client; includes feelings, perceptions, and beliefs

therapeutic communication interaction between nurse and client aimed at gathering information and achievement of client goals

PRETEST

1 Which statement made by the nurse while taking a nursing history would elicit the greatest amount of client data?

1. "Did your pain begin recently?"
2. "You said the pain started yesterday?"
3. "Can you tell me more about how the pain began?"
4. "The pain isn't bad right now, is it?"

2 A nurse is revising the client goals and interventions in the nursing care plan. What information enables the nurse to make relevant revisions?

1. Knowledge of the hospital's standards of care
2. Medical assessment and written prescriptions
3. Health care team conferences
4. Validation of the effectiveness of nursing interventions

3 The nurse would assess for hyperkalemia in a client with which of the following problems?

1. Renal failure
2. Nausea and vomiting
3. Excessive laxative use
4. Loop diuretic use

4 A nurse has been assigned the following clients on the day shift. In updating their plans of care, which client would have both *Risk for Ineffective Breathing Pattern* and *Risk for Impaired Gas Exchange* as priority nursing diagnoses?

1. A newly admitted 32-year-old female with exacerbation of myasthenia gravis
2. A second day postop 66-year-old client who underwent femoropopliteal bypass grafting
3. A 56-year-old client admitted for an appendectomy
4. An 82-year-old client with nonmetastatic prostate cancer

5 The nurse is caring for a client on digoxin (Lanoxin). Which electrolyte abnormality should the nurse be concerned about regarding the risk of digoxin toxicity?

1. Sodium 132 mEq/L
2. Potassium 3.0 mEq/L
3. Magnesium 1.0 mEq/L
4. Calcium 9.2 mEq/L

6 The nurse is preparing the client for an ultrasound of the gallbladder. Which statement would be the most important to prepare the client for the test?

1. "You will have food and fluids restricted for 4 to 8 hours prior to the test."
2. "Stool in the bowel may cause a reporting of inaccurate findings."
3. "There is no special preparation for this procedure. You may eat and drink as usual."
4. "You will be asked to drink a solution of radionuclide 2 hours prior to the procedure."

7 A client has recently returned to the nursing unit following a bronchoscopy and is requesting a glass of water. What should be the nurse's initial assessment before meeting this request?

1. Determine if the client is able to ambulate without assistance.
2. Ensure that the side rails are up on the client's bed.
3. Determine if the client received a local anesthetic during the procedure.
4. Ensure that the call light is within the client's reach.

8 The nurse is caring for a client who had his oxygen dose decreased to 2 L/min by nasal cannula. Shortly after this change, the client reports feeling short of breath (SOB). The nurse determines that the current pulse oximetry reading reveals an oxygen saturation of 71%. What would be the nurse's initial intervention?

1. Closely monitor the client's condition and increase the oxygen concentration to 15 L/min.
2. Place the client in a semi-Fowler's position and continue to monitor.
3. Do nothing; the drop in oxygen concentration is expected with the change in oxygen being delivered.
4. Sit the client up, assess the client's respiratory status, and notify the health care provider immediately.

9 The nurse is caring for a man who was admitted after being found unresponsive at home by his wife. If all of the following assessments and interventions must be completed on this client, place them in order of priority from highest priority to lowest. Place the options in the correct order.

1. Perform a neurological exam.
2. Obtain blood samples.
3. Prepare client for CT scan.
4. Assess and establish airway.

10 The nurse is assisting with prioritization of admission, discharge, and triage of acutely ill clients. Which client would require continued monitoring in the intensive care unit? Select all that apply.

1. Client with terminal cancer in the process of dying
2. Client with congestive heart failure and chronic renal failure who develops an exacerbation of the heart failure
3. Hemodynamically unstable client who requires vasoactive drugs to maintain blood pressure
4. Client with metastatic lung disease who develops a pneumonia
5. Client with a tracheostomy who may require mechanical ventilation

➤ *See pages 35–37 for Answers and Rationales.*

I. THE NURSING PROCESS

    A. Overview of 5 steps (or phases) of nursing process
        1. Assessment is a systematic, comprehensive process of collecting, organizing, and documenting client-specific data gathered from various available sources; it includes medical, personal, social, and environmental status; data is also obtained from a comprehensive or system-specific physical assessment
        2. Diagnosing/analysis involves interpretation of assessment data to identify client specific needs and strengths, and formulation of an appropriate nursing **diagnosis**; it includes both actual and potential identified needs

3. **Planning** utilizes assessment data and diagnoses to formulate client goals (desired outcomes), to prioritize nursing diagnoses, and to identify specific interventions to meet these goals
   a. It is a collaborative effort that assigns achievable and measurable, prioritized short- and long-term goals and appropriate interventions to meet these goals in a specified time frame
   b. Since it is a written plan of care, it allows for continuity and communication among client, family, and health care providers
4. **Implementation** involves carrying out plan of care through direct or appropriately delegated nursing orders; communication, supervision, and collaboration are essential to successful implementation
5. **Evaluation** includes determination of effectiveness of an implemented plan of care and revision of plan as needed to achieve desired client outcomes
   a. Nurse assesses actual outcomes and compares them with desired outcomes
   b. If appropriate, new client goals are identified and reprioritized; appropriate interventions are prescribed; and revised plan of care is implemented
   c. Is an ongoing process throughout client's period of care
B. **Relationships** of steps of nursing process
   1. The **nursing process** is a systematic, problem-solving technique
   2. It is client-oriented and goal-directed to meet identified actual and potential needs of client and family
   3. All 5 steps are adaptable to meet ever-changing client needs and depend upon successful application of critical thinking and human caring skills, open communication, and excellent listening skills
   4. It promotes nurse–client–health care team interaction to effectively determine the appropriate means to meet identified client needs and to achieve desired outcomes (see Figure 1-1)

Figure 1-1

The nursing process is a continual process whose steps overlap to meet the client's changing needs

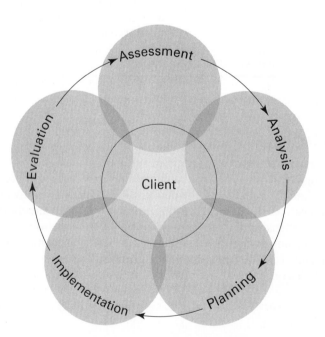

II. ASSESSMENT PHASE

- **A.** *Database* **collection**: client-specific data collected through client health history, physical assessment, and diagnostic test findings
  - **1. Subjective data**
    - **a.** Is a collection of client's symptoms, feelings, or individual perception of problems and needs
    - **b.** Includes health history and chief problem reported by client
    - **c.** Data can also be obtained from client's family, friends, or other health care providers as an interpretation of perceived client needs
  - **2. Objective data**
    - **a.** Is data that can be substantiated by physical examination, laboratory findings, or direct observation
    - **b.** Is measurable against normal reference data or ranges and can be verified by more than one person
- **B. Nursing interview skills**
  - **1.** Establish rapport: the approach used with a client is essential to success of a nursing interview; introduce yourself, your title, and purpose of interview to begin interview process; call client by formal name to show respect and then ask how client wishes to be addressed during interview; this recognition enhances client's sense of being unique
    - **a.** Set up environment to be quiet and undisturbed with controlled lighting and temperature; this reduces distractions and enhances client comfort, which may enhance data collection
    - **b.** Use of good interpersonal skills during interview process affects data collection in a positive way and may increase usefulness of information gathered
      - **1)** Demonstrate a nonjudgmental, accepting attitude toward client when gathering assessment data
      - **2)** Expressing concern, genuine caring, and establishing rapport will place client at ease and facilitate client's comfort to provide accurate and thorough information
  - **2.** Questions are asked during nursing interview to gather information for use in all steps of nursing process; use a combination of types of questions to elicit this information
    - **a.** Formulate questions to gather information about client's health concerns, perceived needs, chief complaint, and symptoms
    - **b.** *Open-ended questions* allow client to provide general information rather than focus on facts and provide client with a sense of control
      - **1)** Client can decide how much information to give and how to say it
      - **2)** Questions such as "What usually causes the onset of this pain?" or "When did these concerns begin?" can be very effective
      - **3)** Open-ended questions require more than a 1- or 2-word response and are useful at beginning of interview when nurse and client are establishing a trusting relationship
      - **4)** Disadvantages are that this type of question can be time consuming and may cause nurse to miss some important information; it is also not useful when interviewing a confused client or in emergent situations
    - **c.** *Closed-ended questions* are directed towards fact finding and are generally used to restrict client's response to specifically focus on a certain area or concern, or to elicit information quickly and efficiently
      - **1)** Questions such as "Are you thinking of hurting yourself or others?" or "Where is the pain now?" will encourage short and to-the-point answers
      - **2)** Closed-ended questions, if overused, may discourage open communication or sharing of valuable information

3. **Therapeutic communication** (a nurse–client interaction aimed at information gathering and client goal achievement) is fundamental to developing a constructive and understanding relationship between client and nurse that is directed toward meeting client's identified needs; the following techniques are helpful:
   a. *Active listening* involves not only hearing client's words but also processing this information to understand what client is communicating; it involves watching client's body language and facial expressions as client conveys a message; use of good listening skills conveys to client a sense that the nurse is accepting, caring, and attentive to client's concerns
   b. *Rephrasing* information stated by client indicates to client that message has been heard by nurse and allows for clarification (if needed), and serves to focus further discussion
   c. *Reflecting* on information shared by client conveys not only an understanding of message and associated feelings, but also encourages further discussion and information sharing; remember that use of reflection should not convey a message of being judgmental or giving advice
   d. *Summarizing* reviews main information gathered during interview and allows client and nurse to identify any information that may have been omitted or to assure that information was interpreted appropriately
4. Compare verbal and nonverbal cues
   a. Be aware that body language and other nonverbal cues expressed by client are frequently just as important as client's verbal information
   b. **Nonverbal communication** (such as appearance, posture, gestures, or facial expressions) can often tell as much about client's health, feelings, and self-image as client's verbalization
   c. Take into consideration cultural differences that may affect a client's nonverbal communication
   d. Always validate your interpretation of nonverbal cues with client to ensure accuracy
5. Terminating the interview is a necessary part of interviewing process; it summarizes and validates information gathered and gives client an opportunity to share any additional information or comments about interview process; it also allows opportunity to plan for future interactions

C. **Organizing data**
1. Utilizing a nursing model: all data must be systematically collected, organized, and documented using an established framework
2. *Human Response Patterns* from North American Nursing Diagnosis Association (NANDA) is one framework that organizes client data into 9 patterns that reflect client's interaction with environment and provides a basis for developing nursing diagnoses (North American Nursing Diagnosis Association (NANDA))
3. Gordon's *Functional Health Patterns* is another commonly used format for organizing data into categories that can be used to develop nursing diagnoses and a plan of nursing care

III. DIAGNOSIS PHASE

A. **Problem identification**
1. Involves critical analysis of assessment data gathered and compares data to standards or established criteria used to recognize quality
2. Identifies client's situation, highlighting his or her actual or potential health care risks or needs
3. Identified needs must be amenable to nursing intervention

    B. **Selecting a diagnosis**
       1. NANDA has developed a universal taxonomy of diagnostic labels that can be individualized to a specific client based upon client's human response pattern
       2. NANDA has defined nursing diagnosis as a clinical judgment about individual, family, or community response to an actual or potential health problem or life process
       3. NANDA has stated that these nursing diagnoses provide the basis for applied interventions
    C. **Writing a diagnostic statement**
       1. Utilize **PES format** (problem, etiology, and signs and symptoms)
       2. Problem identification is based on analysis of subjective and objective assessment data to determine client's response to individual health problem that may respond to nursing intervention
       3. Problem is stated with a NANDA diagnostic label for general area of client need such as Activity Intolerance and Knowledge Deficit
       4. **Etiology** of problem is the probable cause or causes of identified problem (related to [r/t]), for example, related to physical immobility or related to hospitalization
       5. Signs and symptoms (**defining characteristics**) are observable, measured, or reported evidence of diagnosis (as evidenced by)
       6. Sample PES format: Anxiety related to hospitalization as manifested by crying and withdrawal

IV. PLANNING PHASE

    A. **Priority setting** involves establishing a hierarchy of needs
       1. Those needs that are life threatening are usually given highest priority
       2. Determination is based on client's and family's or significant other's input and value/belief system
       3. *Maslow's hierarchy of needs theory* is frequently used in priority setting
       4. Prioritization is also affected by resource availability
       5. Medical plan must also be taken into consideration when prioritizing nursing care plan
    B. **Goals/*outcomes*** are those identifiable client responses that are the result of prescribed nursing orders or interventions
       1. Short-term goals are expected client responses and accomplishments over a brief period of time; they are goals that meet client's immediate needs, for example, "Client will tolerate a clear liquid diet by Monday"
       2. Long-term goals focus on client's long-term health care needs or condition; they may be focused on criteria for discharge, rehabilitation, or self-care promotion, for example, "Client will be able to perform self-tracheostomy suctioning by discharge"
       3. Discharge planning should begin at time of first nurse–client encounter
       4. Nursing orders or interventions that are prescribed to achieve client goals must be client specific, feasible and congruent with approved standards and medical plan, and must be clearly communicated in writing

V. IMPLEMENTATION PHASE

    A. **Nursing plan** of care is carried out using clinical reasoning
    B. **Daily priorities** are set based upon client status
    C. **Activities** may be delegated as appropriate
    D. **Data is collected** as interventions are completed related to client's response
    E. **Continual assessment and documentation,** both written and verbal, are essential
    F. **Nursing care plans** provide a scientific basis or rationale for client care and help to ensure optimal outcomes

VI. EVALUATION PHASE

    A. Determines achievement of client goals and effectiveness of plan of care

        1. Data is collected on an ongoing basis about client's progress and achievement of desired outcomes

        2. Nursing interventions are evaluated for their effectiveness in achievement of desired outcomes

    B. Nursing plan of care is modified or terminated as needed based on results of evaluation

        1. Additional assessment may be needed

        2. Modification to the nursing diagnoses, goals, or interventions may be required

        3. Termination of care plan will occur if goals have been met

VII. DOCUMENTATION

    A. A vehicle for communication

        1. Delineates all steps of nursing process in a clear, concise manner

        2. Facilitates interdisciplinary communication

        3. Provides information for educational purposes, accreditation, and/or reimbursement but must assure a degree of confidentiality

        4. Must be legible and utilize standardized abbreviations and terms

        5. Provides a written record of care and its outcomes

    B. Legal implications

        1. Medical record is a legal document and can be used in court related to care provided and outcomes

        2. Must adhere to professional standards and agency policies

VIII. HISTORY-TAKING AS PART OF PHYSICAL ASSESSMENT

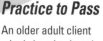

Practice to Pass

An older adult client who is hearing impaired has been scheduled for a routine physical examination. What actions should be taken to enhance the ability to obtain an accurate health history?

    A. Communicating with adult client

        1. Prior to beginning an assessment of adult client, it is essential to gather all necessary client information, medical records, and needed equipment

        2. Create an environment free of obvious interruptions with adequate lighting, temperature, and comfort for the client

        3. When beginning health history–taking and physical review of systems, assure client of purpose and confidentiality of this process

        4. Allow enough time to complete history and physical examination

        5. Use language at a level appropriate for client during history and physical exam

        6. Use proper names unless otherwise agreed upon

        7. Use specific medical terms only if understood by client, and give a full explanation of what to expect during exam

        8. Recognize cultural influences or values that may affect assessment process

        9. Take special care of clients who are older adults, mentally, physically, or socially challenged such as the visually- or hearing-impaired, or those with language difficulties; in these cases, a family member or support person should be included in process if authorized by client

    B. Health history and interview

        1. Health history and interview are the initial steps in physical assessment process and provide subjective information needed to develop an individualized plan of nursing care

        2. Information gathered will serve as basis for understanding client's expectations of this episode of health care, client concerns and needs, and provide a means to identify possible areas for specific physical and laboratory data collection

    C. Outline of client's health history

        1. *Chief complaint/current problem* is the reason client seeks health care; it should be quoted in client's own words; include documentation of history of chief complaint such as onset, location, duration, quality, alleviating and aggravating factors, and associated symptoms

2. *Past medical history* includes a summary of all medical problems that client has experienced during his or her lifetime

   a. It should include all allergies, chronic and acute illnesses, communicable diseases, blood transfusions, major injuries, accidents, or surgeries with dates and where hospitalized

   b. An immunization history should be obtained; particular attention should be paid to hepatitis B and tuberculosis (TB) in at risk populations, varicella in child-bearing women, flu and pneumonia vaccines in older adult and chronically ill populations, and tetanus toxoid in the general population

   c. A list of vitamins, dietary supplements, herbal preparations, over-the-counter (OTC) or prescription medication use is also obtained

3. *Family history* includes a record of health status of client's immediate blood relatives (parents, aunts, uncles, grandparents, siblings, spouse, and children), including age, current health status, known chronic illnesses or links to genetic disease; a *genogram* (see Figure 1-2) is often used to depict this information

Figure 1-2

Interpreting a genogram
A. Standard symbols,
B. Combining symbols to provide additional information,
C. A family genogram.

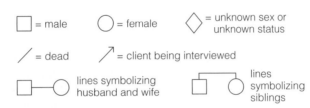

A Genogram symbols

B Combining symbols to provide additional information

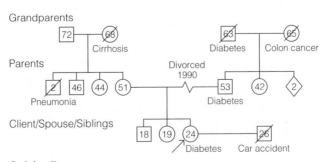

C A family genogram

4. *Personal history* reviews aspects of client's lifestyle that may affect current health or identify risk factors for health problems
   a. Note alcohol use; quantity and frequency of consumption
   b. Note tobacco use, for example, cigarettes, cigars, chewing tobacco, snuff, or pipe smoking; cigarettes are usually calculated in pack-year history (number of packs per day multiplied by number of years smoked)
   c. Document use of illegal drugs or inappropriate use of drugs prescribed, OTC or street drugs, as well as route of use; although this is a sensitive issue, it is vital for appropriately assessing and diagnosing client's needs
   d. Address client's sexual practices in order to identify areas of risk and potential educational needs; include gender preference and mode of sexual contact
   e. Collect information about client's education, financial status, religious and ethnic background, work and home environment, travel history, hobbies, sleep pattern, stress management activities, use of sunscreen and seatbelts, date of last health checkup, safety, and perceived risk of violence

5. *Review of systems* is a detailed history according to body systems
   a. General: assess client's perception of overall health at present and in past; note presence of fatigue, malaise, fever, chills, night sweats, sensitivity to heat and cold, or recent weight or appetite changes
   b. Skin: ask about changes in skin pigmentation, jaundice, rashes, moles, lumps, sores, odors, excessive sweating, changes in hair growth pattern or hair growth in unusual places, changes in skin or nail texture
   c. Head and neck: ask whether client has had recent head trauma, headaches, vertigo, syncope, changes in mental status, pain, tenderness, decreased movement in neck, difficulty swallowing, or swelling in head or neck
   d. Eyes: ask about visual changes, pain, use of glasses, contact lenses, reading devices, double or blurred vision, night blindness, visual halos, flashing lights, blind spots, excessive tearing or drainage, eye irritation, glaucoma, or cataracts
   e. Ears: inquire about use of hearing aids, changes in hearing acuity, discharge, pain, ringing in ears (tinnitus), recent or chronic earaches or infections
   f. Nose and sinuses: ask about recent colds, pain, stuffiness, discharge, polyps, obstructions, nosebleeds, difficulty breathing, or feeling of sinus pressure
   g. Mouth and throat: ask about dentures, toothaches, caries, abscesses, gum bleeding or swelling, changes in appearance of tongue or pain in tongue, chewing difficulties or pain, changes in taste or salivation, hoarseness, new growth or spots in mouth, throat or neck pain, or enlarged thyroid
   h. Breasts: ask male and female clients about any noted pain, tenderness, discharge from nipples, and changes in size or dimpling, or skin changes
   i. Respiratory: ask about any shortness of breath, breathing pattern changes, acute or chronic cough, sputum production or change in color, bloody sputum, wheezing, and date of last chest x-ray
   j. Cardiac: inquire about edema, shortness of breath at night relieved by sleeping on several pillows, exercise or stair climbing tolerance, chest pain, murmurs, palpitations, and date and results of last electrocardiogram (ECG)
   k. Gastrointestinal: ask about changes in appetite or bowel movement, nausea, vomiting, heartburn or indigestion, excessive thirst, diarrhea, constipation, change in stool color, flatulence, hemorrhoids, abdominal pain with location and intensity, or abdominal swelling; include history of eating disorder, noting type
   l. Urinary: inquire about urinary burning or frequency, nocturia, decreased stream of flow, hesitancy, polyuria, bedwetting, incontinence, frequent urinary tract infection, or history of kidney stones

m. Genital
   1) Female client: ask about onset of menarche, date of last menstrual period, any premenstrual symptoms, intermenstrual bleeding, painful periods, vaginal discharges, pain, sexually transmitted infections, sexual activity, use of birth control, safe sex practices, last Pap smear and mammogram, pregnancy history, hormone replacement therapy, and regular practice of self-breast exam
   2) Male client: ask about penile discharge, testicular pain or lumps, sexually transmitted infections, sexual activity, safe sex practices, impotence, infertility, erections, hernias, enlarged prostate, and regular practice of testicular self-exam
n. Peripheral vascular: ask client about any noted varicosities, pain in calf when walking, hand, leg, or foot cramps, blood clots in legs, ankle or hand swelling, and changes in temperature or sensation in fingers or feet
o. Musculoskeletal: inquire about joint or muscle stiffness, pain, decreased range of motion, weakness, swelling, deformities, bone tenderness, gout, arthritis, muscle atrophy, herniated discs, or broken bones or recurrent dislocated joints
p. Neurological: ask about any changes in balance, coordination, sensory perception, changes in speech or thought processes, aphasia, headaches, tremors, seizures, weakness, head injuries, or fainting
q. Hematologic: inquire about bruising, bleeding, anemia, blood type, sickle cell anemia, and history of blood transfusions (and reactions)
r. Endocrine: ask about fatigue, heat or cold intolerance, bulging eyes, weight changes, changes in urine volume, changes in hair distribution, changes in size of head, hands, or feet, swelling in anterior neck, diabetes mellitus (DM), or hormone replacement therapy
s. Psychiatric: inquire about depression, irritability, tension and feeling of excessive stress, suicidal or homicidal ideations, or disturbances in thought processes

D. Impact of cultural and religious beliefs

1. Cultural and religious norms and values will affect client's view and response to illness, need to seek care, and care client believes to be appropriate
2. Nurse must recognize importance of client's beliefs and values, identify specific practices, and incorporate these into plan of care
3. Communication style, both verbal and nonverbal, must be assessed (for example, some Asian cultures value silence and suppression of emotions, and view eye contact as disrespectful); client may require services of a translator or family member (if available and appropriate) to convey his or her needs
4. Family and social relationships must be considered
   a. Family is the center of many cultures, and in some cultures decisions about health care are made by family or a particular family member and not by client
   b. Strong family values and traditions may require that a family member be present at all times while client is receiving care; others may require privacy at all times
5. Health customs and practices, such as the use of complementary or alternative medicine or herbs must be considered; folk healers, ointments, heat, cold, and/or special foods may be essential components of client's care
   a. Make every attempt to allow incorporation of these practices into plan of care
   b. If serious conflicts exist, attempt to collaborate with client
6. Religious beliefs are essential to client's well-being; respect and honor client's belief systems and document any specific spiritual needs and requests of client

Practice to Pass

You are obtaining a health history on a client with a chief complaint of nausea. What information would be important to obtain?

IX. PHYSICAL EXAMINATION TECHNIQUES

A. *Inspection*: observation of client; involves assessment for external signs or gross deviation; this may be visual or olfactory, noting size, shape, symmetry, color, scars, position, and appearance of client or body parts; it can also involve using sense of smell to detect unusual odors or observing movements such as tremors

B. *Palpation*: use of touch to determine characteristics of exposed and underlying tissues and organs; is best performed when client is relaxed

   1. Various parts of hands are used to palpate certain areas of body or gain specific information

      a. Use dorsal surface to assess body temperature because of its increased sensitivity

      b. Use palmar surface finger pads to assess moisture, texture, masses, pulses, crepitus, fine tactile discrimination, and organ size, shape, position, and consistency

      c. Use ulnar surface, ball of hand, and palmar metacarpophalangeal joints to assess using vibrations

   2. Types of palpation

      a. Light palpation: uses superficial, gentle, delicate touch with finger pads for surface assessments of skin and assessment of superficial or enlarged masses, fluid, and tender or guarded areas

      b. Deep palpation: uses fingertips and hand to assess internal organs and structures to a depth of about 2–3 cm or more using either 1 or 2 hands

      c. Ballottement: utilizes fingers to tap around suspected masses floating in a fluid-filled cavity and sense rebound of mass as it returns to its original position

C. *Percussion*: striking of one object against another to cause vibrations that produce a sound

   1. Percussion sounds are assessed according to location, intensity, pitch, duration, and quality; each body part or area percussed has a normal or expected sound and any deviation is further assessed

   2. Percussion produces 5 distinct sounds: flatness, dullness, resonance, hyperresonance, and tympany; each sound is normal in certain areas; there are 2 types of percussion

      a. Direct percussion utilizes fingers or fist of examiner's hand to tap directly on client's skin to elicit a sound, such as when percussing sinus region; a percussion hammer can also be utilized to assess reflexes

      b. Indirect percussion involves nurse tapping finger or fingers of one hand with other hand that is in contact with client's skin, such as when assessing over lung fields

D. *Auscultation*: uses sense of hearing to assess sounds produced by body organs

   1. Auscultated sounds are classified by presence, location, intensity, pitch, quality, and duration

   2. Types of **auscultation**

      a. Direct: involves detection of sounds with ear alone either away from client or with ear in contact with client's skin; wheezing or hyperactive bowel sounds can sometimes be heard with direct auscultation

      b. Indirect or mediated: involves detection of sound with assistance from some type of amplified or nonamplified listening device

         1) Most commonly used device is an acoustic stethoscope, which does not amplify sound but rather blocks out environmental noises

         2) Another type of mediated auscultation device is the Doppler, which will amplify sounds to allow detection and characterization

         3) Note that the order of these techniques may be adjusted depending on client condition; an example is auscultation before palpation and percussion in a client with an abdominal problem

Practice to Pass

You are performing a physical examination on a client who has recently had abdominal surgery. What changes would occur in your physical assessment?

E. Measurement of vital signs, height, and weight

1. Vital signs include temperature, pulse, respirations, and blood pressure (BP); these provide a baseline for client as well as evaluate health status changes or needs

   a. Temperature: measurement of body's balance between heat production and heat loss to environment

   1) Usual sites of measurement are oral, rectal, axillary, or tympanic membrane

   2) Normal temperature for an adult is 98°F (36.7°C) to 98.6°F (37°C)

   3) Factors affecting temperature can include age, exercise, circadian rhythms, hormones, stress, and environment

   4) Note that electronic thermometers are most commonly used; plastic strip thermometers are least accurate

   b. Pulse: a measurement of a wave of blood as generated by left ventricle; includes both rate and rhythm

   1) Most common sites of measurement are radial or apical pulse; however, pulse can also be obtained in temporal, carotid, brachial, femoral, popliteal, posterior tibial, or dorsalis pedis areas; apical pulse is typically the required pulse for medication management

   2) Normal pulse range for an adult is considered to be 60–100 beats per minute but is client specific

   3) Factors affecting pulse rate can include age, gender, medications, exercise, stress, temperature, hemorrhage, position change, and preexisting medical condition(s)

   c. Respirations: measurement of act of breathing characterized by its rate, rhythm, depth, and character

   1) Respirations are normally measured with client at rest

   2) Normal adult respiratory rate (RR) is considered to be 12–20 respirations per minute

   3) Normal respirations are not labored and do not require use of accessory muscles

   4) Factors that may affect RR are exercise, stress, temperature, medication, altitude, brainstem injury, and preexisting medical conditions such as asthma

   d. Blood pressure (BP): measurement of blood flow through arteries; it is recorded as systolic and diastolic pressures

   1) BP is measured in millimeters of mercury (mmHg) and is recorded as a fraction of systolic/diastolic; although usually measured indirectly at brachial artery, it may also be obtained at radial and popliteal arteries with a BP cuff

   2) Normal adult BP is considered to be 120/80 or lower; however, it is more accurate to compare BP to client's baseline when assessing current health status

   3) Age, gender, race, obesity, medications, exercise, stress, time of day, or preexisting medical condition affect BP readings

   4) BP cuff bladder width should be 40% of circumference of extremity and its length should be two-thirds of limb circumference; use of an inappropriate size cuff can cause erroneous BP readings

   5) BP readings may also be obtained directly and continuously using a catheter inserted directly into brachial, radial, or femoral artery, which is then connected to hemodynamic monitoring equipment and displayed on a monitor

2. Height: the client's length; is measured to establish a baseline with which to compare subsequent measurements and serves as an indicator of health status; is often used to assist in identifying hormonal, genetic, or organ system dysfunction

3. Weight: a measure of client's body mass in pounds or kilograms; is measured to establish a baseline for future measurements and to assist in identifying actual or potential health care needs; often height and weight measurements are plotted together on a graph, or combined to calculate body mass index (BMI) in determining established norms of growth, development, and nutritional status

X. COMMON LABORATORY TESTS

A. Blood chemistries

1. Albumin (serum): normal range is 3.5–5.0 grams/dL; represents 52–68% of total protein
    a. Description: a component of protein that is synthesized by liver; is responsible for increasing osmotic pressure to maintain intravascular fluid retention and for transporting hormones, fatty acids, bilirubin, medications, and substances insoluble in water; a decrease in albumin will cause fluid shifts from blood vessels into tissues with edema formation
    b. Clinical problems: *decreased levels* of albumin occur in acute liver failure, liver cirrhosis, malnutrition, malabsorption syndromes, ulcerative colitis, renal disorders, and preeclampsia; *increased levels* may occur in dehydration, severe diarrhea, or vomiting
    c. Medications that may affect albumin levels—*decrease*: aspirin, ascorbic acid, penicillin, and sulfonamides; *increase*: heparin
    d. Nursing implications
        1) No dietary or fluid restrictions prior to blood being drawn
        2) Assess for edema or ascites formation; prevent skin breakdown
2. Ammonia (serum): normal range is 15–45 mcg/dL
    a. Description: a by-product of nitrogen breakdown in protein metabolism; it is normally converted to urea in liver and excreted by kidney
    b. Clinical problems: *decreased levels* may occur in renal failure, and in malignant or essential hypertension; *increased levels* may occur in hepatic failure, hepatic encephalopathy, hepatic coma, cor pulmonale, Reye syndrome, severe heart failure, high-protein diets with liver dysfunction, acidosis, parenteral nutrition, and exercise
    c. Medications that may affect ammonia levels—*decreased levels*: some antibiotics such as neomycin, tetracycline, diphenhydramine, and potassium salt; *increased levels*: ammonium chloride, acetazolamide, isoniazid (INH), and diuretics such as furosemide, thiazides, and ethacrynic acid
    d. Nursing implications
        1) Client should fast prior to blood being drawn
        2) Place specimen in ice and immediately transport to laboratory since ammonia will increase over time
        3) Monitor client for symptoms of hepatic failure such as confusion, lethargy, tremors, or twitching
        4) Monitor clients that receive drugs known to either increase or decrease ammonia levels as well as preparations that are used to intentionally alter intestinal flora or frequency of bowel movements
3. Amylase (serum): normal range is 60–160 Somogyi units/dL; slightly increased in pregnancy and in older adults; urine amylase: 4–37 units/L over 2 hours
    a. Description: an enzyme produced in pancreas, salivary glands, and liver that aids in digestion of complex carbohydrates
    b. Clinical problems: *decreased levels* of amylase can be seen in chronic pancreatitis, acute and subacute liver necrosis, chronic alcoholism, toxic hepatitis, severe burns, severe thyrotoxicosis, or hydration with D_5W IV solution; *increased levels* may occur with acute and chronic pancreatitis, acute cholecystitis, obstruction of pancreatic duct, peptic ulcer perforation, gastric surgery, acute alcohol intoxication, diabetes mellitus (DM), diabetic acidosis, burns, pregnancy, benign prostatic hyperplasia, and renal failure
    c. Medications that may affect amylase levels—*decrease*: citrates, glucose, fluorides, oxalates; *increase*: ACTH, ethyl alcohol, narcotics, salicylates, tetracycline, and thiazide diuretics

Table 1-1   **Acid–Base Disturbances**

Acid–Base Imbalance	pH	PaCO$_2$	HCO$_3$	BE	Clinical Problems
Respiratory acidosis	↓	↑	Normal	Normal	Chronic lung diseases, acute respiratory distress syndrome (ARDS), anesthesia, pneumonia, pneumothorax
Respiratory alkalosis	↑	↓	Normal	Normal	Hyperventilation, anxiety, sepsis, pulmonary emboli, tetany, fever
Metabolic acidosis	↓	Normal	↓	↓	Diabetes mellitus, renal failure, burns, shock, starvation, malnutrition
Metabolic alkalosis	↑	Normal	↑	↑	Excessive bicarbonate intake, severe vomiting, hepatic failure, Cushing's disease, hyperaldosteronism

   d. Nursing implications: restrict food and narcotics for 2 hours prior to blood being drawn

  4. Arterial blood gases (ABGs) from whole blood: normal ranges include pH 7.35–7.45, PaCO$_2$ 35–45 mmHg, PaO$_2$ 80–100 mmHg, HCO$_3$ (bicarbonate) 22–26 mEq/L; base excess (BE) +2 to -2 mEq/L

   a. Description: ABGs are used to assess acid–base imbalances caused by metabolic or respiratory conditions; findings are utilized to detect metabolic acidosis or metabolic alkalosis, or respiratory acidosis or respiratory alkalosis, or a combination of both metabolic and respiratory imbalances

   b. Table 1-1 demonstrates relationship among pH, PaCO$_2$, HCO$_3$ and base excess with each condition

    1) Respiratory acidosis is characterized by a low pH and elevated PaCO$_2$

    2) Respiratory alkalosis is characterized by an elevated pH and decreased PaCO$_2$

    3) Metabolic acidosis is characterized by a low pH, decreased HCO$_3$, and decreased BE

    4) Metabolic alkalosis is characterized by an elevated pH, increased HCO$_3$, and increased BE

    5) Compensation is determined by the normalcy of the pH level

   c. Medications that may affect pH levels—*decreased*: narcotics, barbiturates, ammonium chloride, acetazolamide; *increased*: sodium bicarbonate, antacids, steroids, salicylate overdose, or diuretics

   d. Nursing implications

    1) Monitor vital signs, level of consciousness, respiratory status, and lung sounds frequently to assess acid–base imbalance

    2) Administer IV fluids, medications, and respiratory therapy as prescribed

    3) Advise laboratory personnel to anticipate arrival of ABG specimen for immediate processing

    4) Explain procedure to client

  5. Bicarbonate (serum): normal range is 22–26 mEq/L

   a. Description: an essential *anion* (negatively charged ion) that is part of renal and blood buffer systems; is responsible for maintaining an appropriate acid–base environment for vital biologic processes at tissue and cellular levels; a decrease in bicarbonate leads to an acidic environment while an excess of bicarbonate leads to an alkaline environment within body

   b. Clinical problems: *decreased levels* of bicarbonate occur with renal failure, diarrhea, lactic acidosis, and diabetic ketoacidosis; *increased levels* may occur with excessive bicarbonate or antacid intake, excessive GI suctioning or vomiting, hyperaldosteronism, or diuretic therapy

    c. Medications that affect bicarbonate levels—*increase:* diuretics, OTC antacids, or excessive administration of sodium bicarbonate

    d. Nursing implications: health history data helps determine possible causes of alterations in bicarbonate levels; assessment of respiratory and renal status is important

6. Bilirubin (serum)—normal ranges are total bilirubin 0.1–1.2 mg/dL, direct bilirubin 0–0.3 mg/dL; indirect bilirubin 0.1–1 mg/dL

    a. Description: a breakdown product of hemoglobin in reticuloendothelial system; it is transported in plasma to liver where it is broken down and excreted in bile; there are 2 forms of bilirubin: direct or conjugated (soluble in plasma) and indirect or unconjugated (protein-bound)

    b. Clinical problems: *decreased levels* of direct bilirubin occur with iron-deficiency anemia; *increased levels* of direct bilirubin occur with hepatic disease such as hepatitis, cirrhosis, cancer of liver, obstructions with stones or tumors, and infectious mononucleosis; *increased levels* of indirect bilirubin can be seen with hemolytic anemias, sickle cell anemia, septicemia, transfusion reactions, heart failure, and malaria

    c. Medications that may affect bilirubin levels—*decrease*: aspirin, penicillin, caffeine, and barbiturates; *increase*: antibiotics, barbiturates, diuretics, isoniazid (INH), oral contraceptives, steroids, and vitamins A, C, and K

    d. Nursing implications

        1) Client should not eat a high-fat diet or yellow vegetables immediately before blood draw

        2) Specimen should be protected from light and processed immediately upon arrival in laboratory to reduce effects of light on bilirubin

        3) Monitor client for evidence of jaundice

7. Calcium (serum): normal range is 4.5–5.5 mEq/L or 9–11 mg/dL

    a. Description: an essential *cation* (a positively charged ion), necessary for structure of bones and teeth, contraction of muscles and conduction of nerve impulses, secretion of hormones, blood clotting, and selective transportation across cell membranes

    b. Clinical problems: *decreased levels* of calcium occur in GI malabsorption diseases, decreased calcium and vitamin D intake, hypoparathyroidism, chronic renal failure, infections, pancreatitis, alcoholism, trauma to or removal of parathyroid glands, and pregnancy; *increased levels* may occur with hyperparathyroidism; cancers of bone, breast, lung, kidney, or bladder; multiple fractures; immobility; or renal calculi

    c. Medications that may affect calcium levels—*decrease*: antibiotics, cortisone, heparin, laxatives, insulin, and antacids high in magnesium; *increase*: calcium salts, vitamin D, estrogen preparations, and thiazide diuretics

    d. Nursing implications

        1) No dietary limitations prior to blood being drawn

        2) Assess client for signs of tetany, positive Chvostek or Trousseau sign (occur when calcium level falls below 6 mg/dL), or digoxin toxicity

        3) Do not add calcium to solutions that contain bicarbonate, as it will form a precipitate

8. Carbon dioxide (serum): normal range is 22–30 mEq/L

    a. Description: an important compound used to maintain metabolic acid–base balance; concentration of bicarbonate is closely linked to carbon dioxide concentration in acid–base balance

    b. Clinical problems—*decreased levels*: diabetic ketoacidosis, metabolic acidosis, starvation, dehydration, shock, acute renal failure, and salicylate toxicity; *increased levels*: metabolic alkalosis, severe vomiting, and hypothyroidism

    c. Medications that may affect carbon dioxide levels—*decrease*: antibiotics, diuretics, thiazides, and paraldehyde; *increase*: barbiturates, loop diuretics, and steroids

    d. Nursing implications: assess for signs of metabolic acidosis and alkalosis

Table 1-2	**Cholesterol Levels and Implications**	
Type of Cholesterol	**Value**	**Implications**
Total cholesterol	< 200 mg/dL	Desirable
	200–240 mg/dL	Moderate risk
	> 240 mg/dL	High risk
High-density lipoproteins	29–77 mg/dL	Usual range
	> 60 mg/dL	Very low risk for coronary heart disease (CHD)
	46–59 mg/dL	Low risk for CHD
	35–45 mg/dL	Moderate risk for CHD
	< 35 mg/dL	High risk for CHD
Low-density lipoproteins	60–160 mg/dL	Usual range
	< 130 mg/dL	Low risk for CHD
	130–159 mg/dL	Moderate risk for CHD
	> 160 mg/dL	High risk for CHD
HDL:LDL ratio	3:1	

9. Cholesterol/lipoproteins (serum): for normal ranges see Table 1-2
   a. Description: a blood lipoprotein that is synthesized in liver
      1) Cholesterol assists in formation of bile salts for fat digestion and formation of adrenal, ovarian, and testicular hormones
      2) High-density lipoproteins (HDL) and low-density lipoproteins (LDL) are fractions of lipoproteins that contain varying amounts of cholesterol, protein, triglycerides, and phospholipids
      3) HDLs are primarily composed of protein and have about 20% cholesterol; they are called "good" lipids because they may serve a protective function against coronary heart disease (CHD)
      4) LDLs are primarily composed of cholesterol and are felt to increase risk of CHD
      5) In general, the higher the ratio of HDL: LDL, the lower the risk of CHD
   b. Clinical problems: *decreased levels* of cholesterol will be seen in malnutrition, starvation, and hyperthyroidism; *increased levels* of cholesterol and lipoproteins will be seen with hypercholesterolemia, hyperlipoproteinemia, acute myocardial infarction (MI), diabetes, cirrhosis, nephrotic syndrome, hypothyroidism, pregnancy and eclampsia, and intake of high-fat diets
   c. Medications that may affect lipoprotein levels—*decrease*: estrogen, aspirin, antibiotics, heparin, colchicine, thyroxine; *increase*: oral contraceptives, steroids, phenothiazines, sulfonamides, and phenytoin
   d. Nursing implications: a diet high in fat or cholesterol may raise lipoprotein levels
10. Cortisol: (plasma) normal in morning is 5–23 mcg/dL; afternoon is 3–13 mcg/dL
   a. Description: a glucocorticoid released from adrenal cortex in response to adrenocorticotropic hormone (ACTH) levels
   b. Clinical problems—*decreased levels*: Addison's disease, decreased functioning of anterior pituitary gland, and hypothyroidism; *increased levels*: Cushing's disease, adrenal gland neoplasms, pregnancy, stress, hyperthyroidism, and acute MI
   c. Medications that may affect cortisol levels—*decrease*: androgens, phenytoin; *increase*: estrogen, oral contraceptives, and spironolactone
   d. Nursing implications: client should be NPO and on bedrest immediately prior to blood being drawn due to utilization of cortisol with physical exercise

11. Creatine kinase (serum) normal range is male 5–35 mcg/mL; female 5–25 mcg/mL
    a. Description: an enzyme found in skeletal and heart muscle and brain tissue; has 3 isoenzymes that can be separated to isolate location of enzyme released: CK-MM—skeletal muscle, CK-MB—heart muscle, and CK-BB—brain tissue; differentiation can help determine specific tissue damaged and monitor progression of condition
    b. Clinical problems: *increased levels* of creatine kinase and its isoenzymes are observed in MI, excessive physical activity, skeletal muscle diseases, trauma, surgery, intramuscular (IM) injections, cerebrovascular accident (CVA or stroke), head trauma, seizures, or pulmonary embolism
    c. Medications that may affect creatine kinase levels—*increase*: high-dose aspirin, ampicillin, carbenicillin, or dexamethasone
    d. Nursing implications: withhold IM injections if creatine kinase levels are expected to be drawn; assess clinical signs and symptoms of diseases that may cause elevated CK or CK isoenzyme levels
12. Creatinine (serum) normal range is 0.8–1.6 mg/dL; urine is 1–2 grams/24h
    a. Description: a by-product of muscle catabolism that is excreted by kidney; it is used to determine renal function
    b. Clinical problems: *decreased levels* of creatinine are sometimes seen in females due to their decreased muscle mass; *increased levels* occur in acute and chronic renal failure, neoplasms, heart failure, acute MI, lupus erythematosus, and a diet high in muscle meats
    c. Medications that may affect creatinine levels—*increase:* nephrotoxic antibiotics, lithium, and methyldopa
    d. Nursing implications: clients suspected of having increased serum creatinine and decreased creatinine clearance levels should be monitored for signs and symptoms of renal disease
13. Glucose, fasting (serum): normal range is 70–110 mg/dL
    a. Description: test to determine client's ability to convert glucose to glycogen
    b. Clinical problems: *decreased levels* of glucose may occur with hypoglycemia, adrenal gland hypofunction, malnutrition, alcoholism, liver disease, or malabsorption syndromes; *increased levels* of glucose occur with DM, Cushing's disease, stress, burns, infection, acute pancreatitis, and extensive trauma
    c. Medications that may affect glucose levels—*decrease*: excessive insulin intake; *increase:* anesthetic agents, steroids, ACTH, diuretics, epinephrine, or phenytoin
    d. Nursing implications
       1) Ensure that client has been NPO for at least 12 hours and that all morning insulin has been held prior to blood draw
       2) Observe for signs of hypoglycemia and hyperglycemia
14. Glucose tolerance test (serum) normal range is less than 140 mg/dL
    a. Description: test utilized to detect DM; client ingests a fluid containing 75 grams of glucose after a fasting serum glucose level has been drawn; serum blood specimens are collected every 30 minutes for 2 hours after ingestion
    b. Clinical problems: *increased levels*: impaired glucose tolerance, DM
    c. Medications that may affect glucose levels: *increase*: steroids, phenytoin, diuretics, nicotinic acid
    d. Nursing implications: client should be at rest for length of test and should receive thorough instructions about test, purpose, and what to expect during test
15. Glycosylated hemoglobin A1c (Hgb A1c): normal is 5.5–7% of total Hgb
    a. Description: measures glucose molecules attached to hemoglobin; is used to help diagnose and monitor DM

      b. Clinical problems: *decreased levels*: chronic renal failure, chronic blood loss, anemias and thalassemia; *increased levels:* hemodialysis, pregnancy, alcohol ingestion, and DM

      c. Medication that may affect Hgb A1c level: prolonged used of cortisol, ACTH heparin therapy

      d. Nursing implications: NPO not required but suggested, identify clinical conditions that may affect result; send specimen to lab quickly to prevent hemolysis of specimen; document dose, frequency and adherence to any antiglycemic medications

16. Iron (serum) normal range is 50–150 mcg/dL

      a. Description: iron is necessary for synthesis of hemoglobin in bone marrow

      b. Clinical problems: *decreased levels* of iron occur with iron-deficiency anemia, malabsorption diseases, chronic bleeding disorders, pregnancy, and chronic renal failure; *increased levels* of iron occur with pernicious and hemolytic anemias, liver disease, lead toxicity, and thalassemia

      c. Medications that may affect iron levels—*increase*: iron preparations and oral contraceptives

      d. Nursing implications: monitor for signs of iron-deficiency anemia and avoid hemolysis of blood specimen, which may cause elevated results

17. Lactic dehydrogenase (serum) normal ranges are total LDH 100–190 IU/L; LDH isoenzymes: LDH^1 is 14–26%, LDH^2 is 27–37%, LDH^3 is 13–26%, LDH^4 is 8–16%, LDH^5 is 6–16%

      a. Description: intracellular enzyme important for cellular metabolism; there are 5 isoenzymes of LDH: LDH^1 and LDH^2 are primarily found in cardiac cells, LDH^3 is primarily found in pulmonary cells, and LDH^4 and LDH^5 are primarily found in hepatic cells

      b. Clinical problems: *increased levels* of total LDH and specific isoenzymes can be found in MI, acute hepatic diseases, pulmonary embolus, pulmonary infarction, skeletal muscle diseases, cancers, stroke, anemia, and excessive exercise

      c. Medications that may affect LDH levels—*increase*: narcotics and frequent IM injections

      d. Nursing implications

         1) Assess for signs and symptoms of cardiac, hepatic, musculoskeletal, and pulmonary diseases

         2) Assess levels and trends of LDH values and report them to health care provider as appropriate

         3) Minimize IM injections at least 8 hours prior to blood draw

18. Lipase (serum) normal range is 20–180 IU/L

      a. Description: an enzyme secreted by pancreas that aids in fat digestion

      b. Clinical problems: *elevated levels* of lipase will occur with acute and chronic pancreatitis, pancreatic cancers, acute renal failure, and obstruction of pancreatic duct (because lipase remains in blood for up to 14 days after an episode of acute pancreatitis, it is useful in late diagnosis of this condition)

      c. Medications that may affect lipase levels—*increase*: narcotics and steroids

      d. Nursing implications: client should be NPO except water for 8 hours prior to blood draw

19. Magnesium (serum) normal range is 1.5–2.5 mEq/L

      a. Description: essential cation primarily stored in bones and cartilage; it facilitates muscle contraction, carbohydrate and protein metabolism, and regulation of potassium and calcium

      b. Clinical problems: *decreased levels* of magnesium occur in malabsorption syndromes, cirrhosis, alcoholism, hypokalemia, dehydration, malnutrition, and hypoparathyroidism; *increased levels* of magnesium occur in renal failure, dehydration, and DM

    c. Medications that may affect magnesium levels—*increase*: magnesium-rich antacids and laxatives high in magnesium such as milk of magnesia and magnesium citrate; *decrease*: diuretics, insulin, calcium gluconate, and neomycin

    d. Nursing implications

        1) Monitor for signs and symptoms of magnesium imbalance

        2) Monitor ECG strips for peaked T wave or wide QRS complex that indicate need to evaluate serum magnesium and potassium levels

20. Osmolality normal range (serum) is 280–300 mOsm/kg H_2O; normal range for urine osmolality is 50–1200 mOsm/kg H_2O

    a. Description: measurement of serum and urine concentration as a result of number of particles dissolved in solution

    b. Clinical problems

        1) *Decreased serum osmolality levels* could indicate intravascular fluid overload or syndrome of inappropriate ADH (SIADH)

        2) *Decreased urine osmolality levels* could indicate diabetes insipidus, acute renal failure, or hyponatremia

        3) *Increased serum osmolality levels* could indicate dehydration, hypernatremia, hyperglycemia, or diabetes insipidus

        4) *Increased urine osmolality* could indicate SIADH

    c. Medications that affect osmolality levels—*decrease*: excessive IV fluid infusion of D_5W

    d. Nursing implications

        1) There are no special restrictions before serum collection

        2) Urine osmolality testing requires intake of a high-protein diet for several days prior to urine collection and fluid restriction for 8–12 hours prior to urine collection

        3) The second specimen of the morning is sent for analysis

21. Phosphorus (serum) normal range is 1.7–2.6 mEq/L or 2.5–4.5 mg/dL

    a. Description: an essential intracellular anion stored primarily in bones; it serves to regulate energy transfer as ATP, and assist in metabolism of carbohydrate, fat, and protein

    b. Clinical problems: *decreased levels* occur in malabsorption syndromes, starvation, hyperparathyroidism, hypercalcemia, chronic alcoholism, and diabetic acidosis; *increased levels* occur in hypocalcemia, bone tumors, renal insufficiency and failure, Cushing's disease, and multiple fractures

    c. Medications that may affect phosphorus levels—*decrease*: antacids, insulin, mannitol; *increase*: heparin, phenytoin, and phosphate

    d. Nursing implications: because phosphorus levels are the inverse of calcium levels, check calcium levels and observe for signs of tetany if phosphorus levels are elevated

22. Potassium (serum) normal range is 3.5–5.1 mEq/L

    a. Description: an essential intracellular cation needed for protein synthesis, glucose storage and use, and electrical activity of excitable membranes such as cardiac muscle

    b. Clinical problems: *decreased levels* of potassium occur in dehydration, excessive vomiting and diarrhea, starvation, stress, trauma, burns, metabolic alkalosis, diabetic acidosis, and gastric suctioning; *increased levels* of potassium occur in acute renal failure, excessive use of salt substitutes, metabolic acidosis, oliguria, and anuria

    c. Medications that may affect potassium levels—*decrease*: diuretics (potassium-wasting), sodium polystyrene sulfonate (Kayexalate), lactulose, insulin, aspirin, and laxatives; *increase*: potassium-sparing diuretics, heparin, histamine, antibiotics, and epinephrine

!

  d. Nursing implications
    1) Closely monitor serum potassium levels and signs and symptoms of potassium imbalance
    2) Decreased potassium levels can cause ECG changes such as AV conduction defects, depressed S-T segments, and inverted or flat T waves
    3) Increased potassium levels can cause widened QRS complexes and peaked T waves
    4) Clients with hypokalemia are predisposed to development of digitalis toxicity

23. Prealbumin (antibody assay; serum) normal range is 17–40 mg/dL
  a. Description: test of precursor to albumin, transthyretin, which has a shorter half-life (2–4 days) than albumin and therefore can more easily indicate changes in protein synthesis and catabolism; useful in monitoring nutritional status and effectiveness of total parenteral nutrition (TPN)
  b. Clinical problems: *decreased levels* of prealbumin occur in protein-wasting disease, malnutrition, malignancy, liver disease, zinc deficiency, and chronic illness; *increased levels* of prealbumin are seen in Hodgkin's disease, chronic kidney disease, and adrenal hyperfunction
  c. Medications affecting prealbumin levels: *decreased levels* with estrogen and oral contraceptive administration; *increased levels* with high doses of either steroids or nonsteroidal anti-inflammatory drugs (NSAIDs)
  d. Nursing implications
    1) Usually no need for NPO status before collection of blood sample
    2) Obtain and record nutritional intake history, vital signs, and weight

24. Prostate-specific antigen (PSA) (serum) normal ranges are 1–4 ng/mL; benign prostatic hyperplasia 4–19 ng/mL; prostate cancer 10–120 ng/mL
  a. Description: glycoprotein present in prostate tissue; PSA is a highly sensitive indicator of prostatic cancer and is used to diagnose and monitor treatment effectiveness and prognosis
  b. Clinical problems: *increased levels* of PSA occur in prostatic cancer and benign prostatic hyperplasia
  c. Nursing implications: a thorough client genitourinary history and health assessment helps determine need for this test and monitor progression of disease process; an initial high PSA level requires additional testing

25. Protein (serum and urine) normal ranges are *serum*: total protein = 6–8 grams/dL, albumin = 52–68% of total protein, globulin = 32–48% of total protein; *urine*: normal range is 0–5mg/dL (random); 24-hour urine specimen: 25–150 mg
  a. Protein and its components (albumin and globulin) are essential to maintain colloid osmotic pressure, supply of amino acids, and for immunity to diseases
  b. Clinical problems
    1) *Decreased levels of serum proteins* occur in malnutrition, starvation, malabsorption syndromes, severe burns, chronic renal failure, toxemia, and nephrotic syndromes
    2) *Increased levels of serum proteins* occur with dehydration, nausea, vomiting, diarrhea, and excessive exercise
    3) *Increased levels of urine proteins* occur with glomerulonephritis, nephrotic syndrome, systemic lupus erythematosus, drug toxicities, renal infections, and toxemia of pregnancy
  c. Medications that may affect protein levels—*increased*: supplemental infusions of protein-rich solutions; increased urine proteins may occur with the use of contrast media, nephrotoxic antibiotics, and tolbutamide
! **d.** Nursing implications: monitor nutritional status and start replacement therapies as ordered; continually monitor I & O

26. Sodium (serum) normal range is 135–145 mEq/L
    a. Description: major cation in extracellular fluid responsible for maintaining extra-cellular volume, osmolality, urine concentration, and cardiac and skeletal muscle contraction through sodium-potassium pump
    b. Clinical problems: *decreased levels* of sodium occur in vomiting, diarrhea, gastric suctioning, SIADH, burn injury, and renal failure; *increased levels* occur in diabetes insipidus, congestive heart failure, hepatic failure, severe vomiting, and diarrhea
    c. Medications that may affect sodium levels—*decrease*: diuretics including mannitol and thiazides; *increase*: laxatives, steroids, antibiotics
    d. Nursing implications: closely monitor for signs and symptoms of sodium imbalance (high sodium intake immediately prior to blood draw will affect results)

27. Thyroid hormones (serum) normal ranges: thyroid-stimulating hormone (TSH) is 0.35–5.5 microIU/mL; triiodothyronine (T^3) is 80–200 ng/dL; thyroxine (T^4) is 4.6–11 mcg/dL
    a. Description: TSH is secreted by anterior pituitary gland, which stimulates release of T^3 and T^4 through a negative feedback mechanism; thyroid hormones are responsible for controlling rate of metabolic processes, normal growth and development, and nervous system maturation
    b. Clinical problems: *decreased levels* of thyroid hormones occur in hypothyroidism caused by pituitary malfunction, myxedema, cretinism, renal failure, strenuous exercise, and trauma; *increased levels* of thyroid hormones occur in hyperthy-roidism caused by thyroid malfunction, goiter, Graves' disease, thyroiditis, and thyrotoxic crisis
    c. Medications that may affect thyroid hormone levels: *decrease*: aspirin, steroids, dopamine, phenytoin, and testosterone; *increase*: oral contraceptives, estrogen, potassium iodide, and perphenazine
    d. Nursing implications: closely monitor client for signs of thyroid hormone imbal-ances, particularly tachycardia and cardiovascular changes

28. Triglycerides (serum) normal ranges: 10–140 mg/dL at 12–29 yrs; 20–150 mg/dL at 30–39 yrs; 30–160 mg dL at 40–49 yrs; 40–190 mg/dL at 50 yrs and older
    a. Description: most common blood lipid in body involved in energy production, storage, and insulation; this lipid is a major contributor to development of CHD and other arterial diseases
    b. Clinical problems: *decreased levels* of triglycerides occur in hyperthyroidism, pro-tein malnutrition, congenital lipoproteinemia, and excessive exercise; *increased levels* of triglycerides occur in hyperlipoproteinemia, hypertension, acute MI, nephrotic syndrome, alcoholic cirrhosis, Down syndrome, high-carbohydrate diet, and pregnancy
    c. Medications that may affect triglyceride levels—*decrease*: clofibrate, phenformin, metformin, and ascorbic acid; *increase*: oral contraceptives and estrogen
    d. Nursing implications: client should be NPO for at least 12 hours prior to blood draw; recent alcohol or high-carbohydrate diet intake will elevate triglyceride level

29. Troponin I (serum) normal level is less than 0.1 ng/mL; is diagnostic for MI at greater than 2.2 ng/mL
    a. Description: a cardiac-specific protein marker for myocardial injury; elevation begins 4–6 hours after onset of chest pain and peaks at approximately 12–24 hours making it a useful tool to diagnose myocardial injury
    b. Clinical problems: *increased levels* of Troponin I occur with myocardial injury and MI, may also be seen in clients with heart failure, pulmonary hypertension and long-term kidney disease
    c. Medication that may affect Troponin I levels: none known at present

   d. Nursing implications

    1) A thorough and serial cardiac assessment is essential in monitoring clients with suspected or diagnosed myocardial injury

    2) A screening test for Troponin I is performed at bedside

    3) Be aware of correct test procedures and interpretation of test results, being mindful of client's preexisting conditions

  30. Urea nitrogen (serum) normal range is 8–22 mg/dL; also known as blood urea nitrogen (BUN)

   a. Description: urea is an end product of protein metabolism formed in liver and excreted by kidneys

   b. Clinical problems: *decreased levels* of BUN occur with severe liver disease, malnutrition, overhydration, low protein intake, and pregnancy; *increased levels* of BUN occur with dehydration, renal insufficiency or failure, other kidney diseases, DM, sepsis, GI bleeding, and high-protein diet

   c. Medications that may affect urea nitrogen levels—*decrease*: phenothiazines; *increase*: diuretics, antibiotics, lithium, morphine, propranolol, and methyldopa

   d. Nursing implications: assess for adequate hydration status and monitor intake and output (I & O) if renal disease is suspected

  31. Uric acid (serum) normal range is 3.5–8 mg/dL (male); 2.8–6.8 mg/dL (female)

   a. Description: a by-product of purine metabolism that is normally excreted by kidneys

   b. Clinical problems: *decreased levels* of uric acid occur in acidosis, folic acid anemia, and pregnancy; *increased levels* of uric acid occur with gout, alcoholism, renal failure, leukemias and metastatic carcinomas, hyperlipoproteinemia, DM, stress, and polycythemia

   c. Medications that may affect uric acid levels—*decrease*: allopurinol, warfarin, probenecid, and sulfinpyrazone; *increase*: acetaminophen, ascorbic acid, diuretics, levodopa, methyldopa, aspirin, and theophylline

   d. Nursing implications: monitor urine output and assess for signs of gout and kidney stones

 B. Hematology

  1. Activated partial thromboplastin time (APTT) (serum) normal range is 20–35 seconds; for anticoagulation therapy it is 1.5–2.5 times normal

   a. Description: screening test used to detect clotting deficiencies and to monitor effectiveness of heparin therapy

   b. Clinical problems: *increased levels* occur with clotting factor V, VIII, IX, X, XI, and XII deficiencies, cirrhosis of liver, disseminated intravascular coagulopathy (DIC), leukemia, and Hodgkin's disease

   c. Medications that may affect APTT—*increase*: heparin, salicylates, and enoxaparin

   d. Nursing implications: assess for signs and symptoms of bleeding and report APTT results to prescriber; protamine is antidote to both heparin and enoxaparin

  2. Prothrombin time (PT) (plasma) normal range is 10–13 seconds; anticoagulation therapy range is 1.5–2 times control

   a. Description: measures clotting abilities of fibrinogen, prothrombin, and factors V, VII, and X; is used to monitor effectiveness of oral anticoagulation therapy with warfarin (Coumadin)

   b. Clinical problems: *decreased levels* occur in pulmonary embolism, acute MI, and thrombophlebitis; *increased levels* may occur with alcohol ingestion, liver disease, clotting factor deficiencies, congestive heart failure, erythroblastosis fetalis, and leukemias

   c. Medications that may affect the PT—*decrease*: oral contraceptives, vitamin K, digitalis, diuretics, rifampin, and metaproterenol; *increase*: oral anticoagulants, salicylates, phenytoin, methyldopa, and chlordiazepoxide

   d. Nursing implications
   1) Monitor plasma PT level and report to prescriber
   2) Monitor for signs and symptoms of bleeding
   3) Vitamin K is the antidote for elevated PT levels
   e. The international normalized ratio (INR) may be used instead of PT; therapeutic level is commonly 2–3
3. Erythrocyte sedimentation rate (ESR) normal range: less than 20 mm/hr
   a. Description: measures rate at which red blood cells (RBCs) settle out of unclotted blood; primary influence on ESR is presence of acute phase reactants in presence of inflammation
   b. Clinical problems: *decreased rate* occurs with sickle cell anemia, degenerative arthritis, angina pectoris, and factor V deficiency; *increased rate* occurs with acute infections, inflammatory conditions, systemic lupus erythematosus (SLE), pregnancy, cancers, burns, rheumatoid arthritis, and rheumatic fever
   c. Medications that may affect ESR—*decrease*: aspirin, quinine, and steroids; *increase*: oral contraceptives, dextran, methyldopa, theophylline, and procainamide
   d. Nursing implications: withhold any medications that can affect ESR 4 hours prior to blood draw
4. Hematocrit (Hct) normal range: 40–54% (male); 36–46% (female); slight variations are found in some texts
   a. Description: percent of packed red blood cells (RBCs) per 100 mL of blood
   b. Clinical problems: *decreased levels* may occur with acute blood loss, chronic liver failure, anemias, chronic renal failure, malnutrition, bone marrow deficiencies, SLE, rheumatoid arthritis, and vitamin B and C deficiencies; *increased levels* may occur with hypovolemia, severe diarrhea, burns, trauma, eclampsia, chronic anoxia, diabetic ketoacidosis (from dehydration), and polycythemia
   c. Medications that may *decrease levels*: penicillin and chloramphenicol
   d. Nursing implications: assess change in vital signs; monitor signs and symptoms of anemia, fluid volume status, and output
5. Hemoglobin (Hgb) normal range is male: 13.5–17 grams/dL; female: 12–15 grams/dL; slight variations are found in some texts
   a. Description: oxygen-carrying component of RBC
   b. Clinical problems: *decreased levels* may occur in anemias, renal disease, and over-hydration; *increased levels* may occur in dehydration, chronic pulmonary disease, severe burns, polycythemia, and high altitudes
   c. Medications that may affect hemoglobin levels—*decrease*: antibiotics, aspirin, indomethacin, rifampin, and antineoplastic medications; *increase*: gentamicin and methyldopa
   d. Nursing implications: assess for signs and symptoms of dehydration and anemia
6. Platelet count normal range is 150,000–400,000/mm^3
   a. Description: basic blood element primarily responsible for clotting
   b. Clinical problems: *decreased levels* of platelets may occur in cancer, leukemias, liver disease, kidney disease, DIC, and SLE; *increased levels* of platelets may occur in polycythemia, acute blood loss, splenectomy, and infections
   c. Medications that may affect platelet count—*decrease*: aspirin, chloromycetin, chemotherapeutic agents, thiazide diuretics, and quinidine
   d. Nursing implications: assess for signs and symptoms of bleeding disorders and monitor platelet count in clients undergoing chemotherapy and radiation therapy
7. Reticulocyte count normal level is 0.5–1.5% of all RBCs
   a. Description: immature RBCs released by bone marrow that become mature RBCs in 1–2 days

Practice to Pass

Your client, who was recently started on daily warfarin sodium (Coumadin) therapy, has just received an order from the health care provider to have biweekly prothrombin times (PT) drawn. The client asks you why. What would your response be?

    b. Clinical problems that may affect reticulocyte count: *decreased levels* may occur in anemias, radiation therapy, hypopituitary and hypoadrenal functioning, and excessive alcohol intake; *increased levels* may occur with chronic blood loss, anemias, thalassemia, leukemias, and as an effect of treatment of iron, vitamin B_{12}, and folic acid deficiencies

    c. Nursing implications: monitor effectiveness of anemia therapy

8. White blood cell count (WBC) normal range is 4,500–11,000 cells/mm^3

    a. Description: component of body's defense system; an increase indicates presence of infection or inflammation

    b. Clinical problems: *decreased levels* may occur in anemias, viral infections, malaria, alcoholism, SLE, and rheumatoid arthritis; *increased levels* may occur in acute infections, tissue injury and necrosis, stress, sickle cell anemia, and hemolytic anemia

    c. Medications that may affect WBC—*decrease*: antibiotics, acetaminophen, chemotherapeutic agents, chlordiazepoxide, oral hypoglycemics, indomethacin, rifampin, and phenothiazide; *increase*: aspirin, antibiotics, allopurinol, heparin, digitalis, lithium, and epinephrine

    d. Nursing implications: monitor for signs of inflammation and infection

9. White blood cell differential

    a. Description: there are 5 types of WBCs with each having a specific function in body's defense systems; differential provides specific information about infection and disease process based upon WBC cell type

    b. Clinical problems: see Table 1-3

    c. Nursing implications: assess for signs and symptoms of infection, allergic reaction, and wound healing process

C. Serology and immunology

1. Antinuclear antibody (ANA) (serum): normal finding is negative

    a. Description: measures presence of antibodies that destroy nucleus of cells and cause tissue death; is a screening test for collagen diseases

    b. Clinical problems: *positive or increased levels* may be seen in some collagen diseases such as SLE, scleroderma, rheumatoid arthritis, leukemia, systemic sclerosis, infectious mononucleosis, and myasthenia gravis

Table 1-3	White Blood Cell Differential		
Type	**Normal Value**	**Function**	**Clinical Problems**
Neutrophils	50–70%	First response to tissue injury and inflammation	*Decreased:* viral diseases, anemias, leukemias, and agranulocytosis *Increased:* acute infections, acute appendicitis, inflammation, acute pancreatitis
Eosinophils	1–3%	Response to allergic and parasite conditions	*Decreased:* burns, shock *Increased:* allergies, cancer, phlebitis
Basophils	0.4–1%	Promote healing	*Decreased:* hypersensitivity reaction, stress, pregnancy *Increased:* inflammatory process, wound healing, leukemia
Monocytes	4–6%	Second response to infection	*Decreased:* aplastic anemia *Increased:* viral diseases, cancer, collagen diseases
Lymphocytes	25–35%	Assist in immune response (B and T lymphocytes)	*Decreased:* cancer, leukemia, aplastic anemia, multiple sclerosis, renal failure, nephrotic syndrome, SLE

    c. Medications that affect ANA value—*increase*: antibiotics, antihypertensives, isoniazid, thiazides, diuretics, oral contraceptives, antidysrhythmics, and chlorpromazine

    d. Nursing implications: monitor for signs and symptoms of collagen diseases

2. C-reactive protein (serum): normal finding is negative

    a. Description: is a protein found in blood when there is tissue injury or inflammation in body; elevated levels of C-reactive protein occur with an acute bacterial inflammatory process approximately 6–10 hours after tissue damage has begun and begin to decline approximately 48–72 hours after

    b. Clinical problems: *increased levels* may occur with acute MI, rheumatoid arthritis, rheumatic fever, pyelonephritis, metastatic cancer, inflammatory bowel syndromes, intrauterine devices, and bacterial infections

    c. Medications that may affect C-reactive protein levels—*increase*: oral contraceptives

    d. Nursing implications: client should be NPO except for water for 8–12 hours prior to blood draw; assess client for signs and symptoms of acute inflammatory illness

3. Carcinoembryonic antigen (CEA) (serum): normal in nonsmokers is less than 2.5 ng/dL; in smokers is less than 5.0 ng/dL

    a. Description: used to detect colon and pancreatic carcinoma and monitor effectiveness of treatment

    b. Clinical problems: *increased levels* of CEA occur with carcinomas of GI tract, pancreas, liver, lung, breast, cervix, prostate, bladder, testes, and kidney; leukemia; inflammatory bowel disease; chronic smoking; ulcerative colitis; acute renal failure; acute pancreatitis; and chronic ischemic cardiac disease

    c. Nursing implications: heparin should be withheld for 2 days prior to blood draw; since results are not absolute, give support to client and family while awaiting results

4. Immunoglobulins (Ig)(serum): normal ranges are total Ig = 900–2,200 mg/dL; IgG = 650–1,700 mg/dL; IgA = 70–400 mg/dL; IgM = 40–350 mg/dL; IgD = 0–8 mg/dL; IgE = less than 40 units/mL

    a. Description: specific blood proteins involved in antibody–antigen immune response

      1) IgG: provides early immunity in newborn and results from exposure to antiviral and antibody activity

      2) IgA: protects mucous membranes from bacterial and viral infections

      3) IgM: is responsible for primary immunity from antigen exposure

      4) IgD: unknown

      5) IgE: response to allergic and anaphylactic reactions

    b. Nursing implications: assess client's immunization and vaccination status, infectious disease exposure history, and blood transfusion history

5. Rapid plasma reagin (RPR) (serum) normal finding is nonreactive

    a. Description: RPR test is used to diagnose syphilis

    b. Clinical problems that may affect a false-positive RPR include TB, pneumonia, chickenpox, mononucleosis, rheumatoid arthritis, SLE, hepatitis, and pregnancy

    c. Nursing implications: assess client's sexual history to ensure notification of possible contacts if testing proves positive for syphilis

6. Venereal disease research laboratory (VDRL) (serum) normal finding is nonreactive

    a. Description: VDRL test is used to detect presence of syphilis

    b. Clinical problems that may cause a false positive VDRL include TB, rheumatoid arthritis, SLE, hepatitis, infectious mononucleosis, or recent smallpox vaccine

    c. Nursing implications: assess client's sexual history and obtain a thorough client history to rule out any possible causes of false positive results

> ### Practice to Pass
>
> Your client has told you that he is very concerned that his RPR has been reported as reactant. How would you respond to this client?

Table 1-4 **Normal Urinalysis Results**	
Color	pale yellow
Protein	1–14 mg/dL
Odor	aromatic similar to ammonia
Bilirubin	negative
Turbidity	clear
RBCs	1–2 per high-power field
Specific gravity	1.005–1.030
WBCs	0–5 per high-power field
PH	4.5–8
Casts	none–few
Glucose	< 15 mg/dL
Bacteria	< 1,000
Ketones	negative
Nitrates	negative

D. Urinalysis (UA): normal findings (see Table 1-4)
   1. Description: UA is used to determine presence of renal or urinary tract disorders; it can also be used to determine metabolic dysfunctions
   2. Clinical problems that may affect results of urinalysis can include: contaminated specimen, fluid balance, pregnancy, liver disease, renal disease, presence of bacteria or infection, ingestion of certain foods and medications, trauma, diabetes, or pituitary gland disorders
   3. Medications that may affect urinalysis include: antibiotics, phenytoin, methylene blue, sulfisoxazole-phenazopyridine (Azo-Gantrisin), methocarbanol, iron injections, contrast media, steroids, epinephrine, and anticoagulants
   4. Nursing implications
      a. Assist client in obtaining a clean specimen or obtain a catheterized specimen
      b. Send specimen to the laboratory ASAP
      c. Assess client's fluid status, medications, and foods taken recently
E. Fecal analysis: normal findings for occult blood–negative; ova and parasites–negative; fecal fat less than 7 grams/24 hr
   1. Description: fecal analysis is usually performed to diagnose diseases of GI tract
   2. Clinical problems
      a. Positive stool occult blood can occur with cancer, peptic ulcer disease, ulcerative colitis, or diverticulitis
      b. Presence of ova and parasites indicates infection
      c. Increased findings of fecal fat can occur with malabsorption syndrome, pancreatic diseases, or Crohn's disease
   3. Nursing implications: assist client to obtain a fresh specimen; send specimen to the laboratory as soon as possible for analysis, assess dietary intake in past 24 hours with attention to fatty foods, high fiber or laxative use
F. Cerebrospinal fluid (CSF) analysis: normal findings are clear color; WBCs = 0 to 8/mm^3; protein = 15–45 mg/dL; chloride = 118–132 mEq/L; glucose = 40–80 mg/dL
   1. Description: CSF is obtained by lumbar puncture and fluid analysis is done to diagnose spinal and cerebral diseases and infections

   2. Clinical problems
    a. Color may change because of presence of RBCs or an elevated cell count
    b. Increased cell count may be caused by infection, tumor, or presence of blood
    c. Elevated protein levels may indicate tumor, viral or bacterial infection, or Guillain-Barré syndrome
    d. Elevated glucose levels may occur with some types of meningitis, brain cancer, or leukemia

   3. Nursing implications
    a. Assist with lumbar puncture to obtain specimen
    b. Explain procedure to client, provide comfort during positioning, and answer questions as needed
    c. Ensure that specimens are placed in sterile containers and sent to laboratory for analysis immediately
    d. Monitor client's neuromotor status postprocedure

XI. COMMON DIAGNOSTIC TESTS

A. Computed tomography (CT) scan

1. General description
 a. A noninvasive, diagnostic radiographic procedure that provides cross-sectional images of body to differentiate subtle changes in tissue density of selected structure
 b. CT scans are performed to rule out presence of or evaluate enlarged nodes, lesions, abscesses, hemorrhage, and extent of cancer metastases
 c. X-ray beam scans a thin layer of client's body and transmits that information to a computer that constructs images on a screen for interpretation
 d. Client will lie on a movable scanning table and pass through opening in scanner; client should be reassured that he or she will be visible to radiology staff during procedure
 e. A spiral or helical CT scan can be used for any CT imaging; it requires use of contrast and produces higher resolution images
 f. Nursing implications: check for allergies to contrast media or iodine; note history of decreased renal function or renal failure since kidneys excrete contrast; some relative considerations are needed for clients taking metformin (Glucophage); check for pregnancy if client of child-bearing age

2. CT of head
 a. Client lies on CT scanner table in a supine position with tape or Velcro straps across forehead to prevent any motion
 b. Depending on client's history and health care provider request, contrast media may be administered intravenously
 c. Sedation is given occasionally for restlessness, if necessary
 d. Test can be used to detect aneurysms, presence of blood, fluid, tumors, or structural abnormalities

3. CT of abdomen
 a. Client is required to drink approximately 42 ounces of contrast media prior to test and will also require intravenous (IV) access for administration of contrast media
 b. Contrast media may cause client to become flushed or nauseated, but this reaction is usually transient
 c. Test can be used to determine presence of fluid, lesions, structural malformations, foreign bodies, or hemorrhage

B. Doppler studies

1. General information: a diagnostic, noninvasive exam that uses echoes of an ultrasonic beam to create 3-dimensional oscilloscope pictures or waveform diagrams on a computer screen as beam is "bounced back" to Doppler probe

2. Cardiac (called echocardiogram): a diagnostic test to evaluate cardiac structures and valves; an image is produced on a screen as ultrasound waves emitted from Doppler probe are reflected back to a transducer from cardiac structures; this test is used to evaluate or diagnose cardiac tamponade, heart valve malformation or malfunctioning, left ventricular function, and septal defects; a conductive gel is used to enhance transmission of emitted waves

3. Transesophageal echocardiogram: uses a Doppler probe inserted into esophagus to evaluate cardiac function with more clarity than a noninvasive study; client is NPO prior to study and is usually sedated during procedure

4. Vascular studies: upper- and lower-extremity venous and arterial evaluations can be done to detect presence of thrombus, structural malformation, claudication, and effectiveness of surgical revascularization; a conductive gel is used to enhance transmission of emitted waves

C. Electrocardiography

1. General description: a noninvasive diagnostic exam used to record electrical activity of heart

2. A 12-lead electrocardiogram (ECG): involves placement of electrodes, usually on limbs and anterior chest, to detect electrical impulses that are transposed as waveforms to graphic recorder or monitor screen; it is done to evaluate configuration, duration, rate, and rhythm of these waveforms to detect dysrhythmias or conduction defects that may indicate myocardial abnormality; ST segment depression indicates myocardial ischemia, ST segment elevation indicates acute MI; shortened or prolonged QT interval indicates ischemia or electrolyte imbalance

3. Ambulatory ECG: monitoring of client's cardiac electrical activity while client is engaged in normal or diagnostic activities

   a. Holter monitor: used to record client's ECG (2-leads) over a 24-hour period while performing normal daily activities; is used to correlate client's symptoms to cardiac activity, and to provide information on heart rate, type, and frequency of any dysrhythmias; client is asked to keep a log of activities and any symptoms that develop during the 24-hour period

   b. Graded exercise treadmill test (GXT): a noninvasive test performed on a treadmill to evaluate chest pain, other symptoms of CHD, cardiac functional capacity, or cardiac dysrhythmias that may develop during stress

      1) Electrodes are placed on client's chest and a continuous 12-lead ECG is performed

      2) Client's BP is also continuously monitored throughout testing procedure

      3) During procedure, client is asked to walk on treadmill as speed and elevation of grade is gradually increased until a target heart rate is reached (which is 80–90% of a maximum heart rate based on client's age and level of physical activity)

      4) Certain medications (such as propranolol, a beta-adrenergic blocker) and conditions such as chest pain, fatigue, or peripheral vascular disease may preclude client from reaching his or her target heart rate

      5) Test may be augmented with injection of thallium and scanning of heart before and after exercise

D. Endoscopy

1. General description: an invasive diagnostic procedure during which a long flexible fiberoptic tube is introduced into GI or respiratory tract to visualize tissues; aids in diagnosis of disease, bleeding, or masses

2. Bronchoscopy: an invasive procedure performed to directly visualize bronchi for abnormal color, strictures, abscesses, masses, foreign bodies, and to obtain sputum specimens and tissue biopsies

      a. Procedure requires that client receive a local anesthetic to enhance comfort and to inhibit cough reflex as tube is passed through nasopharynx and oropharynx into trachea

      b. During and immediately postprocedure, client must be monitored for impaired respirations, laryngospasm, and bleeding

      c. Because of impaired gag reflex caused by local anesthetic and sedation caused by medications given during procedure, client should be carefully monitored until awake and gag reflex has returned

   3. Colonoscopy: an invasive procedure performed for direct visualization of large intestine for abnormal color, inflammation, strictures, masses, foreign bodies, or bleeding; biopsy and removal of tumors and polyps can also be performed; since client will probably receive mild sedation during procedure, it is important to monitor carefully vital signs during and after procedure until client is fully awake

   4. Sigmoidoscopy is similar to colonoscopy but evaluates sigmoid colon

   5. Esophagogastroduodenoscopy is similar in principle to other procedures but evaluates upper GI tract by examining esophagus, stomach, and duodenum

E. Magnetic resonance imaging (MRI)

   1. A noninvasive diagnostic tool used to create images of multiple body planes through use of a magnetic field and radiofrequency waves

   2. Its purpose is to detect tissue structures and tears, fluid accumulations, abnormal masses, and neurological and vascular disorders

   3. Is particularly useful in visualizing soft tissue and fluid collections in areas scanned throughout body

   4. Because a magnetic field is used for testing, all metal items must be removed prior to placing client in MRI cylinder

   5. If client requires emergency care, client must be removed from vicinity of MRI scanner for care

   6. Client should be advised that MRI cylinder is narrow and that various noises will be heard while scanner is in use

   7. Client should also be advised that although he or she is in a narrow cylinder, client is able to communicate with technician via an intercom system within cylinder

   8. Mild sedation, relaxation techniques, and earplugs may be useful for client who is anxious about lying in a confined area

   9. Advances in MRI technology have allowed for creation of a less confining open chamber for those clients with severe claustrophobia

  10. Nursing implications: check for presence of metal implants in body or history of claustrophobia

F. Ophthalmoscopy: a noninvasive procedure used to examine inner eye structures of retina, optic disc, blood vessels, fundus, and macula; an ophthalmoscope is used to allow for magnification and directed lighting so examiner can assess for abnormalities in these structures

G. Otoscopic exam: a noninvasive procedure used to examine external auditory canal and tympanic membrane

   1. An otoscope is used to allow magnification, directed lighting, and access through external auditory canal to visualize canal and tympanic membrane

   2. This allows examiner to assess for lesions, obstructions, inflammation, and to visualize foreign bodies within auditory canal

   3. Tympanic membrane is assessed for color and evaluated for lesions or perforations

H. Pulse oximetry: a noninvasive, intermittent or continuous monitor utilized to trend a client's arterial oxygen saturation

   1. A probe, usually attached to client's finger, toe, earlobe, or bridge of nose, passes an infrared light through tissue and measures oxygen saturation of blood

    2. Be aware that result may be affected by abnormal hemoglobin levels and vascular insufficiencies and should be compared to client's ABGs initially

    3. This is often measured at time of respiratory assessment; normal is considered to be greater than 90% or 95%, depending on source used

I. Radiography: diagnostic procedures that use radiation exposure to visualize underlying structures

    1. Chest x-ray: a noninvasive diagnostic procedure used for general screening and diagnosis of lung and bone abnormalities

      a. Can be performed in radiology department or at client's bedside

      b. Precautions to prevent excessive radiation exposure should be taken by staff during procedure, and shielding should be provided for clients who are pregnant or of child-bearing age

      c. Ensure that appropriate views are ordered and taken (anteroposterior [AP] or lateral)

    2. Skull x-ray: a noninvasive, diagnostic radiographic procedure used to examine skull for fractures or abnormalities

      a. Skull fractures, if present, are classified by location and type, for example, depressed, linear, or penetrating

      b. Orbit area is examined for presence of free air indicating sinus bone fracture or fractures of orbits that may indicate potential damage to eyes or extensive brain damage

      c. Client should be advised to lie very still during procedure

    3. KUB: a noninvasive, diagnostic radiographic procedure used to examine kidneys, ureters, and bladder for abnormalities

    4. Upper GI series (barium swallow): a radiographic and fluoroscopic examination of pharynx and esophagus as client swallows a barium sulfate mixture

      a. Results of this procedure are used with other information to diagnose hiatal hernia, esophageal varices or diverticuli, head, neck, or stomach cancer, polyps, strictures, or pharyngeal muscle dysfunctions

      b. Client will be asked to be NPO for 8 hours prior to procedure

      c. During procedure, client will swallow quantities of barium mixture as a radiographic recording of its movement is made

      d. After procedure, it is important that client eliminates barium from GI tract; additional fluids or a mild cathartic may be ordered to aid in its elimination

    5. Lower GI series (barium enema): a radiographic and fluoroscopic examination of large intestine to detect structure abnormalities of large intestine such as tumor, diverticuli, or polyps

      a. It is essential that client's large intestine be free of stool at time of examination

      b. Client will be NPO for 8 hours prior to exam (or after midnight) after a clear liquid diet for 1–2 days preprocedure

      c. Enemas or laxative suppositories will be ordered for evening before and morning of exam to ensure absence of stool

      d. After procedure, it is important that client eliminate barium from GI tract; additional fluids, a laxative, or an enema may be ordered

    6. Ventilation perfusion (VQ) scan

      a. Is performed to diagnose possible pulmonary thrombosis or embolism; involves injecting a radionuclide intravenously and obtaining a series of images to detect areas of decreased radionuclide uptake in lung tissue, indicating decreased blood flow

      b. Ventilation scan involves inhalation of a mixture of air and radioactive gas; a nuclear scan is performed to measure amount of gas exchange

      c. In pulmonary embolism, indications of decreased blood flow will be noted in area but no ventilation abnormality will be noted

     d. During procedure, it is necessary that client have IV access and client is monitored postprocedure for any possible anaphylactic reaction to radionuclide

     e. Because of excretion of radionuclide in urine, use of gloves and thorough handwashing should be performed for 24 hours postprocedure

J. Skin testing: an intradermal (ID) injection or cutaneous scratch of a substance to assess for hypersensitivity to that substance

  1. Allergic reactions: testing involves multiple intradermal injections or cutaneous scratches applied to client's back or forearm and subsequent monitoring for a local or systemic reaction of hypersensitivity

     a. It is necessary to have immediate access to emergency equipment because of potential for anaphylactic reaction whenever allergy testing is performed

     b. Client should be advised to report any symptoms of drowsiness, skin rash, or palpitations during or following testing

     c. Client should also be advised of possibility of repeat or further testing

  2. Purified protein derivative (PPD): this skin test is administered ID to detect presence of TB infection or exposure

     a. A 0.1 mg dose of PPD is planted on inner aspect of forearm using a tuberculin syringe with a 25- to 27-gauge needle

     b. Injection site is usually observed 48–72 hours after administration and result is interpreted based on size of induration

     c. A positive result usually indicates active TB or exposure to someone with TB and requires further testing with a chest x-ray and possible sputum culture

  3. Fungi test: a skin test to detect presence of a fungal infection such as coccidioidomycosis or histoplasmosis

     a. Test involves intradermal injection of fungal material

     b. Positive reactions of erythema and induration will be noted when results are read in 24–48 hours

     c. If positive, blood titers will usually be drawn at 1- to 2-week intervals to monitor titers

     d. A negative blood titer result does not rule out infection, however; client should be advised that repeat testing might be necessary

K. Ultrasound: a noninvasive diagnostic procedure that passes high-frequency sound waves through body that are then reflected by underlying body structures to a transducer; recorded images are created on a computer screen to detect abnormalities or contents of structure; a conductive gel is used to enhance transmission of waves

  1. Abdominal: noninvasive procedure performed to detect presence of fluid (such as ascites), masses, blood, or abnormal structural changes; client should be instructed that he or she may be given enemas or be NPO for a period of time prior to testing because presence of stool, gas, or air can alter recorded images

  2. Gallbladder: a noninvasive procedure used to detect presence of gallstones and detect abnormalities of the gallbladder; client teaching will include taking a low-fat or fat-free diet on day before exam; client will be NPO or have clear liquids for 8–12 hours prior to exam

  3. Hepatobiliary: a noninvasive procedure used to detect cirrhosis, cysts, subphrenic abscesses, tumors, and to visualize biliary ducts; client teaching will include need for bowel cleansing and NPO status prior to procedure

L. Visual acuity

  1. A noninvasive test that uses Snellen chart, a chart with letters of varying sizes and standardized numbers at end of each line

  2. Top number (20) indicates distance, measured in feet, between client and chart

  3. Bottom number is distance, measured in feet, at which a person with normal vision can read the line

4. Each eye is tested individually while covering opposite eye with an occluder
5. Client should be tested with and without corrective lenses as appropriate
6. A reading for each eye should be documented
7. Normal findings are considered to be 20/20
8. Abnormal findings will include absent acuity in an eye, uncorrected acuity of 20/30 or greater in 1 eye, or that vision in both eyes is different by 2 lines or more
9. Alternatives to Snellen chart: an "E" Snellen chart and one with pictures have been developed for use with clients who are unable to read
10. Near vision is tested with a pocket Snellen chart, Rosenbaum card, or any printed material held approximately 14 inches from face; inability to read comfortably at this distance without moving card is considered abnormal and may possibly be caused by aging

M. Gene testing
1. Gene tests (also called DNA-based tests) are used to diagnose a genetic disorder
2. May involve direct examination of DNA molecule and biochemical tests for gene products such as enzymes
3. May also include microscopic examination of chromosome
4. Genetic tests may be used for:
   a. Determining genetic disease carrier status
   b. Prenatal diagnostic testing and preimplantation screening
   c. Predicting adult-onset disorders such as Huntington's disease
   d. Determining risk of developing adult-onset cancers
   e. Predicting genetic risk for developing Alzheimer's disease
   f. Confirmatory diagnosis of a symptomatic client for a specific genetic disorder
   g. Forensic identity testing
5. Nursing implications: determine type of test required and help counsel client as results can leave client with some uncertainties

Case Study

A. S., a 50-year-old male client, has been admitted for a chief complaint of upper abdominal pain, nausea, and vomiting. His primary health care provider is ruling out a medical diagnosis of acute pancreatitis.

1. What questions would you ask during the collection of his health history database pertaining to the chief complaint?
2. What laboratory tests would you anticipate to be ordered?
3. Which diagnostic procedures would you expect to be ordered?
4. What is the client teaching related to these procedures?
5. Identify 3 possible nursing diagnoses that would be appropriate for this client.

For suggested responses, see pages 620–621.

POSTTEST

1 A client has been admitted to the unit for treatment of dehydration. During the initial meeting of the client and nurse, which nursing action is most appropriate?

1. Evaluate client's response to treatment thus far.
2. Establish the outcomes of hospitalization for the client.
3. Tell the client that the provider will explain what to expect in the hospital.
4. Determine preliminary client needs upon discharge.

2 The nurse would perform which activity that relates to the evaluation phase of the nursing process during client care?

1. Ambulate a client 20 feet down the hallway.
2. Question a client about family medical history.
3. Assess a client's progress toward a desired outcome.
4. Assign a nursing diagnosis to an identified need.

3 The nurse is caring for a client who was admitted from the operating room following a traumatic amputation sustained during a motor vehicle crash. The client is awake upon arrival to the nursing unit and is hemodynamically stable at this time. The nurse monitors which elements of the complete blood count as indicators of potential complications? Select all that apply.

1. Total white blood cell count (WBCs)
2. Neutrophils
3. Eosinophils
4. Red blood cells (RBCs)
5. Platelets

4 The nurse is preparing a client for a magnetic resonance imaging (MRI) procedure. Prior to sending the client to radiology, the nurse should take which action that is unique to this test?

1. Empty urinary catheter so drainage is not obstructed during the test.
2. Determine that the plastic name band is in place.
3. Remove client's partial dental plate.
4. Send an extra blanket and a pillow for repositioning during the test.

5 The nurse is caring for a client admitted with a diagnosis of *rule out acute myocardial infarction* (AMI). When reviewing the client's laboratory data, the nurse concludes that which laboratory report is diagnostic for an AMI?

1. Elevations in troponin T and I
2. Elevated total cholesterol
3. Elevated total creatine kinase
4. Decrease in myoglobin

6 The nurse is caring for a client diagnosed with acute renal failure. Which numeric values best represent this client's anticipated arterial blood gas results?

1. pH 7.48, pCO_2 37 mmHg, HCO_3^- 29 mEq/L
2. pH 7.34, pCO_2 49 mmHg, HCO_3^- 23 mEq/L
3. pH 7.27, pCO_2 38 mmHg, HCO_3^- 19 mEq/L
4. pH 7.46, pCO_2 30 mEq/L, HCO_3^- 25 mEq/L

7 The nurse is caring for a client newly diagnosed with renal failure. What serum laboratory value should the nurse use as the most specific indicator of the effectiveness of treatment?

1. Potassium level 5.0 mEq/L
2. Blood urea nitrogen (BUN) 40 mg/dL
3. Creatinine level 3.2 mg/dL
4. Urine specific gravity 1.010

8 A client is scheduled for a colonoscopy and asks the nurse what will be determined from the test. What would be the nurse's best response?

1. "It will evaluate whether there is a tumor or other problem in the large intestine."
2. "It will determine whether there is any blood in the abdominal cavity."
3. "It will evaluate the presence of esophageal varices and provide opportunity to sclerose them."
4. "It will assess the effectiveness of the treatment you had for the peptic ulcer."

9 Which factor should the nurse consider when assessing the medication needs of a client with type 1 diabetes mellitus who is being admitted to the nursing unit? Select all that apply.

1. The client's exercise pattern
2. The client' acute illness condition
3. The nutritional status of the client
4. The length of time the client has been diagnosed with diabetes
5. Allergies previously reported

10 A client presents to the emergency department reporting left arm pain following a fall. What is the first physical examination technique the nurse would use in assessing this client?

1. Palpation for any deformities or areas of tenderness
2. Inspection for any deformities, discoloration, or obvious bone protrusion
3. Palpation of distal pulses
4. Information gathering about the circumstances of the injury

➤ *See pages 37–39 for Answers and Rationales.*

ANSWERS & RATIONALES

Pretest

1 **Answer: 3 Rationale:** Open-ended questions encourage the client to speak freely and to elaborate and clarify answers as needed. Restrictive questions that only require a "yes" or "no" answer do not encourage free exchange of information nor does frequent rephrasing of the client's answer. Leading questions tend to elicit the answer that the nurse anticipated. **Cognitive Level:** Applying **Client Need:** Psychosocial Integrity **Integrated Process:** Communication and Documentation **Content Area:** Fundamentals **Strategy:** As you read each option, place yourself in the client's position and answer the question as you would if you were the client. If your answer to a question is "yes" or "no," the client will likely answer the same way. The option that encourages you to answer at length is likely to elicit the same response in the client. **Reference:** Berman, A. J., & Snyder, S. (2011). *Kozier and Erb's fundamentals of nursing: Concepts, process, and practice* (9th ed.). Upper Saddle River, NJ: Prentice Hall, pp. 289–290. LeMone, P., Burke, K., & Bauldoff, G. (2011). *Medical-surgical nursing:*

Critical thinking in patient care (5th ed.). Upper Saddle River, NJ: Pearson Education, pp. 159, 169.

2 **Answer: 4 Rationale:** It is necessary to know how well the interventions worked in order to revise them appropriately. Medical assessment and written prescriptions are components of the client care but not the focus of the nursing plan of care. The focus of the care plan is to direct the nurse to where the client is in his or her recovery, where he needs to go next, and what the nurse and client need to do to achieve the goal. **Cognitive Level:** Applying **Client Need:** Management of Care **Integrated Process:** Communication and Documentation **Content Area:** Fundamentals **Strategy:** The question is asking you to determine when the client needs additional interventions that have not already been implemented. Differentiate the options that tell you what to do or how to do it from the one that tells you if the intervention was effective. **Reference:** Smith, S., Duell, D., & Martin, B. (2012). *Clinical nursing skills: Basic to advanced skills* (8th ed.). Upper Saddle River, NJ: Pearson Education, pp. 20–24.

3 **Answer: 1** **Rationale:** Renal failure results in the inability of the kidneys to excrete potassium, which leads to hyperkalemia. Nausea, vomiting, excessive laxative use, and loop diuretic all cause excess fluid loss from the body. With this fluid will also be loss of electrolytes, which would lead to hypokalemia rather than hyperkalemia. **Cognitive Level:** Applying **Client Need:** Physiological Adaptation **Integrated Process:** Nursing Process: Assessment **Content Area:** Adult Health **Strategy:** With each option, think about what is happening to the body. Some options cause a loss of electrolytes because of increased elimination, but only one decreases fluids through elimination. **Reference:** LeMone, P., Burke, K., & Bauldoff, G. (2011). *Medical-surgical nursing: Critical thinking in patient care* (5th ed.). Upper Saddle River, NJ: Pearson Education, p. 427.

4 **Answer: 1** **Rationale:** A client with myasthenia gravis may have risk for ineffective breathing pattern because of neuromuscular effects of the disease, and may also have risk for impaired gas exchange because of possible respiratory impairments from the physiological process of this disease. A postoperative client who had surgery more than 24 hours ago may have pain at the surgical site but should not have hypoventilation from anesthesia, as these effects should wear off within 24 hours. A preoperative client in pain may or may not have respirations affected. It is highly unlikely that a client with prostate cancer will experience respiratory difficulty unless there is dysuria or localized pain, which may result in change in breathing pattern. **Cognitive Level:** Analyzing **Client Need:** Physiological Adaptation **Integrated Process:** Nursing Process: Assessment **Content Area:** Adult Health **Strategy:** First determine what the question is asking, and then determine what respiratory alteration may cause both a problem with breathing pattern and a problem with gas exchange. **Reference:** LeMone, P., Burke, K., & Bauldoff, G. (2011). *Medical-surgical nursing: Critical thinking in patient care* (5th ed.). Upper Saddle River, NJ: Pearson Education, p. 1290.

5 **Answer: 2** **Rationale:** A low serum potassium level (normal 3.5–5.1 mEq/L) enhances the action of digoxin (Lanoxin) and predisposes the client receiving the medication to develop toxicity. Hyponatremia, hypomagnesemia, and a normal calcium level do not contribute to digoxin toxicity. **Cognitive Level:** Analyzing **Client Need:** Pharmacological and Parenteral Therapies **Integrated Process:** Nursing Process: Assessment **Content Area:** Adult Health **Strategy:** Think of the primary action of digoxin (Lanoxin), which is to increase myocardial contractility. This is primarily indicated in heart failure where diuretics are given, causing a potassium loss. **Reference:** Adams, M., & Koch, R. (2010). *Pharmacology: Connections to nursing practice.* Upper Saddle River, NJ: Prentice Hall, p. 614. Osborn, K. S., Wraa, C. E., & Watson, A. (2010). *Medical-surgical nursing: Preparation for practice.* Upper Saddle River, NJ: Prentice Hall, pp. 429, 431.

6 **Answer: 1** **Rationale:** The client will be required to have an empty stomach for the procedure to allow visualization of the gallbladder and adjacent structures to accurately rule out tumors, structural abnormalities, or the presence of stones. Since the lower GI tract is not visualized during this procedure, there is no need for the bowel to be empty. Also, ultrasound does not require the use of radioactive isotopes. **Cognitive Level:** Applying **Client Need:** Reduction of Risk Potential **Integrated Process:** Communication and Documentation **Content Area:** Adult Health **Strategy:** Recall that the gallbladder sits below the liver and adjacent to the stomach. If the body is engaged in digestion, the gallbladder will not be visualized and the ultrasound will be of no diagnostic value. **Reference:** LeMone, P., Burke, K., & Bauldoff, G. (2011). *Medical-surgical nursing: Critical thinking in patient care* (5th ed.). Upper Saddle River, NJ: Pearson Education, pp. 356, 574.

7 **Answer: 3** **Rationale:** The administration of a local anesthetic is possible during the procedure to decrease the gag reflex and increase comfort. The nurse should check for the return of the gag reflex to prevent the potential for aspiration. The position of the side rails, the availability of the call light, and the ability to ambulate without assistance are safety concerns but are not related to the specific client request. **Cognitive Level:** Applying **Client Need:** Reduction of Risk Potential **Integrated Process:** Nursing Process: Assessment **Content Area:** Adult Health **Strategy:** Because the bronchoscopy requires a local anesthetic, the oropharynx is anesthetized. This prevents the client from sensing the presence of fluids and closing the larynx to protect the airway. **Reference:** LeMone, P., Burke, K., & Bauldoff, G. (2011). *Medical-surgical nursing: Critical thinking in patient care* (5th ed.). Upper Saddle River, NJ: Pearson Education, p. 356.

8 **Answer: 4** **Rationale:** An oxygen saturation of less than 80% with observable signs of shortness of breath indicates respiratory distress, which requires immediate intervention. A rapid respiratory assessment should be performed and the health care provider advised of the findings immediately. Symptomatic respiratory distress should never be ignored. The repositioning of the client and the receiving of a health care provider's order to increase the rate of oxygen delivery would help increase the oxygen saturation. The client should be continually monitored, but 15 L/min flow rate of oxygen via nasal cannula is excessive. **Cognitive Level:** Analyzing **Client Need:** Reduction of Risk Potential **Integrated Process:** Nursing Process: Diagnosis **Content Area:** Adult Health **Strategy:** In clients with shortness of breath (SOB) and decreased oxygen saturation, immediate intervention is needed. However, the nasal cannula is typically used at a maximum of 6 L/min. Repositioning the client will certainly maximize lung expansion but the health care provider is also needed because of the significant decrease to 70%. **Reference:** Smith, S. F., Duell, D. J., & Martin, B. C.

(2012). *Clinical nursing skills: Basic to advanced skills* (8th ed.). Upper Saddle River, NJ: Pearson Education, pp. 966–967.

9 **Answer: 4, 1, 2, 3** **Rationale:** Airway and respiratory status take priority over all other interventions. After this is established, performing a neurological exam is indicated as the first step in determining if the cause of the unresponsiveness is related to a neurological or metabolic cause. Blood would then be drawn in a general physiologic screening as well as in a toxicology screen to determine the presence of drugs as a cause for the unresponsiveness. If the cause of the unresponsiveness is determined to be neurological in origin, a CT scan would then be done. **Cognitive Level:** Analyzing **Client Need:** Management of Care **Integrated Process:** Nursing Process: Implementation **Content Area:** Adult Health **Strategy:** In emergency situations, apply the ABCs (airway, breathing, and circulation), with airway being first. Then continue with the assessments listed with the least invasive and time consuming to the most time consuming. **Reference:** Smith, S. F., Duell, D. J., & Martin, B. C. (2012). *Clinical nursing skills: Basic to advanced skills* (8th ed.). Upper Saddle River, NJ: Pearson Education, pp. 26–27.

10 **Answer: 2, 3, 4** **Rationale:** Priority is given to acutely ill, unstable clients who require invasive procedures or monitoring that cannot occur outside the intensive care area, and who for all purposes have a good chance of surviving their acute illness. **Cognitive Level:** Analyzing **Client Need:** Physiological Adaptation **Integrated Process:** Nursing Process: Assessment **Content Area:** Adult Health **Strategy:** Consider which clients require the most frequent assessment and care, and who require caregivers with specialized knowledge of therapeutic interventions. This will help you to choose correctly. **Reference:** Wagner, K., Johnson, K., & Hardin-Pierce, M. (2010). *High-acuity nursing* (5th ed.). Upper Saddle River, NJ: Pearson Education, p. 3.

Posttest

1 **Answer: 4** **Rationale:** Discharge planning should begin on admission to the unit and should be an ongoing process. As a rule, clients are not ready to discuss discharge plans on the day of admission; however, planning for appropriate follow-up and coordination of care frequently cannot be achieved on the morning of discharge. The client has just been admitted so there are no fully executed treatments to evaluate. It is the nurse's responsibility to orient the client to the hospital and its routine. All outcomes should be mutually established by the client and nurse. **Cognitive Level:** Applying **Client Need:** Management of Care **Integrated Process:** Nursing Process: Planning **Content Area:** Fundamentals **Strategy:** This is the first meeting with the client, so eliminate any options inconsistent with this timing. Differentiate the provider's role from the nurse's role. Identify the option that is consistent with the goal of promoting independence and

autonomy for the client. **Reference:** Smith, S. F., Duell, D. J., & Martin, B. C. (2012). *Clinical nursing skills* (8th ed.). Upper Saddle River, NJ: Pearson Education, pp. 64–66, 113–114.

2 **Answer: 3** **Rationale:** The evaluation step of the client's plan of care includes the assessment of the client's progress toward a previously identified desired outcome. The desired outcome would have been the result of assessment, planning by establishing nursing diagnoses, and implementation of interventions that promote goal achievement. **Cognitive Level:** Applying **Client Need:** Management of Care **Integrated Process:** Nursing Process: Evaluation **Content Area:** Fundamentals **Strategy:** Eliminate options that reflect any steps in the nursing process unrelated to evaluation. **Reference:** Smith, S. F., Duell, D. J., & Martin, B. C. (2012). *Clinical nursing skills* (8th ed.). Upper Saddle River, NJ: Pearson Education, pp. 20–22.

3 **Answer: 1, 2, 4** **Rationale:** The risk for postoperative infection is high in a traumatic amputation so the WBCs should be monitored as an indicator of a wound infection. The neutrophil count would be monitored as part of the WBC, since these cells respond to pathogens. Because the client has come directly from surgery, the client could have a low RBC count from blood loss at the time of the amputation and during surgery. There is no information about blood transfusions, so the RBC count should be monitored for anemia. Eosinophils and basophils are other types of WBCs that do not respond to acute infection. A low platelet count would put the client at risk for bleeding, but the client is hemodynamically stable so this is not a primary concern. **Cognitive Level:** Analyzing **Client Need:** Reduction of Risk Potential **Integrated Process:** Nursing Process: Assessment **Content Area:** Adult Health **Strategy:** The keys to answering this item are that the client has undergone surgery and that there was a traumatic amputation. Select the options that reflect the greatest dangers of blood loss and infection. **Reference:** LeMone, P., Burke, K., & Bauldoff, G. (2011). *Medical-surgical nursing: Critical thinking in patient care* (5th ed.). Upper Saddle River, NJ: Pearson Education, pp. 1314–1341.

4 **Answer: 3** **Rationale:** Magnetic resonance imaging (MRI) testing involves the use of a magnetic field and radiofrequency waves. Any object that contains metal of any kind will be attracted to the magnetic field, which will affect the diagnostic ability of the test and can potentially harm the client. Plastic and the urinary catheter are not attracted to the magnetic field. In addition, it is standard procedure (not unique) to be sure that clients are wearing an identification bracelet. The MRI suite has devices for positioning that completely immobilize the client, so sending blankets and a pillow for repositioning is unnecessary. **Cognitive Level:** Applying **Client Need:** Reduction of Risk Potential **Integrated Process:** Nursing Process: Planning **Content Area:** Fundamentals **Strategy:** A critical word to guide you in this question is *unique*.

Review the basis of the magnetic resonance imaging (MRI) and the risks associated with the use of a magnet. Then use the process of elimination to discard any option that does not focus on this risk. **Reference:** Kee, J. L. (2010). *Laboratory and diagnostic tests* (8th ed.). Upper Saddle River, NJ: Pearson Education, pp. 506–507.

5 Answer: 1 Rationale: Elevations in troponin T and I are not found in healthy individuals, so any elevation is indicative of an acute cardiac event. While the elevation in the total cholesterol places the client at risk for an acute myocardial infarction (AMI), it is not diagnostic. The total creatine kinase is nonspecific and may indicate brain (CK-BB), myocardial (CK-MB), or skeletal damage (CK-MM). The isoenzyme CK-MB is specific for an AMI. Myoglobin would be increased in AMI, not decreased, but this is a nonspecific finding because myoglobin refers only to muscle tissue. **Cognitive Level:** Analyzing **Client Need:** Reduction of Risk Potential **Integrated Process:** Nursing Process: Assessment **Content Area:** Adult Health **Strategy:** Eliminate components that are nonspecific for myocardial injury. Review the items secreted from the injured myocardial cell. Recall that any item secreted from the cell will increase the serum level of that component. **Reference:** LeMone, P., Burke, K., & Bauldoff, G. (2011). *Medical-surgical nursing: Critical thinking in patient care* (5th ed.). Upper Saddle River, NJ: Pearson Education, p. 937.

6 Answer: 3 Rationale: Clients in acute renal failure have an accumulation of uric acid in the blood that makes them acidotic, and thus the acidosis is of metabolic origin, not respiratory origin. The bicarbonate (HCO_3^-) level is low because it is used trying to neutralize body acid. A low pH (normal 7.35–7.45) would indicate an acidosis, while a high pH indicates alkalosis. An elevated bicarbonate level (normal 22–26 mEq/L) indicates a metabolic cause for alkalosis. A low pCO_2 (normal 35–45) should indicate a respiratory alkalosis. **Cognitive Level:** Analyzing **Client Need:** Reduction of Risk Potential **Integrated Process:** Nursing Process: Assessment **Content Area:** Adult Health **Strategy:** The kidneys eliminate an acid, so if they are not functioning, acid accumulates in the blood, making it acidic. Eliminate any pH that is not acidotic. Then differentiate respiratory acidosis from metabolic acidosis. **Reference:** LeMone, P., Burke, K., & Bauldoff, G. (2011). *Medical-surgical nursing: Critical thinking in patient care* (5th ed.). Upper Saddle River, NJ: Pearson Education, p. 1232.

7 Answer: 3 Rationale: Creatinine levels (normal 0.8–1.6 mg/dL) are more sensitive and specific for renal function than the BUN (normal 8–22 mg/dL). Although the BUN is used to assess renal function, it can also be affected by diet and fluid status and is therefore not the most specific indicator available. The potassium level can be affected by many factors as well, such as tissue damage and adrenal insufficiency; however, this level is normal (range 3.5–5.1 mEq/L). Specific gravity is not a

blood test, but rather is performed on the urine, and the value of 1.010 is within normal range (1.010–1.025). **Cognitive Level:** Analyzing **Client Need:** Reduction of Risk Potential **Integrated Process:** Nursing Process: Assessment **Content Area:** Adult Health **Strategy:** The critical word in the question is *specific*. Eliminate any options that are not directly related to abnormal renal function, including the potassium level at the high end of normal and the normal urine specific gravity. Then eliminate the options that can be abnormal from other causes, which is the BUN. **Reference:** LeMone, P., Burke, K., & Bauldoff, G. (2011). *Medical-surgical nursing: Critical thinking in patient care* (5th ed.). Upper Saddle River, NJ: Pearson Education, p. 760. Osborn, K. S., Wraa, C. E., & Watson, A. (2010). *Medical-surgical nursing: Preparation for practice*. Upper Saddle River, NJ: Pearson Education, pp. 835, 1465.

8 Answer: 1 Rationale: A colonoscopy is the insertion of a flexible tube into the lower GI tract for evaluation and treatment of conditions of the lower bowel. An evaluation of the esophagus and stomach would require an approach from the upper GI tract such as an esophagogastroduodenoscopy (EGD). The presence of blood in the abdominal cavity would require an abdominal ultrasound or other x-ray procedure. **Cognitive Level:** Applying **Client Need:** Reduction of Risk Potential **Integrated Process:** Teaching and Learning **Content Area:** Adult Health **Strategy:** Recall that colonoscopy means direct visualization of the colon. Eliminate any options unrelated to this definition. **Reference:** LeMone, P., Burke, K., & Bauldoff, G. (2011). *Medical-surgical nursing: Critical thinking in patient care* (5th ed.). Upper Saddle River, NJ: Pearson Education, pp. 742–745.

9 Answer: 1, 2, 3 Rationale: A balance between glucose and insulin is needed to maintain homeostasis and stabilize the diabetes. Exercise, acute illness, and nutrition are all instrumental in assessment and determining medication need status. Length of time since diagnosis may give some information as to self-management but is not specific to medication therapy. Allergies that were previously reported are not specific to insulin therapy, especially since the development of human insulin using recombinant DNA technology. **Cognitive Level:** Analyzing **Client Need:** Pharmacological and Parenteral Therapies **Integrated Process:** Nursing Process: Assessment **Content Area:** Adult Health **Strategy:** Review the pathophysiology of diabetes mellitus and determine the factors that contribute to stabilization of insulin in the body. **Reference:** Wagner, K., Johnson, K., & Hardin-Pierce, M. (2010). *High-acuity nursing* (5th ed.). Upper Saddle River, NJ: Pearson Education, p. 801.

10 Answer: 2 Rationale: The first nursing assessment technique utilized to gather data is inspection of the area. Palpation of any area would be attempted after the inspection. Obtaining the client history is not a component of the physical examination. **Cognitive Level:** Applying **Client Need:** Health Promotion and Maintenance **Integrated Process:** Nursing Process: Assessment **Content Area:** Adult Health **Strategy:** Always look at the area of reported problem first for visible signs of an

abnormality. **Reference:** LeMone, P., Burke, K., & Bauldoff, G. (2011). *Medical-surgical nursing: Critical thinking in patient care* (5th ed.). Upper Saddle River, NJ: Pearson Education, pp. 282–284.

References

Berman, A., & Snyder, S. (2012). *Kozier & Erb's fundamentals of nursing: Concepts, process, and practice* (9th ed.). Upper Saddle River, NJ: Pearson Education.

Berman, A. J., Snyder, S., & McKinney, D. S. (2011). *Nursing basics for clinical practice.* Upper Saddle River, NJ: Pearson Education.

D'Amico, D., & Barbarito, C. (2012). *Health & physical assessment in nursing* (2nd ed.). Upper Saddle River, NJ: Pearson Education.

Ignatavicius, D. D., & Workman, M. L. (2013). *Medical-surgical nursing: Critical thinking for collaborative care* (7th ed.) Philadelphia: W. B. Saunders Company.

Kee, J. L. (2010). *Laboratory and diagnostic tests* (8th ed.). Upper Saddle River, NJ: Pearson Education.

Kee, J. L. (2009). *Handbook of laboratory and diagnostic tests with nursing implications* (6th ed.). Upper Saddle River, NJ: Pearson Education.

Lehne, R. (2010). *Pharmacology for nursing care* (7th ed.). St. Louis, MO: Saunders.

LeMone, P., Burke, K., & Bauldoff, G. (2011). *Medical-surgical nursing: Critical thinking in patient care* (5th ed.). Upper Saddle River, NJ: Pearson Education.

Lewis, S., Dirksen, S., Heitkemper, M., Bucher, L., & Camera, I. (2011). *Medical surgical nursing: Assessment and management of clinical problems* (8th ed.). St. Louis, MO: Elsevier.

McCance, K. L., & Huether, S. E. (2010). *Pathophysiology: The biologic basis for disease in adults and children* (6th ed.). St. Louis, MO: Mosby, Inc.

Osborn, K. S., Wraa, C. E., & Watson, A. (2010). *Medical surgical nursing: Preparation for practice.* Upper Saddle River, NJ: Pearson Education.

Smith, S. F., Duell, D. J., & Martin, B. C. (2012). *Clinical nursing skills: Basic to advanced skills* (8th ed.). Upper Saddle River, NJ: Pearson Education.

Wilson, B. A., Shannon, M. T., & Shields, K. M. (2012). *Pearson nurse's drug guide 2012.* Upper Saddle River, NJ: Pearson Education.

ANSWERS & RATIONALES

Chapter Outline

Overview of Anatomy and
  Physiology
Diagnostic Tests and
  Assessments

Common Nursing Techniques
  and Procedures
Nursing Management of Client
  Having Thoracic Surgery

Disorders of the Respiratory
  System

NCLEX-RN® Test Prep

Use the accompanying online resource,
NursingReviewsandRationales, to test
yourself with hundreds of NCLEX®-style
practice questions.

Objectives

➤ Identify basic structures and functions of the respiratory system.
➤ Describe the pathophysiology and etiology of common respiratory
  disorders.
➤ Discuss expected assessment data and diagnostic test findings for
  selected respiratory disorders.
➤ Identify priority nursing problems associated with selected
  respiratory disorders.
➤ Discuss therapeutic management of a client experiencing selected
  respiratory disorders.
➤ Discuss nursing management of a client experiencing a respiratory
  disorder.
➤ Identify expected outcomes for the client experiencing a
  respiratory disorder.

Review at a Glance

acid a substance that is capable
of losing hydrogen ions
acidosis condition of increased
hydrogen ion concentration in blood
alkalosis condition of decreased
hydrogen ion concentration in blood
alveolar ventilation volume of air
that undergoes gas exchange
anatomic dead space portion
of respiratory system from nose to
bronchioles that functions only as an air
pathway; about 25% of air inhaled with
each breath remains here and is unavail-
able for gas exchange
base a substance that is capable of
accepting hydrogen ions
buffer a weak acid or a weak base
that transfers hydrogen ions between
solutions to maintain acid–base
balance

compliance elastic property of lungs
and thorax; also referred to as distensibility
diffusion movement of gas from an
area of higher pressure to an area of
lower pressure
expiration movement of air from
lungs; process is generally passive, but
may become more conscious and forced
with obstructive lung disease
inspiration movement of air from
atmosphere into respiratory system;
process is generally active
oxygen saturation percentage of
oxygen bound to hemoglobin compared
to volume that hemoglobin is capable of
binding
perfusion circulation of blood into
tissues and cells
pH refers to hydrogen ion concentration
of a solution; indicator of ratio of acid and

base in blood; a lower pH value indicates
greater hydrogen ion concentration
and greater acidity; a higher pH value
indicates lower hydrogen ion concentration and higher alkalinity
pulmonary ventilation total
volume of gas exchange between
atmosphere and lungs
respiration mechanical and
metabolic processes involved with
oxygen transport from atmospheric air
into cells and carbon dioxide transport
from cells back into the atmosphere
**ventilation–perfusion
mismatch** clinically significant imbalance between volume of air and volume of
blood circulating to alveoli; average ratio is
4 L of air for every 5 L of blood that flows into
alveoli (ratio of 0.8); also commonly known
as VQ (ventilation quotient) mismatch

PRETEST

1 The nurse is caring for a client in the short procedure unit (SPU) following a bronchoscopy using moderate (conscious) sedation. Prior to discharging the client, the nurse verifies that the client has achieved which priority outcome?

1. Verbalizes symptoms of late complications
2. Demonstrates an intact gag reflex
3. Remains afebrile for up to 2 postop days
4. Reports being thirsty and asks for oral fluids

2 The nurse is caring for a 68-year-old client who is scheduled for discharge later that day. An arterial blood gas (ABG) done the previous morning reveals a PaO_2 of 87 mmHg. The client has a respiratory rate of 22 and clear lungs and reports no shortness of breath. What should be the nurse's response?

1. Call the health care provider to report the PaO_2.
2. Monitor the client more closely because a physiological abnormality is beginning.
3. Do nothing because a PaO_2 of 87 is normal in an older adult.
4. Call the family to tell them to anticipate that the discharge will be cancelled.

3 The nurse is caring for a client diagnosed with right middle lobe pneumonia. The nurse should perform which intervention to mobilize secretions?

1. Administer antibiotics as ordered.
2. Limit fluids to intravenous fluids only.
3. Place the client in a prone position to increase alveolar expansion.
4. Assist client to use incentive spirometer hourly.

4 Which type of transmission-based precaution technique should the nurse implement for the client diagnosed with bacterial meningitis?

1. Standard
2. Airborne
3. Enteric
4. Droplet

5 A postoperative client with emphysema is receiving oxygen at 2 L/min via nasal cannula when the client reports shortness of breath. The spouse asks the nurse to increase the oxygen to help the client breathe easier. Which response by the nurse is appropriate?

1. "I have a better technique; I will switch him to 100% non-rebreather mask."
2. "Higher concentration of oxygen may decrease breathing and cause more difficulty."
3. "I think you should leave for an hour; it's just anxiety, and rest will improve the breathing."
4. "This is an indication that he is in pain; I will treat that."

6 The home health nurse is assessing an adolescent who has frequent school absences because of acute asthma attacks. Assessment reveals mild inspiratory wheezes and current oxygen saturation (SaO_2) of 98%. The client can answer questions in full sentences and accurately demonstrates the use of inhalers. After documenting this data, what would be the next best action by the nurse?

1. Report to home health agency that client has adequate knowledge of how to manage disease.
2. Question family members to determine if they know CPR in event of a respiratory emergency.
3. Perform an environmental assessment to identify asthma triggers.
4. Report the situation to the Department of Youth Services for truancy and possible neglect.

7 The nurse is teaching a client with newly diagnosed emphysema how to manage the disease. The client asks how pursed-lip breathing helps the emphysema. What would be the best response by the nurse?

1. "It prevents air sacs in the lungs from trapping air."
2. "It decreases the pressure in the airways."
3. "The resistance on exhalation increases muscle strength in the diaphragm."
4. "It helps slow the respiratory rate."

8 When teaching a client scheduled for a bedside thoracentesis, what would the nurse explain is the primary purpose for this procedure?

1. It is used to obtain pleural tissue for evaluation.
2. It is used to determine the stage of a lung tumor.
3. It is used to withdraw fluid from the pleural space.
4. It is used to directly examine the pleural space.

9 The nurse is caring for a client who has just had a pleural chest tube inserted for a mixed pneumothorax and hemothorax. In the image, locate the section used to determine that air is leaving the pleural space.

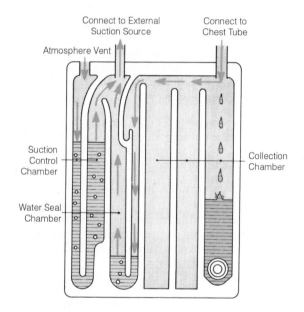

10 The nurse is caring for a client diagnosed with pneumothorax, which is being treated with a chest tube to re-expand the lung. Which actions are appropriate for the nurse to take when caring for this client? Select all that apply.

1. Clamp chest tube when assisting client from bed to chair.
2. Report fluctuations in water seal section of chest drainage system.
3. Maintain an occlusive dressing, such as petrolatum gauze, around chest tube at insertion site.
4. Gently massage chest tubes hourly to promote chest drainage.
5. Encourage client to maintain a high Fowler's position.

➤ *See pages 78–80 for Answers and Rationales.*

I. OVERVIEW OF ANATOMY AND PHYSIOLOGY

    A. Respiratory system structures: anatomic areas include upper and lower respiratory tract, accessory structures, and blood supply; functional areas include conducting airways (**anatomic dead space**) from nose to terminal bronchioles, and gas exchange airways, from respiratory bronchioles to alveoli and alveolar ducts

        1. Upper respiratory tract (conducting airways)

            a. Nose: pathway for air exchange between atmospheric air and respiratory tract; filters, humidifies (requires about 250 milliliters [mL] of fluid daily), and heats inspired air; nasal hairs trap airborne particles in mucus, and cilia propel them into nasopharynx to be expelled by coughing or diverted into gastrointestinal (GI) tract; olfactory nerve receptors are responsible for sense of smell

            b. Paranasal sinuses: air-filled cavities in frontal, maxillary, ethmoid, and sphenoid bones that contribute to mucus production and voice resonance

            c. Pharynx: nasopharynx, laryngopharynx (pathway for air), and oropharynx (pathway for food); adenoids in nasopharynx and tonsils in oropharynx contain lymphatic tissue that contributes to immune function

            d. Larynx: vibration of vocal cords within larynx produces voice; remains open only when air is passing through; epiglottis closes during swallowing to prevent passage of food into trachea

            e. Trachea: pathway between upper and lower respiratory tract; divides into right and left mainstem bronchi

        2. Lower respiratory tract (conducting airways and gas exchange airways)

            a. Bronchi: pathway for air from trachea into lungs through right and left mainstem bronchus (conducting airways); mainstem bronchi branch into smaller bronchioles that terminate in alveoli; right mainstem bronchus is straighter, making it a more common passage for aspirated gastric contents and dislocated endotracheal tubes; terminal bronchioles (gas exchange airways) have a semi-permeable membrane and participate in gas exchange

            b. Alveoli: air-filled sacs in lungs; oxygen diffuses from alveoli (gas exchange airways) into blood across alveolar-capillary membrane (primary site of gas exchange); carbon dioxide diffuses across pulmonary capillary membrane into alveoli; spherical shape of alveoli provides greater surface area for gas exchange

                1) Type I alveolar cells: squamous epithelium cells that participate in gas exchange

                2) Type II alveolar cells: also are epithelial cells; help maintain alveolar integrity and have some macrophage function to help immune system

            c. Lungs: function is air exchange; reoxygenate blood and neutralize some vasoactive substances; right lung is divided into 3 lobes—upper, middle, and lower; left lung is divided into 2 lobes—upper and lower; upper area is called the apex; lower area is called the base

            d. Pleura: 2-layer membrane covering lungs and thoracic cavity; visceral pleura covers external lung surface; parietal pleura lines thoracic cavity; pleural fluid lubricates pleural layers and holds them together during inspiration and expiration

            e. Pleural cavity: air-filled space of thoracic cavity housing lower respiratory tract

        3. Accessory structures: contribute to mechanics of breathing

            a. Rib cage: 12 pairs of ribs and sternum provide skeletal support and protection for heart and lungs

            b. Intercostal muscles: located between ribs, contraction facilitates chest expansion during inspiration by increasing anterior-posterior and lateral diameter of chest

            c. Diaphragm: separates thoracic cavity from abdominal cavity; brain's respiratory center controls contraction of diaphragm via phrenic nerve; flattens during inspiration to allow greater chest expansion during inspiration; an intact nervous system is essential to proper functioning of diaphragm

B. Respiratory system functions: primary function is exchange of gases between external environment and blood; process of respiration involves ventilation, perfusion, diffusion, and nervous system control; **respiration** refers to mechanical and metabolic processes involved with oxygen (O_2) transport from atmospheric air into blood, and carbon dioxide (CO_2) transport from blood back to atmospheric air

1. Ventilation: passage of gases between atmosphere and lungs; ventilation phases include inspiration and expiration; adequacy of ventilation is influenced by respiratory system pressures, respiratory tissue properties, airway resistance, lung volumes and capacities, body position, and disease processes

    a. **Pulmonary ventilation**: total volume of gas exchange between atmosphere and lungs

    b. **Alveolar ventilation**: volume of air that undergoes gas exchange

    c. Ventilation phases

        1) **Inspiration**: nerve impulses travel from brain via phrenic nerve to contract diaphragm, increasing diameter of thoracic cavity; intrapleural pressure decreases, becoming more negative compared to atmospheric air; air moves from area of higher pressure (atmosphere) to lower pressure (respiratory system); air moves through structures of respiratory system to alveoli and pulmonary capillaries where gas exchange occurs

        2) **Expiration**: diaphragm relaxes and pushes upward, decreasing thoracic cavity diameter; intrapleural pressure remains negative compared to atmospheric air, but becomes less negative than during inspiration; intrapulmonic pressure becomes higher than atmospheric pressure, allowing passive air flow from lung through respiratory structures into atmosphere; smaller airways may collapse during expiration, particularly when in supine position

    d. Respiratory system pressures: atmospheric pressure of 760 mmHg serves as reference point for comparison to respiratory pressures

        1) Intrapulmonary pressure: also called intra-alveolar pressure; equals atmospheric pressure when glottis is open and there is no air movement

        2) Intrapleural pressure: negative pressure produced by opposite forces of elastic recoil between lungs and chest wall; with glottis open and alveolar air in communication with atmosphere, it measures negative compared to intrapulmonary pressure; with glottis closed, during coughing or with forced expiration, it measures positive compared to atmospheric air; normally negative intrapleural pressure prevents lung collapse

        3) Intrathoracic pressure: compared to atmospheric air, negative pressure inside thoracic cavity equals intrapleural pressure; with forced expiration against a closed glottis, intrathoracic pressure becomes positive

    e. Respiratory tissue properties: respiratory vessels and airways are implanted in elastic tissues

        1) **Compliance**: elastic property of lung related to elastic and collagen fibers; compliance changes with changes in respiratory system pressures and/or lung fluid content; higher compliance occurs in lung that is more easily distended; lower compliance occurs in lung that is not easily distended

        2) Elastic recoil: ability of lungs to return to original shape after air is expelled; recoil occurs due to opposing forces created by movement of lungs and chest wall

        3) Distensibility: ease of lung inflation made more difficult by increased volume of lung fluid content or consolidation of lung tissue

        4) Stiffness: resistance of lungs to stretch to accommodate air volume; increased lung stiffness lowers compliance

      f. Airway resistance: obstruction to airflow caused by conditions of respiratory system tissues (elastic recoil, compliance), changes in airway diameter (bronchoconstriction, mucous obstruction), and/or pressure differences between atmospheric air and intrapulmonary air

      g. Lung volumes and capacities: lung volumes describe normal individual quantities of air exchanged during specific periods of breathing cycle; lung capacities describe combined quantities of lung volumes during specific periods of breathing cycle (see Box 2-1)

      h. Body position: gravity accounts for greater ventilation in dependent areas of lung; with inspiration and when body is upright, sitting, or standing, airway opening allows for airflow to follow path of least resistance into more compliant lung bases

  2. **Perfusion**: blood flow through pulmonary capillary bed and to respiratory system structures; this circulation includes pulmonary circulation and bronchial circulation

      a. Pulmonary circulation: pulmonary artery carries deoxygenated (venous) blood from right ventricle, branches into pulmonary capillaries, and connects to alveoli; CO_2 is exchanged for O_2 at pulmonary capillary membranes, which merge into pulmonary venules and veins that carry oxygenated blood back to left atrium of heart

      b. Bronchial circulation: bronchial arteries branching from thoracic aorta circulate blood to conducting airways and other respiratory tract tissues; bronchial blood does not circulate to alveoli and is not included in gas exchange; deoxygenated bronchial blood drains through bronchial capillaries and veins into vena cava and right side of heart; deoxygenated blood from small bronchial veins drains into azygos and pulmonary veins into left side of heart, and then combines with oxygenated blood from pulmonary circulation

      c. Characteristics of respiratory system circulation: blood pressure (BP) and resistance to blood flow are lower in pulmonary blood vessels (BVs) compared to systemic BVs; adequacy of pulmonary capillary blood flow depends upon a mean pulmonary arterial pressure (MPAP) that is greater than mean pulmonary venous pressure (MPVP); blood volume in pulmonary capillary bed increases when MPVP exceeds MPAP, causing pulmonary edema; pulmonary BVs constrict in response to hypoxia

---

Box 2-1	• Tidal volume (V_T): total air volume inspired and expired during one breathing cycle.
Lung Volumes and Capacities	• Inspiratory reserve volume (IRV): maximum air volume inspired with forced inspiration (i.e., movement of air from the atmosphere into the respiratory system) following normal inspiration.

- Tidal volume (V_T): total air volume inspired and expired during one breathing cycle.
- Inspiratory reserve volume (IRV): maximum air volume inspired with forced inspiration (i.e., movement of air from the atmosphere into the respiratory system) following normal inspiration.
- Expiratory reserve volume (ERV): air volume that can be expired with force following normal expiration.
- Residual volume (RV): air volume remaining in lungs following forced expiration.
- Total lung capacity (TLC): maximum capacity of air volume of the lungs. TLC = IRV + V_T + ERV + RV
- Inspiratory capacity (IC): maximum air volume that can be inhaled following a normal exhalation. IC = V_T + IRV
- Vital capacity (VC): maximum air volume that can be exhaled after a maximum inhalation. VC = IRV + V_T + ERV
- Functional residual capacity (FRC): residual air volume in lungs after a normal exhalation. FRC = ERV + RV

3. **Diffusion**: movement of gas from an area of higher pressure to lower pressure; O_2 diffuses from atmosphere into alveoli, across pulmonary capillary membrane and into pulmonary capillaries for circulation; CO_2 diffuses out of pulmonary capillaries across capillary membrane and into alveoli to be exhaled; diffusion continues until pressure differences become equal between the 2 areas
   a. Fick's Law: describes process of gas diffusion; it is directly proportional to concentration gradient and surface area of membrane and inversely proportional to distance that air needs to travel
   b. Variables that influence gas exchange (see Table 2-1)
   c. Ventilation–perfusion relationship: adequate gas exchange requires alveolar ventilation of about 4 L/min balanced with alveolar capillary perfusion of about 5 L/min (see Figure 2-1)
      1) Normal ventilation–perfusion (V/Q) ratio: 4:5
      2) V/Q ratio is influenced by partial pressure of O_2 and partial pressure of CO_2
      3) Average normal PaO_2 = 100 mmHg; average normal $PaCO_2$ = 40 mmHg
      4) Partial pressure of gases varies in different lung areas
      5) Under normal conditions and in upright position, ventilation is greater than perfusion in lung apices; ventilation greater than perfusion yields a V/Q ratio greater than 4:5; perfusion greater than ventilation yields a V/Q ratio less than 4:5
      6) Under normal conditions and in upright position, perfusion and ventilation are greater in lung bases
4. Nervous system control of breathing: initiates within medulla oblongata and pons of brainstem
   a. Medulla oblongata: controls inspiration, expiration, and breathing pattern
   b. Pons: controls rate and depth of respiration
   c. Sensory input to brainstem: impulses that influence breathing and respiration are transmitted to brainstem from chemoreceptors, stretch receptors, proprioceptors, baroreceptors, and external environment
      1) Central chemoreceptors in medulla: increased PCO_2 and/or decreased blood pH causes increased alveolar ventilation as a compensatory mechanism to maintain PCO_2 and pH at normal levels
      2) Peripheral chemoreceptors in aortic arch and carotid bodies: increased PCO_2 and/or decreased pH, and/or decreased partial pressure of arterial oxygen (PO_2) causes increased alveolar ventilation
      3) Stretch receptors in alveolar septa, bronchi, and bronchioles: prevent overdistention of lungs when they are inflated
      4) Proprioceptors in muscles and tendons of movable joints: stimulate ventilation with exercise to increase O_2 supply during time of increased O_2 demand

Table 2-1   **Variables That Influence Gas Exchange**

Variable	Example
Partial pressure of the gas	Supplemental oxygen increases partial pressure of inspired air
Surface area	Loss of lung tissue by surgery or disease decreases surface area available for gas exchange
Molecular weight and gas solubility	CO_2 is more soluble in the pulmonary capillary membranes and diffuses more quickly than oxygen
Thickness of membrane	Membrane is thickened by some disease processes such as pneumonia, pulmonary edema; a thicker membrane impedes effective air exchange

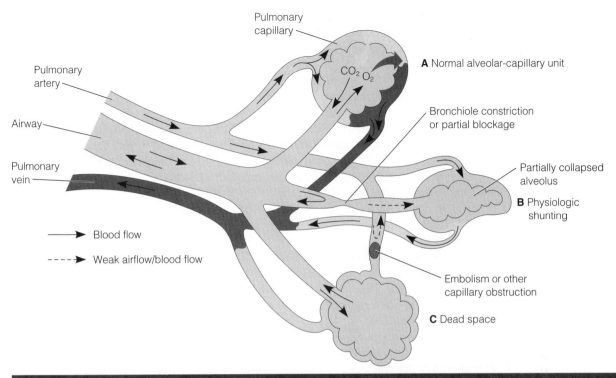

Pulmonary
capillary

Pulmonary
artery

Airway

Pulmonary
vein

CO_2 O_2

A Normal alveolar-capillary unit

Bronchiole constriction
or partial blockage

Partially collapsed
alveolus

B Physiologic
shunting

Embolism or other
capillary obstruction

C Dead space

⟶ Blood flow

---⟶ Weak airflow/blood flow

Figure 2-1

Ventilation-perfusion relationships A. Normal alveolar-capillary unit with an ideal match of ventilation and blood flow. Maximum gas exchange occurs between alveolar wall and blood, B. Physiologic shunting: a unit with adequate perfusion but inadequate ventilation, C. Dead space: a unit with adequate ventilation but inadequate perfusion. In the latter 2 cases, gas exchange is impaired.

5) Baroreceptors in aortic arch and carotid sinus: alter respiration relative to changes in arterial BP; elevated arterial BP lowers respiration; BP below 80 mmHg increases respiration

6) External environment: factors such as cold, physical stress, air pollution, smoking, and pain alter respiration; infection and fever increase respiration caused by increased O_2 demand

d. Nerve impulses travel from brainstem via phrenic nerve to diaphragm and stimulate muscle contraction for breathing

II. DIAGNOSTIC TESTS AND ASSESSMENTS

A. Radiological studies

1. Chest x-ray: performed to visualize structures, fluid, and air in thoracic cavity; anterior-posterior and lateral views are most common; appropriate use of lead shielding reduces overall exposure to x-rays

2. Computed tomography (CT): provides a cross-sectional visualization of examined tissue; identifies slight variations in tissue thickness so it may detect lesions not identified by x-ray

a. Performed with or without contrast (check allergies to iodine if contrast used)

b. Computerized images are greatly enhanced compared to traditional x-rays

     c. Newer technology uses a spiral or helical CT scan, which produces thinner slices and is quicker to perform than typical CT; enhanced data is also a diagnostic benefit

  3. Magnetic resonance imaging (MRI): computerized images similar to CT identify subtle changes in tissue structure; uses body's natural radio frequency impulses; assess client to ensure metal sources are removed; clients with metal implants may be ineligible for MRI

  4. Pulmonary angiogram: provides visualization of pulmonary vasculature; radioactive contrast medium is injected through a central venous catheter into right side of heart and pulmonary artery for visualization of pulmonary circulation pathway; identifies circulation alterations (congenital abnormalities, thromboembolism) and tumor demarcation; assess for iodine allergy

  5. Ventilation–perfusion scan: radioactive isotope injected to identify areas of ventilation and perfusion within lungs

B. Pulse oximetry

  1. Noninvasive test that monitors arterial **oxygen saturation** (percentage of oxygen bound to hemoglobin compared to volume that hemoglobin is capable of binding); a level greater than 95% is considered normal

  2. Uses a light spectroscopy probe attached to a local tissue site such as a finger, earlobe, or nose

  3. Lowered accuracy occurs with diminished peripheral perfusion, brightly lit environment, acrylic fingernails, and dark skin color

C. Pulmonary function test

  1. Uses a spirometer to measure lung volumes and capacities during forced breathing techniques

  2. Identifies normal or abnormal pulmonary functions

  3. Differentiates restrictive versus obstructive alterations of pulmonary function

  4. Assesses effects of bronchodilator therapy

D. Bronchoscopy

  1. Visualizes bronchi and branches using a fiberoptic scope

  2. Is performed for diagnostic and/or therapeutic reasons

  3. Obtains tissue and/or fluid specimens from lung

  4. Removes foreign bodies from lungs

  5. May be performed on clients breathing room air, supplemental oxygen, or receiving mechanical ventilation

  6. Preprocedure care

     a. Client NPO 6–12 hours before procedure

     b. Requires informed consent

     c. Administer analgesia or sedation as ordered

     d. Local or topical anesthesia applied to nasal and pharyngeal areas

  7. Postprocedure care

     a. Priority is airway maintenance

     b. Assess for return of gag reflex and symptoms of laryngeal edema—hoarseness, stridor, dyspnea, vital signs, and chest pain

E. Thoracentesis

  1. Introduces a needle into thoracic cavity to remove fluid from pleural cavity

  2. Is used for diagnostic and/or therapeutic reasons

  3. May be required for microbiology or cytology

  4. Permits drainage of fluid in pleural effusion

F. Laboratory

  1. Arterial blood gases: blood specimen obtained by arterial puncture or drawn from arterial line; identifies acid–base status and compensatory mechanisms

Parameter	Normal Value
pH	7.35–7.45
PCO_2	35–45 mmHg
HCO_3^-	22–26 mEq/L
PO_2	80–100 mmHg
BE	–2– +2 mEq

a. Identification of acid–base status
   1) **Acid**: donates hydrogen ions
   2) **Base**: accepts hydrogen ions
   3) Acid–base balance is classified as normal, acidotic, or alkalotic; acid–base balance can be altered by respiratory or metabolic components, either individually or in combination
b. Check **pH** (first step): reflects concentration of hydrogen ions (H^+) in blood; pH is an overall indicator of acid–base balance or buffering; a **buffer** is a weak acid or a weak base that transfers H^+ between solutions to maintain acid–base balance
   1) pH value less than 7.35 indicates **acidosis** (condition of increased H^+ concentration in blood)
   2) pH value greater than 7.45 indicates **alkalosis** (condition of decreased H^+ concentration in blood)
c. Check PCO_2 (second step): is an indicator of respiratory buffering
   1) PCO_2 less than 35 mmHg indicates alkalosis
   2) PCO_2 greater than 45 mmHg indicates acidosis
   Examples: pH < 7.35 + PCO_2 > 45 mmHg = respiratory acidosis
   pH > 7.45 + PCO_2 < 35 mmHg = respiratory alkalosis
d. Check HCO_3^- (third step): is an indicator of metabolic buffering
   1) HCO_3^- < 22 mEq/L indicates acidosis
   2) HCO_3^- > 26 mEq/L indicates alkalosis
   Examples: pH < 7.35 + HCO_3^- < 22 mEq/L = metabolic acidosis
   pH > 7.45 + HCO_3^- > 26 mEq/L = metabolic alkalosis
e. Base excess (BE) indicates amount of excess or insufficient level of bicarbonate in system and helps in determining cause of imbalance; a negative base excess reflects an acid excess; a value outside of normal range (-2 to +2 mEq) suggests a metabolic cause of abnormality
f. After interpreting pH value as normal, acidotic, or alkalotic, determine whether respiratory or metabolic buffering component matches acid–base component identified by pH
   Example 1: pH of 7.2 = Acidosis
   PCO_2 of 50 mmHg = Acidosis
   HCO_3^- of 24 mEq/L = Normal
   Interpretation: respiratory acidosis
   Example 2: pH of 7.5 = Alkalosis
   PCO_2 of 30 mmHg = Alkalosis
   HCO_3^- of 23 mEq/L = Normal
   Interpretation: respiratory alkalosis
   Example 3: pH of 7.25 = Acidosis
   PCO_2 of 42 mmHg = Normal
   HCO_3^- of 18 mEq/L = Acidosis
   Interpretation: metabolic acidosis

Example 4: pH of 7.55 = Alkalosis
PCO_2 of 38 mmHg = Normal
HCO_3^- of 30 mEq/L = Alkalosis
Interpretation: metabolic alkalosis

Example 5: pH of 7.2 = Acidosis
PCO_2 of 50 mmHg = Acidosis
HCO_3^- of 20 mEq/L = Acidosis
Interpretation: combined respiratory and metabolic acidosis

Example 6: pH of 7.5 = Alkalosis
PCO_2 of 30 mmHg = Alkalosis
HCO_3^- of 30 mEq/L = Alkalosis
Interpretation: combined respiratory and metabolic alkalosis

    g. Identification of acid–base compensation: acid–base balance can be normal, uncompensated, partially compensated, or compensated (see Table 2-2)

    h. In addition to acid–base evaluation, ABGs also evaluate oxygenation status; a decreased PaO_2 occurs when atmospheric oxygen is reduced or when there is hypoventilation, impaired alveolar diffusion (for example, pulmonary edema, pneumonia); administration of supplemental O_2 should cause PaO_2 to rise again to normal or baseline

2. Sputum analysis: specimen obtained for microbiology (gram stain, culture and sensitivity) or cytology; performed to identify infectious organisms and appropriate antimicrobial therapy

    a. Sputum collection procedure: sputum obtained by expectoration, suctioning, saline-induced specimen from airways, thoracentesis, lung needle biopsy, or transtracheal aspiration; for sputum collection from clients who can cooperate, have client rinse mouth prior to attempting to obtain expectorated specimen

        1) Specimens for acid–fast bacilli (mycobacterium tuberculosis) may be collected on 3 different days; specimen collection following a long sleep period (early morning) is desirable because of greater concentration; if unable to obtain a sputum specimen for acid–fast bacilli, gastric specimen may be obtained because mycobacterium tuberculosis is not altered by acidic gastric contents

        2) Specimens for cytology require collection container with a fixative agent

    b. Specimen processing: specimens should be collected in appropriate type of container and sent to laboratory promptly

3. Skin testing: performed to assess for allergic reactions to specified antigens (type I hypersensitivity), exposure to tuberculosis-causing organisms (type IV hypersensitivity), or fungi

    a. Skin test administration: injection must be intradermal

        1) Circle injection site with a long-lasting marker

        2) Diagram the forearm injection site on chart

Table 2-2 Determining Acid–Base Compensation in Arterial Blood Gases

Acid–Base Compensation	Arterial Blood Gas Analysis
Normal	Normal pH, normal PCO_2, and normal HCO_3^-
Uncompensated	Abnormal pH, abnormal PCO_2, or abnormal HCO_3^-
Partially compensated	Abnormal pH, abnormal PCO_2 and HCO_3^-; pH (acidosis or alkalosis) matches either PCO_2 or HCO_3^-, but not both
Compensated	Normal pH, abnormal PCO_2, and abnormal HCO_3^-

      b. Skin test interpretation

          1) Measure area of induration (if present), not reddened areas; size of induration is related to positive result with tuberculin testing; result should be read 48–72 hours after placement

          2) Positive result: client has been exposed to antigen; positive result from tuberculin testing does not mean client has active disease, only that there has been exposure

              a) Induration of 5 mm or greater: indicates recent exposure to infectious tuberculosis, or possible human immunodeficiency virus infection; chest x-ray findings with characteristic Ghon tubercles are likely healed and not active infection sites

              b) Induration of 10 mm or greater: indicates typical finding of active tuberculosis infection in populations with chronic, complicating diseases such as diabetes, end-stage renal disease, gastrointestinal cancer; finding is compatible in high-risk populations such as intravenous drug users, homeless, and residents of high-infection incidence areas

          3) Negative result: indicates no exposure to antigen or tuberculosis; false-negative findings occur with suppression of cell-mediated immunity such as that which occurs with human immunodeficiency virus

III. COMMON NURSING TECHNIQUES AND PROCEDURES

    A. Airway management: goal is to maintain patent airway

      1. Head and jaw position

        a. Upper airway obstruction is often caused by loss of local muscle tone or a foreign object

        b. Open airway using head tilt and anterior chin lift maneuver

        c. In clients with suspected neck injury, open airway by anterior chin displacement and/or jaw thrust; do *not* perform head tilt

        d. Perform abdominal thrusts (previously called Heimlich maneuver) in conscious clients with suspected foreign body obstruction of airway

      2. Artificial airways

        a. Oropharyngeal airway: maintains airway patency by preventing posterior tongue displacement

          1) Oropharyngeal airway is intended only for unconscious clients because of risk for vomiting or laryngeal spasms

          2) Airway must be sized for client; measure from corner of mouth to angle of lower mandible

          3) Assess oral cavity for possible foreign body or vomitus and remove loose dentures prior to insertion

          4) Tongue blade may be needed to temporarily displace tongue during insertion

          5) Insert oral airway with tip pointing towards soft palate, then rotate 180 degrees; flange should rest softly on lips

          6) Head and jaw position must be maintained independent of airway placement

        b. Nasopharyngeal airway: maintains airway patency via nasal route in client who is unconscious or semi-conscious or in whom placement of oropharyngeal airway is not feasible

          1) Airway must be sized for client; a tube that is longer than appropriate may pass into esophagus, causing stomach distention and inadequate ventilation; also estimate airway diameter; an estimate of diameter size is size of client's small finger

2) Assess client for contraindications, such as severe facial injuries or basal skull fracture (including "raccoon eyes" or "Battle's sign")

3) Head and jaw position must be maintained independent of airway placement

c. Endotracheal (ET) intubation: a long, cuffed ET tube is inserted with a laryngoscope by specially trained personnel for long-term airway management or for connection to a mechanical ventilator

1) ET tube must be sized for client

2) Lung auscultation immediately following placement should yield bilaterally equal breath sounds

3) Proper placement is confirmed by chest x-ray as soon as feasible relative to client's location and condition

4) ET tube tip must be located above carina to facilitate ventilation of both lungs

d. Tracheostomy: surgical placement of cuffed airway into trachea by specially trained personnel

1) Ventilation may be spontaneous or via mechanical ventilation

2) Supplemental oxygen can be delivered via a trach collar or mechanical ventilator

e. Cricothyrotomy: emergency surgical opening of cricothyroid membrane to maintain patent airway when other methods fail or are not feasible

3. Techniques for airway clearance

a. Oropharyngeal suctioning: nonsterile procedure to remove secretions from upper airway; alert clients may be taught to do self-suctioning

b. Nasotracheal suctioning: sterile procedure to remove secretions from tracheal area; may be performed to obtain a sterile sputum specimen

c. Tracheobronchial suctioning: sterile procedure using individual suction catheters or in-line suction catheter for clearing secretions via endotracheal tube

B. Body positioning

1. Physiology: fluid shift theory

a. Lung ventilation and perfusion are gravity dependent

b. Changes in body position from supine (0 degrees) to varying degrees of head elevation or lateral positioning activates reflexive cardiovascular changes that produce fluid shifts in lungs and chest vessels

2. Specific conditions

a. Acute respiratory failure

1) Elevate head at least 45 degrees

2) Position increases chest expansion

3) Elevation mobilizes fluid from chest into more dependent areas

b. Unilateral lung disease

1) Place individual with unaffected lung in dependent position ("good lung down"); this may vary when there is surgical removal of lung tissue

2) Position by using gravity to promote ventilation–perfusion matching

c. Acute respiratory distress syndrome (ARDS)

1) Prone positioning may be attempted in clients on maximal mechanical ventilation with unresponsive hypoxemia

2) With position change from supine to prone, previously nondependent air-filled alveoli become dependent, perfusion becomes greater to air-filled alveoli as opposed to previously fluid-filled dependent alveoli, thereby possibly improving ventilation–perfusion matching

3) Oxygenation improves in some clients with ARDS placed in prone position

4) Caution should be used to avoid unintentional dislodgment of ET tube during positioning

Practice to Pass

How should the client with unilateral lung disease be positioned to achieve optimal oxygenation and why?

C. **Oxygen administration**
   1. Nasal cannula
      a. Oxygen dose delivered is related to client's tidal volume and amount of O_2 flow
      b. Typical O_2 flow of 1–6 L/min will provide O_2 concentrations of 24 to 44%
      c. Oxygen concentration increases by about 4% for each 1 L of O_2 flow (room air oxygen concentration is about 21%)
      d. Clients with chronic obstructive pulmonary disease (COPD) should receive low dose of O_2 flow, about 1–2 L/min, to prevent respiratory depression; these clients are used to high CO_2 levels and low O_2 levels, so increased O_2 can cause a loss of respiratory drive
   2. Face mask
      a. Similar to nasal cannula O_2 administration, O_2 dose delivered is diluted by room air
      b. Exhaled CO_2 trapped by mask can be re-breathed
      c. Oxygen flow should be greater than 5 L/min to minimize re-breathing CO_2
      d. Provides O_2 concentration of 40–60%
   3. Face mask with O_2 reservoir
      a. Constant flow of O_2 into attached reservoir bag attached to mask minimizes re-breathing of exhaled CO_2
      b. Typical O_2 dose of 6–10 L/min provides 60–100% O_2 concentration
      c. Delivery system used for clients who require higher O_2 concentrations, but in whom ET intubation is not yet feasible
   4. Venturi mask
      a. Utilizes O_2 delivery device that provides more control over O_2 concentration than previously described delivery systems
      b. Delivers O_2 in concentrations of 24, 28, 35, and 40%
      c. Used in clients with COPD and chronic CO_2 retention
   5. Continuous positive airway pressure (CPAP) and bilevel positive airway pressure (BiPAP): discussed in Chapter 17
   6. Mechanical ventilation: discussed in Chapter 17
D. **Pulmonary hygiene**
   1. Pursed lip breathing
      a. Client exhales through pursed lips
      b. Slows down speed of exhalation and reduces collapse airway, thus enhancing respiration
   2. Coughing
      a. Adequate coughing for airway clearance requires higher airway pressures
      b. Augmented coughing: caregiver places hand below xiphoid process and thrusts downward on abdomen as client ends inspiration
      c. Huff coughing: client attempts sequential coughing while saying "huff"; maneuver keeps glottis open during coughing; beneficial in clients with COPD
   3. Chest physical therapy
      a. Purpose: to mobilize bronchial secretions into larger airways for removal by coughing or suctioning
      b. Indications: greater than 30 mL secretions per day, secretions with artificial airway, and/or atelectasis
      c. Percussion
         1) Client positioned for maximal drainage from appropriate area
         2) Technique involves use of cupped hands alternately percussing indicated area
         3) Contraindications: lung cancer, hemoptysis, and bronchospasm, increased intracranial pressure, or head or neck trauma

Practice to Pass

Why should individuals with chronic lung disease initially be given low concentration (1 to 2 L/min) of supplemental oxygen?

    d. Vibration

        1) Pressure is applied with palm of hand or electrical vibrator over appropriate area of chest

        2) Vibration may be used in some clients when percussion is contraindicated

    e. Postural drainage

        1) Uses gravity to mobilize bronchial secretions

        2) Nebulized bronchodilators may be administered prior to postural drainage

        3) Contraindicated about 1 hour before and within 3 hours after a meal to reduce risk of vomiting and/or aspiration

E. Tracheostomy care

  1. Purpose: temporary or permanent artificial airway

    a. Temporary

        1) Maintains airway when ET intubation is not feasible or possible

        2) Facilitates ventilator management and/or weaning

    b. Permanent

        1) Maintains airway after surgical alteration of head or neck

        2) Tracheostomy tube may be temporary or permanent; stoma may not require tracheostomy tube for long-term patency after surgical tracheostomy tract is healed

  2. Maintain aseptic conditions when suctioning or cleaning tracheostomy

  3. Safety precautions

    a. Keep tracheostomy tube obturator at head of bed for reinsertion in case of accidental dislodgment

    b. Keep manual ventilation bag connected to O_2 source at bedside

    c. Keep a spare unused tracheostomy tube at bedside for emergency use

F. Laryngectomy care

  1. Purpose: excision of larynx as treatment for cancer

  2. Preoperative teaching: client and family must be educated about long-term implications including loss of voice, swallowing difficulties, altered route for nutrition intake, and permanent tracheostomy

  3. Postoperative care

    a. Maintain patent airway

    b. Provide pain management

    c. Provide appropriate nutritional support

    d. Teach client/family how to care for tracheostomy and feeding tube (if applicable)

    e. Provide alternative means of communicating with client, such as writing supplies, picture or word board, or speaking through tracheostomy valve

    f. Provide emotional support to client and family; make appropriate referrals

G. Respiratory isolation

  1. The Occupational Safety and Health Administration (OSHA) mandates that employers provide protective materials to caregivers at risk for exposure to infectious substances (Occupational Safety & Health Administration (OSHA) http://www.osha.gov/)

  2. OSHA Respiratory Protection Standards were last revised in 2006

    a. Standard precautions

        1) Includes handwashing, gloves, and protective face gear utilized for all clients independent of actual or potential risk for infection

        2) Are recommended for all care providers coming in possible contact with blood, mucous membranes, non-intact skin, or parenteral devices of an infected client

Practice to Pass

What are the key safety measures the nurse must maintain for the client with a tracheostomy?

b. Transmission-based precautions: airborne, droplet, and/or contact precautions

    1) Are methods used for clients with known or suspected infections that require isolation measures in addition to Standard Precautions; airborne and droplet are used to limit spread of organisms that cause respiratory infections

    2) Airborne precautions

        a) Organisms spread through airborne routes use small particulates that are dispersed widely by air currents and may be inhaled by anyone within same room or even over a greater distance

        b) Infections include respiratory tuberculosis, rubeola, *varicella*, and disseminated zoster

        c) Special air handling and ventilation are needed to prevent airborne transmission

        d) Client is in a monitored negative air pressure room with door closed

        e) Anyone entering room of a client with respiratory tuberculosis wears respiratory protection including a fit-tested N95 respirator

        f) Susceptible or non-immune persons entering room of a client with rubeola or *varicella* will also wear an N95 respirator

        g) Client transport is minimized but when transport is necessary, the client will wear a surgical mask

    3) Droplet precautions

        a) Organisms spread by droplets use those larger particles usually generated when an infected client coughs, sneezes, or talks, but may be dispersed during procedures such as suctioning or bronchoscopy; droplets do not remain suspended in air and require close contact between source and recipient for spread

        b) Infections include *B. pertussis*, influenza virus, adenovirus, rhinovirus, *N. meningitides*, and *group A streptococcus*

        c) Masks are worn when working within 3 feet of client

        d) Equipment and furniture is disinfected before removal from infected client's environment

        e) When transport is necessary, client will wear a surgical mask

        f) Special air handling is not necessary, and door to room may remain open

        g) Clients with an active infection with same microorganism but without other infections may be cohorted (grouped) in same room if necessary

IV. NURSING MANAGEMENT OF CLIENT HAVING THORACIC SURGERY

A. Preoperative period

    1. Reduce anxiety through preoperative teaching about procedure and postoperative course and care

    2. Assess client's support systems and ability to care for self after surgery

    3. Administer preoperative medications, such as antibiotics, opioid analgesics, and anti-anxiety agents as prescribed

    4. Obtain baseline vital signs, oxygenation status, and mental status for comparison postoperatively

    5. Teach postoperative expectations, including chest tube management and incentive spirometry

B. Postoperative period

    1. Perform baseline assessments for vital signs, oxygenation status, and cognitive status as for all postoperative clients

    2. Maintain patent airway; administer supplemental O_2 as prescribed

3. Position client for optimal ventilation and perfusion; note any specific surgeon's orders for positioning; be prepared to initiate respiratory support (intubation, emergency tracheostomy, mechanical ventilation) as needed

4. Maintain water seal drainage if chest tube present

5. Maintain sterility of operative dressing

6. Maintain client safety

7. Administer antibiotics, bronchodilators, corticosteroids, inhalation agents, or other medications as ordered

8. Administer analgesics as ordered; adequate pain management facilitates chest expansion and optimal ventilation

9. Encourage position change, use of incentive spirometer, and coughing and deep-breathing exercises to maintain airway patency and reduce risk of atelectasis

10. Assess for possible surgical complications that should be reported immediately to maintain oxygenation
    a. Change in level of consciousness (LOC) ranging from restlessness and agitation to lethargy or unresponsiveness (may indicate hypoxemia)
    b. Increase in respiratory rate, unequal chest expansion, decreased breath sounds, and/or use of accessory muscles for breathing
    c. Loss of water seal drainage in closed chest drainage system
    d. Greater than desired volume of chest drainage (75–100 mL drainage over 1 hour is an average acceptable upper limit); orders should specify volume of acceptable chest tube drainage

11. Teach client and family about postdischarge home care and follow-up; include smoking cessation if applicable

12. Refer to community health resources for assistance with postdischarge care if needed

C. **Care of client with a chest tube**

1. Purpose of chest tube: to reestablish negative intrathoracic pressure following equalization of pressure between chest and atmosphere due to surgery, trauma, or pneumothorax and/or to provide drainage of blood, fluid, or air

2. Routine postprocedural care
    a. Maintain occlusive dressing at chest tube insertion site
    b. Monitor client's respiratory status
    c. Secure all chest tube and suction tubing connections with tape
    d. Keep collection apparatus below level of chest to allow gravity to promote chest drainage
    e. Milk chest tube to maintain tube patency *only if ordered*; milking chest tube can cause tissue damage
    f. Chest tube is not clamped when client is mobile and is never clamped without a health care provider order and/or according to agency policy
    g. In some types of disposable drainage apparatus, the water column fluctuates with breathing (also called *tidaling*); check manufacturer's product description to verify
    h. Maintain indicated amount of water in water seal chamber; below-normal water volume creates higher suction than may be desired, contributing to pleural tissue damage
    i. Monitor for bubbling in water seal chamber; intermittent bubbling is expected if client has pneumothorax; continuous bubbling means an air leak is present and must be found and fixed
    j. Monitor level of fluid in the suction control chamber (if fluid is used to maintain suction) to ensure it is at proper level; fluid level in this chamber directly corresponds to amount of suction pressure exerted on system

!

    k. Monitor hourly chest tube drainage output (health care provider usually specifies hourly volume of drainage that is acceptable)

    l. Monitor respiratory status: pneumothorax can enlarge or reoccur even in presence of a patent chest tube drainage system

3. Types of closed chest drainage collection systems for chest tubes (Figure 2-2)

    a. Sterile plastic disposable collection units are used to apply intrathoracic suction and to collect chest tube drainage

    b. Closed chest drainage collection systems have three chambers

        1) Drainage chamber: collects drainage and can be marked once per shift or more frequently to track amounts of drainage over time

!

        2) Water seal chamber: prevents air in drainage tubing and collection container from flowing back into chest; chamber is filled to the 2-cm mark with sterile water to maintain underwater seal; it is imperative that this seal not be interrupted; fluctuation can be seen here as client breathes

        3) Suction control chamber: helps to reestablish negative intrathoracic pressure; chamber can be filled with water to proper level to regulate amount of suction—most commonly 20 cm (such as Pleurevac 4000); some systems use "dry" suction (such as Pleurevac 6000) in which a knob is turned to appropriate level; both types are connected to low wall suction with a connecting tube

    c. One-way valve (Heimlich valve)

        1) Purpose: performed for emergency treatment of tension pneumothorax during conditions of life-threatening cardiovascular collapse

        2) Catheter-over-needle is inserted in 2nd intercostal space, midclavicular line to relieve a tension pneumothorax

        3) Catheter remains in chest after needle removal; audible hissing sound confirms presence of tension pneumothorax

        4) Intrathoracic air escapes into atmosphere via chest catheter; procedure actually creates a simple pneumothorax

        5) Further treatment includes placement of thoracostomy tube and connection to negative pressure drainage collection apparatus as soon as feasible

Practice to Pass

What nursing measures are used to prevent recurrence of pneumothorax?

Figure 2-2

Closed chest drainage system

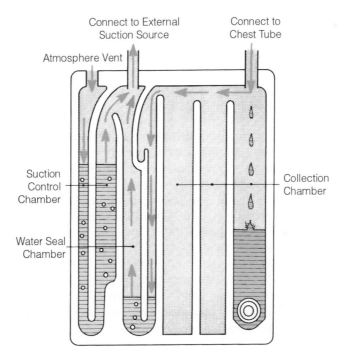

D. **Positioning client after lung surgery**: orders should specify turning parameters for specific client

1. Lobectomy: positioning includes lying on back or turned to either side
2. Segmental resection: positioning includes lying on back and turned onto nonoperative side; positioning on operative side may place tension on sutures and promote bleeding
3. Pneumonectomy
   a. Positioning includes lying on back and tilted toward operative side
   b. Client may be turned temporarily slightly toward nonoperative side, but should not remain in this position
   c. Turning client with operative side in a dependent position promotes desired consolidation of fluid in pleural space previously occupied by removed lung and prevents heart and remaining lung from shifting into operative side
   d. Positioning client with operative side dependent facilitates ventilation and perfusion
   e. Avoid complete lateral turning to either side, which will change pressure dynamics within chest and could lead to mediastinal shift

V. DISORDERS OF THE RESPIRATORY SYSTEM

A. Obstructive pulmonary diseases

1. Emphysema
   a. Description
      1) Progressive destruction of alveoli related to chronic inflammation
      2) Decreased surface area of respiratory bronchioles, alveoli, and alveolar ducts available for gas exchange
      3) Airway collapse due to loss of elasticity in respiratory system tissues
      4) A chronic form of obstructive pulmonary disease (COPD)
         a) A major characteristic of emphysema is airflow restriction
         b) Common symptom includes difficulty with exhalation caused by airways obstructed by edema or excessive mucus production
         c) Lung hyperinflation causes alveolar air trapping and leads to frequent pulmonary infections
         d) Symptoms may be reversible in asthma, but are typically progressive with emphysema, chronic bronchitis, and cystic fibrosis
   b. Etiology and pathophysiology
      1) Cigarette smoking is the primary etiology associated with emphysema
      2) Contributing factors include chronic respiratory inflammation from air pollution or long-term exposure to coal, glass, asbestos, and some chemical fumes
      3) Diagnosis in young and middle-aged adults may be associated with hereditary deficiency of alpha1–antitrypsin, an enzyme that prevents breakdown of lung tissue protein
      4) Air trapping in respiratory bronchioles, alveoli, and alveolar ducts leads to repeated infections and characteristic barrel chest appearance
      5) Work of breathing requires more energy and greater use of accessory muscles
   c. Assessment
      1) Clinical manifestations: most classic symptom is shortness of breath
         a) "Pink puffer" is a classic clinical description characterized by barrel chest, pursed-lip breathing (caused by forced exhalation), obvious use of accessory muscles when breathing, and underweight appearance
         b) Exertional dyspnea progresses with advancing disease

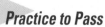

Practice to Pass

How should the nurse position the client who had a pneumonectomy in the postoperative phase and why?

c) Persistent tachycardia is related to inadequate oxygenation

d) Lung auscultation yields overall diminished breath sounds, and wheezes or crackles may be present

2) Diagnostic and laboratory test findings

a) ABG analysis reveals slightly decreased PO_2; PCO_2 is not elevated until later stages

b) Chest x-ray indicates hyperinflated lungs with a flattened diaphragm; heart size is normal or small

c) Pulmonary function tests demonstrate low vital capacity and forced expiratory volume (FEV_1)

d. Therapeutic management

1) Goals of therapy are to improve ventilation and promote patent airway by removal of secretions

2) Remove environmental pollutants and encourage smoking cessation where applicable

3) Bronchodilator therapy

4) Beta-adrenergic agonists

5) Corticosteroid therapy

6) Oxygen therapy and nebulization therapy

7) Chest physiotherapy

8) Intermittent positive pressure breathing (IPPB)

9) Adequate fluid intake

10) Oral care

11) Mechanical ventilation

12) Surgical procedures include bullectomy, lung volume reduction surgery, and lung transplantation

e. Priority nursing problems: alterations in gas exchange or respiratory pattern, risk for infection, insufficient nutrients for bodily needs, inability to endure exercise or activity, inadequate knowledge, nonadherence to smoking cessation

f. Planning and implementation

1) Provide education and referrals for clients with behaviors that increase risk for development of emphysema and other chronic obstructive pulmonary diseases

2) Refer clients to a structured pulmonary conditioning program and provide reinforcement as appropriate

3) Teach clients to avoid pulmonary irritants

4) Teach client breathing techniques that reduce CO_2 retention such as pursed lip breathing

5) Assist clients to develop appropriate nutritional plans to provide adequate calories

6) Teach importance of adequate fluid intake to assist with liquefaction of secretions

7) Teach importance of oral care to reduce infection

8) Administer supplemental low-flow oxygen as necessary; be prepared to initiate mechanical ventilation support

9) Administer and teach clients about antibiotic therapy

10) Administer and teach clients about bronchodilator therapy and use of measured-dose (metered dose) inhalants

11) Position clients to optimize and maintain airway and effective breathing patterns, usually with head elevated according to comfort

Practice to Pass

How does emphysema alter gas exchange?

g. Medication therapy

   1) Immunization against pneumonia (every 5 years) and influenza

   2) Antibiotics as needed for concurrent respiratory infection (yearly)

   3) Bronchodilators: controversial use in COPD, but maintenance therapy may be used to reduce dyspnea and attempt to increase FEV_1

   4) Beta-adrenergic agonists: used as bronchodilators in COPD and administered by nebulizer or metered dose inhaler (MDI)

   5) Anticholinergics: ipratropium (Atrovent) administered as maintenance therapy by inhaler; considered one of the most effective bronchodilators for COPD

   6) Long-acting theophylline: controversial use in COPD but may be beneficial to strengthen diaphragm contractility and decrease work of breathing

   7) Corticosteroids: controversial use in COPD but may be beneficial for clients with asthma history or with frequent exacerbations unresponsive to therapy with beta agonists

h. Client education

   1) Smoking cessation

   2) How to avoid occupational or environmental pollutants

   3) Maintenance of adequate nutrition with emphasis on higher calorie intake

   4) Energy conservation techniques

i. Evaluation of expected outcomes

   1) Activity tolerance is optimized

   2) Pulmonary irritants such as smoking, air pollution, or occupational exposure are avoided

   3) Pulmonary infections are reduced in number and severity

   4) Nutritional intake is adequate but not excessive for individual energy needs

2. Chronic bronchitis

a. Description

   1) A disorder of chronic airway inflammation; is a form of COPD

   2) Chronic productive cough lasting at least 3 months during 2 years

b. Etiology and pathophysiology

   1) Cigarette smoking is the primary etiology of chronic bronchitis

   2) Contributing factors include chronic respiratory inflammation from air pollution or occupational substances such as coal, glass, asbestos, and chemical fumes

   3) Chronic inflammation of airways produces hyperplasia of mucous glands, resulting in excessive sputum production

   4) Cilia disappear, and their airway clearance function is lost

   5) Goblet cells develop in abnormal sites of terminal bronchioles, also increasing sputum production

   6) Mucosal edema and increased production of thick mucus progressively obstructs airflow

   7) Work of breathing increases with progressive airway obstruction

   8) Repeated pulmonary infections result from increased sputum production with ineffective airway clearance

   9) Polycythemia develops as a compensatory response to chronic hypoxemia

c. Assessment

   1) Clinical manifestations

     a) Frequent cough, with or without (foul-smelling) sputum

     b) Frequent pulmonary infections

     c) Dyspnea and activity intolerance occurs as disease progresses

     d) Classic appearance of "blue bloater" includes tendency for obesity and bluish-red skin discoloration from cyanosis and polycythemia

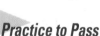

Practice to Pass

What is the primary lifestyle change that the nurse should teach the client with chronic bronchitis?

        e) Increased anterior–posterior chest diameter

        f) Occasional wheezing may occur

    2) Diagnostic and laboratory test findings

        a) Lung auscultation; note that in some clients the sounds may be normal

        b) Blood test: elevated RBC count in CBC and elevated hemoglobin and hematocrit in later stages

        c) ABGs may be required depending on the severity; results will generally show respiratory acidosis

        d) Chest x-ray reveals enlarged heart, congested lung fields, and normal or flattened diaphragm

        e) Pulmonary function indicates increased residual volume, decreased vital capacity, FEV_1, and FEV_1:FVC ratio

        f) Pulse oximetry will reveal O_2 saturation readings less than 95%

d. Therapeutic management

    1) Includes measures previously described in section on emphysema

    2) Antimicrobials

e. Priority nursing problems: alteration in gas exchange, ineffective cough, risk for infection, excess nutrients above bodily needs, inability to endure exercise or activity, inadequate knowledge

f. Planning and implementation

    1) Provide education or referrals to clients with behaviors that increase risk of developing emphysema and other chronic obstructive pulmonary diseases

    2) Refer clients to a structured pulmonary conditioning program and provide reinforcement as appropriate

    3) Teach clients how to avoid pulmonary irritants

    4) Assist clients to develop appropriate nutritional plans that provide adequate calories but maintain ideal weight

    5) Provide adequate fluid intake (2 liters) daily to assist with liquefaction (unless contraindicated by another condition)

    6) Provide oral care to reduce risk of infection

    7) Administer supplemental low-flow O_2 as necessary; be prepared to initiate mechanical ventilation

    8) Administer and teach clients about antibiotic therapy

    9) Surgical interventions include bullectomy, lung volume reduction surgery, and lung transplantation

g. Medication therapy

    1) Immunization; pneumococcal (single dose or every 5 years), influenza (yearly)

    2) Antibiotics

    3) Bronchodilators: controversial use in COPD, but maintenance therapy may be used to reduce dyspnea and attempt to increase FEV_1

    4) Beta-adrenergic agonists: used as bronchodilators in COPD and administered by nebulizer or MDI

    5) Anticholinergics: ipratropium (Atrovent) administered as maintenance therapy by inhaler; considered one of the most effective bronchodilators for COPD

    6) Long-acting theophylline: controversial use in COPD but may be beneficial to strengthen diaphragm contractility and decrease work of breathing

    7) Corticosteroids: controversial use in COPD but may be beneficial for clients with history of asthma or with frequent exacerbations unresponsive to beta-agonist medications

h. Client education

    1) Smoking cessation

    2) Avoiding occupational or environmental pollutants

        3) Nutritional therapies for adequate energy needs and weight management

        4) Importance of adequate fluid intake

        5) Need for oral care

    i. Evaluation of expected outcomes

        1) Activity tolerance is optimized

        2) Pulmonary irritants, such as smoking, air pollution, and occupational exposure are minimized

        3) Frequency and severity of pulmonary infections are minimized

        4) Weight is normalized

        5) Client and/or family describe appropriate lifestyle changes to optimize health

3. Asthma

    a. Description

        1) Chronic inflammation of airways leads to intermittent obstruction

        2) Severity and duration of symptoms are unpredictable

        3) Progressive airway obstruction that is unresponsive to treatment leads to status asthmaticus, a medical emergency

        4) Is sometimes considered a form of COPD

    b. Etiology and pathophysiology

        1) Intrinsic etiologies: uncertain causes; physical or psychological stress; exercise induced

        2) Extrinsic etiologies: antigen-antibody (allergic) reaction to specific irritants; common triggers include air pollutants, sinusitis, cold and dry air, medications, food additives, hormonal influences, and gastroesophageal reflux

        3) Characterized by widespread spasms of bronchiole smooth muscle with airway edema

        4) Excessive secretion of thick mucus contributes to airway obstruction

        5) Lungs become hyperinflated and alveolar air trapping occurs

        6) Gas exchange becomes impaired as ventilation–perfusion mismatching occurs

    c. Assessment

        1) Clinical manifestations

           a) Severe dyspnea

           b) Wheezing with expiration; intensity of wheezing is not related to severity of airway obstruction; clients with severe airway obstruction may not be able to move enough air to produce wheezing sound

           c) Cough

           d) Feelings of chest tightness

           e) Prolonged expiration is noted

           f) Mild to greatly diminished breath sounds upon auscultation; diminished or absent breath sounds may be related to atelectasis or pneumothorax

           g) Hyperresonant sound on percussion

           h) Increased heart rate and BP

           i) Extreme restlessness, anxiety, agitation

           j) Tachypnea with use of accessory muscles

         2) Diagnostic and laboratory test findings (during an episode or "attack")

           a) ABG reveals decreased PO_2, mild respiratory alkalosis

           b) Blood count reveals elevated eosinophil count

           c) Pulmonary function test reveals increased residual volume, decreased vital capacity, decreased forced expiratory volume, and peak expiratory flow rate

           d) Oxygen saturation level may be decreased below normal

    d. Therapeutic management

        1) Identify asthma signs or symptoms that require emergency intervention such as symptoms worsening or not improving with routine treatment, and decreasing LOC

        2) Acute episodes are managed with inhaled beta agonists, bronchodilators, anti-inflammatory agents, corticosteroids, and oxygen therapy; in severe cases, mechanical ventilation may be instituted

        3) Chronic management includes administration of drugs described in the medication section

        4) Decrease exposure to asthma triggers

  e. Priority nursing problems: ineffective cough or respiratory pattern, risk for infection, fear or anxiety

  f. Planning and implementation

        1) Assess respiratory and oxygenation status

        2) Administer supplemental oxygen as needed

        3) Administer bronchodilators as prescribed

        4) Observe characteristics of sputum

        5) Identify, avoid, and remove precipitating factors

        6) Teach client relaxation techniques during nonacute periods

        7) Provide emotional support to client and family

        8) Be prepared to establish IV access

        9) Be prepared to initiate mechanical ventilation if indicated

        10) Diagnostic testing during nonacute period includes chest x-ray, pulmonary function studies, allergy skin testing, and serum eosinophil and IgE levels

        11) Long term treatment may include allergy desensitization therapy if appropriate

  g. Medication therapy

        1) Short-acting beta-agonist inhaler: used for mild symptoms occurring twice weekly or less; also used for intermittent symptomatic relief and may be combined with long-acting medications

        2) Anti-inflammatory inhaler: used for mild symptoms occurring daily

        3) Anti-inflammatory inhaler plus medium-dose corticosteroid inhaler: used for moderate symptoms occurring daily or more often

        4) Anti-inflammatory inhaler plus long-acting bronchodilator plus oral corticosteroid: used for severe symptoms occurring daily or more often

        5) If appropriate, allergy desensitization therapy

  h. Client education

        1) Identify asthma triggers

        2) Teach proper use of metered-dose inhaler with reservoir

        3) Use peak flow meter for daily self-assessment of asthma status

        4) Identify asthma symptoms requiring emergency intervention

  i. Evaluation of expected outcomes

        1) Absence of dyspnea, chest tightness, wheezing

        2) Respiratory rate 12–20 breaths per minute

        3) Oxygen saturation and ABG values within normal range

        4) Bilaterally clear and equal breath sounds

        5) Afebrile

        6) Adequate airway clearance of clear, thin secretions

        7) Absence/resolution of anxiety

        8) Clear chest x-ray or return to client's usual baseline

        9) Normal or improved pulmonary function tests and peak flow volumes

B. Restrictive pulmonary disease: pleural effusion, empyema, and chylothorax

  1. Pleural effusion

    a. Description: is an accumulation of fluid in pleural space that indicates underlying pulmonary disease or abnormality; is a form of restrictive lung disease

    b. Etiology and pathophysiology

        1) Transudative pleural effusion
           a) Pleural fluid contains a small quantity of protein
           b) Fluid moves from capillaries into pleural space
           c) Most common cause is increased hydrostatic pressure, such as what occurs with heart failure
           d) Decreased oncotic pressure caused by an inadequate albumin level occurs more frequently with chronic renal and liver disease
        2) Exudative pleural effusion
           a) Pleural fluid contains a large quantity of protein
           b) Inflammatory response causes increased capillary permeability with fluid shift out of capillaries
           c) Exudation is associated with pulmonary tumors, pulmonary infections, pulmonary emboli, pancreatitis, and ruptured esophagus
           d) Obstruction of mediastinal lymphatic vessels draining parietal pleural space may be caused by tumors that frequently metastasize to those nodes such as lung and breast cancers, lymphomas

2. Empyema
    a. Pleural fluid containing pus
    b. Associated with infectious processes such as pneumonia, lung abscess, and tuberculosis

3. Chylothorax
    a. A type of pleural effusion caused by disruption of pulmonary lymph vessels
    b. Typically results from surgery or trauma

4. Assessment of restrictive pulmonary diseases
    a. Clinical manifestations
        1) Worsening dyspnea
        2) Diminished or absent breath sounds on affected side
        3) Dullness to percussion on affected side
        4) Chest wall pain
        5) Fever, persistent cough, night sweats, and weight loss with empyema
    b. Diagnostic and laboratory test findings
        1) Chest x-ray with visible fluid accumulation of greater than 250 mL
        2) Thoracentesis to differentiate source of pleural fluid

5. Therapeutic management
    a. Goal is to treat underlying cause
    b. Thoracentesis for drainage of pleural cavity
    c. Antibiotic therapy
    d. Surgical procedure may include decortication, or separation of pleural membranes

6. Priority nursing problems: alterations in respiratory pattern or gas exchange, pain, risk for infection, risk for fever

7. Planning and implementation
    a. Monitor respiratory and oxygenation status
    b. Assist health care provider with thoracentesis or thoracotomy if indicated
    c. Treat underlying cause
    d. Provide supplemental oxygen if indicated
    e. Provide adequate nutrition with focus on adequate protein intake

8. Medication therapy: analgesics, antipyretics, and if chylothorax present, intravenous lipids

9. Client education
    a. Explain underlying cause of specific type of pleural effusion
    b. Monitor for changes in respiratory and oxygenation status
    c. Instruct about purpose of thoracentesis or thoracotomy

Practice to Pass

What nutritional alterations are necessary for the client with pleural effusion caused by chylothorax?

10. Evaluation of expected outcomes
    a. Resolution or reduction of accumulated pleural fluid
    b. Afebrile
    c. Control of chest wall pain
    d. Adequate protein intake
    e. Respiratory rate 12–20 breaths per minute

C. **Pneumothorax and hemothorax**
   1. Description
      a. Pneumothorax: air accumulation in pleural space
         1) Spontaneous: rupture of air-filled bleb allows pathway for air movement between respiratory system and pleural space; collapse of involved tissue may seal leak with minimal client symptoms; air leak may progress until pressure between thoracic cavity and atmosphere equalizes and client is symptomatic
            a) Primary: spontaneous rupture of bleb in otherwise healthy client; occurs more often in tall, slender males aged 20–40
            b) Secondary: rupture of overly distended alveolus or alveoli; occurs in clients with known COPD; severity of symptoms varies with size of pneumothorax
         2) Tension: disruption of chest wall or lungs causes air accumulation in pleural space; pressure on mediastinum causes pressure on other lung and interrupts venous return to heart; is a medical emergency that requires emergency placement of chest tube to relieve increasing pressure in thoracic cavity to restore adequate cardiac output
         3) Traumatic: disruption of pleura, bronchi, or lung tissue caused by blunt or penetrating trauma with air accumulation in pleural space
         4) Iatrogenic: disruption of pleura, bronchi, or lung tissue during instrumentation for central venous line placement, lung biopsy, or thoracentesis; produces unintentional air leak within respiratory system; clinical manifestations and treatment are same as for spontaneous pneumothorax
      b. Hemothorax: blood accumulation in pleural space; clinical manifestations and treatment are same as for pneumothorax
   2. Etiology and pathophysiology
      a. Normal intrapleural pressure is negative compared to atmospheric air pressure
      b. Pressure difference between thoracic cavity and atmosphere is one stimulus for breathing
      c. Disruption of pleura causes air accumulation within pleural space
      d. Intrapleural pressure equalizes with atmospheric air, removing one stimulus for breathing
      e. Lung collapses as pressure increases in thoracic cavity
      f. Excessive pressure is placed on chest organs and great vessels
      g. Preload decreases and cardiac output is compromised
   3. Assessment
      a. Clinical manifestations
         1) Dyspnea
         2) Tracheal deviation toward unaffected side
         3) Diminished breath sounds on affected side
         4) Percussion dullness on affected side
         5) Unequal chest expansion (reduced on affected side)
         6) Crepitus over chest
      b. Diagnostic and laboratory test findings
         1) Chest x-ray reveals pneumothorax
         2) ABG shows decreased PO_2

4. Therapeutic management
   a. Includes antibiotics if infection is suspected; in mild cases, no chest tube is required; if pneumothorax is significant, a chest tube is inserted
   b. Placement of chest tube with water seal drainage
   c. Spontaneous pneumothorax: in otherwise healthy client, may resolve without invasive treatment
   d. If spontaneous pneumothorax occurs repeatedly, may require pleurodesis or sclerotherapy, an instillation of an agent (such as talc) or doxycycline in pleural spaces to allow pleura to adhere together; other procedures include partial pleurectomy, stapling, or laser pleurodesis for pleural sealing
   e. Analgesic may be needed
5. Priority nursing problems: alterations in gas exchange or respiratory pattern, potential for infection or injury, potential for reduced cardiac output, pain, fear or anxiety
6. Planning and implementation
   a. Care of client with a chest tube: previously discussed in this chapter (see Section IV C, p. 56)
   b. Monitor respiratory and oxygenation status
   c. Provide supplemental oxygen as indicated
   d. Maintain infection control practices
7. Medication therapy: analgesics and antibiotics
8. Client education
   a. Purpose of chest tube
   b. Activity limitations
   c. Pain management
9. Evaluation of expected outcomes
   a. Absence or resolution of dyspnea
   b. Afebrile
   c. Oxygen saturation or ABG results within normal range
   d. Control of pain
   e. Bilaterally clear and equal breath sounds
   f. Client is able to participate in activities of daily living

D. **Atelectasis**
   1. Description
      a. Collapsed alveoli
      b. Common complication in postoperative or immobilized clients
   2. Etiology and pathophysiology
      a. Pulmonary secretions and/or exudates contribute to airway obstruction
      b. Airway obstruction increases intra-alveolar pressure, causing alveolar collapse
      c. Surface area available for gas exchange is decreased
   3. Assessment
      a. Clinical manifestations
         1) Low-grade fever
         2) Breath sounds diminished or absent in affected area
         3) Diminished rate and depth of respiration
         4) Physical inactivity caused by immobility or pain
      b. Diagnostic and laboratory test findings: chest x-ray reveals area of collapse
   4. Therapeutic management
      a. Primary goal is prevention of atelectasis
      b. Chest physical therapy and general pulmonary hygiene measures
      c. Intermittent positive pressure breathing treatments
      d. Supplemental oxygen as indicated

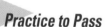

Practice to Pass

How can tension pneumothorax cause life-threatening condition?

5. Priority nursing problems: alterations in gas exchange or respiratory pattern, ineffective cough, potential for fever

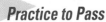

6. Planning and implementation

  a. Monitor respiratory and oxygenation status

  b. Deep-breathing and coughing exercises

  c. Incentive spirometry

  d. Frequent position change

  e. Ambulation as soon as feasible with client condition

  f. Maintain adequate hydration and nutrition

  g. Assist with incisional splinting in surgical client

7. Medication therapy: analgesics and antipyretics

8. Client education

  a. Diaphragmatic and abdominal breathing techniques

  b. Nonpharmacologic pain control measures

9. Evaluation of expected outcomes

  a. Maintenance of airway

  b. Effective cough with clear, thin secretions

  c. Afebrile

  d. Absence or resolution of dyspnea

  e. Respiratory rate 12–20 breaths per minute

  f. Oxygen saturation or ABG results return to normal range or client's baseline

  g. Bilaterally clear and equal breath sounds

  h. Client participates in activities of daily living

Practice to Pass

What nursing measures are utilized to prevent atelectasis?

E. Pneumonia

1. Description

  a. Acute inflammation of lung parenchyma (alveoli and respiratory bronchioles)

  b. Classified as viral versus bacterial, community-acquired versus hospital-acquired, atypical, or pneumocystis

2. Etiology and pathophysiology

  a. Causative agent can be infectious (bacteria, viruses, fungi, and other microbes) or noninfectious (aspirated or inhaled substances)

  b. Most common organism for both community-acquired and hospital-acquired is gram-positive bacteria, *Streptococcus pneumoniae*, *staph aureus*, and *varicella*

  c. Other common organisms associated with community-acquired pneumonia include *Klebsiella pneumoniae*, *Pseudomonas aeruginosa*, *chlamydia*, *Escherichia coli*, *haemophilus influenzae* and other influenzae viruses, and *pneumocystis jiroveci (carinii)*

  d. Spread of microbes in alveoli activates inflammatory and immune response

  e. Antigen–antibody response damages mucous membranes of bronchioles and alveoli, resulting in edema

  f. Microbe cellular debris and exudate fill alveoli and can impair gas exchange

3. Assessment

  a. Viral

    1) Fever: low grade

    2) Cough: nonproductive

    3) White blood cell count: normal to low elevation

    4) Chest x-ray: minimal changes evident

    5) Clinical course: less severe than pneumonia of bacterial origin

  b. Bacterial

    1) Fever: high

    2) Cough: productive

    3) White blood cell count: high elevation

        4) Chest x-ray: obvious infiltrates

        5) Clinical course: more severe than pneumonia of viral origin

   4. Therapeutic management

    a. Antibiotic therapy, analgesics, antipyretics

    b. Oxygen therapy to treat hypoxemia

  5. Priority nursing problems: alterations in gas exchange or respiratory pattern, ineffective cough, insufficient nutrients for bodily needs, inability to endure activity or exercise, pain, anxiety, potential for fever

  6. Planning and implementation

    a. Maintain patent airway

     b. Monitor respiratory and oxygenation status

    c. Provide supplemental O_2 as indicated

    d. Be prepared to initiate mechanical ventilatory support

    e. Administer antimicrobials as prescribed

    f. Provide pain management

     g. Provide nutritional support and increased fluids via appropriate route

    h. Provide adequate opportunities for physical rest

    i. For all hospitalized clients, take measures to prevent spread of pneumonia

        1) Maintain standard precautions and appropriate infection control measures

        2) Maintain adequate nutrition and increased fluid intake

        3) Activate aspiration precautions

        4) Oral hygiene

        5) Encourage activity and mobility as soon as feasible

  7. Medication therapy

    a. Antibiotics or other antimicrobials as indicated

    b. Analgesics and antipyretics

   8. Client education

    a. Immunization against influenza and pneumococcal pneumonia (the latter if immunocompromised or 65 years or older)

    b. Activity limitations and importance of rest

    c. Effects and dosages of medications

    d. Avoid pollutants and irritants such as smoke

    e. Symptoms to report to health care provider (return of fever, worsening respiratory status)

  9. Evaluation of expected outcomes

    a. Absence of respiratory distress

    b. Breath sounds clear to auscultation with adequate air exchange

    c. Effective coughing with expectoration of sputum if indicated

    d. Decreased or absent chest pain

    e. Resolution of fever

    f. Maintenance of normal body weight

    g. Client participates in care with decreased or no activity intolerance

F. Pulmonary tuberculosis

  1. Description

    a. Lung infection caused by *Mycobacterium tuberculosis*

    b. Any tissue can be infected, but tuberculosis is often found in lung

  2. Etiology and pathophysiology

    a. *Mycobacterium tuberculosis* is an acid-fast, gram-positive bacillus with transmission via airborne droplets

    b. Infection usually results from frequent close contact with an infected individual

    c. Inhaled bacilli inhabit respiratory bronchioles and alveoli

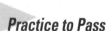

Practice to Pass

How do assessment findings differ among clients with viral versus bacterial origin of pneumonia?

       d. Bacilli travel through lymph circulation and may spread throughout body before cell-mediated immunity can contain its movement

       e. Eventual activation of cell-mediated immunity produces a granuloma lesion

       f. Liquefied necrotic material from Ghon tubercle portion of granuloma lesion results in passage of infectious particles into major airways where they can be exhaled into air

3. Assessment

       a. Clinical manifestations

         1) Frequent cough with copious frothy, pink sputum; nonproductive cough early in morning develops first as an early symptom

         2) Night sweats

         3) Anorexia

         4) Weight loss

         5) Fever

       b. Laboratory and diagnostic test findings

         1) Positive tuberculin skin test (indicated exposure)

         2) Appearance of characteristic Ghon tubercle on chest x-ray

         3) Positive acid-fast bacillus sputum cultures (provides definitive diagnosis of infection)

4. Therapeutic management: see medication therapy below

5. Priority nursing problems: alterations in respiratory pattern, insufficient nutrients for bodily needs, fever, pain, inability to endure activity or exercise, inability to maintain health

6. Planning and implementation

       a. Monitor respiratory and oxygenation status

       b. Provide adequate nutrition and hydration

       c. Institute standard precautions (Centers for Disease Control Tier 1) and airborne precautions (Tier 2, transmission-based precautions)

         1) Use a private room with negative air pressure that has 6–12 full air exchanges per hour and is vented to outside or has its own air filtration system

         2) Wear specially fitted mask (N95 respirator) whenever entering client's room; fit-test mask with each use

         3) Provide visitors with appropriate masks

         4) Wear gown and masks if client does not reliably cover mouth during coughing or sneezing to reduce risk of transmission to others

         5) Provide client with a surgical mask if it is necessary to bring client to another department; choose shortest and least busy route and alert that department ahead of time about client's status; schedule tests for less busy times of day

       d. Administer antimicrobial therapy as prescribed

       e. Provide supplemental O_2 as indicated

       f. Obtain periodic sputum cultures after onset of antimicrobial therapy

       g. Identify possible source of exposure

7. Medication therapy

       a. Antibiotic prophylaxis: for people exposed to clients with active disease

       b. Isoniazid (INH) drug of choice for 6 months if no clinical evidence of disease

       c. INH drug of choice for 12 months if abnormal chest x-ray or high-risk population such as with human immunodeficiency virus (HIV) or drug-induced immunosuppression

       d. Active disease: treatment options prescribed by Centers for Disease Control (CDC)

         1) Option 1: INH, rifampin (Rifadin), pyrazinamide (Tebrazid), and ethambutol (Myambutol) or streptomycin given daily or 2–3 times weekly (if therapy verified); if cultures report sensitivity to rifampin or isoniazid, ethambutol or streptomycin can be stopped; minimal 6 months drug therapy; drug therapy continues for at least 3 months after first negative sputum culture obtained

   2) Option 2: INH, rifampin, pyrazinamide, and ethambutol or streptomycin given daily for 2 weeks, then 2 times weekly for 6 weeks, then 2 times weekly isoniazid and rifampin for 16 weeks

   3) Option 3: INH, rifampin, pyrazinamide, and ethambutol or streptomycin 3 times weekly for 6 months

   4) Option 4: active TB with HIV; option 1, 2, or 3 for minimum of 9 months and to continue for at least 6 months after first negative sputum culture

8. Client education

   a. Infection control measures, including handwashing, coughing into tissues and disposing of them in a closed bag

   b. No special precautions need to be taken with clothing, books, personal objects, or eating utensils because inanimate objects do not easily spread these bacteria

   c. Teach client, family, and close contacts about mechanisms of transmission and antimicrobial therapy, including need to take medication for full course of therapy to prevent recurrence and/or development of drug-resistant organisms

   d. Teach client about adverse effects of medications, including but not limited to the following:

      1) INH: hepatotoxicity that requires assessment of onset of jaundice, periodic monitoring of liver function tests, peripheral neuritis (numbness and tingling) that can be minimized with intake of vitamin B_6, hematologic effects (anemia, agranulocytosis, bleeding), or hypersensitivity

      2) Rifampin: relatively low toxicity, but monitor CBC, liver function tests, and renal status; medication causes orange discoloration of body fluids

      3) Pyrazinamide: primarily causes hepatotoxicity and elevates uric acid levels; periodic monitoring of blood levels is indicated and assessment of jaundice and symptoms of gout (joint pain); clients should be monitored for hyperglycemia

      4) Ethambutol: causes optic neuritis; obtain baseline vision screening and periodic eye exams (changes can include loss of visual acuity and red/green color discrimination)

      5) Streptomycin: primarily causes ototoxicity and nephrotoxicity (similar to other aminoglycoside antibiotics); monitor hearing ability and renal function; maintain fluid intake of 2.5–3 liters of fluid per day

   e. Maintain good nutrition and provide adequate rest periods for healing and to minimize fatigue, adequate fluid intake to approximately 2 liters per day

9. Evaluation of expected outcomes

   a. Adherence to prescribed medication therapy

   b. Resolution of productive cough

   c. Afebrile

   d. Respiratory rate 12–20 breaths per minute

   e. Oxygen saturation or ABG results within normal range or client's baseline

   f. Maintenance of appropriate body weight

   g. Resolution of active infectious phase

   h. Prevention of spread to contacts

G. Pulmonary embolism (PE)

1. Description

   a. Emboli lodge in pulmonary vasculature and obstruct adequate blood flow through pulmonary capillaries

Practice to Pass

What therapies are used as tuberculosis prophylaxis for individuals who have been exposed to an individual with active disease?

        b. Ventilation–perfusion mismatch: a clinically significant imbalance between volume of air and volume of blood circulating to gas exchange area of lungs; causes impaired gas exchange

        c. PE is a frequent complication of hospitalized clients

2. Etiology and pathophysiology

        a. Most common sites for origin of emboli include venous thromboses in deep veins of lower extremities, pelvis, or right side of heart

        b. Risk factors for PE include immobility, hypercoagulability, trauma to endothelial layer of BVs, long bone fractures, and pregnancy (amniotic fluid embolism during labor and delivery)

        c. Dislodgment of venous thromboses occurs with movement into pulmonary vasculature; fat emboli travel from site of long bone fractures and traumatized vessels

        d. Emboli obstruct small to large areas of pulmonary vasculature, preventing adequate perfusion and gas exchange

        e. A massive area of obstructed tissue leads to pulmonary infarction

        f. Severe impairment of gas exchange can be rapidly fatal

3. Assessment

        a. Clinical manifestations

            1) Restlessness, anxiety, agitation, mental status changes, and decreasing LOC

            2) Shortness of breath

            3) Chest pain

            4) Hemoptysis

            5) Cyanosis

            6) Recent history of thromboembolism and/or long bone fractures

            7) Lung crackles upon auscultation

            8) Vital signs: tachycardia, tachypnea, hypotension, fever

        b. Diagnostic and laboratory test findings

            1) Possible atrial fibrillation

            2) Chest x-ray may be normal

            3) Spiral or helical CT scan demonstrates obstruction to pulmonary vasculature

            4) Ventilation–perfusion scan indicates areas of mismatch

            5) Abnormal ABGs and decreased oxygen saturation

            6) Pulmonary angiogram reveals PE

4. Therapeutic management

        a. Oxygen therapy

        b. Anticoagulant therapy

        c. Embolectomy

        d. Thrombolytic therapy

        e. To prevent future pulmonary emboli, an intracaval filter may be inserted into inferior vena cava to trap emboli from a known source

5. Priority nursing problems: alterations in gas exchange or respiratory pattern, anxiety, pain, reduced mobility

6. Planning and implementation

        a. Maintain patent airway and provide supplemental O_2

        b. Be prepared to initiate mechanical ventilation

        c. Maintain IV access

        d. Circulatory support as indicated

        e. Placement of vena cava filter

        f. Pain management

        g. Pulmonary embolectomy

7. Medication therapy

        a. Thrombolytic or anticoagulant therapy

      b. Opioid analgesics

      c. Antianxiety agents

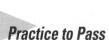

  8. Client education

      a. Prevention of thromboembolism

      b. Avoid immobility as much as feasible

      c. Signs and symptoms of venous occlusion

      d. Anticoagulant therapy (as indicated), with PT, PTT, and/or INR blood level monitoring

      e. While on anticoagulant therapy, avoid activity that can lead to bruising or bleeding and avoid variable intake of foods containing vitamin K (for warfarin [Coumadin] therapy)

Practice to Pass

What nursing measures are indicated for prevention of pulmonary emboli?

  9. Evaluation of expected outcomes

      a. Respiratory rate 12–20 breaths per minute

      b. Oxygen saturation and ABG results within normal range or client's baseline

      c. Alert and oriented mental status

      d. Absence or resolution of chest pain

      e. Absence or resolution of anxiety

      f. Prevention of further thromboembolic phenomena

      g. Prevention of complications

H. Bronchogenic carcinoma

  1. Description

      a. Lung cancer is the leading cause of death from malignancy

      b. Five-year survival rate is less than 15%

      c. Greater than 90% of lung cancers originate in bronchus epithelium

  2. Etiology and pathophysiology

      a. Leading cause is cigarette smoking; cancer risk increases with length of smoking exposure

      b. Contributing factors include inhaled environmental substances such as air pollution, arsenic, asbestos, iron, radon, and aromatic hydrocarbons

      c. Some clients have a genetic predisposition to bronchogenic carcinoma

      d. Tumor growth commonly begins in bronchus then migrates to upper lobes of lungs

      e. Nonspecific inflammatory cellular changes lead to excessive mucus production, desquamation, metaplasia of epithelium, and slow-growing bronchogenic carcinoma

      f. Tumor types include small cell and non-small cell

      g. Metastasis occurs by direct contact and transport in blood and lymph

  3. Assessment

      a. Clinical manifestations

         1) Asymptomatic until mass has spread to pleura or chest wall and is often late in course of disease

         2) Persistent cough (progressively increases) with or without hemoptysis

         3) Localized chest pain

         4) Dyspnea

         5) Unilateral wheeze upon auscultation

         6) Swallowing difficulty

         7) Anorexia and weight loss

         8) Enlarged neck lymph nodes

      b. Diagnostic and laboratory test findings

         1) Mass visible on chest x-ray

         2) CT scan or MRI of chest may better differentiate mass

         3) Sputum for cytology reveals tumor cells

         4) Bronchoscopy for direct biopsy or washings for cytology reveal tumor cells

4. Therapeutic management
    a. Surgical resection
        1) Pneumonectomy: removal of an entire lung
        2) Lobectomy: removal of a lobe of lung
        3) Segmentectomy (segmental resection): removal of a segment or segments of a lung
        4) Wedge resection: dissection and removal of a defined area in the lung
        5) Note that small cell carcinoma is typically inoperable
    b. Chemotherapy and radiation therapy: see Chapter 12
    c. Laser therapy
    d. Immunotherapy
5. Priority nursing problems: anticipatory grief, anxiety, pain, inadequate knowledge, alterations in gas exchange or respiratory pattern, ineffective cough, loss of hope or power
6. Planning and implementation
    a. Provide psychosocial support for client and family
    b. Provide preoperative and postoperative care for client having surgery
    c. Administer O_2 therapy as prescribed
    d. Assist client with pain management
    e. Position to optimize oxygenation according to surgical procedure
    f. Provide care of chest tubes as previously discussed
7. Medication therapy
    a. Opioid analgesics
    b. Chemotherapy
    c. Immunotherapy
    d. Antiemetics
8. Client education
    a. Treatment plan, including discussion of medication side effects
    b. Assistance with coping skills
    c. Pain management
9. Evaluation of expected outcomes
    a. Pain control
    b. Effective airway clearance
    c. Effective breathing pattern
    d. Coping skills, realistic personal goals

I. **Cancer of the larynx**
1. Description
    a. Most laryngeal tumors are benign
    b. Most common form of malignant laryngeal cancer is squamous cell carcinoma
2. Etiology and pathophysiology
    a. Primary etiologies for laryngeal cancer include long-term cigarette smoking and alcohol ingestion
    b. Contributing factors include chronic laryngeal irritation caused by singing, air pollution, and environmental hazards
    c. Tumor growth occurs in glottis, supraglottis, and subglottis; symptoms are specific to site of tumor
    d. Chronic laryngeal irritation leads to precancerous lesions, leukoplakia, and erythroplakia
    e. Carcinoma may develop at site of precancerous lesions
    f. Lungs are most common site for laryngeal metastasis

3. Assessment

   a. Clinical manifestations

     1) Persistent hoarseness

     2) Palpable jugular nodes

     3) Sore throat

     4) Pain when swallowing

     5) Unexplained earache

   b. Diagnostic and laboratory test findings

     1) Tissue biopsy finding

     2) X-ray visualization

     3) MRI, CT with mass detected

     4) Barium swallow visualization

4. Therapeutic management

   a. Choice of treatment depends on stage of disease and general condition of client

   b. Radiation therapy or brachytherapy; brachytherapy involves placement of a radioactive source next to tumor site

   c. Chemotherapy

   d. Laryngectomy

   e. Radical neck dissection

5. Priority nursing problems: inability to communicate verbally, ineffective cough, pain, anxiety, inadequate knowledge, insufficient nutrients for bodily needs, reduced swallowing ability

6. Planning and implementation

   a. Biopsy of laryngeal lesions and other diagnostic tests, such as CT scan, MRI of head and neck, chest x-ray

   b. Maintain patent airway (tracheostomy performed with laryngectomy)

   c. Pain management

   d. Provide adequate hydration and nutrition (temporary or permanent altered route for nutrition)

   e. Provide alternate means for communication as previously discussed and plan for permanent means of communication (artificial larynx or esophageal speech)

   f. Monitor respiratory and oxygenation status

   g. Provide O_2 supplementation as indicated

7. Medication therapy: opioid analgesics and antipyretics

8. Client education

   a. Smoking cessation

   b. Changes in body image

   c. Care of tracheostomy

   d. Use of artificial larynx

   e. Supraglottic swallowing for voice production (esophageal speech)

   f. Nutritional access device if indicated

   g. Pain management

   h. Signs of tumor spread

9. Evaluation of expected outcomes

   a. Absence of cancer spread

   b. Effective communication

   c. Appropriate body weight maintained

   d. Absence or resolution of pain

   e. Demonstration of self-care

   f. Psychological adjustment to permanent loss of natural means of communication

J. Thoracic trauma
1. Description: alteration of breathing mechanics and/or gas exchange caused by respiratory system trauma
    a. Blunt trauma: injury to chest wall without disruption of pleura
        1) Rib fractures
        2) Flail chest
        3) Soft tissue rupture: diaphragm, trachea, bronchi, and major BVs
        4) Tension pneumothorax
        5) Contusion of lungs or heart
    b. Penetrating trauma: injury involves disruption of pleura
        1) Internal wounds communicate with external atmosphere
        2) Open air-sucking wounds
        3) Pneumothorax and/or hemothorax
        4) Tissue wounds: heart, lungs, major blood vessels
2. Etiology and pathophysiology
    a. Blunt trauma: mechanism of injury commonly involves motor vehicle collisions, falls, and assaults
    b. Penetrating trauma: mechanism of injury commonly involves firearms, motor vehicle collisions, falls, or assaults
    c. Pathophysiology varies related to specific injury: rib fracture is most common type of chest trauma
        1) Flail chest
            a) Rib fractures in at least 2 places (separated from bony skeleton)
            b) Chest wall unstable with paradoxical chest expansion (flail segment moves inward with inhalation and outward with exhalation)
            c) Ventilation–perfusion mismatch
            d) Possible underlying lung injury
        2) Rupture of diaphragm
            a) Abdominal contents dislocate upward into thoracic cavity
            b) Decrease in diaphragmatic control of breathing
3. Assessment
    a. Clinical manifestations
        1) Chest pain, may be severe such as with flail chest
        2) Shallow breathing with splinting
        3) Possible unequal chest expansion
        4) Tachycardia, tachypnea, hypotension
        5) Crepitus over chest
    b. Diagnostic and laboratory test findings
        1) Chest x-ray findings show white opacifications
        2) ABGs reveal hypoxemia
4. Therapeutic management: same as pneumothorax and hemothorax (see earlier in chapter Section V C, pp. 62–63)
5. Priority nursing problems: pain, alterations in respiratory pattern or gas exchange, ineffective cough, reduced cardiac output, inability to endure exercise or activity
6. Planning and implementation
    a. Ventilation support
    b. Prepare to initiate mechanical ventilation if needed
    c. Maintain IV access
    d. Placement of chest tube with water seal drainage may be indicated
    e. Provide pain management
7. Medication therapy: opioid analgesics, epidural analgesia may be appropriate

8. Client education
   a. Techniques for pulmonary hygiene
   b. Pain management: patient-controlled analgesia may be appropriate
   c. Prevention of thromboembolic phenomena
   d. Measures to decrease anxiety
9. Evaluation of expected outcomes
   a. Adequate ventilation and perfusion
   b. Control/relief of pain
   c. Oxygen saturation and ABG results within normal range
   d. Respiratory rate 12–20 breaths per minute with normal depth

Case Study

A 62-year-old client with a history of COPD is admitted to the hospital with an acute exacerbation and left-sided pneumonia. The nurse observes increased anterior–posterior diameter of the chest, reddish-blue skin tone, and prolonged expiratory phase when breathing. Admission vital signs: temperature 101.5°F (oral), blood pressure 154/92, heart rate 110, and respiratory rate 26 breaths/minute.

1. Which nursing diagnosis is the priority for this client?

2. During the initial physical assessment of the client, the client exhibits a frequent cough with copious purulent secretions expectorated. This assessment finding is compatible with which etiology of pneumonia?

3. What should the nutritional plan for this client include?

4. To optimize oxygenation for this client with left-side pneumonia, what body position should be encouraged?

5. The client reports feeling slightly "short of breath." What is the appropriate choice in initiating supplemental oxygen in this client?

For suggested responses, see page 621.

POSTTEST

1 The nurse is caring for a client just admitted with a diagnosis of pulmonary cystic fibrosis (CF). What would be the priority goal when planning care for this client?

1. Improving airway clearance
2. Removing allergens from the environment
3. Eliminating foods that are known to cause intolerance
4. Preparing client for the CF-specific sweat test

2 Which arterial blood gas (ABG) report would the nurse expect in a client with advanced chronic obstructive pulmonary disease (COPD)?

1. pH 7.55, $PaCO_2$ 30 mmHg, PaO_2 80 mmHg, HCO_3^- 24 mEq/L
2. pH 7.40, $PaCO_2$ 40 mmHg, PaO_2 94 mmHg, HCO_3^- 22 mEq/L
3. pH 7.38, $PaCO_2$ 45 mmHg, PaO_2 88 mmHg, HCO_3^- 24 mEq/L
4. pH 7.30, $PaCO_2$ 60 mmHg, PaO_2 70 mmHg, HCO_3^- 30 mEq/L

3 The nurse considers that which concept should have priority for discussion during discharge teaching for a client who has chronic bronchitis?

1. Fluid restriction
2. Smoking cessation
3. Avoidance of crowds
4. Side effects of drug therapy

4 A client with a diagnosis of HIV has returned to the clinic 72 hours after a tuberculin skin test was given and there is an induration of 6 mm at the administration site. The client is visibly upset and states, "I can't believe I have TB!" Which statement by the nurse is most appropriate?

1. "Don't worry, this is a good result. At least it is not 10 mm."
2. "The doctor will prescribe isoniazid for you to take for the next 3 months."
3. "This finding does not confirm TB; it may indicate a recent exposure to tuberculosis."
4. "We'll need to do a chest x-ray. This may be false positive because of your history of HIV."

5 The nurse is caring for a client with a tracheostomy tube. The nurse keeps which concept in mind while caring for this client?

1. Client must be suctioned as needed using clean technique.
2. Tracheotomy tube must be capped to allow client to eat by mouth.
3. The oxygen or air needs to be humidified.
4. Saline can be inserted into the tracheotomy tube before suctioning if secretions are thick.

6 The registered nurse (RN) has an unlicensed assistive person (UAP) assigned to help with the clients. Which task can the RN delegate to the UAP? Select all that apply.

1. Perform a routine measurement of a client's peak expiratory flow rate.
2. Switch supplemental oxygen from face mask to nasal cannula as ordered.
3. Teach the client how to use the incentive spirometer.
4. Administer a nebulizer treatment for the client with recurrent asthma exacerbation.
5. Ambulate a client who has had a chest tube removed 8 hours ago.

7 A client has a right chest tube post-thoracotomy. When assisting the client to ambulate, the nurse should use what measure to maintain functioning of the closed chest drainage system?

1. Keep collection device below the level of the chest.
2. Clamp chest tube before assisting the client out of bed.
3. Milk chest tube when client returns to bed to re-establish patency.
4. Connect collection device to a portable suction machine.

8 A client is brought to the emergency department after his motor vehicle crashed into a tree. Which finding suggests to the nurse that the client has experienced a tension pneumothorax?

1. Tachypnea
2. Hypotension
3. Tracheal deviation
4. Unilateral wheezing

9 The nurse is assessing a client on admission who reports a gradual increase in shortness of breath over at least the past 6 months. If the client denies a history of smoking, why would the nurse ask about exposure to secondhand smoke?

1. Clients with secondhand smoking exposure typically present with difficulty breathing.
2. Secondhand smoke causes acute airway obstruction.
3. This form of smoking is more likely to cause lung cancer.
4. The nurse wants to estimate the risk for smoke inhalation within the client's immediate environment.

10 When auscultating breath sounds in the client with an acute asthma exacerbation, the nurse uses which pieces of information to help interpret and plan for the severity of asthma? Select all that apply.

1. The presence or absence of a cough
2. The presence or absence of bilateral wheezing
3. The presence or absence of unilateral wheezing
4. The duration of the expiratory phase
5. The rate of the respirations

➤ *See pages 80–82 for Answers and Rationales.*

ANSWERS & RATIONALES

Pretest

1 **Answer: 2** **Rationale:** An intact gag reflex indicates that topical sedation has lost its effect and the client is able to swallow (a major safety consideration prior to discharging the client from the health care facility). The ability to swallow precedes consumption of oral intake and coincides with the return of the cough and gag reflex. Knowing symptoms to report to the health care provider following discharge is important but the physiological condition following a bronchoscopy takes priority in this case. Fever, if present, may take hours to days to resolve, may be unrelated to the bronchoscopy, and may have been present at the onset of the procedure. **Cognitive Level:** Analyzing **Client Need:** Reduction of Risk Potential **Integrated Process:** Nursing Process: Evaluation **Content Area:** Adult Health **Strategy:** Note that a critical word in the question is *priority*. This tells you that more than one option may be a correct nursing action but that one is more important than the others. Apply the ABCs (airway, breathing, and circulation). Recall that an intact airway always takes precedence over other assessments. **Reference:** Berman, A. J., & Snyder, S. (2012). *Skills in clinical nursing* (7th ed.). Upper Saddle River, NJ: Pearson Education, p. 1188.

2 **Answer: 3** **Rationale:** The PaO$_2$ normally drops as the individual ages and can be as low as 83 in a 90-year-old (adult normal 80 to 100). The client's assessment is normal. Since the client reports no distress, there is no reason to call the health care provider for a normal finding. There is no need to anticipate an untoward event or anticipate canceling the discharge. **Cognitive Level:** Analyzing **Client Need:** Reduction of Risk Potential **Integrated Process:** Nursing Process: Implementation **Content Area:** Adult Health **Strategy:** To answer this question, you need to understand the normal changes associated with aging and the normal values for arterial blood gases (ABGs). These 2 content areas will enable you to determine that there is no need for any corrective therapeutic action. **Reference:** Berman, A. J., & Snyder, S. (2011). *Kozier and Erb's fundamentals of nursing: Concepts, process, and practice* (9th ed.). Upper Saddle River, NJ: Pearson Education, pp. 1474–1477.

3 **Answer: 4** **Rationale:** Helping clients deep breathe or use the incentive spirometer promotes maximum lung expansion, mobilizes secretions, and encourages cough. Antibiotics are given for bacterial pneumonia to eradicate the infecting organism; however, they do not mobilize secretions. Fluids and humidification liquefy secretions, making them easier to mobilize; there is no reason to avoid oral fluids, since there is no indication that there is a problem with swallowing. Clients with pneumonia are placed in the Fowler's position to maximize lung expansion; the prone position may be used in clients with adult respiratory distress syndrome (ARDS) and refractory hypoxemia. **Cognitive Level:** Applying **Client Need:** Physiological Adaptation **Integrated Process:** Nursing Process: Implementation **Content Area:** Adult Health **Strategy:** Review the indications for each of the options. The answer selected must have a primary purpose of mobilizing or liquefying secretions. **Reference:** LeMone, P., Burke, K., & Bauldoff, G. (2011). *Medical-surgical nursing: Critical thinking in patient care* (5th ed.). Upper Saddle River, NJ: Pearson Education, p. 1182.

4 **Answer: 4** **Rationale:** According to the Centers for Disease Control, some diseases require precautions to limit the risk of infection to others. Standard precautions are required for all clients and include hand hygiene. Communicable diseases that are transferred by small air particles require airborne precautions. Enteric precautions is an older term that refers to precautions used with coming into possible contact with gastrointestinal secretions such as stool. This terminology has been largely replaced with contact precautions, which addresses any form of contact with contaminated objects. Droplet precautions are required for conditions such as pertussis and meningitis that are transmitted on large particle droplets typically transmitted through the oropharynx. **Cognitive Level:** Analyzing **Client Need:** Physiological Adaptation **Integrated Process:** Nursing Process: Planning **Content Area:** Adult Health **Strategy:** First identify the source and mode of infections, then determine how to control them based on established Centers for Disease Control (CDC) guidelines. **Reference:** LeMone, P., Burke, K., & Bauldoff, G. (2011). *Medical-surgical nursing: Critical* *thinking in patient care* (5th ed.). Upper Saddle River, NJ: Pearson Education, pp. 300–301.

5 **Answer: 2** **Rationale:** Carbon dioxide level is one of the primary stimuli for breathing in clients with chronic obstructive pulmonary disease (COPD), who adjust to higher than normal carbon dioxide levels. Abrupt elevation of the oxygen level will depress the stimulus for breathing and can produce respiratory arrest. Administration of 100% oxygen to the client with COPD who is not receiving mechanical ventilation is highly likely to lead to depressed breathing and respiratory arrest. The spouse's presence may be providing comfort and support for the client. Psychological distress caused by the spouse's absence may worsen the dyspnea. Pain medication may depress breathing and should only be used to alleviate pain, not dyspnea. **Cognitive Level:** Applying **Client Need:** Physiological Adaptation **Integrated Process:** Communication and Documentation **Content Area:** Adult Health **Strategy:** This item requires an understanding of the physiology of emphysema and chronic obstructive pulmonary disease (COPD) as well as principles of oxygen therapy. In addition, recall knowledge of the implications of the side effects of analgesia and emphysema are needed. **Reference:** LeMone, P., Burke, K., & Bauldoff, G. (2011). *Medical-surgical nursing: Critical thinking in patient care* (5th ed.). Upper Saddle River, NJ: Pearson Education, pp. 1241–1245.

6 **Answer: 3** **Rationale:** Asthma is an inflammatory process of the airways that is triggered in response to allergens or nonallergic irritants. Frequently, the triggers are in the environment, particularly down pillows, dust mites in mattresses, or pets. An environmental assessment would enable the nurse to identify the triggers that provoke the inflammatory response and offer interventions that could minimize asthmatic attacks. It is insufficient to report the client's adequate knowledge base without attempting to determine a reason for the frequent attacks. Emergency management of status asthmaticus requires hospitalization and intravenous fluids, bronchodilators, and possibly mechanical ventilation. Asthma is a chronic condition that is precipitated by multiple triggers. Acute exacerbations may be frequent but are not necessarily a sign of neglect. **Cognitive Level:** Analyzing **Client Need:** Health Promotion and Maintenance **Integrated Process:** Nursing Process: Implementation **Content Area:** Adult Health **Strategy:** Recall the link between environmental exposure to an allergen and the development of symptoms in asthma. Recall that the first step of the nursing process is assessment, and this is needed to determine possible etiologies for the client's frequent exacerbations. **Reference:** LeMone, P., Burke, K., & Bauldoff, G. (2011). *Medical-surgical nursing: Critical thinking in patient care* (5th ed.). Upper Saddle River, NJ: Pearson Education, p. 1230.

7 **Answer: 1** **Rationale:** Pursed-lip breathing is a technique used by individuals with chronic obstructive pulmonary

disease (COPD) where clients exhale through pursed lips. This increases airway pressure, delays the airway compression that occurs with exhalation, and reduces air trapping in the alveoli. The potential slowing of the respiratory rate is incidental and unrelated to why it is used. **Cognitive Level:** Applying **Client Need:** Physiological Adaptation **Integrated Process:** Teaching and Learning **Content Area:** Adult Health **Strategy:** The core issue of the question is knowledge of the pathophysiology of emphysema and how pursed-lip breathing is helpful in the management of this disease. Visualize this respiratory pattern and compare each option to the mental picture of the effect on the lungs. **Reference:** LeMone, P., Burke, K., & Bauldoff, G. (2011). *Medical-surgical nursing: Critical thinking in patient care* (5th ed.). Upper Saddle River, NJ: Pearson Education, p. 1238.

8 **Answer: 3** **Rationale:** Thoracentesis is used to withdraw fluids or air from the pleural space for diagnosis or therapeutic purposes. Although it may be used to help determine the stage of cancer, this is not the primary purpose in this case, because there is no specific reference to cancer in the question. Obtaining pleural tissue for evaluation occurs with tissue biopsy, which can be done if there are abnormal findings upon evaluation of pleural fluid. Thoracentesis does not involve direct visualization of the pleural cavity. **Cognitive Level:** Applying **Client Need:** Reduction of Risk Potential **Integrated Process:** Teaching and Learning **Content Area:** Adult Health **Strategy:** Recall what thoracentesis is and the procedural technique used. Then recall that it removes air or fluid to make the correct selection. **Reference:** LeMone, P., Burke, K., & Bauldoff, G. (2011). *Medical-surgical nursing: Critical thinking in patient care* (5th ed.). Upper Saddle River, NJ: Pearson Education, p. 1206.

9 **Answer:**

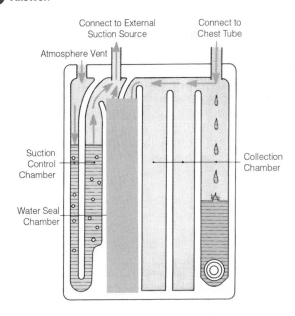

ANSWERS & RATIONALES

Rationale: Going from right to left (facing the page) the disposable chest drainage system is modeled on the 3-bottle system for chest drainage. The chamber connected to the client (chest tube) collects the chest drainage. The middle chamber is the water seal and it protects the lung from collapse. This chamber contains water that allows air from the pleural space to escape but prevents this air from reentering the system. The chamber on the left determines the amount of suction applied to the system. **Cognitive Level:** Applying **Client Need:** Physiological Adaptation **Integrated Process:** Nursing Process: Assessment **Content Area:** Adult Health **Strategy:** Recall the elements of the typical chest drainage system. When a client has a pneumothorax, the chest tube allows for the escape of air from the pleura and prevents air from entering the pleura. Recall that the escape of air is indicated by the bubbling in the water seal chamber to help you choose correctly. **Reference:** Smith, S. F., Duell, D. J., & Martin, B. C. (2012). *Clinical nursing skills* (8th ed.). Upper Saddle River, NJ: Pearson Education, pp. 123–126.

10 Answer: 3, 5 Rationale: Chest tubes are inserted into the pleural space to drain fluids or air from the pleural space and promote lung re-expansion. If the drainage system is occluded in any way, re-expansion can be prevented or fluid and air can accumulate and cause a tension pneumothorax. Fluctuations in the water seal are normal and represent normal inspiration and expiration. The chest tube has tiny holes at the tip to promote drainage. Respiration can cause the tube to slide in and out of the insertion site, which could potentially cause one of the small holes to be located on the outside of the thoracic wall and re-collapse the lung. For that reason, placing an occlusive dressing around the chest tube keeps the holes sealed and prevents possible re-collapse. An upright position facilitates the chest expansion. Milking the chest tube can change intrathoracic pressure and cause lung injury. **Cognitive Level:** Applying **Client Need:** Reduction of Risk Potential **Integrated Process:** Nursing Process: Implementation **Content Area:** Adult Health **Strategy:** Review the purpose for each chamber in a closed chest drainage system. Next, consider that clamping or milking the chest tube changes the pressure within the system. Finally, recall the benefits associated with maintaining a proper dressing and client position. **Reference:** Smith, S. F., Duell, D. J., & Martin, B. C. (2012). *Clinical nursing skills: Basic to advanced skills* (8th ed.). Upper Saddle River, NJ: Pearson Education, p. 1217.

Posttest

1 Answer: 1 Rationale: Ineffective airway clearance is the major challenge for persons with cystic fibrosis (CF). Irritants in the environment can trigger exacerbations in these clients, but is not the priority in this situation. Malabsorption syndrome is common in clients with GI-associated CF condition. Although the sweat test is the standard diagnostic measure for CF diagnosis, this choice is not appropriate because this client has already been diagnosed. **Cognitive Level:** Applying **Client Need:** Physiological Adaptation **Integrated Process:** Nursing Process: Planning **Content Area:** Adult Health **Strategy:** Note that the client has already been diagnosed and the type of CF is identified. Focus then on the option that addresses the main problem of this condition. **Reference:** Osborn, K. S., Wraa, C. E., & Watson, A. (2010). *Medical surgical nursing: Preparation for practice*. Upper Saddle River, NJ: Pearson Education, p. 968.

2 Answer: 4 Rationale: During the later stages of chronic obstructive pulmonary disease (COPD), arterial blood gas (ABG) findings indicate low pH (less than 7.35), elevated pCO_2 (greater than 45 mmHg), low pO_2 (less than 80 mmHg), and elevated HCO_3^- (greater than 26 mEq/L). Variations in the CO_2 level are an indication of the body's attempt to compensate for chronically low pH. These clients typically do not have normal ABG levels. **Cognitive Level:** Analyzing **Client Need:** Reduction of Risk Potential **Integrated Process:** Nursing Process: Assessment **Content Area:** Adult Health **Strategy:** Review the pathophysiology of chronic obstructive pulmonary disease (COPD). Eliminate any answer choices that do not indicate an acidosis. Then eliminate answer choices that do not indicate CO_2 retention. **Reference:** LeMone, P., Burke, K., & Bauldoff, G. (2011). *Medical-surgical nursing: Critical thinking in patient care* (5th ed.). Upper Saddle River, NJ: Pearson Education, pp. 226–227.

3 Answer: 2 Rationale: Cigarette smoking is the primary etiology of chronic bronchitis so cessation is the priority for the client. Avoidance of crowds to lower the risk of pulmonary infections is a recommendation that is individualized and less common than the need for smoking cessation. Teaching the client about potential side effects of any prescribed medications should be included in all discharge teaching. Fluids are often increased to liquefy secretions and prevent mucous plugs. **Cognitive Level:** Applying **Client Need:** Health Promotion and Maintenance **Integrated Process:** Nursing Process: Planning **Content Area:** Adult Health **Strategy:** The core issue of the question is being able to prioritize items needed in discharge teaching for a client with bronchitis. Recall that smoking is a key ongoing risk factor to lung tissue to place this as highest priority. **Reference:** Osborn, K. S., Wraa, C. E., & Watson, A. (2010). *Medical surgical nursing: Preparation for practice* (Vol. Combined). Upper Saddle River, NJ: Pearson Education, p. 935.

4 Answer: 3 Rationale: In HIV-positive clients, an induration of 5 to 10 mm after a tuberculin skin test indicates exposure to an individual infected with mycobacterium tuberculosis. History of HIV is not related to false positive tuberculin skin test, but is related to a positive result at measurements of greater than 5 mm. These clients are often immunocompromised, placing them at greater risk of infection. **Cognitive Level:** Applying **Client Need:** Physiological Adaptation **Integrated Process:** Communication and Documentation **Content Area:**

Adult Health **Strategy:** Differentiate exposure to the tuberculosis (TB) bacilli from active infection. Eliminate items that infer that the client is actively infected or is unrelated to TB. The medical diagnosis of being immune deficient is most important in the interpretation of the findings. **Reference:** Osborn, K. S., Wraa, C. E., & Watson, A. (2010). *Medical surgical nursing: Preparation for practice.* Upper Saddle River, NJ: Pearson Education, p. 946.

5 **Answer: 3** **Rationale:** Because the tracheostomy bypasses the normal airway's humidification, supplemental humidification is needed to keep the airways moist and prevent mucous plugs and airway occlusion from occurring. The tracheotomy is capped and the balloon deflated to enable clients to speak. This is done periodically to help prevent tracheal erosion. Clients should be suctioned using sterile technique to prevent introduction of bacteria. Saline should not be inserted into the trachea prior to suctioning for the same reason. **Cognitive Level:** Analyzing **Client Need:** Basic Care and Comfort **Integrated Process:** Nursing Process: Planning **Content Area:** Adult Health **Strategy:** Since the tracheostomy bypasses the oropharynx, select the answer choice that replaces the functions of the oropharynx. **Reference:** Berman, A. J., Snyder, S., & Jackson, C. (2009). *Skills in clinical nursing* (6th ed.). Upper Saddle River, NJ: Pearson Education, p. 632.

6 **Answer: 1, 5** **Rationale:** The RN is ultimately responsible for the care of the client; however, assisting stable clients with routine needs is within the scope of practice for an unlicensed assistive personnel (UAP). Measurement of peak expiratory flow is a task-based activity and is within the scope of the UAP. The duties of a UAP should not include client teaching, assessing clients, client teaching, or medication administration. The RN is ultimately responsible for the care of the client. **Cognitive Level:** Analyzing **Client Need:** Management of Care **Integrated Process:** Nursing Process: Implementation **Content Area:** Adult Health **Strategy:** Determine which roles can be performed by the unlicensed assistive person (UAP) and eliminate the incorrect answer choices. **Reference:** Berman, A. J., Snyder, S., & Jackson, C. (2009). *Skills in clinical nursing* (6th ed.). Upper Saddle River, NJ: Pearson Education, pp. 18, 32, 606, 630.

7 **Answer: 1** **Rationale:** Keeping the drainage system below the level of the chest maintains the water seal and prevents backflow of air and fluid into the chest. The chest tube should never be clamped as this may cause a pneumothorax. "Milking" the tube increases negative pressure in the thorax and can cause lung injury. When ordered, the chest drainage system is attached to wall suction rather than portable suction. **Cognitive Level:** Applying **Client Need:** Physiological Adaptation **Integrated Process:** Nursing Process: Implementation **Content Area:** Adult Health **Strategy:** Recall principles of chest tube management. Since the question is asking what should be done, eliminate options that are not recommended,

such as those that create pressure inside the tubing (which could be harmful to the client). Also use knowledge of gravity as an aid to drainage to help make a selection. **Reference:** Osborn, K. S., Wraa, C. E., & Watson, A. (2010). *Medical surgical nursing: Preparation for practice.* Upper Saddle River, NJ: Pearson Education, pp. 990–991.

8 **Answer: 3** **Rationale:** Tension pneumothorax is a life-threatening condition, so the nurse must recognize potential indicators. Sudden deviation of the trachea toward the unaffected side occurs due to increased pressure within the pleural cavity; this occurs only with a tension pneumothorax. Increasing pressure on the great vessels in the chest decreases cardiac output, which can be fatal. Hypotension and tachypnea occur with pneumothorax but are also related to numerous other conditions and are therefore nonspecific. Unilateral wheezing is indicative of narrowing of the airways. **Cognitive Level:** Applying **Client Need:** Physiological Adaptation **Integrated Process:** Nursing Process: Assessment **Content Area:** Adult Health **Strategy:** Define tension pneumothorax and recall that the air that cannot be displaced creates pressure that puts the other structures in the thorax at risk. Eliminate answer choices that are nonspecific findings. The answer choice that is specific for a tension pneumothorax remains. **Reference:** Osborn, K. S., Wraa, C. E., & Watson, A. (2010). *Medical surgical nursing: Preparation for practice.* Upper Saddle River, NJ: Pearson Education, p. 989.

9 **Answer: 4** **Rationale:** Exposure to secondhand smoke has been found to cause similar deleterious effects as when cigarettes are used directly. A variety of respiratory signs or symptoms, not just difficulty breathing, can be present because of exposure to secondhand smoke. The changes are gradual; if the client presents with acute obstruction, the nurse should suspect another cause. Exposure to secondhand smoke is not more likely to cause lung cancer than smoking directly. **Cognitive Level:** Applying **Client Need:** Physiological Adaptation **Integrated Process:** Nursing Process: Assessment **Content Area:** Adult Health **Strategy:** First, recall smoking and secondhand smoke are considered risk factors for pulmonary diseases, especially cancer, Next, use a true or false technique to eliminate the incorrect answers. **Reference:** LeMone, P., Burke, K., & Bauldoff, G. (2011). *Medical-surgical nursing: Critical thinking in patient care* (5th ed.). Upper Saddle River, NJ: Pearson Education, p. 344.

10 **Answer: 2, 5** **Rationale:** Asthmatic symptoms are produced by an inflammation of airways bilaterally. If there is unilateral wheezing, this indicates an airway obstruction from another cause. Asthmatic symptoms are produced by an inflammation of airways bilaterally. The respiratory rate will be increased in respiratory distress, which gives valid information in addition to the other findings when determining the severity of asthma. It is common for a cough to accompany the distress of an asthma attack due to bronchial irritation; however, the cough does not indicate the severity of the asthma. Breath sounds are prolonged in the expiratory phase with asthma, but this factor does not alter the plan of care. **Cognitive Level:** Applying **Client Need:** Physiological Adaptation **Integrated Process:** Nursing Process: Assessment **Content Area:** Adult Health **Strategy:** To determine the correct options, recall the pathophysiology of asthma. Remember that airway inflammation can be so severe that the client moves minimal air (which increases respiratory effort) and that the changes are bilateral. **Reference:** LeMone, P., Burke, K., & Bauldoff, G. (2011). *Medical-surgical nursing: Critical thinking in patient care* (5th ed.). Upper Saddle River, NJ: Pearson Education, pp. 1230–1235.

References

Berman, A., & Snyder, S. (2012). *Kozier & Erb's fundamentals of nursing: Concepts, process, and practice* (9th ed.). Upper Saddle River, NJ: Pearson Education.

Berman, A. J., Snyder, S., & McKinney, D. S. (2011). *Nursing basics for clinical practice.* Upper Saddle River, NJ: Pearson Education.

D'Amico, D., & Barbarito, C. (2012). *Health & physical assessment in nursing* (2nd ed.). Upper Saddle River, NJ: Pearson Education, Inc.

Ignatavicius, D. D., & Workman, M. L. (2013). *Medical-surgical nursing: Critical thinking for collaborative care* (7th ed.) Philadelphia: W. B. Saunders Company.

Kee, J. L. (2010). *Laboratory and diagnostic tests* (8th ed.). Upper Saddle River, NJ: Pearson Education.

Kee, J. L. (2009). *Handbook of laboratory and diagnostic tests with nursing implications* (6th ed.). Upper Saddle River, NJ: Pearson Education.

Lehne, R. (2010). *Pharmacology for nursing care* (7th ed.). St. Louis, MO: Saunders.

LeMone, P., Burke, K., & Bauldoff, G. (2011). *Medical-surgical nursing: Critical thinking in patient care* (5th ed.). Upper Saddle River, NJ: Pearson Education.

Lewis, S., Dirksen, S. Heitkemper, M., Bucher, L., & Camera, I. (2011). *Medical surgical nursing: Assessment and management of clinical problems* (8th ed.). St. Louis, MO: Elsevier.

McCance, K. L., & Huether, S. E. (2010). *Pathophysiology: The biologic basis for disease in adults and children* (6th ed.). St. Louis, MO: Mosby, Inc.

Osborn, K. S., Wraa, C. E., & Watson, A. (2010). *Medical surgical nursing: Preparation for practice* (Vol. Combined). Upper Saddle River, NJ: Pearson Education.

Smith, S. F., Duell, D. J., & Martin, B. C. (2012). *Clinical nursing skills: Basic to advanced skills* (8th ed.). Upper Saddle River, NJ: Pearson Education.

Wilson, B. A., Shannon, M. T., & Shields, K. M. (2012). *Pearson nurse's drug guide 2012.* Upper Saddle River, NJ: Pearson Education.

Cardiac Disorders

Chapter Outline

Overview of Anatomy and
  Physiology of Heart
Diagnostic Tests and Assessments
Common Nursing Techniques
  and Procedures

Myocardial Infarction (MI)
Heart Failure
Endocarditis (Infective,
  Subacute Bacterial)
Valvular Disorders

Cardiomyopathy
Pericarditis

Objectives

➤ Identify basic structures and function of the heart.
➤ Describe the pathophysiology and etiology of common
  cardiac disorders.
➤ Describe expected assessment data and diagnostic test findings for
  selected cardiac disorders.
➤ Identify priority nursing problems for selected cardiac disorders.
➤ Discuss therapeutic management of selected cardiac disorders.
➤ Prioritize nursing management of the client experiencing a
  cardiac disorder.
➤ Identify expected outcomes for the client experiencing a
  cardiac disorder.

 NCLEX-RN® Test Prep

Use the accompanying online resource,
NursingReviewsandRationales, to test
yourself with hundreds of NCLEX®-style
practice questions.

Review at a Glance

afterload resistance that ventricles must overcome to eject blood into systemic circulation; directly related to arterial blood pressure

angina pectoris chest pain resulting from restricted blood flow to myocardium

bradycardia heart rate less than 60 beats per minute

cardiac cycle one complete heartbeat; includes 2 phases: systole (ventricular contraction) and diastole (ventricular relaxation and refilling)

cardiac output (CO) volume of blood in liters ejected by heart each minute; indicator of pump function of heart; normal adult CO is 4–8 L/min; $CO = HR \times SV$

contractility strength of contraction regardless of preload; decreased by hypoxia and some drugs (beta blockers

and calcium channel blockers); increased by drugs (digoxin and dopamine)

coronary heart disease (CHD) buildup of atherosclerotic plaque in coronary arteries that restricts blood flow to heart muscle

cor pulmonale right-sided failure and enlarged right atrium caused by chronic pulmonary hypertension

dysrhythmia an irregular heart rate or rhythm; irregularity may involve atria, ventricles, or both

ejection fraction (EF) portion of blood ejected during systole compared to total ventricular filling volume; normal EF is 55–65% in adults

ischemia decreased supply of oxygenated blood to heart muscle

infarction myocardial tissue injury from lack of oxygenation

jugular venous distention (JVD) increased pressure in jugular veins, visible more than a few millimeters above clavicle with client supine with head of bed raised to 45-degree angle

preload degree of myocardial fiber stretch at end of ventricular diastole; influenced by ventricular filling volume and myocardial compliance

pulmonary edema significant fluid overload in lungs with acute exacerbation of left heart failure

regurgitation improper or incomplete closure of heart valves, resulting in back flow of blood

stenosis condition in which heart valve leaflets are fused together, have a narrow opening, are stiff, or unable to open or close properly

stroke volume (SV) volume of blood ejected from left ventricle each cardiac cycle

tachycardia heart rate greater than 100 beats per minute

tamponade life-threatening medical emergency resulting from excess fluid collection in pericardial sac; interferes with heart filling and severely decreases cardiac output;

if left untreated will lead to cardiac arrest and possible death

PRETEST

1 When assessing a client who underwent pericardiocentesis, the nurse notes a decreased blood pressure, distended neck veins, and clear lungs. The nurse suspects that the client has developed which of the following?

1. Heart failure
2. Cardiac tamponade
3. Pericarditis
4. Cardiomyopathy

2 A 54-year-old male client was recently diagnosed with subacute bacterial endocarditis (SBE). The nurse determines that the client understands the discharge teaching when he makes which statement?

1. "I need a referral to a dietician to understand a low-sodium diet."
2. "I have to call my doctor so I can get antibiotics before seeing the dentist."
3. "Can I take the antibiotics as a pill now?"
4. "If I quit smoking, it will help the endocarditis."

3 The nurse on a cardiac unit is caring for a client admitted with an acute exacerbation of heart failure. The nurse concludes that the client's condition is worsening after noting which client data during assessment? Select all that apply.

1. Normal sinus rhythm that becomes sinus tachycardia
2. Urine drainage is increased in amount
3. Onset of a cough with pink, frothy sputum
4. Presence of dyspnea at rest
5. Falls asleep when not disturbed

4 A client is scheduled for coronary angiography. In reviewing the client's record, what significant finding would the nurse report to the health care provider before the diagnostic procedure?

1. Client reported an allergy to iodine.
2. Client's electrocardiogram shows atrial fibrillation.
3. Potassium level is 4.0 mEq/L.
4. Client has a history of chronic renal failure.

5 The nurse is implementing a discharge teaching plan for a client newly diagnosed with heart failure. When discussing fluid status with the client, the nurse would explain the importance of doing which of the following?

1. Restricting fluid intake to approximately 800 mL per day
2. Taking a single extra dose of diuretic if there is decreased urination for several days
3. Recording body weight every day before breakfast and report a weight gain of 3 or more pounds in a week
4. Keeping track of daily output and calling health care provider if it is less than 1 liter on any day

6 The nurse is caring for a client with complete heart block who is being prepared to have a temporary transvenous pacemaker inserted. In briefly explaining the blockage to the cardiac conduction system to the client, the nurse would point out which area on the diagram shown? Select the affected area.

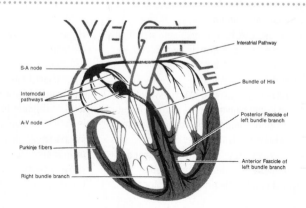

7 A client is getting ready to go home after acute myocardial infarction (AMI). The client is asking questions about the prescribed medications, and wants to know why metoprolol (Lopressor) was prescribed. The nurse's best response would be which of the following?

1. "Your heart was beating too slowly, and metoprolol (Lopressor) increases your heart rate."
2. "Lopressor helps to increase the blood supply to the heart by dilating your coronary arteries."
3. "Lopressor helps make your heart beat stronger to supply more blood to your body."
4. "Lopressor slows your heart rate and decreases the amount of work it has to do so it can heal."

8 A client is taking digoxin (Lanoxin) and furosemide (Lasix) for heart failure. The nurse approves of which of the following client selections that is the best menu choice for this client?

1. Chicken with baked potato and cantaloupe
2. Ham and cheese omelet with low-cholesterol egg substitute
3. Grilled cheese sandwich and pan-browned potatoes
4. Pizza with low-fat mozzarella cheese and pepperoni

9 The nurse is caring for a newly admitted client with a diagnosis of restrictive cardiomyopathy. When planning this client's care, which of the following would be the most appropriate nursing diagnosis?

1. Fear related to new onset of symptoms
2. Hopelessness related to lack of cure and debilitating symptoms
3. Deficient Knowledge related to medication regime
4. Activity Intolerance related to decreased cardiac output

10 The nurse working on a cardiac telemetry unit prepares to use an external pacemaker after noting that an assigned client has a blood pressure of 70/52 and has developed which cardiac dysrhythmia that is amenable to this therapy? Select all that apply.

1. Ventricular fibrillation
2. Atrial fibrillation
3. Ventricular tachycardia
4. Second-degree heart block
5. Third-degree heart block

➤ *See pages 110–111 for Answers and Rationales.*

I. OVERVIEW OF ANATOMY AND PHYSIOLOGY OF HEART

A. Structures of heart

1. Heart is a hollow muscular organ enclosed in a protective sac, divided into 4 chambers
2. Heart wall has 3 layers: *epicardium,* fibrous outside protective layer; *myocardium,* middle layer of specialized cardiac muscle; *endocardium,* endothelial lining of chambers
3. *Pericardium:* protective sac encasing heart; 2 fibrous layers with small amount of serous fluid separating layers for lubrication
4. Chambers
   a. Heart has 4 hollow chambers divided by a septum into right and left sides
   b. Each side has an upper chamber (*atrium*) and a lower chamber (*ventricle*)
      1) Atria are smaller than ventricles
      2) Blood flows from body into right atrium and from lungs into left atrium
      3) With atrial contraction, blood is pumped from atria into ventricles
      4) With ventricular contraction, blood is pumped from right ventricle into pulmonary artery (PA) and lungs, and from left ventricle into aorta and arterial circulation
5. Valves of heart
   a. Atrioventricular (A-V) valves separate atria from ventricles; they control blood flow between atria and ventricles
      1) Tricuspid valve, between right atrium and right ventricle, has 3 leaflets
      2) Mitral valve, between left atrium and left ventricle, has 2 leaflets

      3) Leaflets of A-V valves are connected to papillary muscles by chordae tendonae to prevent backflow

      4) S_1 (first heart sound) is heard when A-V valves close

    b. Semilunar valves separate cardiac chambers from great vessels and control blood flow out of cardiac chambers

      1) Pulmonic valve is between right ventricle and pulmonic artery, and deoxygenated blood flows through this valve to lungs

      2) Aortic valve is between left ventricle and aorta, and oxygenated blood is pumped from heart through this valve into systemic circulation

      3) Each semilunar valve has 3 cusps that prevent backflow

      4) S_2 (second heart sound) is heard when semilunar valves close

B. Function of heart

  1. Circulation (see Figure 3-1): each side of heart acts as a pump to circulate blood through lungs or through body to perfuse tissues

    a. Double pump: right side responsible for pulmonary circulation; left side responsible for systemic circulation

Figure 3-1

Circulation through the heart

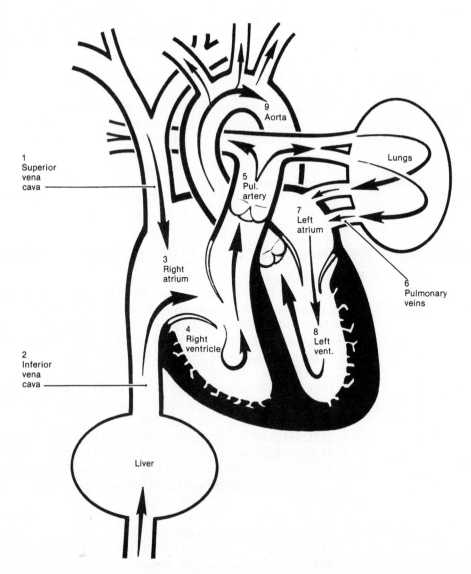

    b. Right heart circulation—deoxygenated blood:
Venous system (1 and 2) ⇒ right atrium (3) ⇒ right ventricle (4) ⇒ lungs for oxygenation via pulmonary artery (5)

    c. Left heart circulation—oxygenated blood:
Lungs via pulmonary veins (6) ⇒ left atrium (7) ⇒ left ventricle (8) ⇒ aorta (9) ⇒ systemic circulation for tissue perfusion

    d. Coronary arteries branch off aorta to supply oxygenated blood to heart

2. Cardiac conduction system (see Figure 3-2): a series of pathways that conduct electrical impulses through heart, stimulate depolarization and resulting muscle contraction of chambers in a specific sequence, and initiate pumping action of heart

    a. Conduction takes place because of special electrophysiologic properties of specialized cells in conduction system

    b. These properties include *automaticity* (ability to initiate an electrical impulse), *excitability* (ability of a cell to respond to a stimulus), and *conductivity* (ability to transmit impulses from one cell to another)

    c. Components of cardiac conduction system are as follows:

        1) Sinoatrial (SA) node: natural pacemaker; concentration of cells responsible for initiating conduction impulse in a healthy heart; located in right atrium at juncture with superior vena cava; rate 60–100 beats per minute (bpm) in adult

        2) Internodal pathways: carry impulse from SA node to AV node through both right and left atria; impulse initiates process of depolarization in both atria; depolarization results in myocardial contraction of both atria

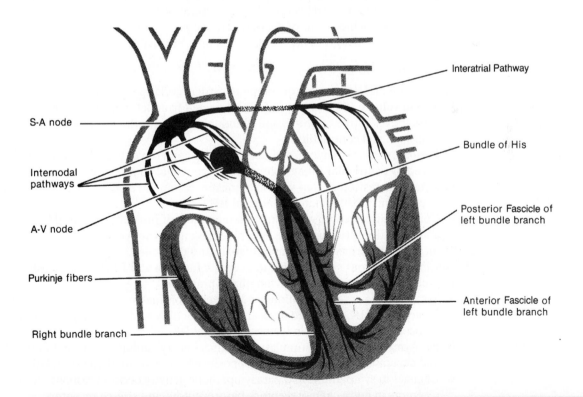

Figure 3-2

The normal conduction system of the heart

3) Atrioventricular (AV) node: located at base of atrial septum; slows impulse; allows atria to fully empty before initiating depolarization of ventricles; when SA node is not functioning, can initiate an impulse at rate of 40–60 beats per minute in an adult

4) Bundle of His: short branch of conductive cells connecting AV node to bundle branches at intraventricular septum

5) Bundle branches: right (RBB) and left (LBB) split off on either side of intra-ventricular septum; carry impulse to Purkinje fibers

6) Purkinje fibers: diffuse network of conduction pathways; are terminal branches of conduction system; conduct impulses rapidly throughout ventricles; initiate rapid depolarization wave throughout myocardium and resulting ventricular contraction; when SA and AV nodes fail, can initiate impulses at rate of 20–40 beats per minute in an adult

3. Cardiac cycle: each cardiac cycle is one complete heartbeat; includes 2 parts—systole (ventricular contraction) and diastole (relaxation and ventricular refilling)

a. Systole: portion of cardiac cycle when ventricles depolarize and contract to pump blood into pulmonary and systemic circulation; begins with closure of AV valves; ends with closure of semilunar valves

b. Diastole: portion of cardiac cycle when ventricles repolarize and refill with blood; begins with closure of semilunar valves; ends with closure of AV valves

c. Atrial systole (depolarization and contraction) is part of late ventricular diastole and atrial diastole occurs during ventricular systole

4. Cardiac output (CO): volume of blood in liters ejected by heart each minute; indicator of pump function of heart; normal adult CO is 4–8 L/min; CO is measured directly by PA catheter (for example, Swan-Ganz) in a critical care setting or indirectly using $ScvO_2$ (central venous oxygen saturation); clinical indicators of decreased CO include signs of decreased tissue perfusion such as a change in level of consciousness (early), and decreased blood pressure (BP) (late)

$$CO = HR \times SV$$

a. Heart rate (HR): number of complete cardiac cycles per minute

b. Stroke volume (SV): volume of blood ejected from left ventricle with each cardiac cycle; stroke volume and ultimately CO are influenced by preload, afterload, and contractility

c. Preload: degree of myocardial fiber stretch at end of ventricular diastole; influenced by ventricular filling volume and myocardial compliance

d. Afterload: resistance that ventricles must overcome to eject blood into systemic circulation; directly related to arterial BP

e. Contractility: strength of contraction regardless of preload; decreased by hypoxia and some drugs (for example, beta blockers and calcium channel blockers); increased by drugs (for example, digoxin and dopamine)

5. Autonomic nervous system: regulates cardiac function and BP; balance exists between sympathetic and parasympathetic branches

a. Sympathetic nerve stimulation produces epinephrine and norepinephrine; results in increased HR, increased myocardial contractility, and increased peripheral vasoconstriction; results in increased arterial BP

b. Parasympathetic nerve stimulation produces acetylcholine, results in lowered HR and decreased contractility; is the opposite effect of sympathetic stimulation

c. Changes in sympathetic and parasympathetic activity occur in response to sensory receptors in body, chemoreceptors, baroreceptors, and stretch receptors

1) Chemoreceptors: located in aortic arch and carotid bodies; sense chemical changes in blood, primarily hypoxia and to a lesser degree hypercapnia; respond by inducing vasoconstriction

2) Baroreceptors: provide a rapid response to changes in pressure; sensation of low pressure initiates sympathetic stimulation, resulting in increased HR, vasoconstriction, and consequently increased pressure; sensation of increased pressure sends impulses to medulla, decreasing HR and BP (vagal response)

II. DIAGNOSTIC TESTS AND ASSESSMENTS

A. Laboratory tests

1. Client preparation: the following blood tests involve simple phlebotomy, following agency procedure
2. Postprocedure nursing care: apply pressure and small dressing to site; assess for bleeding
3. Serum enzymes: increased in blood with heart damage; evaluates myocardial tissue **infarction** (damage to myocardium from decreased oxygenation); serial testing over time detects trend and determines peak time and extent of injury and cell death

   a. Creatine kinase (CK): formerly known as creatine phosphokinase (CPK), elevation indicates muscle injury; CK-MB is isoenzyme specific to myocardial muscle; rises within 6 hours of injury, peaks at 18 hours postinjury and returns to normal in 2–3 days; is useful for early diagnosis of myocardial infarction (MI)

   b. Troponin: onset is before CK-MB in MI, peaks at 24 hours and returns to normal around 2 weeks; provides early sensitivity, extended blood levels, and is more specific to cardiac injury for diagnosis of MI with an uncertain timeframe (refer to Chapter 1 for more details)

   c. Lactic dehydrogenase (LDH): is found in many body tissues; cardiac origin is confirmed with analysis of isoenzymes (L_1 is greater than L_2; "flipped" from normal levels); elevation is detected within 24–72 hours after MI, peaks in 3–4 days, and returns to normal around 2 weeks; is useful in delayed diagnosis of MI

   d. Brain natriuretic peptide (BNP): is a hormone found in left ventricle; elevated in heart failure (normal 0–99 ng/L), but may be higher with aging and in women; question results if creatinine level is also elevated

4. Drug levels: blood tests to detect toxic levels of cardiac medications

   a. Digoxin: therapeutic range is 0.5–2 ng/mL; early signs of toxicity include nausea, vomiting, anorexia; abdominal pain, **bradycardia** (HR less than 60 beats/minute), other **dysrhythmia** (irregular HR or rhythm involving atria, ventricles, or both), and visual disturbances (yellow/green halos) may occur

   b. Quinidine: therapeutic range is 2–6 mcg/mL; signs of toxicity include tinnitus, hearing loss, visual disturbances, nausea, dizziness, widened QRS, ventricular dysrhythmias

5. Electrolytes: normal levels are essential for proper cardiac function; some medications, renal or cardiac conditions may contribute to electrolyte imbalance

   a. Potassium (K^+): normal 3.5–5.1 mEq/L

   1) Hypokalemia can occur with diuretic therapy (especially loop diuretics such as furosemide); cardiac effects include increased risk of digoxin toxicity, ventricular dysrhythmias, flattening and inversion of T wave or presence of U wave

   2) Hyperkalemia is usually related to renal dysfunction or intake of excess potassium dietary supplements; cardiac effects include ventricular dysrhythmias, tall peaked T waves on ECG, and asystole

   b. Sodium (Na^+): normal 135–145 mEq/L

   1) Hyponatremia with long-term diuretic therapy

   2) Hypernatremia may result in dehydration

   3) Hypo- or hypernatremia may result in **tachycardia** (HR greater than 100 beats per minute)

      c. Calcium (Ca^{++}): normal 9–11 mg/dL or 4.5–5.5 mEq/L

          1) Blood levels are affected by hormonal imbalances, renal failure, and several medications

          2) Cardiac effects of hypocalcemia include ventricular dysrhythmias, prolonged QT interval, and cardiac arrest

          3) Hypercalcemia shortens QT interval and causes AV block, digoxin hypersensitivity, and cardiac arrest

      d. Magnesium (Mg^{++}): normal 1.5–2.5 mg/dL

          1) Cardiac effects of decreased Mg^{++} include ventricular tachycardia and fibrillation

          2) Cardiac effects of increased Mg^{++} include bradycardia, hypotension, prolonged PR and QRS intervals

   6. Serum lipid profile: aid to determine risk of developing atherosclerosis

      a. Total serum lipids normal value: 400–800 mg/dL

      b. Triglycerides: lipids stored in fat tissue, readily available for energy production; normal serum value is 10–190 mg/dL, (without elevated cholesterol, up to 250 mg/dL may be acceptable)

      c. Cholesterol: main lipid associated with atherosclerotic disease; normal is less than 200 mg/dL in adults

      d. Lipoproteins: proteins in blood to transport cholesterol, triglycerides, and other fats; refer again to Chapter 1 for normal lipoprotein ranges

          1) High-density lipoproteins (HDL): transport cholesterol to liver for excretion; HDL/total cholesterol ratio should be at least 1:5, 1:3 more ideal

          2) Low-density lipoproteins (LDL): transport cholesterol to peripheral tissues, associated with increased risk of coronary heart disease

      e. Preprocedure nursing care: instruct to fast for 12–14 hours before testing to ensure accurate results

B. Electrocardiography

   1. Is a graphic recording of electrical activity of heart; cardiac complex consists of P wave (represents atrial depolarization; normal duration 0.12–0.2 second), QRS complex (represents ventricular depolarization; normal duration less than 0.12 second), ST segment, T wave, and U wave represent ventricular repolarization; each QRS complex should be preceded by a P wave

   2. Resting or 12-lead electrocardiogram (ECG): represents a recording of electrical activity of heart from 12 different views (leads), including 3 bipolar limb leads (I, II, and III), 3 unipolar limb leads (avL, avR, avF), and 6 chest leads (V1–V6); used to determine cardiac rhythm, as well as ischemia, injury, infarction, hypertrophy, electrolyte imbalance, and drug effects (such as digoxin and quinidine), depending on types of changes seen and location by leads

      a. Client preparation: secure electrodes to appropriate locations on chest and extremities; instruct to remain still during test; reassure client that he or she will not receive any electrical shock or impulses

      b. No postprocedure nursing care

   3. Holter monitoring: continuous ambulatory ECG monitoring over time (usual 24 hours) with small, timed, portable ECG recording device

      a. Client preparation: secure electrodes to appropriate locations on chest; instruct to continue normal activity and maintain a log of activities and any symptoms

      b. No postprocedure nursing care

   4. Stress test: continuous multilead ECG monitoring during controlled and supervised exercise, usually on treadmill; for clients who cannot tolerate exercise, cardiac stress can be drug induced with Dobutamine (Dobutrex)

      a. Client preparation: obtained written consent; explain procedure, instruct to eat a light meal 1–2 hours before exam (no caffeine, alcohol, or smoking), wear comfortable clothing and rubber-soled walking shoes

       b. Nursing care during procedure: secure electrodes to appropriate locations on chest, obtain and record baseline BP and ECG tracing; instruct client to exercise as instructed and report any pain, weakness, dizziness, shortness of breath, or other symptoms immediately; monitor ECG continuously, record at frequent intervals and with any symptoms or changes in vital signs (pulse or BP), ST segments, or cardiac rhythm

       c. Postprocedure nursing care: continue to monitor ECG and BP until client returns completely to baseline and is symptom free

C. Echocardiography

    1. Is an ultrasound of heart to evaluate structure and function of chambers and valves

    2. Client preparation: instruct to remain still during test; secure electrodes for simultaneous ECG tracing; explain that it is typically painless, however, lubricant placed on skin may be cool

    3. Postprocedure nursing care: cleanse lubricant from chest wall

D. Phonocardiography

    1. Is a graphic recording of heart sounds with simultaneous ECG

    2. Client preparation: instruct to remain quiet and still during test; secure electrodes for simultaneous ECG tracing; explain that there will be no pain or electrical shocks

    3. No postprocedure nursing care

E. Coronary angiography/arteriography

    1. Is an invasive procedure during which cardiologist injects dye into coronary arteries and immediately records a series of x-ray films (using fluoroscopy) to assess structure of arteries

    2. Client preparation: obtain written consent; explain procedure, assess for history of allergies to contrast dye or iodine; initiate IV access; begin fluids as prescribed

    3. Postprocedure nursing care: same as for cardiac catheterization (see section below)

F. Cardiac catheterization

    1. Is insertion of a catheter into heart and surrounding blood vessels to obtain diagnostic information about structure and function of heart

    2. Can be performed on right or left side of heart

    3. Client preparation, nursing care during procedure, and postprocedure nursing care are outlined in Box 3-1

G. Radionuclide tests

    1. Are safe methods of evaluating left ventricular muscle function and coronary artery blood distribution; can provide some of the same information as radiographic angiography with less risk to client

       a. Client preparation: obtain written consent if required; explain procedure, instruct that fasting may be required for a short period before the exam; radioisotope contrast will be injected through a venipuncture; it will be necessary to alternately change position and remain still during exam; there is no associated pain or discomfort

       b. Nursing care during procedure: none; is performed in nuclear medicine department

       c. Postprocedure nursing care: drinking fluids will facilitate excretion of radioisotope; use standard precautions to handle body secretions; assess venipuncture site for bleeding or hematoma; if stress test was performed, assess BP and HR at frequent intervals; maintain continuous ECG monitoring as indicated

    2. Allows visualization of ventricles through several cardiac cycles; calculates **ejection fraction (EF)** (portion of blood ejected during systole, compared with total ventricular filling volume); normal EF is 55–65%

    3. MUGA (gated pool imaging or multigated acquisition) scan: a quick and safe way to assess heart size, ventricular wall motion and ejection fracture using red blood cells (RBCs) tagged with radioactive technetium 99; when RBCs enter atria and ventricles, scan can provide views of heart chambers; these images are then combined to make a film of heart beating

Box 3-1	**Client Preparation**

Care of Client Undergoing Cardiac Catheterization

Client Preparation
- Obtain written consent
- Assess client history of allergies to iodine or contrast dye or media.
- Ensure preprocedure labs are drawn as prescribed: serum blood urea nitrogen (BUN) and creatinine (these assess kidney function for excretion of contrast), and activated partial thromboplastin time (aPTT) and possibly prothrombin time (PT) or International Normalized Ratio (INR), since client will receive heparin during procedure.
- Explain that client will be awake and may experience various sensations during procedure, including flushing sensation as dye is injected, or fluttering feeling as catheter passes through heart.
- Explain postprocedure routine (see postprocedure nursing care).
- Prepare insertion site by shaving or clipping and cleansing with antiseptic.
- Nothing by mouth (NPO) except sips of water with cardiac medications as indicated for 6–8 hours.
- Initiate IV site with fluids as ordered.
- Administer preprocedure medications as prescribed.

Nursing Care During Procedure
- Procedure is performed in catheterization lab by cardiologist; nurse monitors ECG and vital signs continuously, administers moderate (conscious) sedation as ordered, and provides emotional support.

Postprocedure Nursing Care
- Maintain client on bedrest for 4–6 hours.
- Keep affected extremity straight; after 1–2 hours head may be elevated less than 30° for those who had femoral artery insertion site.
- Maintain pressure dressing at insertion site.
- Monitor BP, HR, distal pulses, color and temperature of extremity, and assess for signs of bleeding at site (with leg site, check under client for bleeding) according to agency schedule, (routinely q 15 min for 1 hour, q 30 min for 2 hours, q hour for 4 hours, or q 8 hours for associated procedure of percutaneous transluminal coronary angioplasty [PTCA]).
- Report signs of chest pain, dysrhythmias, bleeding, hematoma formation, or other changes; significant changes in vital signs, pulses, color, or temperature of extremity should be reported immediately to physician; bleeding may be reported by client as a feeling of warmth in insertion area.
- If bleeding occurs, restore manual pressure to site.
- Maintain IV and encourage oral fluids as ordered to eliminate dye as soon as possible; contrast medium can be nephrotoxic.
- Monitor I & O to determine whether client is becoming dehydrated from increased urine output because of dye excretion.

4. Thallium imaging: used to assess myocardial **ischemia** (decreased supply of oxygenated blood) during stress testing
5. PET (positron emission tomography) scan: evaluates cardiac metabolism and assesses tissue perfusion

H. **Hemodynamic monitoring**
   1. Is measurement of pressures in heart and calculation of hemodynamic parameters
   2. Central venous pressure (CVP) monitoring: appropriate for clients who require accurate monitoring of fluid volume status do not require more invasive PA pressure monitoring
      a. Tip of CVP catheter lies in superior vena cava at juncture with right atrium
      b. Measures right heart filling pressure and provides data about right ventricular preload; is not a satisfactory method of determining left heart pressures

    c. Normal CVP is 2–8 cm H_2O or 2–6 mmHg; decreased CVP indicates decreased circulating volume; increased CVP indicates increased blood volume or right heart failure

3. PA pressure monitoring: appropriate for critically ill clients requiring more accurate assessments of left heart pressures, including those undergoing cardiac surgery, in shock or with serious MI

    a. PA (Swan-Ganz) catheter has tip in pulmonary artery

    b. Pressure measurement is obtained after catheter tip is wedged in a pulmonary capillary, and is called pulmonary capillary wedge pressure or PCWP; indicates left ventricular end diastolic pressure (LVEDP), which is left ventricular preload

    c. Allows calculation of actual CO and other hemodynamic parameters at frequent intervals in critically ill clients

        1) Client preparation: obtain consent according to policy; insertion is under strict sterile technique, usually at bedside; explain that sterile drapes may cover face (with an internal jugular or subclavian insertion site); assist to position client flat or slight Trendelenburg as tolerated and instruct client to remain still during procedure

        2) Nursing care during insertion procedure: assist provider in maintaining a sterile field; administer medications as ordered; monitor and document HR, BP, and ECG during procedure; reassure client through procedure

        3) Postprocedure nursing care: monitor vital signs (VS), continuous ECG monitoring postinsertion; maintain client on bedrest and avoid unnecessary movements; follow policy to maintain patency and sterility of catheter

        4) Nursing responsibilities in hemodynamic monitoring: position transducer at level of right atrium (left midaxillary line, fourth intercostal space, which is called phlebostatic axis); level the CVP or PA catheter (Swan-Ganz) transducer to this point at regular intervals according to policy (usually each shift) and before each measurement; maintain patency of catheter with a constant small amount of fluid delivered under pressure; vigilantly assess wave form to ensure catheter tip is in PA and *not* wedged in capillary unless PCWP is being measured (could lead to pulmonary infarction)

III. COMMON NURSING TECHNIQUES AND PROCEDURES

A. Dysrhythmia monitoring

1. Continuous ECG monitoring with portable telemetry unit; indicated for clients requiring surgery at risk for life-threatening conditions, with cardiac and noncardiac comorbid diseases, and those undergoing procedures and pharmacological therapies affecting heart

2. Lead placements (ECG continuous monitors have 3 or 5 color-coded leads)

    a. Placement of leads with 3-lead monitor

        1) Below right clavicle (right arm; white)

        2) Below left clavicle (left arm; black)

        3) Lowest rib, left midclavicular line (left leg; red)

    b. Placement of leads with 5-lead monitor includes same as 3-lead (above) with 2 additional placements:

        1) Lowest rib, right midclavicular line (right leg; green)

        2) Fifth lead on 1 of 6 chest leads (1 of V leads on 12-lead ECG; brown)

3. Preparation of client: explain procedure and reassure that procedure is painless; identify proper placement, cleanse skin with soap and water, shave hairy areas, use alcohol or skin prep according to agency policy, dry with cloth or gauze, and apply fresh electrodes

4. Interpretations of ECG patterns originating in sinus node (see Table 3-1)

Table 3-1	ECG Characteristics of Selected Cardiac Rhythms and Dysrhythmias	
Rhythm/ECG Appearance	**ECG Characteristics**	**Management**
Sinus Rhythms		
Normal sinus rhythm (NSR)	Rate: 60–100 bpm Rhythm: Regular P:QRS: 1:1 PR interval: 0.12–0.20 sec QRS: 0.06–0.10 sec	None; normal heart rhythm.
Sinus tachycardia	Rate: 101–150 bpm Rhythm: Regular P:QRS: 1:1 (P wave may be hidden in preceding T wave with fast rate) PR interval: 0.12–0.20 sec QRS: 0.06-0.10 sec	Treat only if client is symptomatic or is at risk for myocardial damage. Treat underlying cause (e.g., hypovolemia, fever, pain). Beta blockers or verapamil may be used.
Sinus bradycardia	Rate: less than 60 bpm Rhythm: Regular P:QRS: 1:1 PR interval: 0.12–0.20 sec QRS: 0.06–0.10 sec	Treat only if client is symptomatic Intravenous atropine and/or pacemaker therapy may be used.
Sinus arrhythmia	Rate: 60–100 bpm Rhythm: Irregular, varies with respirations P:QRS: 1:1 PR interval: 0.12–0.20 sec QRS: 0.06–0.10 sec	Generally none; considered a normal rhythm in very young and very old.
Atrial Rhythms		
Premature atrial contractions (PAC)	Rate: Variable Rhythm: Irregular; underlying normal rhythm interrupted by early atrial ectopic beats P:QRS: 1:1 PR interval: 0.12–0.20 sec, but may be prolonged QRS: 0.06–0.10 sec	Usually require no treatment. Advise client to reduce alcohol and caffeine intake, to reduce stress, and to stop smoking.
Paroxysmal supraventricular tachycardia (PSVT)	Rate: 100–280 bpm (usually 150–200 bpm) Rhythm: Regular P:QRS: P waves often not identifiable PR interval: Not measured QRS: 0.06–0.10 sec	Treat if client is symptomatic; may include vagal maneuvers (Valsalva, carotid sinus massage); oxygen therapy; adenosine, verapamil, procainamide, propranolol, and esmolol; and synchronized cardioversion.
Atrial flutter	Rate: Atrial 240–360 bpm; ventricular rate depends on degree of AV block and usually is less than 150 bpm Rhythm: Atrial regular, ventricular usually regular P:QRS: 2:1, 4:1, 6:1; may vary PR interval: Not measured QRS: 0.06–0.10 sec	Synchronized cardioversion; drugs to slow ventricular response such as a beta blocker, calcium channel blocker (verapamil), or amiodarone, followed by quinidine, procainamide, flecainide.
Atrial fibrillation	Rate: Atrial 300–600 bpm (too rapid to count); ventricular 100–180 bpm in untreated clients Rhythm: Irregularly irregular P:QRS: Variable PR interval: Not measured QRS: 0.06–0.10 sec	Synchronized cardioversion; drugs to convert rhythm (amiodarone) or reduce ventricular response rate (verapamil, propranolol, digoxin); anticoagulant to reduce risk of clot formation and stroke.

Rhythm/ECG Appearance	ECG Characteristics	Management
Junctional escape rhythm	Rate: 40–60 bpm (junctional tachycardia 60–140 bpm) Rhythm: Regular P:QRS: P waves may be absent, inverted and immediately before or after QRS complex, or may be hidden in QRS complex PR interval: less than 0.10 sec if P wave is before QRS complex QRS: 0.06–0.10 sec	Treat cause if client is experiencing symptoms.
Atrioventricular Conduction Blocks		
First-degree AV block	Rate: Usually 60–100 bpm Rhythm: Regular P:QRS: 1:1 PR interval: greater than 0.20 sec QRS: 0.06–0.10 sec	None required. Continue to monitor client.
Second-degree AV block, type I (Mobitz I, Wenckebach)	Rate: 60–100 bpm Rhythm: Atrial regular, ventricular irregular P:QRS: 1:1 until P wave blocked with no QRS complex following PR interval: Progressively and regularly lengthens QRS complex: 0.06–0.10 sec; sudden absence of QRS complex when P wave blocked	Monitoring and observation; atropine or isoproterenol if client is experiencing symptoms.
Second-degree AV block, type II (Mobitz II)	Rate: Atrial 60–100 bpm; ventricular less than 60 bpm Rhythm: Atrial regular; ventricular irregular P:QRS: Typically 2:1, may vary PR interval: Constant for each conducted beat QRS: 0.06–0.10 sec	Atropine or isoproterenol; pacemaker therapy.
Third-degree AV block (Complete heart block)	Rate: Atrial 60–100 bpm; ventricular 15–60 bpm Rhythm: Atrial regular; ventricular regular P:QRS: No relationship between P waves and QRS complexes; independent rhythms PR interval: Not measured QRS complex: 0.06–0.10 sec if junctional escape rhythm; greater than 0.12 sec if ventricular escape rhythm	Immediate pacemaker therapy.
Ventricular Rhythms		
Premature ventricular contractions (PVC)	Rate: Variable Rhythm: Irregular; PVC interrupts underlying rhythm and is followed by compensatory pause P:QRS: No P wave PR interval: Absent with PVC QRS complex: Wide (greater than 0.12 sec) and bizarre appearance; differs from normal QRS complex	Treat if client is experiencing symptoms. Advise against stimulant use (caffeine, nicotine). Drug therapy includes intravenous lidocaine, procainamide, quinidine, propranolol, phenytoin, and bretylium.
Ventricular tachycardia (VT or V tach)	Rate: 100–250 bpm Rhythm: Regular P:QRS: P waves usually not identifiable PR interval: Not measured QRS complex: 0.12 sec or longer; bizarre shape	Treat if VT is sustained or if client is symptomatic. Treatment includes procainamide, amiodarone, or lidocaine and/or immediate defibrillation if client is unconscious or unstable.
Ventricular fibrillation (VF, V fib)	Rate: Too rapid to count Rhythm: Grossly irregular P:QRS: No identifiable P waves PR interval: None QRS: Bizarre, varying in shape and direction, wavelike	Immediate defibrillation.

a. Four possible rhythms include sinus rhythm, sinus tachycardia (HR greater than 100), sinus bradycardia (HR less than 60), and sinus arrhythmia (irregular)

b. Nursing and therapeutic interventions: with sinus arrest, tachycardia, or bradycardia, assess for signs of inadequate CO and tissue perfusion, including changes in BP, activity tolerance, and level of consciousness; identify and treat cause of sinus tachycardia; medical treatment is appropriate for symptomatic client or with long-term high rates (greater than 150) or extreme low rates (less than 50)

5. ECG patterns originating in atria (refer again to Table 3-1)

a. Include premature atrial contractions (PAC)—atrial ectopic beats superimposed on an underlying rhythm, atrial tachycardia, atrial flutter, and atrial fibrillation

b. Nursing and therapeutic interventions: carotid massage, synchronized cardioversion, pacing, anti-dysrhythmia medications including beta blockers and calcium channel blockers (diltiazem), and digoxin; anticoagulant therapy to reduce the risk of thrombus development

6. ECG patterns originating from AV node (refer again to Table 3-1)

a. Junctional (nodal) escape rhythm (ventricular rate less than 60 bpm) or tachycardia (60–140 bpm)

b. AV blocks including first-degree heart block, second-degree heart block (Mobitz type I or Wenckebach and Mobitz type II) and third-degree (complete) heart block

c. Nursing and therapeutic interventions

1) Monitoring and observation

2) Atropine or isoproterenol or pacemakers for symptomatic heart block

3) *Pacemakers*: permanent pacemakers are inserted in operating room or special cardiac procedures room to treat permanent conduction deficits

4) For temporary conduction deficits, provider inserts temporary pacemakers in a critical care unit through a catheter or nurses may apply an external (transthoracic) pacemaker to stimulate heart with an electrical impulse through chest wall

7. ECG patterns originating from ventricles (refer again to Table 3-1)

a. Include premature ventricular contractions (PVC)—ventricular ectopic beats superimposed on an underlying rhythm, ventricular tachycardia (VT), and ventricular fibrillation (VF)

b. Nursing and therapeutic interventions: for PVCs, monitor for symptoms of decreased CO; instruct to avoid caffeine or nicotine; with VT, assess level of consciousness (LOC) immediately and whether BP and pulse are stable; if stable, treat with lidocaine, procainamide, and finally synchronized cardioversion or defibrillation, depending on rhythm, if client becomes unconscious or unstable; pulseless VT and VF both require immediate defibrillation

8. Asystole

a. Lack of cardiac impulse resulting in absence of atrial or ventricular activity and thus no CO

b. Nursing and therapeutic interventions: initiate cardiopulmonary resuscitation (CPR) including oxygenation and circulatory support; establish or initiate IV access and intubation; drug therapy using advanced cardiac life support (ACLS) protocol; anticipate treatment with atropine sulfate, epinephrine, and vasopressors

B. **Cardiac surgery or endovascular interventions**

1. Percutaneous transluminal coronary angioplasty (PTCA): procedure to increase coronary artery blood flow by inserting a balloon-tipped catheter into narrowed segment of affected artery, inflating balloon to expand arterial lumen (may be done more than once) and removing catheter; may also include insertion of an expandable intracoronary stent (inserted over balloon; remains in place after catheter removed)

Practice to Pass

The nurse is discharging a client from the hospital with a new diagnosis of atrial fibrillation. What would the nurse include in the client and family teaching?

a. Client preparation, nursing care during procedure, and postprocedure nursing care are as outlined in Box 3-1

b. In addition, administer anticoagulants as ordered to prevent thrombus formation, and monitor coagulation studies as indicated

c. Because of anticoagulation during procedure, site may have a vice-type pressure device applied requiring a longer period of hourly site checks; monitor closely for any changes in ECG or signs of chest pain (even minor changes may be indicators of ischemia); obtain a 12-lead ECG and notify provider of any complications

2. Coronary artery bypass grafting (CABG): surgical treatment of CHD for clients with more than 50% occlusion in left main coronary artery or severe blockage in several vessels; diseased arteries are "bypassed" with saphenous veins, mammary arteries, or less frequently, artificial grafts; indicated for myocardial ischemia that cannot be managed by medical treatment; client may be maintained on cardiopulmonary bypass during surgery; newer, less invasive therapies are continuously being investigated

   a. Client preparation

   1) Ensure that all consents are signed

   2) Instruct in routine preoperative teaching, including turning and deep breathing (vigorous coughing is discouraged because it may increase intrathoracic pressure and cause instability in sternal area), incentive spirometry to prevent respiratory complications, and leg exercises to prevent emboli formation

   3) Explain client status in immediate postoperative period, including respiratory support on a ventilator with an endotracheal tube; suctioning; surgical incisions, chest tubes, multiple intravenous lines, tubes, drains, and monitors with alarms and noises; pain management, communication techniques, visiting policies, and expected length of hospitalization and recovery period

   b. Postprocedure nursing care: critical care nurses manage complex nursing care of cardiac surgical client (CABG and valvular repair/replacement) in immediate postoperative period in special cardiac surgical units; tamponade is a life-threatening postoperative complication; within 1–2 days client is transferred to a step-down/telemetry unit where care includes the following:

   1) Monitor client for signs of decreased CO, continuous ECG monitoring; I & O; full assessments with lung sounds and heart sounds at regular intervals (every 4 hours initially, then at least every 8 hours)

   2) Assess and treat postoperative pain

   3) Monitor indicators of CO with increasing activity

   4) Monitor respiratory status and encourage deep breathing and incentive spirometry

   5) Monitor surgical wounds and treating as needed

   6) Explain new medication regime, activity plan for home, cardiac rehabilitation, resumption of sexual activity (may resume sexual activity when client can walk up 2 full flights of stairs without shortness of breath or chest pain; client should be rested, not after a heavy meal or alcohol consumption)

   7) Teach symptoms to report to provider upon discharge, including chest pain, shortness of breath, decrease in activity tolerance, fever, redness, swelling, or drainage from surgical incisions

   8) Explain that clinical depression occurs in about 20% of clients up to 6 months after cardiac surgery; client should notify provider because antidepressants are very effective; include family in teaching and planning for discharge

3. Valvular surgery repair or replacement of dysfunctional valve

   a. Repair

   1) *Valvuloplasty*: reconstruction including repair or removal of calcification or vegetation

  2) *Annuloplasty*: narrowing a dilated valve with a prosthetic ring or purse-string sutures, or enlarging a stenosed valve with a balloon

  3) Repair is the preferred option, because of reduced incidence of postsurgical complications or mortality compared with valve replacement

 b. Replacement: valve is completely replaced

  1) Mechanical valves: more durable and longer lasting; subject to mechanical failure; require lifetime anticoagulation with warfarin (Coumadin) and infections are harder to treat; an example is St. Jude Medical valve

  2) Tissue valves: may deteriorate; frequent replacement is required; not associated with thrombus formation, no long-term anticoagulation; infections are easier to treat

 c. Client preparation and postprocedure nursing care

  1) May vary depending on surgical approach—laparoscopy, endoscopy, or percutaneous surgery through skin, or robot-assisted surgery

  2) Provide general perioperative cardiac surgical care as noted in preceding cardiac surgery section

  3) Provide instructions about preventing infection, which might include prophylactic antibiotics before invasive procedures including dental care; gentle oral care to prevent bacteria from entering bloodstream through gums; and management of anticoagulation therapy if appropriate

4. Permanent pacemakers: are inserted in an electrophysiology or special cardiac procedures lab or operating room to treat permanent cardiac conduction defects; pacemakers may be single chamber (atrial or ventricular, with ventricular being most common) or dual chamber (pacing both atria and ventricles)

 a. Client preparation: obtain consent; instruct that bedrest will be required for 24 hours to prevent dislodgement of leads and activity will gradually be increased

 b. Postprocedure nursing care

  1) Monitor ECG continuously to ensure that pacing beats are being captured and that intrinsic heartbeats are sensed; see Figure 3-3 for example of rhythm with a ventricular demand pacemaker, showing a combination of ventricular paced beats and absence of pacing when client's underlying rhythm is sensed

  2) Monitor for and report issues with pacemaker function, including failure to pace (doesn't fire), failure to capture (fires but doesn't cause ventricular depolarization), runaway pacemaker (continuous rapid firing), or hiccups (lead positioned near diaphragm)

  3) Monitor pacemaker site for signs of bleeding or infection; dressing should remain clean and dry with no temperature elevation, swelling, redness, or tenderness

  4) Explain that client should minimize arm and shoulder movements immediately postprocedure on affected side to ensure that pacemaker wire stays in contact with ventricular wall until fibrotic tissue develops in 2–3 days (which helps anchor lead wire in myocardial wall); maintain bedrest for 24 hours or as prescribed

Figure 3-3

Ventricular demand pacemaker rhythm showing a combination of paced and sensed beats

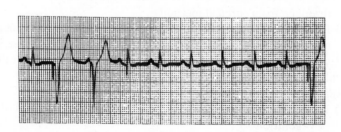

5) Home care: teach client to measure pulse daily and report if lower than pacemaker's preset rate; notify provider of dizziness, light-headedness, or weakness; avoid heavy lifting for 2 months and avoid contact sports permanently (to avoid damaging generator); avoid tight clothing over pacemaker site; avoid holding or using electrical devices over pacemaker site; alert security officials about pacemaker before walking through security scanners; carry MedicAlert identification and pacemaker identification card at all times

IV. MYOCARDIAL INFARCTION (MI)

A. **Description**: myocardial injury from sudden restriction of blood supply to a portion of heart; is a potentially life-threatening condition

B. **Etiology and pathophysiology**

1. Main cause is **coronary heart disease (CHD)**, the buildup of atherosclerotic plaque in coronary arteries that restricts blood flow to heart
   a. Nonmodifiable risk factors include age, gender, family history, and ethnic background
   b. Modifiable risk factors include smoking, obesity, stress, elevated cholesterol, diabetes, and hypertension
2. Coronary artery blood flow is blocked by atherosclerotic narrowing, thrombus formation or (less frequently) persistent vasospasm; myocardium supplied by the arteries is deprived of oxygen; persistent ischemia may rapidly lead to tissue death
3. **Angina pectoris** is chest pain resulting from this restricted blood flow; it is relieved by rest and/or nitroglycerine; it may occur in the following forms:
   a. *Stable angina*, a predictable response to increased activity
   b. *Unstable angina*, with unpredictable occurrence and increasing severity
   c. *Prinzmetal angina*, caused by arterial spasm and often awakening client from sleep; is treated with calcium channel blockers
   d. Angina pectoris may change in character and may progress to MI

C. **Assessment of MI**

1. Chest pain unrelieved by nitroglycerine or rest; may be crushing substernal pain; may radiate to jaw, neck, back, or left arm (some clients describe pain as indigestion and some report no pain—especially diabetic clients who have neuropathy)
2. Other symptoms may include diaphoresis, nausea, fear, anxiety, dyspnea, dysrhythmias
3. ECG (12-lead): ST elevation, accompanied by T-wave inversion; and later new pathologic Q wave in leads that reflect area of damage; note there may be ST elevation MI (STEMI) or non ST elevation MI (non-STEMI)
4. Lab findings: elevated CK with MB isoenzymes greater than 5% (early diagnosis); elevated troponin (early to late diagnosis); or elevated LDH with "flipped" isoenzymes (late diagnosis)

D. **Priority nursing problems**: pain, insufficient cardiac perfusion, reduced cardiac output, anxiety, fear

E. **Planning and implementation**

1. Assess pain status frequently using pain scale or other appropriate tool; pain is usually the first presenting sign of new or extended MI
2. Assess hemodynamic status including BP, HR, LOC, skin color, and temperature frequently (every 5 minutes during episodes of pain; every 15 minutes postpain) during acute phase to evaluate CO; continue to monitor frequently (every 1–2 hours) for first 24 hours post-MI
3. Monitor continuous ECG to detect dysrhythmias (PVCs and tachycardia common)
4. Perform 12-lead ECG immediately with new pain or changes in level or character of pain to identify ischemia and injury
5. Monitor respirations, breath sounds, and I & O to detect early signs of heart failure

6. Monitor O_2 saturation and administer O_2 (usually via nasal cannula at 2–4 L/min) as prescribed to increase oxygen supply to heart
7. Provide for physiological rest to decrease oxygen demands on heart
8. Keep client NPO or progress to liquid diet as ordered; maintain IV access for medications as needed
9. Provide a calm environment and reassure client and family to decrease stress, fear, and anxiety
10. Report significant changes immediately to provider to ensure rapid treatment of complications
11. Interventions in recovery phase: maintain bedrest (with commode) for 24–36 hours and gradually increase activity as prescribed while closely monitoring CO, ECG, and pain status; reinforce importance of reporting new pain immediately; progress diet from liquids to low-sodium, low-fat diet as ordered
12. Monitor and document levels of troponin and CPK-MB levels

F. **Medication therapy**
1. Tip: anticipate MONA: Morphine, Oxygen, Nitroglycerine, and Aspirin as standard treatment for MI
2. Administer morphine sulfate as ordered to relieve chest pain
3. Administer supplemental oxygen to increase to minimize hypoxic myocardial damage
4. Administer nitroglycerine as prescribed to dilate coronary vessels and increase blood flow; sublingual nitroglycerine may be given 1 tablet every 5 minutes up to 3 times to relieve chest pain; IV nitroglycerine is used to dilate coronary arteries and increase coronary blood flow; do not expose nitroglycerine to heat or light; keep sublingual nitroglycerine in a dark glass container, away from heat and discard tablets that are not used in 6 months; tablets should tingle or sting under tongue if potent
5. Administer anticoagulants (IV heparin) and aspirin (antiplatelet) as ordered to prevent additional clot formation, monitor PTT to maintain heparin at therapeutic level
6. Administer thrombolytic therapy (alteplase recombinant [Activase], tissue plasminogen activator [t-PA], or streptokinase [Streptase]) as ordered to dissolve clot, stop progress of MI, and decrease myocardial damage; monitor frequently for signs of bleeding
7. Monitor neurological status frequently for changes; alteplase recombinant and streptokinase are not clot-specific and will dissolve other clots—can cause thrombolytic (hemorrhagic) CVA, a life-threatening complication
8. Administer beta blockers post-MI as ordered to decrease cardiac work and decrease oxygen demands on the heart
9. Administer antidysrhythmic drugs as prescribed or by emergency protocol for dysrhythmias

G. **Surgical interventions**: PTCA, CABG (see previous discussion)
H. **Client education**
1. Include appropriate family members whenever possible
2. Explain cardiac rehabilitation program if prescribed
3. Explain modifiable risk factors and develop a plan with client including supportive resources to decrease lifestyle risk factors (includes low-fat, low-sodium diet, aerobic exercise, smoking cessation, glucose control in diabetes, BP control)
4. Explain medication regimen as prescribed; identify side effects to report (provide written instructions for later reference)
5. Stress importance of immediately reporting chest pain, nausea, dizziness, or shortness of breath
6. Instruct about bleeding precautions if anticoagulant therapy is prescribed: use soft toothbrush, electric razor, avoid trauma or injury; wear or carry medical alert identification

I. Expected outcomes/evaluation
1. Client reports absence of chest pain and decreased anxiety or fear
2. Client has CO within client's normal range and absence of life-threatening dysrhythmias and complications
3. Client identifies modifiable risk factors and develops a plan including family and community supports to decrease risk

V. HEART FAILURE

A. Description
1. Heart failure (HF) is inability of heart to pump adequate blood to meet metabolic needs of body
2. Formerly called congestive heart failure, or CHF

B. Etiology and pathophysiology
1. Multiple causes include myocardial damage from MI, incompetent valves, inflammatory conditions of heart, cardiomyopathy, pulmonary hypertension (causes right-sided HF, called **cor pulmonale**)
2. Compensatory phase (early): CO falls ⟹ sensed by baroreceptors ⟹ stimulate SNS ⟹ release epinephrine and norepinephrine ⟹ increase in HR and vasoconstriction ⟹ increased in filling pressures ⟹ increase in SV and CO (because CO = HR 3 SV, CO is increased); compensatory mechanisms increase cardiac metabolic demands and in time decrease cardiac function and ability to compensate
3. Depending upon cause, HF presents initially as right-sided HF or left-sided HF; as it progresses, the other side becomes affected
   a. Right HF: right ventricle has reduced capacity to pump blood into pulmonary circulation causing stasis or "backup" of blood into venous circulation
   b. Left HF: left ventricle has reduced capacity to pump blood into systemic circulation causing decreased CO and stasis or "backup" of blood into pulmonary circulation
4. Onset of heart failure
   a. Acute, with significant overload in lungs (**pulmonary edema**, characterized by acute restlessness, anxiety, increased crackles, tachypnea, tachycardia, pink frothy sputum, decreased SO_2 and PO_2)
   b. Chronic, with fatigue and activity intolerance as main features; clients with advanced chronic HF require careful management to prevent acute exacerbations

C. Assessment
1. Presenting symptoms
   a. Left HF: dyspnea on exertion (often first clinical sign), orthopnea, paroxysmal nocturnal dyspnea, new S_3 (ventricular gallop), crackles; pulmonary edema is acute life-threatening left HF, as previously described
   b. Right HF: edema of lower extremities; **jugular venous distention (JVD)** is visible more than a few centimeters above clavicle with the client lying at a 45-degree angle; abdominal discomfort and nausea occur from fluid congestion in abdominal organs
   c. Both sides: unexplained fatigue, decreased exercise tolerance, unexplained altered mental status
2. Diagnostic findings
   a. Chest x-ray may show cardiomegaly or vascular congestion
   b. Echocardiogram shows decreased ventricular function and decreased EF
   c. CVP elevated in right HF
   d. PA pressure monitoring may be used to guide treatment in serious case of pulmonary edema

Practice to Pass

A client is admitted to the emergency room with chest pain and is being evaluated for a possible MI. What assessments would the nurse make?

D. Priority nursing problems: reduced cardiac output, fluid overload, alteration in gas exchange, inability to tolerate activity or exercise, inadequate knowledge

E. Planning and implementation

  1. Acute phase

    a. Monitor and record BP, pulse, respirations, ECG, and CVP or PCWP (if appropriate) to detect changes in CO

    b. Maintain client in sitting position to decrease pulmonary congestion and facilitate improved gas exchange

    c. Auscultate heart and lung sounds frequently: increasing crackles or dyspnea, decreasing lung sounds, or new S_3 heart sound indicate worsening HF

    d. Administer O_2 as prescribed to improve gas exchange and increase oxygenation of blood; monitor SO_2 and arterial blood gases (ABG) as prescribed to assess oxygenation

    e. Administer prescribed medications on accurate schedule

    f. Monitor serum electrolytes to detect hypokalemia secondary to diuretic therapy

    g. Monitor accurate intake and output (I & O) to evaluate fluid status; may require indwelling urinary catheter to allow for accurate measurement of urine output

    h. If fluid restriction is prescribed, allocate fluid throughout day to reduce thirst

    i. Encourage physical rest and organized activities with frequent rest periods to reduce cardiac workload

    j. Provide a calm reassuring environment to decrease anxiety; this decreases oxygen consumption and decreases demands on heart

    k. Maximize client independence (note that Centers for Medicare and Medicaid in the United States has listed outcomes of HF as an indicator of competent standard care)

  2. Chronic HF

    a. Establish baseline assessment for fluid status and functional abilities: it is baseline ("normal") for some clients with HF to have bilateral crackles in bases, some level of peripheral edema, or to be unable to walk more than a specific number of feet before tiring

    b. Monitor daily weights to evaluate changes in fluid status

    c. Assess at regular intervals for changes in fluid status or functional activity level

F. Medication therapy

  1. Angiotensin-converting enzyme (ACE) inhibitors to reduce afterload and consequently increase CO (primarily used in ongoing management); monitor for hypotension, especially orthostatic

  2. Angiotensin II receptor blockers (ARBs) interrupt vasoconstrictor andaldosterone-secreting effects of angiotensin II; prescribed for similar reasons as ACE inhibitors

  3. Diuretics (often loop diuretics such as furosemide [Lasix]) to decrease preload and pulmonary congestion, which decreases cardiac work and increases CO; carefully monitor potassium levels with diuretic therapy except for potassium-sparing diuretics (important in acute and chronic treatment of HF)

  4. Vasodilators including nitroglycerine to reduce preload; monitor for hypotension

  5. Morphine to sedate and vasodilate, decreasing cardiac workload; monitor for hypotension or respiratory depression (acute pulmonary edema)

  6. Digoxin (Lanoxin) to improve contractility and correspondingly increase stroke volume and CO; take apical pulse for 1 full minute and withhold dose if HR is below 60 or above 120

  7. Other inotropic agents, dopamine (Intropin) and dobutamine (Dobutrex), are used in critical care when decompensation of CO leads to hypotension; monitor BP and IV site frequently

G. Client education

1. Include family members or others in teaching as appropriate

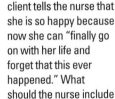

2. Weight monitoring: explain importance of measuring and recording daily weights (in same amount of clothing at same time of day, often early morning after voiding) and report unexplained increase of 3–5 pounds—most sensitive indicator of increased fluid overload

3. Diet: sodium restriction to decrease fluid overload and increased potassium-rich foods to replenish loss from potassium-wasting diuretics; do not restrict water intake unless directed (this will not decrease fluid retention)

4. Medication regime: explain importance of following all medication instructions; remind client that although frequent urination is bothersome, regular diuretic therapy prevents fluid overload and acute exacerbation; instruct to count radial pulse for 1 full minute before taking digoxin and to withhold dose and call prescriber if <60 or >120

5. Activity: help client plan paced activity to maximize available CO

6. Symptoms: report chest pain, new onset of dyspnea on exertion, or paroxysmal nocturnal dyspnea to provider

7. Other: report even minor changes to provider or home care nurse, as they may be an early sign of decompensation

H. Expected outcomes/evaluation

1. CO, BP within client's normal limits; client maintains optimal level of function

2. Minimal edema with weight at optimal level

3. Client maintains medication schedule and prescribed diet, and monitors daily weight

VI. ENDOCARDITIS (INFECTIVE, SUBACUTE BACTERIAL)

A. Description: inflammation of inner layer of heart; usually involves cardiac valves

B. Etiology and pathophysiology

1. Caused by microorganisms in blood; risk factors include IV drug use, structural defects in heart or valves (which increase platelets and fibrin strands in endothelium)

   a. Acute endocarditis: sudden onset with *Staphylococcus aureus* as most common organism

   b. Subacute endocarditis: gradual onset with *Streptococcus viridans* or other less virulent bacteria

2. Microorganisms in bloodstream colonize on fibrin and platelet strands in endothelium, multiply, and develop new strands; seen as "vegetation" attached to endothelium, particularly valves, causing valve damage; segments of vegetation may break off and travel to extremities, manifested as petechiae

C. Assessment

1. Acute: high fever with chills, signs of heart failure, and WBC elevation

2. Subacute: fever of unknown origin, cough, dyspnea, anorexia, malaise, normal WBC, anemia, and elevated erythrocyte sedimentation rate (ESR)

3. Both: positive blood cultures; new cardiac murmur or change in existing murmur; embolic complications from segments of vegetation circulating to organs and extremities including petechiae, splinter hemorrhages in nail beds, Roth spots (retinal hemorrhages with white or pale-colored centers from coagulated fibrin)

D. Priority nursing problems: potential for injury related to thrombus formation, inadequate knowledge related to prevention of repeated infection

E. Planning and implementation

1. Manage IV therapy; assess for any signs of infection

2. Assess appropriateness of home infusion therapy; client may require in-patient treatment in a subacute care facility if home infusion therapy is contraindicated (such as with IV drug abuse)

Practice to Pass

The home care nurse is caring for a client with heart failure who reports that she skips her diuretics several times a week because she can't go out of the house after she has taken them. What should the nurse explain to this client?

Practice to Pass

A client is completing her antibiotic treatment for subacute bacterial endocarditis (SBE). The client tells the nurse that she is so happy because now she can "finally go on with her life and forget that this ever happened." What should the nurse include in a response?

3. Provide for periods of rest and moderate periods of exercise to prevent venous stasis
4. Use anti-embolism stockings to prevent thrombus formation
5. Provide for diversional activity; client should not resume normal activity for 4–6 weeks
F. **Medication therapy**: consists of antibiotics given by the IV route for 6 weeks
G. **Client education**
   1. Client and family role in home infusion therapy; care of IV access site
   2. After an episode of endocarditis, client is susceptible to repeated infections because of lesions on endocardium
   3. Symptoms to report to provider, such as fever, anorexia, malaise
   4. Need for gentle, thorough oral care because infectious organisms can easily enter bloodstream through gums with vigorous brushing or oral treatments
   5. Use of prophylactic antibiotics, as prescribed, before invasive procedures and routine dental care
H. **Expected outcomes/evaluation**: client is free from signs of infection, maintains IV therapy at home (if appropriate), describes signs and symptoms to report, and obtains prophylactic antibiotic therapy before invasive procedures as indicated

VII. VALVULAR DISORDERS

A. **Description**
   1. Defects in cardiac valve structure or function that interfere with proper cardiac circulation
   2. Two major categories
      a. **Stenosis**: heart valve leaflets are fused together, opening is narrow, stiff, and unable to open or close properly
      b. **Regurgitation**: there is improper or incomplete closure of heart valves, resulting in backflow of blood
B. **Etiology and pathophysiology**
   1. Multiple causes including rheumatic heart disease (most common), congenital, MI, and endocarditis
   2. Calcium deposits or scar tissue from endocarditis or MI may cause stiffening of valves in stenosis
   3. Congenital malformations, scar tissue from MI, or fibrin strands from endocarditis may cause regurgitation
   4. Right heart valve dysfunction usually develops in relation to other cardiac structural problems and pulmonic defects are primarily congenital
C. **Assessment**
   1. Heart sounds: each valve dysfunction produces characteristic changes in heart sounds (see Table 3-2)
   2. Symptoms and severity depends on extent of valve dysfunction (from asymptomatic to signs of severe HF)
   3. Symptoms vary depending on the type of valve dysfunction (see Table 3-2)
D. **Priority nursing problems**: reduced cardiac output, potential for thrombus formation or infection, inadequate knowledge, inability to endure exercise or activity (with late-stage dysfunction)
E. **Planning and implementation**
   1. Interventions depend upon the severity of the symptoms and type of dysfunction (refer again to Table 3-2)
   2. Monitor heart sounds to assess for changes
   3. With signs of decreased CO, manage or restrict activity to decrease demands on the heart
   4. Monitor for signs of endocarditis
   5. Report changes to health care provider

Table 3-2	Valvular Disorders

Valve Disorder	Specific Assessment	Planning and Implementation
Mitral stenosis	Murmur: low pitched rumbling diastolic Common in young women Atrial dysrhythmias, especially atrial fibrillation (A-fib)	Monitor closely during pregnancy. Administer diuretics and digoxin as prescribed. Maintain sodium-restricted diet. Anticoagulant therapy if A-fib present. Prepare for surgery.
Mitral regurgitation (insufficiency)	Murmur: high-pitched blowing systolic Usually asymptomatic A-fib common with low incidence of embolization	Administer diuretics, nitrates, and ACE inhibitors as prescribed. Maintain sodium-restricted diet.
Mitral prolapse	Murmur: systolic click Most clients asymptomatic May have PVCs and palpitations, syncope, weakness, and anxiety	Administer beta blockers as prescribed for syncopy and palpitations. Monitor for signs of infective endocarditis. Administer prophylactic antibiotics, if prescribed, with invasive procedures.
Aortic stenosis	Murmur: harsh systolic Late course symptoms: angina; S_3 and S_4; syncope	In symptomatic client, restrict activity to decrease myocardial oxygen consumption. Monitor for signs of infective endocarditis. Administer prophylactic antibiotics, if prescribed, with invasive procedures. Prepare for surgery: symptomatic aortic stenosis has poor prognosis without surgical intervention.
Aortic regurgitation (insufficiency)	Murmur: blowing diastolic Widened pulse pressure Palpitations; tachycardia and PVCs	Medical management same as aortic stenosis. Prepare for surgery, which is the only effective long-term therapy for aortic regurgitation. Note all clients with irregular HR or rhythm should have IV access.

Practice to Pass

A client has had a valve repair surgery and has a new prescription for warfarin (Coumadin). What would the nurse include in the client teaching?

F. **Medication therapy**
   1. Is determined by symptoms
   2. Antidysrhythmic and anticoagulant therapy if atrial fibrillation present
   3. Antibiotic therapy if appropriate for endocarditis
   4. Medication regime to treat heart failure if appropriate
G. **Surgical interventions**: valve replacement
H. **Client education**
   1. Management of anticoagulation therapy to prevent thrombus formation with warfarin (Coumadin) if appropriate
      a. Monitor PT/INR values regularly because the effects of warfarin are influenced by physiological changes in the body, diet changes, or changes in medication
      b. Maintain consistent amount of food containing vitamin K in the diet including green leafy vegetables; variations may alter the effects of warfarin (Coumadin)
   2. Relationships between valve disorders or surgical valves and increased risk for bacterial endocarditis
   3. Methods to prevent endocarditis
I. **Expected outcomes/evaluation**: client reports no signs of endocarditis, describes signs and symptoms to report to MD, obtains prophylactic antibiotic therapy before invasive procedures, and (in a client with a more advanced valve disorder) maintains optimal level of function

VIII. CARDIOMYOPATHY

A. Description: an abnormality of the heart muscle that leads to functional changes in heart

B. Etiology and pathophysiology

1. Cause is unknown; however, in some cases is associated with viral infections, chronic alcohol abuse, or pregnancy

2. Three types: dilated, hypertrophic, and restrictive

    a. Dilated cardiomyopathy (most common): enlargement of all 4 chambers, starting with enlarged ventricles, followed by decreased contractility; CO progressively decreases

    b. Hypertrophic cardiomyopathy: unexplained progressive thickening of ventricular muscle mass causing increased pulmonary and venous pressures; CO progressively decreases

    c. Restrictive cardiomyopathy (least common): excessively rigid ventricular walls do not stretch during diastolic filling, creating back pressure and right HF, as well as reduced stroke volume and, consequently, lowered CO

C. Assessment

1. Fatigue with all types

2. Dilated: weakness, signs of left HF, and S_3 and S_4 heart sounds

3. Hypertrophic: exertional dyspnea, syncope, angina, signs of HF, S_4 heart sound, sudden death is often first sign in asymptomatic clients

4. Restrictive: dyspnea, right-sided HF, S_3 and S_4 heart sounds, and emboli formation

D. Priority nursing problems: reduced cardiac output, inability to endure exercise or activity

E. Planning and implementation

1. Monitor indicators of level of heart failure (vital signs, lung sounds, edema, dyspnea, activity tolerance, and BNP level)

2. Encourage rest and minimize stressful situations to reduce workload on heart

3. Provide counseling and psychological support because of poor prognosis

F. Medication therapy

1. There is no medical therapy to cure or prevent cardiomyopathy except for heart transplant; medical regime is intended to treat symptoms

2. Medications are used to treat signs of HF (see section on medications for heart failure earlier in chapter)

3. Anticoagulation therapy is used with restrictive cardiomyopathy to prevent emboli

G. Client education

1. Avoid alcohol consumption because of its cardiac depressant effects

2. Pace activities to reduce cardiac workload

3. Medication and diet therapy for management of HF

4. Anticoagulation therapy and monitoring if appropriate to prevent emboli formation

H. Expected outcomes/evaluation: client maintains optimal level of activity, has clear lung sounds, has vital signs within normal limits (WNL), shows decreased peripheral edema, follows medication regime, and follows a low-sodium, potassium-rich diet

Practice to Pass

The nurse has a new admission with a diagnosis of restrictive cardiomyopathy. What signs of heart failure would the nurse expect to observe in this client?

X. PERICARDITIS

A. Description: inflammation of pericardium

B. Etiology and pathophysiology

1. Acute pericarditis: may have multiple causes including infectious processes (viral is most common), post-MI (*Dressler's syndrome*) status, neoplasms, trauma, uremia, connective tissue diseases, or endocrine diseases

2. Chronic pericarditis: chronic pericardial inflammation causes fibrous thickening of pericardium, constricting cardiac wall movement and restricting diastolic filling

C. Assessment
   1. Acute: substernal pain, radiating to neck, aggravated by breathing (particularly during inspiration) or coughing; friction rub (scratchy high-pitched sound on auscultation); elevated WBC; fever; malaise; ECG changes including ST and T wave elevations, followed by inverted T waves when ST returns to baseline
   2. Chronic restrictive pericarditis: increasing dyspnea, fatigue leading to progressive signs of HF

D. Priority nursing patterns: pain, risk for reduced cardiac output, risk for alteration in respiratory pattern because of pain

E. Planning and implementation
   1. Assess and manage pain
   2. Administer oxygen as ordered and monitor SO_2
   3. Monitor for complications, especially cardiac **tamponade** (medical emergency resulting from excess fluid collection in pericardial sac that interferes with heart filling and function); signs include:
      a. Jugular venous distention (JVD) with clear lungs
      b. Elevated CVP
      c. Narrowing pulse pressure
      d. Decreased CO
      e. Muffled heart sounds
   4. Report significant changes to provider immediately
   5. Position for comfort: high Fowler's, sitting, or side lying
   6. Provide for periods of rest and limit activity to decrease cardiac workload

F. Medication therapy
   1. Analgesics for pain
   2. Nonsteroidal anti-inflammatory medications (NSAIDs) initially, followed by steroids if inflammation does not respond to NSAIDs
   3. Avoid anticoagulants because of risk of tamponade
   4. Antibiotic therapy if inflammation is caused by bacterial microbes

G. Other medical interventions
   1. Pericardiocentesis: procedure to remove fluid from pericardial sac, performed for diagnostic analysis of fluid to determine cause or as emergency treatment for tamponade
   2. Dialysis for inflammation caused by uremia
   3. Radiation to treat neoplasms

H. Client education
   1. Explanation of inflammatory process to reduce anxiety
   2. Medication management, especially course of anti-inflammatory drugs, dosages, and side effects
   3. Take anti-inflammatory drugs with food, milk, or antacids to reduce gastric distress
   4. Risk for repeated episodes of pericarditis; report symptoms (similar pain or dyspnea) promptly to health care provider

I. Expected outcomes/evaluation: client reports no pain, describes signs and symptoms to report to health care provider, follows medication regime, and has an EF that remains within normal range

---

Practice to Pass

The nurse is caring for a client with pericarditis. What is a life-threatening complication of this diagnosis, and what would the nurse recognize as signs of this complication?

Case Study

J. L. is a 62-year-old male who is scheduled to have coronary artery bypass surgery. His father died of a myocardial infarction (MI) at 65 years of age. J. L. has recently quit smoking. His cholesterol is 220 mg/dL with an HDL of 40 mg/dL. You are the nurse caring for J. L.

1. What will you do to prepare J. L. for surgery?

2. What assessments will you perform for J. L. when he is awaiting surgery?

3. What nursing diagnoses are appropriate in the postoperative period?

4. Following transfer out of critical care, for what complications will you monitor J. L.?

5. What discharge teaching is appropriate when J. L. is ready to go home after surgery?

For suggested responses, see page 621.

POSTTEST

1 A client is prescribed sublingual nitroglycerine for the treatment of angina pectoris. The nurse concludes that what response from the client indicates understanding of this medication?

1. "My health care provider gave me a year's supply of nitroglycerine tablets."
2. "I will carry my nitroglycerine tablets in the inside pocket of my jacket, so they are always close."
3. "I usually take 3 of my nitroglycerine tablets at the same time. I find that they work better that way."
4. "I have a small metal labeled case for a few nitroglycerine tablets that I carry with me when I go out."

2 The nurse is caring for a client with a diagnosis of first-degree heart block. The nurse anticipates that the client's cardiac rhythm strip will reveal which of the following? Select all that apply.

1. Number of QRS complexes are half the number of P waves.
2. PR interval is consistent.
3. QT interval is prolonged.
4. P wave rate is usually slower than the QRS rate.
5. PR interval is prolonged.

3 The nurse is caring for a client who has just returned from the cardiac catheterization lab following a percutaneous transluminal coronary angioplasty (PTCA). The client is receiving a continuous infusion of heparin. The urine is now tea colored. What action should the nurse take next?

1. Notify the health care provider and ask for an order for an aPTT.
2. Monitor the urine for any additional change in color.
3. Assess the insertion site for bleeding and measure pulse and blood pressure.
4. Ask the client if there is any chest pain.

4 The nurse is caring for a client being discharged after valve replacement surgery using a St. Jude mechanical valve. The nurse is reviewing the instructions for the client's follow-up care and determines that the client understands the instructions when the client makes which statement?

1. "I will take warfarin (Coumadin) for 2 months and get my blood drawn every week until I stop taking the drug."
2. "I will remind the doctor to give me a prescription for anticoagulant medication every time I go to the dentist."
3. "I will need to take anticoagulant medication for the rest of my life."
4. "I won't take any anticoagulant medication or blood thinners because they may cause a problem with my new valve."

5 The nurse is caring for a client on the second postoperative day after coronary artery bypass (CABG) surgery. The client has a nursing diagnosis of Impaired Gas Exchange. Which action would the nurse take to best assist the client with this diagnosis?

1. Assist client with deep breathing and vigorous coughing every hour.
2. Ensure that client uses the incentive spirometer every hour.
3. Premedicate client before ambulation.
4. Auscultate lungs once a shift.

6 A client who just underwent cardiac catheterization insists on getting up to go to the bathroom to urinate immediately after returning to his room. What would be the nurse's best response?

1. "You can't walk yet. You may be too weak after the procedure and may fall."
2. "If you bend your leg, you will risk bleeding from the insertion site. It is an artery, and it could lead to complications."
3. "If you get out of bed, you may have an arrhythmia from the catheterization. Your heart has to rest after this procedure."
4. "The doctor has ordered that you stay on bed rest for the next 6 hours. It is important that you follow these orders."

7 The nurse is caring for a client admitted to the emergency department (ED) with chest pain. He reports that chest pain developed while mowing the lawn and he stopped and rested on the sofa, as is typical for him. This time the pain was not relieved by rest so he came to the ED. The chest pain is relieved following administration of 2 sublingual nitroglycerine tablets. The nurse draws which conclusion about this client's status?

1. Client most likely has stable angina.
2. Client has a knowledge deficit because he did not take his sublingual nitroglycerine.
3. Client most likely has unstable angina.
4. Client most likely has acute myocardial infarction.

8 The nurse is assessing a client at 7:30 in the morning on a day when the client has a cardiac stress test scheduled for 11:30. The client reports that no breakfast was delivered this morning and the client is hungry. What is the nurse's best action?

1. Bring client coffee and toast.
2. Explain that client should have no food the morning of a cardiac stress test.
3. Call nutrition department and get the client's regular full breakfast.
4. Have nursing assistant get the client cereal with milk and orange juice.

9 A hospitalized client has continuous electrocardiographic (ECG) monitoring, and the monitor shows that the rhythm has suddenly changed to ventricular tachycardia (VT). Upon entering the room, the nurse notes the client is awake and alert and speaks to the nurse. What are priority actions that the nurse should take? Select all that apply.

1. Administer intravenous lidocaine according to emergency protocol.
2. Obtain the defibrillator and defibrillate the client.
3. Quickly assess the client's blood pressure and pulse.
4. Administer a precordial thump.
5. Ask the unit secretary to telephone the client's family.

10 The physician has diagnosed acute myocardial infarction (AMI) on the basis of electrocardiogram (ECG) changes for a client in the emergency department (ED). The nurse assesses the client frequently, and notes that the client seems forgetful, and periodically asks the nurse to explain the ECG and noninvasive blood pressure monitors. The nurse concludes that the client's response is most likely due to which of the following reasons?

1. Client is showing signs of very early Alzheimer's disease.
2. Client is showing signs of fear and anxiety.
3. Nurses in the emergency room are busy and provide explanations that are too short.
4. Memory lapses are common with clients experiencing myocardial infarction.

➤ *See pages 112–113 for Answers and Rationales.*

ANSWERS & RATIONALES

Pretest

1 **Answer: 2** **Rationale:** Cardiac tamponade results from accumulation of fluid in the pericardial sac. This restricts filling of the cardiac chambers and thus reduces stroke volume, cardiac output, and blood pressure. Because the right atrium is also affected, jugular venous distention (JVD) occurs and the lungs are clear. In heart failure, the cardiac chambers are dilated, and the increase in volume and pressure is reflected back to the lungs causing crackles to develop as an early sign. Although pericarditis is one cause of cardiac tamponade, signs of pericarditis include a temperature elevation, chest pain and a pericardial friction rub. Cardiomyopathy may cause heart failure with the development of crackles. **Cognitive Level:** Analyzing **Client Need:** Physiological Adaptation **Integrated Process:** Nursing Process: Assessment **Content Area:** Adult Health **Strategy:** Review the indications for a pericardiocentesis. Compare the indications to the constellation of symptoms presented in the stem. Alternatively, list the major symptoms for each distracter and compare them to those in the stem. **Reference:** LeMone, P., Burke, K., & Bauldoff, G. (2011). *Medical-surgical nursing: Critical thinking in patient care* (5th ed.). Upper Saddle River, NJ: Pearson Education, p. 998.

2 **Answer: 2** **Rationale:** Once a client is diagnosed with subacute bacterial endocarditis (SBE), he or she is at risk for repeated episodes. Taking prophylactic antibiotics prior to dental care is an important activity to prevent further infections. There is no routine sodium restriction with SBE unless heart failure develops. Antibiotic treatment for SBE is given by the IV route for the entire course. Although stopping smoking will decrease his risk factor for coronary heart disease, it does not affect the SBE. **Cognitive Level:** Applying **Client Need:** Health Promotion and Maintenance **Integrated Process:** Teaching and Learning **Content Area:** Adult Health **Strategy:** Differentiate the immediate damage to the valve that occurs as a result of subacute bacterial endocarditis (SBE) from heart failure and CAD. The appropriate route for the administration is determined by the timing in the course of the disease. **Reference:** LeMone, P., Burke, K., & Bauldoff, G. (2011). *Medical-surgical nursing: Critical thinking in patient care* (5th ed.). Upper Saddle River, NJ: Pearson Education, p. 994.

3 **Answer: 1, 3, 4** **Rationale:** In heart failure, the heart is unable to pump blood effectively, resulting in an increase in the volume and pressure of blood in the heart, which is reflected back to the pulmonary vasculature. As the pressure increases fluid moves from the pulmonary capillaries into the alveoli causing increased crackles, tachypnea, tachycardia, pink frothy sputum, and decreased SpO_2 and paO_2. As the cardiac output falls, the glomerular filtration rate drops and causes a decrease in urine output. The amount and severity of symptoms indicates the severity of the disease. The client in heart failure presents with

acute restlessness and anxiety, and is unable to fall asleep when acutely short of breath with dyspnea. As the cardiac output falls from heart failure, the sympathetic nervous system becomes activated, which causes anxiety and tachycardia. **Cognitive Level:** Analyzing **Client Need:** Physiological Adaptation **Integrated Process:** Nursing Process: Assessment **Content Area:** Adult Health **Strategy:** The critical word in the question is *worsening*. Compare the expected findings seen with heart failure with the findings indicated in the answer choices. Then note the choices that illustrate a worsening state. **Reference:** LeMone, P., Burke, K., & Bauldoff, G. (2011). *Medical-surgical nursing: Critical thinking in patient care* (5th ed.) Upper Saddle River, NJ: Pearson Education Inc., pp. 975–977.

4 **Answer: 1** **Rationale:** The contrast medium or dye typically used for cardiac angiography is iodine based. The client with a known allergy to iodine is at risk for anaphylaxis and requires the use of an alternate (hypoallergenic) contrast medium. Atrial fibrillation and chronic renal failure are not contraindications to cardiac angiography. A value of 4.0 mEq/L is normal value for potassium. **Cognitive Level:** Applying **Client Need:** Reduction of Risk Potential **Integrated Process:** Nursing Process: Planning **Content Area:** Adult Health **Strategy:** The core issue of the question is knowledge of possible risks to a client undergoing angiography. Evaluate each answer choice and determine which one might put the client at risk for an adverse event during coronary angiography. **Reference:** LeMone, P., Burke, K., & Bauldoff, G. (2011). *Medical-surgical nursing: Critical thinking in patient care* (5th ed.). Upper Saddle River, NJ: Pearson Education, p. 886.

5 **Answer: 3** **Rationale:** Daily weight is the most sensitive indicator of changes in fluid status. A daily weight recorded at the same time of day before eating and after voiding enables comparisons from day to day. A weight gain of 3 pounds or more per week should be reported as it likely indicates fluid retention. Recording a daily weight is more accurate for a client at home than recording urine output. A fluid restriction may be recommended for a client with advanced heart failure, but it is not a method of monitoring fluid status. The client should never adjust the dose of his or her medications independently. **Cognitive Level:** Analyzing **Client Need:** Health Promotion and Maintenance **Integrated Process:** Nursing Process: Planning **Content Area:** Adult Health **Strategy:** To answer this question, imagine yourself as the client. Compare the answer choices to what a reasonable person would be able to do at home on a routine basis. Think of what is safe for a client to do. Adjusting medications is never recommended because something else may be occurring that needs investigation by the physician. The critical issue is knowledge of weight as an accurate and reliable gauge to fluid status. **Reference:** LeMone, P., Burke, K., & Bauldoff, G. (2011). *Medical-surgical* *nursing: Critical thinking in patient care* (5th ed.). Upper Saddle River, NJ: Pearson Education, p. 985.

6 Answer:

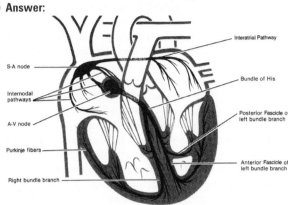

S-A node

Internodal pathways

A-V node

Purkinje fibers

Right bundle branch

Interatrial Pathway

Bundle of His

Posterior Fascicle of left bundle branch

Anterior Fascicle of left bundle branch

Rationale: Atrioventricular (AV) node heart block occurs because of conduction abnormalities at AV node. First-degree block indicates a slowed AV nodal conduction (PR interval greater than 0.2 second duration). Second-degree indicates intermittent AV nodal block that can be either Mobitz Type 1 or Type 2. Third-degree block (complete heart block) indicates a complete dissociation between atrial and ventricular conduction fibers because of a loss of impulse transmission through the AV node. The other areas are unaffected. **Cognitive Level**: Applying **Client Need**: Physiological Adaptation **Integrated Process**: Teaching and Learning **Content Area**: Adult Health **Strategy**: Recall the components of the conduction system and the rhythms that originate within each segment. Use baseline nursing knowledge and the process of elimination to determine the area for selection. **Reference**: LeMone, P., Burke, K. & Bauldoff, G. (2011). *Medical-surgical nursing: Critical thinking in patient care* (5th ed.) Upper Saddle River, NJ: Pearson Education Inc., p. 953.

7 Answer: 4 **Rationale**: Metoprolol (Lopressor) is a beta-adrenergic blocker that slows the heart rate and decreases myocardial contractility. These actions reduce cardiac workload and allow the heart to heal after an AMI. Metoprolol (Lopressor) will not speed up the heart, make the heart beat stronger, or dilate coronary arteries. Nitroglycerine is a drug that dilates the coronary arteries. **Cognitive Level**: Applying **Client Need**: Pharmacological and Parenteral Therapies **Integrated Process**: Teaching and Learning **Content Area**: Adult Health **Strategy**: To answer this question, integrate the normal cardiac physiology, changes that occur with an acute myocardial infarction, and the mechanism of action and side effects of beta blockers. **Reference**: LeMone, P., Burke, K. & Bauldoff, G. (2011). *Medical-surgical nursing: Critical thinking in patient care* (5th ed.) Upper Saddle River, NJ: Pearson Education Inc., p. 938.

8 Answer: 1 **Rationale**: Furosemide (Lasix) is a loop diuretic that causes a loss of serum potassium. When taken concurrently with digoxin (Lanoxin), it can potentiate digoxin toxicity. For clients who are taking a diuretic regularly, especially with concurrent digoxin,

they should be instructed to eat foods high in potassium and low in sodium to prevent additional fluid overload with heart failure and prevent excess potassium loss. Chicken, potato, and cantaloupe are all potassium-rich foods. A ham and cheese omelet, grilled cheese sandwich, and pepperoni pizza are higher in sodium, which may worsen fluid retention. In addition, a grilled cheese sandwich and pepperoni pizza are higher in fat. **Cognitive Level**: Analyzing **Client Need**: Health Promotion and Maintenance **Integrated Process**: Nursing Process: Evaluation **Content Area**: Foundational Sciences **Strategy**: Knowledge of heart failure, digoxin (Lanoxin), furosemide (Lasix), and their connection to the electrolyte content of foods is needed to answer this question. Review each diet selection with these content areas in mind to determine the best choice. **Reference**: LeMone, P., Burke, K. & Bauldoff, G. (2011). *Medical-surgical nursing: Critical thinking in patient care* (5th ed.) Upper Saddle River, NJ: Pearson Education Inc., pp. 981–982.

9 Answer: 4 **Rationale**: All clients with cardiomyopathy have some decrease in their cardiac output and corresponding activity intolerance. The experiences of fear, hopelessness, or deficient knowledge are client specific and must be evaluated on an individual basis. Any or all of these may be present, but more data would be needed to determine whether the other nursing diagnoses apply. **Cognitive Level**: Analyzing **Client Need**: Physiological Adaptation **Integrated Process**: Nursing Process: Diagnosis **Content Area**: Adult Health **Strategy**: Understanding what is happening physiologically helps in selecting the correct option. Note that the focus of the question is a new onset diagnosis. Use Maslow's hierarchy of needs theory to determine that physiological needs must be addressed first. As the disease progresses or more information is learned by the client, the other distracters may become relevant. **Reference**: LeMone, P., Burke, K., & Bauldoff, G. (2011). *Medical-surgical nursing: Critical thinking in patient care* (5th ed.) Upper Saddle River, NJ: Pearson Education Inc., pp. 985–986.

10 Answer: 4, 5 **Rationale**: The client with severe bradycardia, third-degree or complete heart block, or second-degree heart block (which has a high potential to progress to complete AV block) are those who are most likely to need an external pacemaker as a temporary therapy until definitive treatment can be given. Defibrillation is the only effective and definitive treatment for a client who is in ventricular fibrillation. A client in rapid atrial fibrillation and unstable ventricular tachycardia may require synchronized cardioversion to terminate the abnormal rhythm. **Cognitive Level**: Applying **Client Need**: Physiological Adaptation **Integrated Process**: Nursing Process: Planning **Content Area**: Adult Health **Strategy**: Think about the indications for an external pacemaker. Compare the indication to each of the distracters, noting that the term pacemaker implies trying to stimulate cardiac conduction. **Reference**: LeMone, P., Burke, K., & Bauldoff, G. (2011). *Medical-surgical nursing: Critical thinking in patient care* (5th ed.) Upper Saddle River, NJ: Pearson Education Inc., pp. 946–953.

ANSWERS & RATIONALES

Posttest

1 **Answer: 4** **Rationale:** Nitroglycerine tablets are light sensitive and should be stored in a dry, dark container. Nitroglycerine loses potency over time and should be replaced every 6 months or sooner as needed. Exposure to moisture, light, or to heat, as in the pocket of a jacket, may decrease the effectiveness of the tablet. One nitroglycerine tablet should be taken at a time 5 minutes apart; taking more than 1 tablet at a time can actually cause severe hypotension. **Cognitive Level:** Applying **Client Need:** Pharmacological and Parenteral Therapies **Integrated Process:** Nursing Process: Evaluation **Content Area:** Pharmacology **Strategy:** The core issue of the question is knowledge of the proper use and storage of nitroglycerin tablets. Recall the proper dosage sequence and drug storage requirements. **Reference:** LeMone, P., Burke, K., & Bauldoff, G. (2011). *Medical-surgical nursing: Critical thinking in patient care* (5th ed.). Upper Saddle River, NJ: Pearson Education, p. 923.

2 **Answer: 2, 5** **Rationale:** In first-degree heart block, the PR interval is prolonged (greater than 0.20 second) but consistent in length from complex to complex. The number of P waves and QRS complexes are equal in number. The QT segment could become prolonged because of the effects of some antidysrhythmic drugs. **Cognitive Level:** Analyzing **Client Need:** Reduction of Risk Potential **Integrated Process:** Nursing Process: Assessment **Content Area:** Adult Health **Strategy:** Review the characteristics of the various forms of heart block. The critical words *first-degree* are essential to answering the question. Keep in mind that this form of heart block is mildest to help make the correct selections. **Reference:** Lemone, P., Burke, K., & Bauldoff, G. (2011). *Medical-surgical nursing: Critical thinking in patient care* (5th ed.). Upper Saddle River, NJ: Pearson Education, p. 949.

3 **Answer: 3** **Rationale:** Heparin is an anticoagulant that is given following a PTCA to prevent clot formation at the site of the PTCA. If the therapeutic level of heparin is exceeded, the client may bleed. Tea-colored urine is a sign of blood in the urine and additional assessment data is needed regarding other possible sources of bleeding or hypovolemia due to hemorrhage. Once this additional important data is gathered quickly, the health care provider would be notified. Further observation of the color of the urine could potentially worsen the bleeding as the coagulation profile would be further prolonged. While the nurse will ask the client if chest pain is present after an angioplasty because of the risk of coronary spasm, there is no relationship between tea-colored urine and chest pain. **Cognitive Level:** Analyzing **Client Need:** Reduction of Risk Potential **Integrated Process:** Nursing Process: Implementation **Content Area:** Adult Health **Strategy:** The core issue of this question is knowledge of the side effects of heparin therapy and appropriate additional assessments that are needed. The critical word in the question is *next.* Consider that the nurse does not report a single data point to the health care provider without gathering additional data to

enable you to choose correctly. **Reference:** LeMone, P., Burke, K., & Bauldoff, G. (2011). *Medical-surgical nursing: Critical thinking in patient care* (5th ed.). Upper Saddle River, NJ: Pearson Education, p. 1053.

4 **Answer: 3** **Rationale:** A mechanical valve requires life-long anticoagulation therapy to decrease the risk of thrombus formation. If a valve is replaced with a tissue valve, anticoagulation may be required during the immediate postoperative period but is not necessarily life-long. Anticoagulants will not contraindicate for prosthetic valves. It is recommended to take antibiotics prior to dental care. **Cognitive Level:** Analyzing **Client Need:** Reduction of Risk Potential **Integrated Process:** Nursing Process: Evaluation **Content Area:** Adult Health **Strategy:** Remember that foreign bodies in the vascular system increase the risk of thrombus formation. **Reference:** LeMone, P., Burke, K., & Bauldoff, G. (2011). *Medical-surgical nursing: Critical thinking in patient care* (5th ed.). Upper Saddle River, NJ: Pearson Education, pp. 1007–1011.

5 **Answer: 2** **Rationale:** Atelectasis is the number one complication in the postop CABG client. Incentive spirometry and deep breathing are the preferred techniques for lung expansion. Vigorous coughing is discouraged for post-CABG clients because it may increase intrathoracic pressure and cause instability in the sternal area. Premedication before ambulation will facilitate activity tolerance by reducing pain but will not directly affect gas exchange. Auscultating lungs will detect adventitious lung sounds resulting from the ineffective breathing pattern, but it is an assessment, not an action to encourage effective breathing. In addition, performing lung assessment only once per shift is insufficient in the early postoperative period. **Cognitive Level:** Analyzing **Client Need:** Reduction of Risk Potential **Integrated Process:** Nursing Process: Planning **Content Area:** Adult Health **Strategy:** Eliminate all answer choices that are not an intervention or directly related to breathing. **Reference:** LeMone, P., Burke, K., & Bauldoff, G. (2011). *Medical-surgical nursing: Critical thinking in patient care* (5th ed.). Upper Saddle River, NJ: Pearson Education, p. 932.

6 **Answer: 2** **Rationale:** Bed rest is prescribed to allow the arterial puncture to seal and reduce the risk of bleeding. Explaining the rationale to the client is the best way to facilitate the client's cooperation. Getting out of bed after a cardiac catheterization will not cause dysrhythmias. Telling the client that bed rest is required because the physician has ordered it does not provide information about how bed rest helps prevent vascular complications after a cardiac catheterization. Although some clients may be weak after a cardiac catheterization, this does not address how bed rest helps prevent the more serious complication of bleeding at the femoral artery puncture site. **Cognitive Level:** Applying **Client Need:** Reduction of Risk Potential **Integrated Process:** Communication and Documentation **Content Area:** Adult Health **Strategy:** Integrate knowledge of how the cardiac catheter is performed with homeostasis. Recall that any vascular invasion requires time to allow for clot formation. **Reference:** LeMone, P.,

Burke, K., & Bauldoff, G. (2011). *Medical-surgical nursing: Critical thinking in patient care* (5th ed.). Upper Saddle River, NJ: Pearson Education, p. 886.

7 **Answer: 3** **Rationale:** When the character of chest pain changes or it is unrelieved by the usual measures the client has unstable angina and is correct to go to the ED. Stable angina is described as chest pain that occurs in a similar manner, with similar precipitating events, and is relieved with the same intervention (either rest and/or nitroglycerine). There is no information that indicates the client already has a current nitroglycerine prescription, and since the pain is usually relieved, he still should have come to the emergency department. The diagnosis of an acute myocardial infarction requires diagnostic testing such as a 12-lead EKG and measurement of cardiac biomarkers. **Cognitive Level:** Analyzing **Client Need:** Physiological Adaptation **Integrated Process:** Nursing Process: Diagnosis **Content Area:** Adult Health **Strategy:** Define the types of angina and determine which type of angina is represented in the question. **Reference:** LeMone, P., Burke, K., & Bauldoff, G. (2011). *Medical-surgical nursing: Critical thinking in patient care* (5th ed.). Upper Saddle River, NJ: Pearson Education, p. 920.

8 **Answer: 4** **Rationale:** The client should have a light meal with no caffeine before a cardiac stress test and should refrain from eating or drinking for 2 to 3 hours before the test. It is not necessary to make the client NPO until 8:30 a.m. The client should eat a light meal instead of a regular full breakfast. Caffeine may cause sympathetic nervous system stimulation resulting in an increase in heart rate and blood pressure. This could make the results of the test difficult to determine. **Cognitive Level:** Applying **Client Need:** Reduction of Risk Potential **Integrated Process:** Nursing Process: Implementation **Content Area:** Adult Health **Strategy:** Recall that a stress test evaluates the cardiac circulation in relation to cardiac workload. Select the distracter that minimizes cardiac workload but prevents the client from becoming weak or dehydrated prior to the test. **Reference:** LeMone, P., Burke, K., & Bauldoff, G. (2011). *Medical-surgical nursing: Critical thinking in patient care* (5th ed.). Upper Saddle River, NJ: Pearson Education, pp. 886–888.

9 **Answer: 1, 3** **Rationale:** The best first action is to assess the client's level of consciousness and assess if the ventricular tachycardia (VT) is perfusing the body by measuring the BP and pulse. If the client is in a pulseless ventricular tachycardia, immediate defibrillation is performed by an ACLS certified nurse. If the client has a good BP and pulse and is awake and alert, the nurse may administer intravenous lidocaine as ordered. A precordial thump is not part of current basic life support protocol. Telephoning the family may or may not be necessary, but would not be a priority action in this circumstance. **Cognitive Level:** Analyzing **Client Need:** Management of Care **Integrated Process:** Nursing Process: Planning **Content Area:** Adult Health **Strategy:** First, recall that there are 2 forms of presentation with ventricular tachycardia (VT) and the underlying perfusion to the brain and vital organs is a key differentiating factor. Determine actions that are important in this potential emergency situation to choose correctly. **Reference:** LeMone, P., Burke, K., & Bauldoff, G. (2011). *Medical-surgical nursing: Critical thinking in patient care* (5th ed.). Upper Saddle River, NJ: Pearson Education, pp. 948, 951–952.

10 **Answer: 2** **Rationale:** Anxiety and fear are common responses to a diagnosis of myocardial infarction because of the possibility of death. This prevents the client and family from absorbing the detailed explanations about the care being provided. Memory lapses are not a common symptom of myocardial infarction. There is not adequate information to determine that this memory lapse is associated with Alzheimer's disease, and this would not be the best time to make that determination. Nurses in the ED are able to explain procedures well to their clients. **Cognitive Level:** Analyzing **Client Need:** Psychosocial Integrity **Integrated Process:** Nursing Process: Diagnosis **Content Area:** Adult Health **Strategy:** To select the correct option, understand the typical response to acute myocardial infarction and the effects of anxiety. **Reference:** LeMone, P., Burke, K., & Bauldoff, G. (2011). *Medical-surgical nursing: Critical thinking in patient care* (5th ed.). Upper Saddle River, NJ: Pearson Education, p. 942.

References

Berman, A., & Snyder, S. (2012). *Kozier & Erb's fundamentals of nursing: Concepts, process, and practice* (9th ed.). Upper Saddle River, NJ: Pearson Education.

D'Amico, D., & Barbarito, C. (2012). *Health & physical assessment in nursing* (2nd ed.). Upper Saddle River, NJ: Pearson Education, Inc.

Ignatavicius, D. D., & Workman, M. L. (2013). *Medical-surgical nursing: Critical thinking for collaborative care* (7th ed.) Philadelphia: W. B. Saunders Company.

Kee, J. L. (2010). *Laboratory and diagnostic tests* (8th ed.). Upper Saddle River, NJ: Pearson Education.

Lehne, R. (2010). *Pharmacology for nursing care* (7th ed.). St. Louis, MO: Saunders.

LeMone, P., Burke, K., & Bauldoff, G. (2011). *Medical-surgical nursing: Critical thinking in patient care* (5th ed.). Upper Saddle River, NJ: Pearson Education.

Lewis, S., Dirksen, S., Heitkemper, M., Bucher, L., & Camera, I. (2011). *Medical surgical nursing: Assessment and management of clinical problems* (8th ed.). St. Louis, MO: Elsevier.

McCance, K. L., & Huether, S. E. (2010). *Pathophysiology: The biologic basis for disease in adults and children* (6th ed.). St. Louis, MO: Mosby, Inc.

Osborn, K. S., Wraa, C. E., & Watson, A. (2010). *Medical surgical nursing: Preparation for practice.* Upper Saddle River, NJ: Pearson Education.

Smith, S. F., Duell, D. J., & Martin, B. C. (2012). *Clinical nursing skills: Basic to advanced skills* (8th ed.). Upper Saddle River, NJ: Pearson Education.

Wilson, B. A., Shannon, M. T., & Shields, K. M. (2012). *Pearson nurse's drug guide 2012.* Upper Saddle River, NJ: Pearson Education.

ANSWERS & RATIONALES

4 Peripheral Vascular Disorders

Chapter Outline

Overview of Anatomy
  and Physiology
Diagnostic Tests and
  Assessments
Common Nursing Techniques
  and Procedures: Blood
  Pressure Measurement

Primary Hypertension
Peripheral Arterial Disease
Arterial Embolism
Buerger's Disease
  (Thromboangiitis Obliterans)
Raynaud's Disease
Aortic Aneurysm

Thrombophlebitis
Venous Insufficiency
Varicose Veins

NCLEX-RN® Test Prep

Use the accompanying online resource,
NursingReviewsandRationales, to test
yourself with hundreds of NCLEX®-style
practice questions.

Objectives

➤ Identify basic structures and functions of the peripheral vascular
  system.
➤ Describe the pathophysiology and etiology of common peripheral
  vascular disorders.
➤ Discuss expected assessment data and diagnostic findings for
  selected peripheral vascular disorders.
➤ Identify priority nursing problems for selected peripheral vascular
  disorders.
➤ Discuss therapeutic management of selected vascular disorders.
➤ Discuss nursing management of a client experiencing a peripheral
  vascular disorder.
➤ Identify expected outcomes for the client experiencing a peripheral
  vascular disorder.

Review at a Glance

atherosclerosis local accumulation
of lipid and fibrous tissue along intimal
layer of an artery
endarterectomy opening of artery
and removal of obstructing plaque
Homan's sign pain on dorsiflexion of
foot when leg is raised
intermittent claudication
ischemic muscle pain precipitated by a
predictable amount of exercise and
relieved by rest

Korotkoff sounds sounds heard in
auscultation of blood pressure
neurovascular status
color, motion, sensation, temperature,
and presence of distal peripheral pulses
orthostatic hypotension
a drop in systolic blood pressure of 10 to
20 mmHg with upright posture
rest pain pain while resting that may
even awaken client at night; pain is
usually in distal portion of extremity

(toes, arch, forefoot, heel) and is relieved
when foot is placed in dependent position
sympathectomy surgical dissection
of nerve fibers that allows vasoconstriction
to occur
vasodilation widening of a
blood vessel

PRETEST

1 A client with hypertension has a blood pressure of 158/90 after 6 months of intensive exercise and diet modifications. The nurse makes which appropriate statement to the client at this time?

1. "Continue the current treatment plan as your blood pressure is being adequately controlled."
2. "Your current treatment plan is ineffective and will be discontinued; medications will be required instead."
3. "Try to double your exercise time and maintain dietary modifications to continue to reduce your blood pressure."
4. "Medication therapy will likely need to be started along with continuing your exercise and diet program."

2 The nurse has been caring for a client with peripheral arterial disease. The nurse would assess for which outcome as evidence of increased arterial blood supply to the extremity?

1. Reduced muscle pain
2. Reduced sensation to touch
3. Increased rubor
4. Decreased hair on the extremity

3 In teaching a hypertensive client about the side effects of propranolol (Inderal) the nurse plans to include which side effect of this medication therapy?

1. Hypokalemia
2. Constipation
3. Bronchospasm
4. Tachycardia

4 The nurse is doing an assessment on a client during the first postoperative day after abdominal surgery. Which manifestations should the nurse report immediately?

1. Decreased bowel sounds
2. Mild abdominal distention
3. Inability to void immediately after urinary catheter is removed
4. Leg swelling and calf pain

5 The nurse concludes that the hypertensive client taking furosemide (Lasix) demonstrates understanding of the drug when the client states the importance of increasing intake of which beverage?

1. Milk
2. Cranberry juice
3. Orange pekoe tea
4. Orange juice

6 The nurse is caring for a preoperative client diagnosed with abdominal aortic aneurysm (AAA). The client reports the onset of severe back pain. What action should the nurse take next?

1. Call the health care provider immediately.
2. Provide comfort measures to relieve the back discomfort.
3. Monitor the client for one-half hour to see if it continues.
4. Determine if hoarseness or dysphagia is present.

7 The nurse is caring for a client with a diagnosis of deep vein thrombosis (DVT) who is being treated with a continuous infusion of heparin. Which laboratory result should the nurse report immediately?

1. Prothrombin time (PT) of 12
2. Activated partial thromboplastin time (aPTT) of 150
3. International Normalized Ratio (INR) of 2
4. Platelet count of 150,000

8 The nurse is preparing an assignment for a nurse orientee. Because the new nurse has not cared for a client having a Greenfield filter inserted, which clients may be selected for the new nurse's assignment as possible candidates for a Greenfield filter? Select all that apply.

1. 30-year-old woman pregnant with twins
2. 60-year-old man with pelvic fractures, compound femur fracture, and unknown history
3. 54-year-old admitted with acute respiratory distress syndrome (ARDS) with a history of deep vein thrombosis (DVT)
4. 25-year-old with fractured wrist and radius accompanied by soft tissue injury
5. 58-year-old woman following laparoscopic cholecystectomy

9 The nurse is caring for a client diagnosed with hypertension who is being treated with a bumetanide (Bumex) and enalapril (Prinivil). Which item should the nurse include in this client's discharge instructions?

1. Sit up and get out of bed slowly to prevent dizziness.
2. Take all blood pressure readings when lying down.
3. Take blood pressure readings in both arms.
4. Do not take nitroglycerin within 1 hour of these medications.

10 When educating the client with essential hypertension, the nurse instructs the client to do which of the following? Select all that apply.

1. Have regular eye exams.
2. Take antihypertensive medications when blood pressure is elevated.
3. Have blood pressure measured annually.
4. Avoid foods with concentrated sugars.
5. Maintain a program of regular exercise.

➤ *See pages 137–139 for Answers and Rationales.*

I. OVERVIEW OF ANATOMY AND PHYSIOLOGY

A. Structure and function of blood vessels
1. Blood vessels are channels through which blood is distributed to body tissues
2. Walls of an artery or vein consist of three layers: tunica intima, tunica media, and tunica adventitia; wall thickness and amount of connective tissue and smooth muscle depend on amount of pressure the vessel must endure
3. They are divided into arterial system and venous system
   a. Arterial system (Figure 4-1): consists of high-pressure vessels (largest of which is aorta); some branch into arterioles, which measure less than 0.5 mm in diameter; functions to deliver blood to various tissues for nourishment and contribute to tissue temperature regulation
   b. Venous system (Figure 4-2): consists of large diameter, thin-walled vessels that are under much less pressure; some veins (most commonly in legs) contain valves to regulate one-way flow; functions to return blood from capillaries to right atrium for circulation and acts as a reservoir for blood volume

B. Circulation and dynamics of blood flow
1. Blood flow is amount of fluid moved per unit of time through a vessel, organ, or throughout entire circulatory system; adequate flow is necessary to transport nutrients and oxygen to cells and tissue; regulated by:
   a. Pressure: a pressure differential exists between arterial and venous vessels, with blood flowing from arterial "side" of capillaries to lower pressure venous side
   b. Resistance: opposition to blood flow; increased resistance leads to decreased blood flow; peripheral vascular resistance is determined by blood viscosity, length of vessel, and diameter of vessel

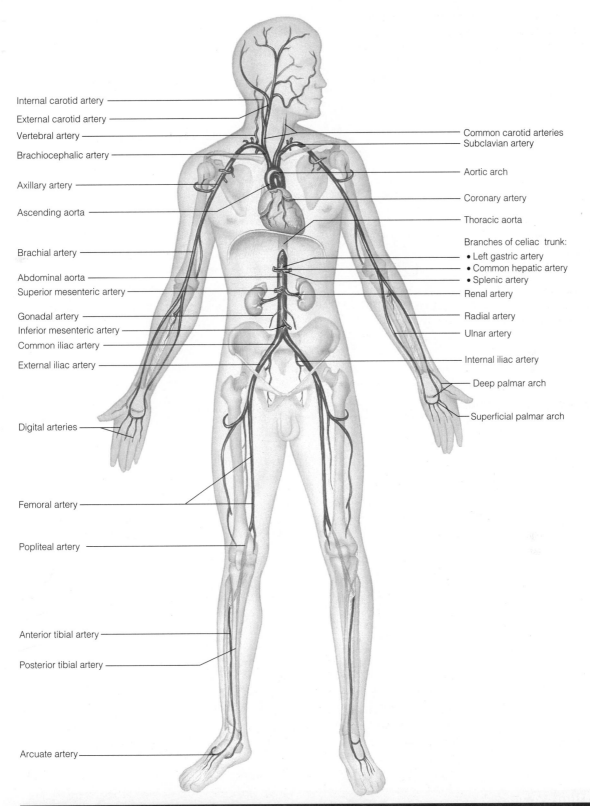

Internal carotid artery

External carotid artery

Vertebral artery

Brachiocephalic artery

Axillary artery

Ascending aorta

Brachial artery

Abdominal aorta

Superior mesenteric artery

Gonadal artery

Inferior mesenteric artery

Common iliac artery

External iliac artery

Digital arteries

Femoral artery

Popliteal artery

Anterior tibial artery

Posterior tibial artery

Arcuate artery

Common carotid arteries

Subclavian artery

Aortic arch

Coronary artery

Thoracic aorta

Branches of celiac trunk:
- Left gastric artery
- Common hepatic artery
- Splenic artery

Renal artery

Radial artery

Ulnar artery

Internal iliac artery

Deep palmar arch

Superficial palmar arch

Figure 4-1

Major arteries of the systemic circulation

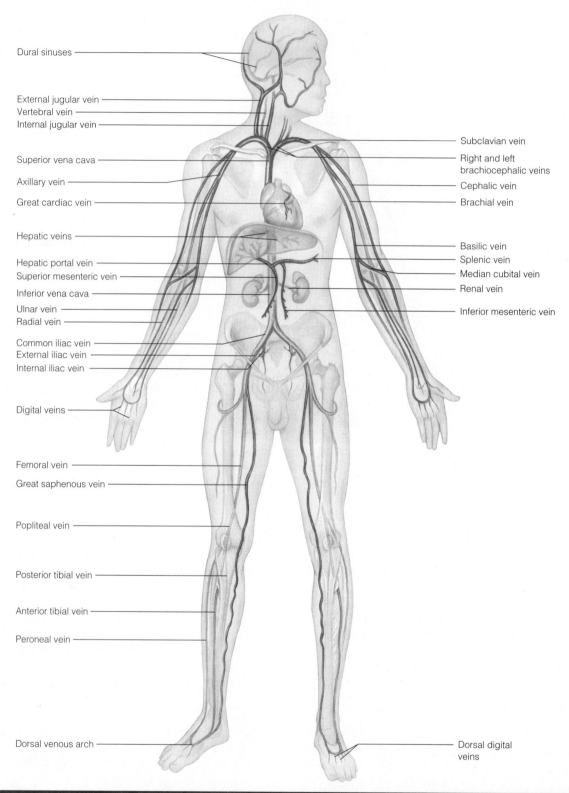

Dural sinuses

External jugular vein
Vertebral vein
Internal jugular vein

Superior vena cava

Axillary vein

Great cardiac vein

Hepatic veins

Hepatic portal vein
Superior mesenteric vein

Inferior vena cava

Ulnar vein
Radial vein

Common iliac vein
External iliac vein
Internal iliac vein

Digital veins

Femoral vein

Great saphenous vein

Popliteal vein

Posterior tibial vein

Anterior tibial vein

Peroneal vein

Dorsal venous arch

Subclavian vein
Right and left
brachiocephalic veins
Cephalic vein
Brachial vein

Basilic vein
Splenic vein
Median cubital vein
Renal vein

Inferior mesenteric vein

Dorsal digital
veins

Figure 4-2

Major veins of the systemic circulation

       c. Velocity: distance blood must travel in a unit of time

       d. Compliance: increase in volume that a vessel can accommodate for with a given increase in pressure; veins are much more compliant than arteries and thus can serve as storage areas in circulatory system

  C. Blood pressure (BP) control: BP is pressure of blood against vessel walls; it is controlled by several factors

    1. Autonomic nervous system (NS)

       a. Sympathetic NS: increases heart rate (HR), speed of impulse conduction through atrioventricular (AV) node, and force of atrial and ventricular contractions

       b. Parasympathetic NS: causes a decrease in HR by action of sinoatrial (SA) node and slows conduction through AV node

    2. Baroreceptors: stimulation of these receptors located in aortic arch and carotid sinus causes information to be sent to vasomotor center in brain stem to enhance parasympathetic NS, causing a decrease in HR and peripheral **vasodilation**, or widening of blood vessels

    3. Chemoreceptors: areas stimulated by decreased arterial oxygen pressure, increased carbon dioxide pressure, and decreased plasma pH to stimulate vasomotor center and increase cardiac activity

    4. Antidiuretic hormone (ADH): a decrease in total blood volume leads posterior pituitary gland to release ADH, causing reabsorption of water by kidneys, resulting in increased blood plasma volume and increased BP

    5. Renin–angiotensin–aldosterone system: in response to sympathetic NS stimulation or decreased renal blood flow, kidneys produce renin that generates angiotensin I, which is converted to angiotensin II; these powerful vasoconstrictors stimulate release of aldosterone from adrenal glands, allowing for sodium retention in kidneys and then suppression of renin

    6. Other factors that may affect BP control: include temperature (cold = vasoconstriction), substances such as nicotine (vasoconstrictor) or alcohol (vasodilator), diet (sodium and fat intake), and factors such as genetics, age, gender, weight, physical health, and emotional state

II. DIAGNOSTIC TESTS AND ASSESSMENTS

  A. Doppler ultrasound: measures velocity of blood flow through a vessel and emits an audible signal; when arterial palpation is difficult or impossible because of occlusive disease, a Doppler can help determine blood flow; a palpable pulse and a Doppler pulse are not equivalent and should not be used interchangeably

  B. Plethysmography: records biologic changes in blood volume in an area of body associated with cardiac contractions or in response to pneumatic venous occlusion; can detect and quantify vascular disease based on changes in pulse contour, BP, or arterial or venous blood flow

  C. Intravenous digital subtraction angiography (IV-DSA): utilizes computer technology to isolate arteries for better visualization of these blood vessels using IV injection of contrast material

  D. Venography: injection of radiopaque dye into veins; serial x-rays are taken to detect deep vein thrombosis and incompetent valves

  E. Angiography: injection of radiopaque dye into arteries to detect plaques, occlusions, injury, etc.

  F. Ankle-brachial index (ABI): most commonly used parameter for overall evaluation of extremity status; ankle pressure normally is same or slightly higher than brachial systolic pressure; expected ABI is 0.8 to 1.0

G. **Computed tomography**: allows for visualization of arterial wall and its structures; used in diagnosis of abdominal aortic aneurysm (AAA) and postoperative vascular complications such as graft occlusion and hemorrhage

H. **Magnetic resonance imaging (MRI)**: uses magnetic fields rather than radiation; used with angiography to detect abnormalities, especially in people who have contraindication to use of contrast dye

III. COMMON NURSING TECHNIQUES AND PROCEDURES: BLOOD PRESSURE MEASUREMENT

A. **Blood pressure** is primarily a function of cardiac output (CO) and systemic vascular resistance (SVR); arterial BP = CO × SVR

B. **Proper technique**

1. Client should be seated with arm bared, supported, and at heart level, with feet resting comfortably on floor or supported

2. Client should not have smoked or ingested caffeine 30 minutes prior
3. BP should be taken in both arms initially
4. Appropriate sized cuff must be used: rubber bladder should at least encircle arm by 80%
5. After palpating brachial or radial pulse, inflate cuff 30 mmHg above level at which pulse disappears
6. Record systolic and diastolic sounds—known as **Korotkoff sounds** (disappearance of sound is the diastolic reading)
7. Two or more readings separated by 2 minutes should be averaged
8. If client's arms are inaccessible, you can obtain readings from thigh or calf, auscultating popliteal or posterior tibial arteries, respectively; cuff size must be adjusted for larger extremity

IV. PRIMARY HYPERTENSION

A. **Description**

1. A disorder characterized by BP that consistently exceeds 140 systolic and 90 diastolic, confirmed on at least 2 visits; onset is primarily in people 25–55 years old
2. Consists of stages: prehypertension (systolic BP 120–139 or diastolic BP 80–89), Stage 1 HTN (systolic BP 140–159 or diastolic BP 90–99), and Stage 2 HTN (systolic BP greater than or equal to 160 or diastolic BP greater than or equal to 100)
3. Hypertensive crisis occurs when systolic BP is 180 mmHg or higher or diastolic BP is 120 mmHg or higher; can be life threatening

B. **Etiology and pathophysiology**

1. Hypertension (HTN) can be primary (essential) or secondary; primary HTN accounts for 90–95% of all cases; secondary HTN results from an underlying and identifiable illness; in primary HTN there is no known cause but risk factors include:
   a. Positive family history
   b. Ethnicity (highest incidence is in African Americans)
   c. High dietary sodium intake
   d. Inactivity and obesity
   e. Excessive alcohol intake
2. Pathophysiology
   a. For arterial BP to rise there must be an increase in either CO or SVR; later in course of disease SVR continues to rise as CO stabilizes
   b. There is no single cause for primary HTN

C. **Assessment**
  1. Subjective data
     a. Past history of cardiovascular, cerebrovascular, renal, or thyroid diseases, diabetes, smoking, or alcohol use
     b. Family history of HTN or cardiovascular disease
     c. Possible absence of symptoms
     d. Reports of fatigue, nocturia, dyspnea on exertion, palpitations, angina, headaches, weight gain, edema, muscle cramps, or blurred vision; symptoms may be caused by target organ damage rather than high BP itself
  2. Objective data
     a. BP consistently greater than 140 mmHg systolic and greater than 90 mmHg diastolic; prehypertension category of at-risk population is systolic BP greater than 130 or diastolic greater than 80
     b. Peripheral edema, retinal vessel changes, diminished or absent peripheral pulses, bruits, murmurs, and S_3 and S_4 heart sounds
  3. Diagnostic tests
     a. Abnormal potassium level (may be low if taking loop diuretics or high if taking potassium-sparing diuretics)
     b. Elevated blood urea nitrogen (BUN), creatinine, glucose, cholesterol, and triglycerides
     c. Abnormal urinalysis
     d. Cardiomegaly on x-ray
     e. Abnormal ECG showing left ventricular hypertrophy
D. **Priority nursing problems**: reduced cardiac output, risk for nonadherence, inability to maintain health
E. **Planning and implementation**
  1. Inform client of numeric BP readings so client can keep an on-going record, compare to target BP goal, and recognize levels that would be of concern
  2. Inform client that HTN is usually asymptomatic, and symptoms will not reliably indicate BP levels
  3. Explain that long-term medical followup and therapy are necessary
  4. Accurately record intake and output and daily weights of hospitalized clients
F. **Medication therapy**
  1. Stepped care approach to HTN is used for medication management
  2. After lifestyle changes prove inadequate for BP control, or if client presents with very high BP, then drug therapy is started
  3. In Stage 1 HTN, initial drug choice often is a thiazide-type diuretic although another type of drug may be considered by provider
  4. A 2-drug combination is often used in Stage 2 hypertension, often combining a thiazide-type diuretic with an angiotensin-converting enzyme (ACE) inhibitor or angiotensin II receptor blocker (ARB), beta blocker (BB), or calcium channel blocker (CCB); see Table 4-1
  5. Choice of drugs and drug dosages are tailored according to response to therapy; aim is to reach desired BP with fewest side effects; other vasodilators may also be used as needed (see Table 4-1 again)
G. **Client education**
  1. Lifestyle modifications
     a. Sodium restriction in diet
     b. DASH (dietary approaches to stop hypertension) diet: includes prescribed number of servings of food in these categories: grains and grain products; vegetables; fruits; low-fat or nonfat dairy foods; meats, poultry, and fish; nuts, seeds, and legumes; fats and oils; and sweets

Table 4-1	Medications Commonly Used to Treat Peripheral Vascular Diseases		
Drug Class and Name: Generic (Trade)	**Therapeutic Use(s)**	**Mechanism of Action**	**Nursing Responsibilities**
Alpha-Adrenergic Blockers Prazosin hydrochloride (Minipress) Doxazosin (Cardura) Terazosin (Hytrin)	Hypertension	Act by blocking alpha$_1$ receptors on arterioles and veins to cause vasodilation	Minipress may cause a "first dose" effect: may result in syncope 30–60 min after first dose • Give first dose at bedtime. • Remain in bed at least 3 hours after first dose. • Avoid driving for at least 24 hours. Assess BP regularly—monitor BP in lying, standing, and sitting positions to detect orthostatic hypotension. Orthostatic hypotension most common side effect; teach client to • change positions slowly. • take med at bedtime when possible. • avoid hazardous activities. Other side effects include light-headedness, impotence in men, reflex tachycardia, and nasal congestion.
Angiotensin-Converting Enzyme (ACE) Inhibitors Benazepril (Lotensin) Captopril (Capoten) Enalapril (Vasotec) Lisinopril (Zestril, Prinivil) Ramipril (Altace) Quinapril (Accupril)	Hypertension Raynaud's disease Congestive heart failure	Inhibits conversion of Angiotensin I to Angiotensin II (a potent vasoconstrictor) Reduces peripheral resistance without changing cardiac output (CO)	Monitor vital signs and compare with baseline. Teach side effects: loss of taste, dry cough, and orthostatic hypotension (especially after first dose). Teach client: • Aspirin and NSAIDs may impair hypotensive effects. • Take 1 hour before meals. • Always consult MD before discontinuing. • Can cause fetal morbidity or mortality in pregnant women.
Beta-Adrenergic Blockers Acebutolol (Sectral) Atenolol (Tenormin) Betaxolol (Kerlone) Metoprolol (Lopressor) Nadolol (Corgard) Propranolol (Inderal)	Hypertension Myocardial infarction Dysrhythmias	Decrease BP by decreasing CO response to sympathetic nerve impulses and renin secretion by kidneys; reduces systemic vascular resistance	Monitor vital signs and compare with baseline. Assess client for heart failure and heart block by checking pulse regularly. Avoid in clients with COPD. Teach client • to always consult MD before discontinuing. • about adverse side effects: orthostatic hypotension, bronchospasm, nightmares, hallucinations.
Angiotensin II Receptor Blockers (ARBs) Candesartan (Atacand) Eprosartan (Teveten) Irbesartan (Avapro) Losartan (Cozaar) Olmesartan (Benicar) Telmisartan (Micardis) Valsartan (Diovan)	Hypertension alone or with left ventricular hypertrophy, nephropathy in type 2 diabetes mellitus	Block vasoconstrictor and aldosterone-secreting effects of angiotensin II	Monitor • vital signs and compare to baseline. • electrolyes, especially K, Na, Cl. • peripheral edema. • skin turgor. • postural hypotension. Take without concern about meal timing. Decreased antihypertensive effect with phenobarbital, rifampin Increased antihypertensive effect with fluconazole Many possible interactions with herbal remedies

(continued)

Table 4-1	Medications Commonly Used to Treat Peripheral Vascular Diseases (Continued)		
Drug Class and Name: Generic (Trade)	**Therapeutic Use(s)**	**Mechanism of Action**	**Nursing Responsibilities**
Calcium Channel Blockers Amlodipine (Norvasc) Diltiazem (Cardizem) Felodipine (Plendil) Isradipine (Dynacirc) Nifedipine (Procardia) Verapamil (Isoptin)	Hypertension	Decrease BP by blocking movement of calcium in cells of smooth muscles, which decreases peripheral resistance	Teach client side effects: • nausea • headaches • orthostatic hypotension • edema Avoid use in clients with CHF. Procardia is given sublingually except when rapid drop in BP is required and then it is chewed.
Centrally Acting Adrenergic Blockers Clonidine (Catapres) Methyldopa (Aldomet)	Hypertension	Act within CNS to reduce sympathetic nerve stimulation of blood vessels and heart, resulting in dilation of arteries and veins	Teach side effects: • dry mouth • sedation • impotence • constipation • severe rebound hypertension if stopped quickly Teach client: use sugarless gum or hard candy for dry mouth; alcohol increases CNS depression

Diuretics
 Thiazides
 Chlorothiazide (Diuril)
 Chlorthalidone (Hygroton)
 Hydrochlorothiazide (HydroDiuril)
 Indapamide (Lozol)
 Metolazone (Zaroxolyn)
	Edema
	 Hypertension
		Depress ability of convoluted tubules to reabsorb sodium and chloride. "Where water goes, so goes sodium."	Teach client:
			 • side effects of electrolyte imbalance:
			    • muscle weakness
			    • dizziness
			 • to take diuretic in morning.
			 • to take with food if GI upset occurs.
			 • to weigh self every morning—report weight gain of more than 2–3 lb.
			 • to eat foods high in potassium (oranges, bananas, broccoli, tomato juice, apricots, etc.).
			 • to avoid alcohol.
			 • to avoid black licorice (may precipitate hypokalemia).
			 • drug increases lithium toxicity.

Loop Bumetanide (Bumex) Furosemide (Lasix)	Potent diuretic for significant diuresis with edema.	Inhibit reabsorption of sodium and chloride in the proximal and distal tubules and loop of Henle	Explain that this type of drug is very fast acting. Teach client to • take diuretic in morning. • take with food or milk. • avoid orthostasis. • use sunscreen (photosensitivity may occur). • take potassium supplement as ordered. • weigh self daily and report increases of 2–3 lb.
Potassium-Sparing Amiloride (Midamor) Spironolactone (Aldactone)	Used with thiazide diuretics to prevent/ correct hypokalemia.	Block sodium-potassium exchange mechanism in the distal portion of the tubule; prevent sodium reabsorption and retain potassium	Teach client to • take with food or milk. • weigh self daily and report a gain of 2–3 lb. • avoid salt substitutes and foods high in potassium. Adverse side effects include gynecomastia and decreased libido.

(continued)

Table 4-1	Medications Commonly Used to Treat Peripheral Vascular Diseases (Continued)		
Drug Class and Name: Generic (Trade)	**Therapeutic Use(s)**	**Mechanism of Action**	**Nursing Responsibilities**
Vasodilators Hydralazine (Apresoline) Sodium nitroprusside (Nipride) Nitroglycerin (Tridil)	Apresoline: arterial vasodilation Nipride: direct action in hypertensive emergencies Tridil: venous vasodilation	All will work to lower BP by acting on smooth muscle of vascular system to cause vasodilation	Apresoline: • Administer IV or IM for hypertensive crisis. • Take oral medication with food. • Monitor daily weights. Nipride: • Protect drug from light, heat, and moisture. • Cover IV bag and tubing with foil. • Discard solution that is not light brown in color. • Administer with sodium thiosulfate to reduce risk of cyanide toxicity. Tridil: • IV infusion only. • Use only glass bottle and administration set provided. • Gradually wean off IV dose.
Other Cilostazol (Pletal)	Intermittent claudication	Not fully understood; inhibits platelet aggregation and allows for vasodilation	Minimal side effects Take with meals. Do not use in clients with CHF. Do not take with grapefruit juice.
Pentoxifylline (Trental)	Intermittent claudication	Decreases viscosity of blood, resulting in increased blood flow to microcirculation	Take with meals. Initial effects may not be noticed for 6–8 weeks. Minimal side effects

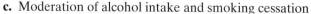

    c. Moderation of alcohol intake and smoking cessation
    d. Exercise and weight reduction
    e. Relaxation techniques for stress reduction
  2. Managing potential side effects of drug therapy
    a. Supplement potassium if taking loop diuretics
    b. Prevent **orthostatic hypotension** (a drop in BP of 10–20 mmHg with upright posture) by rising out of bed or chair slowly
    c. Avoid hot baths and strenuous exercise within 3 hours of taking vasodilators
  3. Importance of adhering to treatment plan; treatment can reduce risk of target organ damage even if there are no symptoms
 H. **Expected outcomes**: decrease in BP to less than 140/90; no target organ damage (kidneys, heart, NS, eyes); client describes how to manage HTN

V. PERIPHERAL ARTERIAL DISEASE

  A. **Description**: disorders that interrupt or impede arterial peripheral blood flow due to vessel compression, vasospasm, and/or structural defects in vessel wall
  B. **Etiology and pathophysiology**
    1. Peripheral arterial occlusive disease is primarily caused by **atherosclerosis** (local accumulation of lipid and fibrous tissue along the intimal layer of an artery), but also may be caused by trauma, embolism, thrombosis, vasospasm, inflammation, or autoimmunity

Practice to Pass

Your client with newly diagnosed hypertension has been advised to follow a DASH diet. What teaching will you include when explaining the DASH diet to the client?

2. By the time symptoms appear, vessel is about 75% narrowed
3. The femoral-popliteal area most commonly affected site in clients without diabetes mellitus; clients with diabetes mellitus most often develop disease in arteries below knees
4. Chronic arterial obstruction leads to inadequate oxygenation of tissues causing **intermittent claudication** (ischemic muscle pain precipitated by a predictable amount of exercise and relieved by rest)

C. **Assessment**
1. Subjective
   a. Client reports aching, cramping, fatigue or weakness in legs that is relieved by rest (claudication); this is an early indication of disease
   b. Client reports **rest pain**, which is pain that occurs while resting; may even awaken client at night; pain is usually in distal portion of extremity (toes, arch, forefoot, heel) and is relieved when foot is placed in dependent (downward) position; this indicates more advanced disease
   c. Client reports coldness or numbness in lower extremities
2. Objective
   a. Extremities may be cool and pale with a cyanotic color on elevation
   b. Bruits may be auscultated
   c. Peripheral pulses may be diminished or absent
   d. Nails may be thickened and opaque (trophic change)
   e. Skin on the legs may be shiny with sparse hair growth (trophic change)
   f. Ulcers may be present on lower extremities in areas with reduced circulation; ulcers have deep pale base, demarcated edges, and are painful
3. Diagnostic testing: includes intravenous digital subtraction angiography (IV-DSA), angiography, Doppler ultrasound, and plethysmography

D. **Priority nursing problems**: reduced tissue perfusion, interrupted skin integrity, pain

E. **Planning and implementation**
1. Goal: adequate tissue perfusion
   a. Assess and record strength of pulse
   b. Encourage client to stop smoking as nicotine causes vasoconstriction and hypercoagulability of blood
   c. Teach client to change position at least hourly and avoid crossing legs at ankles or knees
   d. Encourage client to exercise and walk until onset of pain; explain to stop walking when pain occurs to decrease oxygen demand in affected area and to resume when pain has stopped in order to build tolerance to exercise and stimulate growth of collateral circulation
   e. Teach client to avoid restrictive clothing, including girdles, garters, and socks
2. Goal: relief of pain
   a. Assess pain on a 1–10 scale and provide analgesics as ordered
   b. Teach relaxation techniques because stress increases vasoconstriction
   c. Keep feet warm and in a dependent position; do not elevate feet if pain is present
3. Goal: intact, healthy skin on extremities
   a. Teach client skills in skin care and recommend daily inspection of feet
   b. Teach client to always wear shoes or slippers and avoid trauma to feet; bath water should be checked with hands, not feet, to prevent burns to tissue at high risk for injury that may also have decreased sensation
   c. Teach client to have toenail care performed by a professional
   d. Teach client to seek care if an ulcer develops, as healing will be slow unless arterial blood flow to affected limb is improved through a surgical revascularization procedure

4. If surgery is indicated, provide appropriate postoperative care

    a. Angioplasty

        1) Monitor **neurovascular status** (color, motion, sensitivity, temperature, and presence of distal peripheral pulses) to affected extremity every 15 minutes for 1 hour, every 30 minutes for 2 hours, then q1–4h after sheath removed or per the provider or institution protocol

        2) Notify provider if client experiences weak or thready pulses, and/or coolness, numbness, or tingling in extremity

        3) Monitor sheath site for signs of external and subcutaneous bleeding at same time as neurovascular assessment

        4) Instruct client to notify nurse and apply manual pressure to site if a sensation of warmth or wetness is felt at site (this may indicate external bleeding at procedural site); if bleeding occurs, reinforce initial dressing but do not remove it

        5) Maintain immobilization of affected extremity for at least 6 hours by reminding client to keep extremity still or lightly immobilize ankle with sheet tucked under both sides of mattress

        6) Maintain a pressure dressing and sand bag (or other occlusive device) at site

    b. Bypass grafting

        1) Provide standard postoperative care and frequently monitor neurovascular status

        2) Use bed cradle to keep weight of linens off newly vascularized tissue, which is still friable; use sheepskin under feet as well

        3) Maintain head of bed at 15–20 degrees or lower as prescribed to avoid hip flexion, which could reduce blood flow through newly grafted area

        4) Assess for occlusion of graft by assessing for severe ischemic pain, loss of pulses, decreasing ankle-brachial index, numbness or tingling in extremity, coolness and pallor of extremity

    c. **Endarterectomy** (opening artery and removing obstructing plaque) or amputation in severe cases; use same principles of care

    d. Amputation may be necessary if tissue becomes necrotic or gangrenous; see Chapter 9 for care of client undergoing amputation

F. Medication therapy

  1. Pentoxifylline (Trental) decreases blood viscosity to increase blood flow to microcirculation and tissues of extremities

  2. Cilostazol (Pletal) inhibits platelet aggregation and enhances vasodilation

  3. Aspirin and clopidogrel (Plavix) inhibit platelet aggregation

  4. If preparing client for surgery or other invasive procedure, nurse should assess for and document any prescribed platelet aggregate inhibitors client may be taking

G. Client education

  1. Promote vasodilation: provide warmth (never by direct heat to limb) and prevent long periods of exposure to cold; avoid use of restrictive clothing

  2. Proper positioning: keep feet dependent to increase blood flow to legs; may elevate feet at rest but not above heart level; never cross legs or ankles; following bypass surgery, may keep legs level with rest of body

  3. Stop smoking

  4. Meticulous foot care as should be performed by clients with diabetes mellitus

  5. Trental and Plavix should be taken with food; and expect any effects may take 6–8 weeks for a therapeutic effect

  6. Notify providers of any current prescribed or over the counter medications

  7. Institute provider-approved exercise program with goal for client to be at optimal weight

  8. See Box 4-1 for a summary of client education points for managing peripheral arterial disease

Practice to Pass

You are assigned a client scheduled for angiography. What will you tell your client about this procedure? What are the nursing implications?

Box 4-1	• Stop smoking.

Client and Family Education for Peripheral Arterial Disease

- Stop smoking.
- Lose weight and eat a low-fat diet.
- Avoid crossing legs while sitting.
- Elevate feet at rest, but not above heart level.
- Do not stand or sit for long periods of time.
- Do not wear restrictive clothing.
- Keep affected extremity warm but never apply direct heat.
- Inspect feet daily and keep them clean and dry.
- Avoid walking barefoot; wear properly fitting shoes.
- Avoid mechanical or thermal injury to the legs and feet.
- Begin and maintain an exercise and walking program.
- Notify health care provider of any changes in color, sensation, temperature, or pulses in extremities.

H. **Expected outcomes**: client has improved peripheral tissue perfusion (manifested by palpable or audible pedal pulses and absence of claudication), absence of arterial ulcers, and improved activity tolerance

VI. ARTERIAL EMBOLISM

A. **Description**: arterial emboli usually arise from thrombi that develop in heart as a result of atrial fibrillation, myocardial infarction (MI), prosthetic valves, or HF

B. **Etiology and pathophysiology**
   1. Thrombi become detached and are carried from left side of heart into arterial system where they may lodge and cause obstruction
   2. Symptoms may be abrupt and depend on size and location of embolus
   3. Ischemia will progress to necrosis and gangrene within hours

C. **Assessment: the "six Ps"**
   1. Pain
   2. Pallor (pale color)
   3. Polar (cool temperature of skin)
   4. Pulselessness (diminished or absent pulses)
   5. Parasthesias (altered local sensation)
   6. Paralysis (weakness or inability to move extremity)

D. **Priority nursing problems**: reduced perfusion to peripheral tissues, pain

E. **Planning and implementation**
   1. Assess peripheral pulses and neurovascular status every 2–4 hours
   2. Place affected extremity in a neutral position with no restrictive bedding or clothing; keep extremity warm
   3. Assess level of pain using a 0 to 10 scale
   4. Change position every 2 hours to increase or improve collateral circulation
   5. Assess for and report unusual bleeding from anticoagulant therapy
   6. Monitor lab values, including APTT, PT, and INR levels
   7. If necrosis is present, surgical treatment is required; an emergency embolectomy needs to be performed within 4–5 hours of embolism to prevent necrosis and permanent damage to extremity

F. **Medication therapy (if no necrosis present)**: thrombolytic therapy with streptokinase, t-PA or heparin; warfarin therapy at home

G. **Client education**
   1. Pre- and postoperative teaching if embolectomy is performed
   2. Measures to promote peripheral circulation and maintain tissue integrity (see Box 4-1 again)

H. **Expected outcomes**
1. Strong bilateral peripheral pulses
2. No tissue damage or necrosis
3. Therapeutic lab values for anticoagulant therapy within normal limits
   a. If on warfarin: monitor INR value (normal 0.75–1.25; therapeutic 2–3)
   b. If on heparin: monitor PTT value (therapeutic value 1.5–2.5 times the control)

VII. BUERGER'S DISEASE (THROMBOANGIITIS OBLITERANS)

A. **Description**: an inflammatory disease of small- and medium-sized veins and arteries accompanied by thrombi and sometimes vasospasm of arterial segments; may occur in upper or lower extremities but is most common in leg or foot

B. **Etiology and pathophysiology**
1. Cause of Buerger's disease is unknown, but since it occurs mostly in young men who smoke, it is currently thought to be a reaction to something in cigarettes and/or to have a genetic or autoimmune component
2. Inflammation occurs; microthrombi form; these can lead to vasospasm and this process ultimately obstructs blood flow

C. **Assessment**
1. Initial signs and symptoms are usually a bluish discoloration to a toe or finger and a feeling of coldness in affected limb
2. Since nerves are also inflamed, there may be severe pain and constriction of small blood vessels controlled by them; rest pain is common
3. Overactive sympathetic nerves also may cause feet to sweat excessively, even though they feel cold
4. As blood vessels become blocked, intermittent claudication and other symptoms similar to those of chronic obstructive arterial disease often appear
5. Ischemic ulcers and gangrene are common complications of progressive Buerger's disease

D. **Priority nursing problems**: reduced perfusion to peripheral tissues, pain

E. **Planning and implementation**
1. Arrest progress of disease by smoking cessation
2. Take measures to promote vasodilation (similar to other arterial disorders)
3. Provide for pain relief
4. Provide emotional support

F. **Medication therapy**: analgesic pain medications, calcium channel blockers to reduce vasospasm, pentoxifylline (Trental) to reduce blood viscosity

G. **Client education**
1. Stop smoking
2. Take measures to promote peripheral circulation and maintain tissue integrity (see again Box 4-1)

H. **Expected outcomes**: absence of ulcers and/or impaired skin integrity; pain is relieved; smoking cessation achieved

VIII. RAYNAUD'S DISEASE

A. **Description**: localized, intermittent episodes of vasoconstriction of small arteries of hands and less commonly feet, causing color and temperature changes

B. **Etiology and pathophysiology**
1. A vasospastic disorder of unknown origin that primarily affects young women
2. Vasospastic attacks tend to be bilateral and manifestations usually begin at tips of digits causing pallor, numbness, and a sensation of cold
3. Attacks are triggered by exposure to cold, emotional stress, caffeine, and tobacco use

Practice to Pass

Acute arterial occlusion may be caused by a thrombus or an embolus. What is the difference between the 2 causes? Are there any differences in treatment?

C. **Assessment**
   1. Symptoms usually appear in hands after exposure to cold and/or stress; are bilateral and symmetrical
   2. Classic triphasic color changes (pallor, cyanosis, and rubor) in hands with accompanying reduction in skin temperature
   3. Intensity of pain increases as disease progresses
   4. Skin of fingertips may thicken and nails may become brittle
D. **Priority nursing problems**: reduced perfusion to peripheral tissues, pain
E. **Planning and implementation**
   1. Keep hands warm and free from injury
   2. Avoid stressful situations
   3. In severe cases, a **sympathectomy** (surgical dissection of nerve fibers that allows vasoconstriction to occur) may be performed to relieve symptoms associated with vasospasm
   4. Encourage regular health checks to monitor for coexisting autoimmune illness (commonly occurs with this condition)
F. **Medication therapy**
   1. Analgesics for pain
   2. Vasodilators may provide some relief of symptoms, as well as vascular smooth muscle relaxants and calcium channel blockers
G. **Client education**
   1. Keep hands warm: wear gloves when out of doors, in air-conditioned environments, or when handling cold food
   2. Avoid injury to hands
   3. Lifestyle changes: stop smoking; employ stress relief, such as biofeedback
H. **Expected outcomes**: decrease in or absence of attacks; no injury to hands and/or wounds heal quickly

IX. AORTIC ANEURYSM

A. **Description**: a localized dilation or outpouching of a weakened area in aorta that is classified by region (thoracic or abdominal), size, and as dissecting or nondissecting
B. **Etiology and pathophysiology**
   1. Aorta is particularly susceptible to aneurysm formation because of constant stress on vessel wall; incidence increases with age
   2. Most aneurysms are found in abdominal aorta below level of renal arteries
   3. Growth rate of an aneurysm is unpredictable
   4. Half of all aneurysms larger than 6 cm in size will rupture within 1 year
   5. Major risk factor is atherosclerosis
   6. Major complication is death from internal bleeding
C. **Assessment**
   1. Thoracic aneurysms are often asymptomatic with the first indication being a rupture
      a. Symptoms may include pain in back, neck, and substernal area that may only occur when lying supine
      b. Client may experience dysphagia and dyspnea, stridor, or cough when aneurysm presses on esophagus or laryngeal nerve
   2. Abdominal aneurysms may also be asymptomatic until rupture
      a. Client may report a "heartbeat" in abdomen when lying down
      b. A pulsating abdominal mass may be present
      c. Moderate to severe abdominal or lumbar back pain may be present (severe pain may be a sign of impending rupture)
      d. Client may experience claudication

   e. Cool or cyanotic extremities may be noted
   f. Systolic bruit may be heard

 3. Dissecting aneurysms present with sudden, severe, and persistent pain described as "tearing" or "ripping" in anterior chest or back
   a. Pain may extend to shoulder, epigastric area, or abdomen
   b. Pallor, sweating, and tachycardia are present
   c. Initially client may have an elevated BP that may differ in each arm
   d. Possible syncope and/or paralysis of lower extremities may be present

D. Priority nursing problems: reduced perfusion to peripheral tissues, pain, fear

E. Planning and implementation
   1. Diagnostic tests that may be ordered include chest x-ray, transesophageal echocardiography, aortography, ultrasound, CT scan, and MRI
   2. Overall goals for a client with an aneurysm include the following:
      a. Normal tissue perfusion
      b. Intact motor and neurologic function
      c. Reduction in anxiety
      d. No complications of surgical repair
   3. Surgical care
      a. Surgery may be performed on an emergency or elective basis (surgery not usually performed on aneurysms less than 4–5 cm in size)
      b. Emergency surgery is the only treatment option for a ruptured aneurysm
      c. Development of hematoma in scrotum, perineum, flank, or penis indicates retro-peritoneal rupture
      d. Once aorta ruptures anteriorly into peritoneal cavity, death is almost certain
      e. Surgical technique involves excision of aneurysm with replacement of excised segment with a graft
      f. Preoperatively, nurse marks and assesses all peripheral pulses for comparison postoperatively
      g. Postoperatively, nurse assesses for complications, which may include:
         1) Graft occlusion
         2) Hypovolemia/renal impairment
         3) Respiratory distress
         4) Cardiac dysrhythmias
         5) Paralytic ileus
         6) Musculoskeletal paralysis

F. Medication therapy
   1. Goal of nonsurgical management is to maintain BP at a normal level to reduce risk of rupture; antihypertensives and diuretics may be prescribed
   2. Pulsatile flow may be reduced by drugs that reduce cardiac contractility
   3. Postoperatively, clients will be placed on heparin (Liquaemin) or enoxaparin (Lovenox) for anticoagulation while hospitalized and warfarin (Coumadin) when discharged to home

G. Client education
   1. Encourage clients who do not undergo operative repair to have routine physical exams to monitor status of aneurysm
   2. Teach signs and symptoms of impending rupture (as previously described)
   3. Teach client to self-monitor BP and report any increases immediately
   4. Prepare client to self-manage anticoagulant therapy (see Box 4-2)
   5. For operative clients, teach routine perioperative care
      a. Reinforce compliance with prophylactic antibiotics for clients who will receive graft; may also require this before invasive procedures
      b. Monitor incision site for bleeding or infection

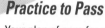
Practice to Pass

Your plan of care for a client postrepair of an aortic aneurysm includes monitoring the graft site and preventing hypovolemic or hemorrhagic shock. What specifically will be included in your plan of care?

Box 4-2	
Client and Family Education for Anticoagulant Therapy	• Wear a medical identification bracelet. • Take medication at approximately the same time each day. • Stress the importance of routine lab work. • Do not use aspirin-containing products or nonsteroidal anti-inflammatory drugs (NSAIDs). • Do not take herbal medicines without recommendation by the clinician. • Avoid trauma. • Shave with an electric razor. • Use a soft toothbrush. • Report possible adverse side effects immediately to health care provider: • Any bleeding that does not stop within several minutes • Unusual bleeding from gums, skin, vagina, rectum, or nose • Weakness or dizziness

        c. Assess neurovascular status of extremities and presence of pulses

        d. Include restrictions on lifting, limited for 4–6 weeks after surgery (no heavy lifting at all)

   H. Expected outcomes: client has normal tissue perfusion; aneurysm does not rupture; surgical clients are free of postoperative complications and maintain normal tissue perfusion after surgical grafting

X. THROMBOPHLEBITIS

   A. Description: formation of a thrombus (clot) in association with inflammation of vein; classified as superficial or deep

   B. Etiology and pathophysiology

     1. Etiology: Virchow's triad (at least 2 of 3 present for thrombosis to occur)

       a. Stasis of venous flow

       b. Damage to inner lining of vein (endothelial layer)

       c. Hypercoagulability of blood

     2. Pathophysiology

       a. RBCs, WBCs, and platelets adhere to form a thrombus (usually in valve cusps of veins)

       b. As thrombus enlarges it eventually occludes lumen of vein

       c. If only partial occlusion of vein occurs, blood flow continues and thrombotic process stops; if detachment does not occur, it will become firmly organized and attached within 24–48 hours

       d. If detachment occurs, emboli form which generally flow through venous system, back to the cardiopulmonary circulation

   C. Assessment

     1. Subjective: history of thrombophlebitis, pelvic/abdominal surgery, obesity, neoplasm (hepatic and pancreatic), congestive heart failure (CHF), atrial fibrillation, prolonged immobility, MI, pregnancy and/or postpartum period, IV therapy, hypercoagulable states (polycythemia, dehydration/malnutrition)

     2. Objective: signs vary according to thrombus size, location, and adequacy of collateral circulation

       a. Superficial

         1) Palpable, firm, subcutaneous, cordlike vein

         2) Surrounding area warm, red, tender to touch

         3) Edema may or may not be present

         4) Most common cause in arms is IV therapy; in legs it is often related to varicose veins

Practice to Pass

The wife of a 57-year-old client admitted for thrombophlebitis rushes into the hall stating, "My husband can't breathe. It happened all of a sudden." On assessment, the client is experiencing severe dyspnea, tachycardia, and chest pain. What is occurring? What nursing actions should be implemented?

   b. Deep

   1) Unilateral edema
   2) Pain
   3) Warm skin and elevated temperature
   4) If inferior vena cava is involved, both legs will be edematous
   5) If superior vena cava is involved, both upper extremities, neck, back, and face may become edematous or cyanotic
   6) If calf is involved, **Homan's sign** may be present (pain when client dorsiflexes own foot, especially when leg is raised)
3. Diagnostic studies
   a. Venous duplex scanning
   b. Doppler ultrasonic flowmeter
   c. D-dimer, a product of fibrin degradation, indicates fibrinolysis (that occurs as a reaction to thrombosis)
   d. Venography and plethysmography, former "gold standards" for diagnosis, are rarely used today
   e. MRI
   f. Lung scan
D. Priority nursing problems: pain, reduced perfusion to peripheral tissues, risk for interrupted skin integrity
E. Planning and implementation
   1. Educate client about diagnostic tests that may be performed
   2. Provide for relief of pain: assess pain on a scale of 0 to 10 and provide analgesics as prescribed

   3. Decrease edema
      a. Apply warm, moist compresses, intermittent or continuous, to affected extremity
      b. Elevating affected leg above heart level to promote venous drainage
      c. Measure and monitor leg or arm circumference when edema is present
      d. Monitor status of peripheral pulses
   4. Prevent skin ulceration
      a. Keep bed covers from touching affected limb by using an overbed cradle
      b. Do not allow use of restrictive clothing
   5. Prevent pulmonary emboli

      a. Maintain strict bedrest, usually enforced until anticoagulant therapy is therapeutic
      b. Never massage affected extremity
      c. Instruct client to report any pink-tinged sputum and monitor for tachypnea, tachycardia, shortness of breath, chest pain, and apprehension, which may indicate a pulmonary embolism
      d. Prepare client for vena cava filter (Greenfield filter) placement
F. Medication therapy
   1. Anticoagulant therapy
      a. Inhibits clotting factors that would extend thrombus formation
      b. Will not induce thrombolysis but prevents clot extension
      c. Heparin: intravenously or subcutaneous while hospitalized
      d. Warfarin: home therapy for 2–4 months
   2. Thrombolytics
      a. Dissolve blood clots by imitating natural enzymatic processes
      b. Approved drugs include streptokinase (Streptase) and alteplase (Activase)
      c. Are usually effective in less than 72 hours
      d. Higher risk for hemorrhage exists than when using heparin therapy
   3. Analgesics: NSAIDs are usually prescribed to reduce pain and relieve inflammation
   4. Stool softeners are usually prescribed for clients on anticoagulants to prevent constipation

G. Client education
1. Prevention
   a. Early ambulation postoperatively
   b. Use of compression stockings or sequential compression device
   c. Low-dose anticoagulant therapy
   d. Avoid prolonged standing or sitting; avoid sitting with crossed legs
   e. Avoid restrictive clothing
   f. Stop smoking
2. Provide education about anticoagulant therapy (see Box 4-2)

H. Expected outcome: free of pain, edema, or tenderness; skin integrity is intact; is free of embolus

XI. VENOUS INSUFFICIENCY

A. Description: inadequate venous return over a long period of time that causes pathologic changes from ischemia in vasculature, skin, and supporting tissues

B. Etiology and pathophysiology
1. Venous insufficiency occurs after prolonged venous hypertension, which stretches veins and damages valves, preventing blood return
2. Venous insufficiency also occurs after thrombus formation or when valves are not functioning correctly, which may result from:
   a. Prolonged standing or sitting (teachers, waitresses, health care personnel, office workers)
   b. Pregnancy and obesity
3. With time, stasis results in edema of lower limbs, discoloration to skin of legs and feet, and venous stasis ulceration

C. Assessment
1. Subjective
   a. Past history of thrombophlebitis, hypertension, varicosities, or diabetes mellitus
   b. Past history of long periods of sitting and/or standing
2. Objective
   a. Edema of lower legs, may extend to knee
   b. Thick, coarse, brownish skin around ankles ("gaiter" area) and feet
   c. Stasis ulcers, usually in malleolar area (ruddy base, uneven edges)
3. See Table 4-2 for a general comparison of manifestations of arterial and venous disorders

Table 4-2 **Comparison of Arterial and Venous Vascular Disease**

Assessment	Arterial Disease	Venous Disease
Color	Pale	Ruddy; cyanotic if dependent
Edema	None or minimal	Usually present
Nails	Thick and brittle	Normal
Pain	Worse with elevation and exercise; may be sudden or severe; rest pain; claudication	Better with elevation; positive Homan's sign, dullness or heaviness or aching pain that increases throughout day
Pulses	Decreased, weak, or absent	Normal
Temperature of extremity	Cool	Warm
Ulcers	Dry and necrotic	Moist; malleolar

   D. Priority nursing problems: interrupted skin integrity, potential for infection, body image alterations, reduced tissue perfusion
   E. Planning and implementation
   1. Increase venous blood return, decrease venous pressure
       a. Bed rest
       b. Keep legs elevated above heart level
       c. Avoid long periods of standing
       d. Wear elastic support or compression stockings
           1) Apply stockings *before* getting out of bed and placing leg in a dependent position
           2) Wear stockings during day and evening; remove at night
           3) Never push stockings down around leg—they will further impair circulation
           4) Handwash stockings daily and air dry; machine washing or drying will damage elastic fibers
   2. Treat venous stasis ulcer(s)
       a. Open lesions are typically treated with a hydrocolloid dressing and compression wraps; a topical ointment, such as low-dose hydrocortisone, zinc oxide, or an antifungal may also be indicated
       b. Ulcers may be treated with an Unna Boot or other compression wrap that is changed every 1–2 weeks and is usually applied over a base dressing
       c. Severe ulcers may need surgical debridement
   F. Medication therapy
   1. Topical agents to skin ulcers, such as hydrocortisone, antifungals, or zinc oxide, may be prescribed
   2. Oral or IV antibiotics may be prescribed when ulcers become infected or cellulitis occurs
   3. Sclerosing agents (called sclerotherapy) may be used to occlude blood flow in a small vein, causing disappearance of varicosity; this may be followed up with use of compression bandage for a short period of time
   G. Client education
   1. Elevate legs for at least 20 minutes 4 times a day
   2. Keep legs above heart level when in bed
   3. Avoid prolonged sitting or standing
   4. Do not cross legs when sitting
   5. Do not wear tight, restrictive pants, socks, or boots; avoid girdles and garters that restrict circulation in the upper leg
   6. Wear support stockings as instructed above
   H. Expected outcomes: reduced edema and healing or prevention of stasis ulcers

XII. VARICOSE VEINS

   A. Description: a vein or veins in which blood has pooled, producing distended, tortuous, and palpable vessels
   B. Etiology and pathophysiology
   1. Worldwide, 1 in 5 people will develop varicosities
   2. Risk factors include being a woman over age 35 years, obesity, positive family history of varicosities, and prolonged standing over long periods of time
   3. Varicose veins may develop after trauma or damage to a vein or valve or from gradual venous distension, which diminishes action of calf muscle as a pump, and increases pull of gravity on blood within legs

    4. As vein swells, increased hydrostatic pressure pushes plasma through stretched vessel walls and edema of surrounding tissue may occur

C. Assessment

    1. Subjective: client may report aching, heaviness, tightness, itching, swelling and an unsightly appearance to leg(s)

    2. Objective

        a. Dilated, tortuous superficial veins will be seen along upper and lower leg

        b. Superficial inflammation may develop along path of varicose vein

        c. Positive Trendelenburg test (done to evaluate valve competence)

            1) Client is placed in a supine position with elevated legs

            2) As client sits up, veins would normally fill from distal end

            3) If there are varicosities, veins fill from proximal end

D. Priority nursing problems: pain, reduced perfusion to peripheral tissues, risk for interrupted skin integrity

E. Planning and implementation

    1. Assess pain on a scale of 0 to 10 and provide analgesics as needed for pain relief

    2. Improve venous circulation

        a. Assess pulses and neurovascular status of lower extremities

        b. Apply support stockings and teach client how to use

        c. Instruct to avoid prolonged sitting and standing and never cross legs; encourage walking

        d. Have client elevate feet above heart level when lying down

    3. Prevent skin breakdown; teach proper skin care and importance of avoiding trauma to legs

    4. Teach preoperative and postoperative care if surgery is chosen

        a. Sclerotherapy involves injecting a sclerosing agent into varicosed vein, usually in physician's office

            1) Procedure is palliative but not curative

            2) Elastic bandages may need to be worn for up to 6 weeks

        b. Vein ligation surgery involves ligation (tying off) of entire vein (usually saphenous) and dissection and removal of incompetent tributaries

            1) Perform hourly circulation checks postoperatively

            2) Elevate extremity to a 15-degree angle to prevent stasis and edema

            3) Apply compression gradient stockings from foot to groin

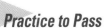

Practice to Pass

A 53-year-old teacher is seen in the ambulatory care center with complaints of leg pain from varicose veins. She asks you why the varicosities cause pain. How do you respond?

F. Medication therapy: possible low dose aspirin therapy to reduce platelet aggregation and subsequent clot development

G. Client education: prevention

    1. Avoid sitting or standing for long periods

    2. Change position often

    3. Avoid constrictive clothing or shoes

    4. Elevate legs when sitting to promote venous return

    5. Maintain ideal body weight

H. Expected outcomes: relief of discomfort; improved circulation; avoidance of complications such as thrombophlebitis and ulcerations

Case Study

Mr. B. comes into the community health clinic with a large, weeping ulcer on the malleolus of the right foot that he claims is not painful. He has 2+ edema in both feet. Vital signs are within normal limits. Lab results are remarkable for a WBC of 12,300/mm³. He states that his occupation is a collector in a tollbooth, he stands most of the time, and he reports often working 10- and 12-hour shifts. He denies taking any medication other than an occasional acetaminophen (Tylenol) for headache.

1. What is the likely cause of the ulcer on Mr. B.'s foot?

2. What are the usual signs and symptoms for this disorder?

3. State three nursing diagnoses appropriate for this client.

4. What are the primary nursing interventions?

5. On Mr. B.'s followup appointment in 2 months, what would you look for to evaluate your nursing care?

For suggested responses, see page 622.

POSTTEST

❶ The nurse is performing an assessment on a 50-year-old male cashier at a local store, who often stands 6 to 8 hours at a time. The nurse should inspect the client for which of the following?

1. Delayed capillary refill
2. Buerger's disease
3. Varicose veins
4. Aneurysms

❷ The nurse is conducting a screening clinic for hypertension in the community. The nurse should pay particular attention to the blood pressure of which client?

1. Caucasian, adult female
2. Hispanic adult male
3. Asian adult male
4. African American adult male

❸ When assessing an older adult client, the nurse determines the capillary refill time to be 5 seconds. The nurse determines the client may be experiencing which of the following?

1. Normal signs of aging
2. Impending stroke
3. Decreased cardiac output
4. Hypokalemia

❹ The nurse is caring for a client who has just returned from the cardiac catheterization laboratory following a percutaneous transluminal coronary angioplasty (PTCA). Which of the following problems is a priority during the *immediate* postprocedure care of this client?

1. Impaired Tissue Perfusion: Cardiac related to presence of atherosclerotic plaque
2. Potential for Internal Hemorrhage related to sodium warfarin (Coumadin) therapy
3. Alteration in INR related to aspirin therapy
4. Potential Complication: Chest Pain related to coronary artery spasm/reocclusion

❺ The nurse is caring for a client diagnosed with hypertension. The nurse concludes that which outcomes indicate successful treatment for this client? Select all that apply.

1. End-organ damage has not developed
2. Return of blood pressure to within normal range
3. No further increase in blood pressure
4. Compliance with medication management
5. Stable systolic blood pressure of 140 mmHg

6 A hypertensive client taking spironolactone (Aldactone) reports onset of diarrhea and stomach cramping. The cardiac monitor shows tall, tented T waves. The nurse suspects which drug-related electrolyte imbalance?

1. Hyponatremia
2. Hypercalcemia
3. Hyperkalemia
4. Hypernatremia

7 The nurse explains to a client that the goal of anticoagulant therapy in a client with a deep vein thrombosis is to do which of the following? Select all that apply.

1. Prevent additional thrombus formation.
2. Dissolve the clot.
3. Allow immediate ambulation.
4. Prevent infection.
5. Interfere with enlargement of existing clot.

8 A client reports leg pain and cramping after short periods of walking that stop when he rests. The nurse concludes that this client's manifestations are consistent with which of the following?

1. Arterial-venous shunting
2. Phlebitis
3. Intermittent claudication
4. Raynaud's disease

9 The nurse anticipates that which medication is likely to be prescribed on a daily basis to a newly hospitalized client with a history of peripheral arterial disease?

1. Acetaminophen (Tylenol)
2. Ibuprofen (Motrin)
3. Aspirin
4. Heparin

10 Which client statement would indicate a positive outcome of discharge teaching for a client newly diagnosed with chronic arterial occlusive disease?

1. "I will keep my feet elevated above the level of my heart when I sleep."
2. "I will wear my compression stockings when awake."
3. "I will keep walking even when I feel pain in my legs to increase circulation."
4. "I will check the temperature of my bathwater with my hands before getting into the water."

➤ *See pages 139–141 for Answers and Rationales.*

ANSWERS & RATIONALES

Pretest

1 Answer: 4 Rationale: Blood pressure should be consistently below 140/90. Lifestyle modification is used in all hypertensive clients with or without medication therapy. Even though the client will be encouraged to continue lifestyle modifications, if they are not effective in lowering the blood pressure after 6 months, antihypertensive medications are begun. **Cognitive Level:** Applying **Client Need:** Physiological Adaptation **Integrated Process:** Communication and Documentation **Content Area:** Adult Health **Strategy:** To answer this question, recall recommended blood pressure readings as well as the protocol for managing hypertension. If nonpharmacologic interventions are going to be effective, it will be evident within the 6 months reported by the client in this question. **Reference:** LeMone, P., Burke, K., &

Bauldoff, G. (2011). *Medical-surgical nursing: Critical thinking in patient care* (5th ed.). Upper Saddle River, NJ: Pearson Education, pp. 1022–1024.

2 Answer: 1 Rationale: The pain of arterial occlusive disease is related to a reduction in blood flow, which causes tissue hypoxia, specifically in the muscle. When treatment is effective, the blood supply is increased and the client's ischemic pain is reduced. Reduced sensation, increased rubor, and hair loss on the extremity are additional manifestations of peripheral arterial disease. **Cognitive Level:** Applying **Client Need:** Physiological Adaptation **Integrated Process:** Nursing Process: Evaluation **Content Area:** Adult Health **Strategy:** Successful interventions achieve desired outcomes. A desired outcome is typically a return as close as possible to the pre-illness level of functioning. Differentiate the answer choices that

...ns.

...2011).

...tient care

...ducation,

...4 Peripheral Vascular Disorders

137

...blocking agent

...a blocker, which

...nervous system

...cts the periphery,

...ult, a potential side

...ta-blocking effect on the

...rather than raising it.

...t of therapy with some of the
calciu... ...s, while hypokalemia may occur
with some... ...increases risk of digitalis toxicity.
Cognitive Level: ...ng **Client Need:** Pharmacological and
Parenteral Therapies **Integrated Process:** Nursing Process:
Planning **Content Area:** Pharmacology **Strategy:** Recall that
propranolol belongs to the drug class of beta-adrenergic
blockers, which interrupt the effects of the sympathetic
nervous system (SNS). Then systematically evaluate
each option looking for one that would be the opposite
of SNS stimulation as the answer to the question.
Reference: LeMone, P., Burke, K., & Bauldoff, G. (2011).
Medical-surgical nursing: Critical thinking in patient care
(5th ed.). Upper Saddle River, NJ: Pearson Education,
pp. 1025–1026.

4 **Answer: 4** **Rationale:** Clients with pelvic or abdominal
procedures are at an increased risk of developing deep
vein thrombosis (DVT). Unilateral edema and calf pain
are signs that are consistent with DVT and must be
reported immediately so treatment can begin to prevent
pulmonary embolus. It is not uncommon for a client to
have absent or decreased bowel sounds for the first or
second postoperative day. This is related to the
anesthesia and inactivity and typically will resolve as
activity levels increase. Abdominal distention is also
common initially following abdominal surgery and will
resolve as the client increases activity and passes flatus.
It is not uncommon for a client to have difficult voiding
immediately after a catheter is removed. As the volume
of urine in the bladder increases and pressure is exerted
on the urinary meatus, the urge to void returns. The
client has 6 to 8 hours to void following a catheter
removal. **Cognitive Level:** Analyzing **Client Need:** Reduction
of Risk Potential **Integrated Process:** Nursing Process:
Assessment **Content Area:** Fundamentals **Strategy:** Review
the care of the postoperative client. Differentiate what is to
be expected (or normal) during the first 24 hours after
surgery from what is an abnormal finding. Then reason
that unexpected findings need to be reported. **Reference:**
LeMone, P., Burke, K., & Bauldoff, G. (2011).
Medical-surgical nursing: Critical thinking in patient care
(5th ed.). Upper Saddle River, NJ: Pearson Education,
pp. 1050–1051.

5 **Answer: 4** **Rationale:** Furosemide is a loop diuretic that
wastes potassium. Thus, the client needs to increase

intake of potassium in the daily diet. Orange juice is an
excellent source of potassium. Tea that is not decaffeinated
can adversely elevate blood pressure and contributes no
vital nutrients. Milk is high in sodium. Cranberry juice is
not as high in potassium as orange juice and would be
helpful for clients who need to acidify the urine. **Cognitive
Level:** Applying **Client Need:** Pharmacological and Parenteral Therapies **Integrated Process:** Teaching and Learning
Content Area: Pharmacology **Strategy:** Two areas of information need to be understood to respond to this question:
the common side effects of furosemide and foods high
in potassium. Consider that the correct option must
replace the electrolyte lost in the urine to choose
correctly. **Reference:** LeMone, P., Burke, K., & Bauldoff, G.
(2011). *Medical-surgical nursing: Critical thinking in
patient care* (5th ed.). Upper Saddle River, NJ: Pearson
Education, pp. 1050–1051.

6 **Answer: 1** **Rationale:** The primary symptom of a dissecting aneurysm is sudden, severe pain commonly located
in the back. This is an emergency, and the client must be
taken to surgery immediately as a life-saving measure,
not continue to be observed. Hoarseness and dysphagia
may be present with an aneurysm but are not indicative
of dissection. Comfort measures for this client will not
relieve the pain. **Cognitive Level:** Analyzing **Client Need:**
Reduction of Risk Potential **Integrated Process:** Nursing
Process: Implementation **Content Area:** Adult Health
Strategy: The critical words in the question are *back pain*.
Recall the risks associated with abdominal aortic
aneurysm (AAA), and the classic manifestations of
those risks, to make the appropriate selection.
Reference: LeMone, P., Burke, K., & Bauldoff, G. (2011).
Medical-surgical nursing: Critical thinking in patient care
(5th ed.). Upper Saddle River, NJ: Pearson Education,
p. 1036.

7 **Answer: 2** **Rationale:** Anticoagulants, such as intravenous
heparin, are given to prevent clot extension and reduce
the risk of subsequent pulmonary embolism. The dosage
is adjusted to maintain the activated partial thromboplastin time (aPTT) at approximately twice the control
or normal value which is approximately 25 to 39 seconds.
An aPTT of 150 is well over this limit and should be
reported to the health care provider immediately. The
prothrombin time and International Normalized Ratio
are tests used to monitor warfarin (Coumadin) therapy.
A platelet count of 150,000 is within normal limits.
Cognitive Level: Applying **Client Need:** Reduction of Risk
Potential **Integrated Process:** Nursing Process: Implementation **Content Area:** Pharmacology **Strategy:** Review the
indications and therapeutic effects of heparin as well as
the recommended dosing protocol to monitor therapeutic
effect. **Reference:** LeMone, P., Burke, K., & Bauldoff, G.
(2011). *Medical-surgical nursing: Critical thinking in
patient care* (5th ed.). Upper Saddle River, NJ: Pearson
Education, pp. 1052–1053.

8 **Answer: 2, 3** **Rationale:** The 60-year-old client has a very
high likelihood of prolonged immobility, which

increases his risk for deep vein thrombosis (DVT). Because of the unknown past medical history and need for imminent surgical intervention, the risk is compounded, and the filter may be inserted to prevent pulmonary embolism (PE). The filter inserted in the inferior vena cava will trap emboli that travel from the legs before they can cause PE. The 54-year-old is at risk for a DVT and subsequent PE because of a previous history of DVT. The new onset acute respiratory distress syndrome (ARDS) indicates a probable lengthy hospitalization so the filter may be inserted prophylactically. The other clients are not as at great risk for DVT and would not benefit from prophylactic filter insertion. Although pregnancy is a risk factor for deep venous thrombosis, it is usually managed with less invasive measures. **Cognitive Level:** Analyzing **Client Need:** Physiological Adaptation **Integrated Process:** Nursing Process: Implementation **Content Area:** Adult Health **Strategy:** Select answer choices where the client is at risk for the development of deep vein thrombosis (DVT). Use knowledge of pathophysiology and complications as you use the process of elimination in evaluating each option. **Reference:** LeMone, P., Burke, K., & Bauldoff, G. (2011). *Medical-surgical nursing: Critical thinking in patient care* (5th ed.). Upper Saddle River, NJ: Pearson Education, pp. 1050–1054.

9 **Answer: 1 Rationale:** Bumetanide (Bumex) is a diuretic and enalapril is an antihypertensive of the angiotensin-converting enzyme (ACE) inhibitor type. Clients being treated with these drugs are at risk for orthostatic hypotension when they change position too rapidly. This could lead to dizziness and possible falls and injury. Taking the blood pressure in both arms is a nursing intervention and not a discharge instruction for the client. The nurse should take the blood pressure while the client is sitting, lying, and standing to determine if orthostatic hypotension is present. There is no evidence that the client is taking nitroglycerine. **Cognitive Level:** Analyzing **Client Need:** Pharmacological and Parenteral Therapies **Integrated Process:** Teaching and Learning **Content Area:** Pharmacology **Strategy:** Review the mechanism of action for both angiotensin-converting enzyme (ACE) inhibitors such as enalapril (Prinivil) and diuretics such as bumetanide (Bumex). Compare those actions with the common side effects of each drug. Integrate this information and focus teaching on how to avoid the combined or augmented effects. **Reference:** LeMone, P., Burke, K., & Bauldoff, G. (2011). *Medical-surgical nursing: Critical thinking in patient care* (5th ed.). Upper Saddle River, NJ: Pearson Education, p. 1025.

10 **Answer: 1, 5 Rationale:** A common complication of hypertensive disease is target organ disease, including retinal damage to the eye. The appearance of the retina can provide important information about the severity of the hypertensive process. Monitoring of the blood pressure annually is insufficient in the client being treated for hypertension. Clients with diabetes (not hypertension) need to avoid foods high in concentrated sugars. The antihypertensive medications need to be taken every day even when the blood pressure is under control. Regular exercise is a lifestyle modification that may help in controlling blood pressure in addition to diet and medication. **Cognitive Level:** Applying **Client Need:** Physiological Adaptation **Integrated Process:** Nursing Process: Implementation **Content Area:** Adult Health **Strategy:** Eliminate all answer choices that are not directly related to hypertension. Keep in mind the implications of hypertension on multiple body systems and the dynamic nature of the disease to aid in eliminating the other answer choices. **Reference:** LeMone, P., Burke, K., & Bauldoff, G. (2011). *Medical-surgical nursing: Critical thinking in patient care* (5th ed.). Upper Saddle River, NJ: Pearson Education, pp. 1020–1021, 1030–1032.

Posttest

1 **Answer: 3 Rationale:** A major risk factor for varicose veins is standing in one place for long periods of time. Delayed capillary refill and aneurysms both reflect the arterial system and are unrelated to standing in one position. Buerger's disease affects arteries and veins, but smoking is the major risk factor for this disorder, which tends to affect young adult males to a greater extent than others. **Cognitive Level:** Applying **Client Need:** Health Promotion and Maintenance **Integrated Process:** Nursing Process: Assessment **Content Area:** Adult Health **Strategy:** Eliminate options that are arterial in nature as this is a high-pressure system. This question is related to the man standing for extended periods of time and therefore is about the low-pressure venous system. **Reference:** LeMone, P., Burke, K., & Bauldoff, G. (2011). *Medical-surgical nursing: Critical thinking in patient care* (5th ed.). Upper Saddle River, NJ: Pearson Education, p. 1060.

2 **Answer: 4 Rationale:** Primary or essential hypertension is more common in African Americans than in people of other ethnic backgrounds. For this reason, this client should be carefully evaluated. **Cognitive Level:** Applying **Client Need:** Health Promotion and Maintenance **Integrated Process:** Nursing Process: Assessment **Content Area:** Adult Health **Strategy:** This question is asking for identification of the population at highest risk for hypertension. Specific knowledge is needed to make a selection, so review this information now if you have the need. **Reference:** LeMone, P., Burke, K., & Bauldoff, G. (2011). *Medical-surgical nursing: Critical thinking in patient care* (5th ed.). Upper Saddle River, NJ: Pearson Education, p. 1021.

3 **Answer: 3 Rationale:** Blanching of the nails for more than 3 seconds after release of pressure may indicate reduced arterial capillary perfusion, which may be an indication of decreased cardiac output. Changes in capillary refill time are not associated with normal changes of aging. Hypokalemia may cause prolongation of the cardiac cycle but does not affect capillary refill. A client with an impending stroke would be more likely to experience central nervous system alterations than cardiovascular symptoms. **Cognitive Level:** Analyzing **Client Need:** Health Promotion and Maintenance **Integrated Process:** Nursing Process: Assessment **Content Area:** Adult Health **Strategy:** This item requires knowledge of what capillary refill time represents and a normal finding. Memorize the number 3 as the time limit for capillary refill. **Reference:** LeMone, P., Burke, K., & Bauldoff, G. (2011). *Medical-surgical nursing: Critical thinking in patient care* (5th ed.). Upper Saddle River, NJ: Pearson Education, p. 258.

4 Answer: 4 Rationale: After percutaneous transluminal coronary angioplasty (PTCA), there is a risk for the blood vessel to go into spasm and/or to reocclude. If this happens, the client will experience chest pain and would be the priority for treatment. The atherosclerotic plaque is compressed against the intimal surface of the coronary artery during the PTCA and is therefore less likely to be directly responsible for decreased perfusion postprocedure. However, because of the continued risk for reocclusion, this problem could be considered to be second in importance. The client is on heparin immediately after the procedure, not sodium warfarin (Coumadin). Sodium warfarin would prolong the International Normalized Ratio (INR) rather than aspirin therapy. **Cognitive Level:** Analyzing **Client Need:** Reduction of Risk Potential **Integrated Process:** Nursing Process: Planning **Content Area:** Adult Health **Strategy:** Note the critical word *immediate* in the stem of the question. This question is related to the timing of specific complications and selected interventions. Eliminate answer options that are likely prior to the procedure or where the pharmacologic intervention is not appropriate. **Reference:** LeMone, P., Burke, K., & Bauldoff, G. (2011). *Medical-surgical nursing: Critical thinking in patient care* (5th ed.). Upper Saddle River, NJ: Pearson Education, p. 928.

5 Answer: 1, 2, 4 Rationale: Whether a client is managed with lifestyle modification or pharmacotherapy, successful treatment is the achievement of a normal blood pressure, compliance with medications, and prevention of end-organ damage. Both the systolic and diastolic blood pressures are relevant to the diagnosis and treatment of hypertension, with acceptable values being lower than 130/88. As long as the BP is elevated, the client is at risk for end-organ damage such as renal failure or ventricular hypertrophy. **Cognitive Level:** Applying **Client Need:** Physiological Adaptation **Integrated Process:** Nursing Process: Evaluation **Content Area:** Adult Health **Strategy:** Review the complications that occur with unmanaged hypertension. Select answer options that can prevent them. **Reference:** LeMone, P., Burke, K., & Bauldoff, G. (2011). *Medical-surgical nursing: Critical thinking in patient care* (5th ed.). Upper Saddle River, NJ: Pearson Education, p. 1020.

6 Answer: 3 Rationale: Spironolactone is a potassium-sparing diuretic. Hyperkalemia (potassium greater than 5.5 mEq/L) is a possible side effect and could lead to the manifestations that the client in the question is experiencing. Hyponatremia can result from excessive use of high ceiling diuretics. Hypercalcemia may occur with the use of thiazide diuretics. Hypernatremia is more likely to occur in dehydration than diuretic use. **Cognitive Level:** Analyzing **Client Need:** Pharmacological and Parenteral Therapies **Integrated Process:** Nursing Process: Diagnosis **Content Area:** Pharmacology **Strategy:** There are 2 content areas that must be known to correctly answer this item: the mechanism of action for spironolactone and manifestations of hyperkalemia. **Reference:** LeMone, P., Burke, K., & Bauldoff, G. (2011). *Medical-surgical nursing: Critical thinking in patient care* (5th ed.). Upper Saddle River, NJ: Pearson Education, p. 981.

7 Answer: 1, 5 Rationale: Anticoagulant therapy is used for deep vein thrombosis to prevent development of new clots or the enlargement of the existing clot. Heparin does not dissolve the clot; a thrombolytic must be given to achieve that effect. Even with anticoagulation, the client is maintained on bedrest to prevent embolization of a portion of the clot to the lungs. Heparin has no effect on infection because it is an anticoagulant rather than an anti-infective. **Cognitive Level:** Applying **Client Need:** Pharmacological and Parenteral Therapies **Integrated Process:** Nursing Process: Implementation **Content Area:** Pharmacology **Strategy:** This question is actually asking the mechanism of action for heparin. The presence of deep vein thrombosis provides a context but is additional but unnecessary data. Recall what heparin does in the body to make the correct selection. **Reference:** LeMone, P., Burke, K., & Bauldoff, G. (2011). *Medical-surgical nursing: Critical thinking in patient care* (5th ed.). Upper Saddle River, NJ: Pearson Education, p. 1052.

8 Answer: 3 Rationale: Intermittent claudication caused by muscle ischemia is a primary symptom of peripheral arterial disease. Pain occurs with activity but is relieved with rest. Raynaud's disease is associated with vasospasm, a functional disorder rather than a structural one. Phlebitis may cause pain, but it is unrelated to activity. Arterial venous shunting describes a joining of arterial and venous circulation. **Cognitive Level:** Applying **Client Need:** Physiological Adaptation **Integrated Process:** Nursing Process: Diagnosis **Content Area:** Adult Health **Strategy:** Eliminate any answer choices that imply venous disease. Among those that remain, compare and contrast the meaning of the option with the question. **Reference:** LeMone, P., Burke, K., & Bauldoff, G. (2011). *Medical-surgical nursing: Critical thinking in patient care* (5th ed.). Upper Saddle River, NJ: Pearson Education, p. 1040.

9 Answer: 3 Rationale: Aspirin prevents platelet aggregation, which is the first step in clot formation. Heparin is an anticoagulant that would be used following an angioplasty or while awaiting surgery in a client with advanced disease. Acetaminophen (Tylenol) and ibuprofen (Motrin) have no therapeutic benefit in arterial disease, although they are helpful as analgesics, and ibuprofen is a nonsteroidal anti-inflammatory agent (NSAID). **Cognitive Level:** Analyzing **Client Need:** Pharmacological and Parenteral Therapies **Integrated Process:** Nursing Process: Diagnosis **Content Area:** Pharmacology **Strategy:** Recall first the categories of the various drugs listed in the options. Eliminate all options that are unrelated to arterial circulation. Then examine the question again to determine the severity of the disease. **Reference:** LeMone, P., Burke, K., & Bauldoff, G. (2011). *Medical-surgical nursing: Critical thinking in patient care* (5th ed.). Upper Saddle River, NJ: Pearson Education, p. 1041.

10 **Answer: 4 Rationale:** Sensation in the feet may be diminished in clients with arterial occlusive disease.

Teach the client to check the bathwater with the hands to prevent the risk of a burn injury. The client should stop and rest when pain is experienced to relieve the ischemia. Elevating the feet and wearing compression stockings are useful treatments for venous disease to prevent or decrease venous stasis. **Cognitive Level:** Analyzing **Client Need:** Health Promotion and Maintenance **Integrated Process:** Nursing Process: Evaluation **Content Area:** Adult Health **Strategy:** The critical words in the question are *arterial occlusive disease*. Since the question is about arterial blood flow, eliminate any options that may compromise arterial flow or are related to venous disease. **Reference:** LeMone, P., Burke, K., & Bauldoff, G. (2011). *Medical-surgical nursing: Critical thinking in patient care* (5th ed.). Upper Saddle River, NJ: Pearson Education, pp. 1042–1043.

References

Berman, A., & Snyder, S. (2012). *Kozier & Erb's fundamentals of nursing: Concepts, process, and practice* (9th ed.). Upper Saddle River, NJ: Pearson Education.

D'Amico, D., & Barbarito, C. (2012). *Health & physical assessment in nursing* (2nd ed.). Upper Saddle River, NJ: Pearson Education, Inc.

Ignatavicius, D. D., & Workman, M. L. (2013). *Medical-surgical nursing: Critical thinking for collaborative care* (7th ed.) Philadelphia: W. B. Saunders Company.

Kee, J. L. (2010). *Laboratory and diagnostic tests* (8th ed.). Upper Saddle River, NJ: Pearson Education.

Lehne, R. (2010). *Pharmacology for nursing care* (7th ed.). St. Louis, MO: Saunders.

LeMone, P., Burke, K., & Bauldoff, G. (2011). *Medical-surgical nursing: Critical thinking in patient care* (5th ed.). Upper Saddle River, NJ: Pearson Education.

Lewis, S., Dirksen, S. Heitkemper, M., Bucher, L., & Camera, I. (2011). *Medical surgical nursing: Assessment and management of clinical problems* (8th ed.). St. Louis, MO: Elsevier.

McCance, K. L., & Huether, S. E. (2010). *Pathophysiology: The biologic basis for disease in adults and children* (6th ed.). St. Louis, MO: Mosby, Inc.

Osborn, K. S., Wraa, C. E., & Watson, A. (2010). *Medical surgical nursing: Preparation for practice.* Upper Saddle River, NJ: Pearson Education.

Smith, S. F., Duell, D. J., & Martin, B. C. (2012). *Clinical nursing skills: Basic to advanced skills* (8th ed.). Upper Saddle River, NJ: Pearson Education.

Wilson, B. A., Shannon, M. T., & Shields, K. M. (2012). *Pearson nurse's drug guide 2012.* Upper Saddle River, NJ: Pearson Education.

5 Neurological Disorders

Chapter Outline

Overview of Anatomy and Physiology of Nervous System

Diagnostic Tests and Assessments of Nervous System

Acute Disorders of Nervous System

Chronic Disorders of Nervous System

NCLEX-RN® Test Prep

Use the accompanying online resource, NursingReviewsandRationales, to test yourself with hundreds of NCLEX®-style practice questions.

Objectives

➤ Identify basic structures and functions of the neurological system.
➤ Describe the pathophysiology and etiology of common neurological disorders.
➤ Discuss expected assessment data and diagnostic test findings for selected neurological disorders.
➤ Identify priority nursing problems for selected neurological disorders.
➤ Discuss therapeutic management of selected neurological disorders.
➤ Discuss nursing management of a client experiencing a neurological disorder.
➤ Identify expected outcomes for a client experiencing a neurological disorder.

Review at a Glance

agnosia inability to recognize familiar subjects; it may be visual, auditory, or tactile

aphasia difficulty in interpreting language

apraxia inability to carry out motor pattern (i.e., drawing a figure, getting dressed) even with strength and coordination

autonomic hyperreflexia an exaggerated sympathetic response that occurs in clients with spinal injuries at or above T-6; response is seen after spinal

shock occurs when stimuli cannot ascend cord, a stimulus such as urge to void or abdominal discomfort triggers massive vasoconstriction below injury, vasodilation above injury, and bradycardia

bradykinesia slow movements caused by muscle rigidity

Broca's area motor control of speech in temporal lobe of dominant hemisphere

dysarthria defective articulation of speech

dysphagia difficulty swallowing

hemianopsia loss of half of visual field in one or both eyes

intrathecal through theca of spinal cord into subarachnoid space

paraplegia paralysis of lower extremities

tetraplegia formerly called quadriplegia; is generalized paralysis affecting both arms and legs

Wernicke's area section of temporal lobe responsible for primary auditory reception area and auditory association areas of speech

PRETEST

1 The nurse is observing a student nurse perform oral hygiene on a client who is unconscious. The nurse decides to intervene when which action by the student nurse is observed?

1. Swabs the client's mouth using toothettes
2. Brushes the teeth with a soft bristle toothbrush
3. Positions the client to one side or the other
4. Uses an alcohol-based mouthwash to rinse the client's mouth

2 A nurse is monitoring a client who has sustained a head injury for signs of increasing intracranial pressure (ICP). The nurse concludes that which vital sign trends are consistent with increasing ICP?

1. Increased temperature, decreased pulse, increased respirations, decreased BP
2. Decreased temperature, increased pulse, decreased respirations, increased BP
3. Decreased temperature, increased pulse, increased respirations, decreased BP
4. Increased temperature, decreased pulse, decreased respirations, increased BP

3 The client with elevated intracranial pressure has been intubated and placed on a mechanical ventilator for the purpose of hyperventilation. Which carbon dioxide value indicates that the optimal amount of hyperventilation has been achieved?

1. $PaCO_2$ 18 mmHg
2. $PaCO_2$ 30 mmHg
3. $PaCO_2$ 38 mmHg
4. $PaCO_2$ 46 mmHg

4 The nurse is encouraging self-care in a client who experienced a thrombotic stroke and who now has right-sided hemiparesis. The nurse knows that the best way to accomplish this goal is to place personal hygiene items in which area?

1. On the overbed table on the right side
2. On the overbed table on the left side
3. One foot away from the bed on the right side
4. One foot away from the bed on the left side

5 A client with a spinal cord injury is experiencing autonomic hyperreflexia. The nurse should carefully monitor this client for which manifestations? Select all that apply.

1. Severe, throbbing headache
2. Warm, moist skin of the head and neck
3. Hypertension
4. Tachycardia
5. Hot, sweaty skin below the level of injury

6 The nurse is assessing a pain response on a client who was admitted with a diagnosis of cerebrovascular accident (CVA or stroke) 3 days ago. The nurse notes that the client responds by extending the arms and rotating them internally and documents that the client is exhibiting which neurological manifestation?

1. Decerebrate posturing
2. Decorticate posturing
3. Kernig's sign
4. Babinski reflex

7 The nurse is teaching a client with Parkinson's disease about safety and mobility. The nurse concludes that teaching has been successful when the client makes which statements? Select all that apply.

1. "I will rock back and forth when I am getting up out of a chair."
2. "I will get shoes with Velcro fasteners."
3. "I will plan to do my exercises in the evening before I go to bed."
4. "I will sit in my soft recliner when I watch television."
5. "I will wear clothes with buttons to help with my physical therapy."

8 The nurse is caring for a client diagnosed with Stage 2 of Alzheimer's disease and assesses the client's problem of memory impairment. Which intervention should the nurse plan to address this problem?

1. Ensure that the client is wearing an ID badge.
2. Place client in a bright, stimulating environment.
3. Write a note on cover of chart asking for prn order for restraints.
4. Instruct ancillary caregivers to assess client's level of consciousness (LOC) hourly.

9 A client newly diagnosed with trigeminal neuralgia asks the nurse to explain why it hurts so much when an episode occurs. What is the best response by the nurse?

1. "The nerve is stimulated by temperature or pressure, which creates the pain."
2. "When your blood glucose decreases, it irritates the nerve, which in turn causes the pain."
3. "The adrenalin your body releases when you are scared irritates the nerve."
4. "It is caused by an immune system reaction to the flu virus."

10 A client is scheduled for an electroencephalogram (EEG) early in the morning. The nurse working the night shift prior to the procedure should plan to implement which action in the early morning on the day of the test?

1. Instruct client to refrain from washing hair.
2. Withhold daily dose of antiepileptic drug.
3. Place client on NPO status.
4. Reinforce client teaching that the test is only mildly uncomfortable.

➤ *See pages 175–177 for Answers and Rationales.*

I. OVERVIEW OF ANATOMY AND PHYSIOLOGY OF NERVOUS SYSTEM

A. Basic structure and function of cells in nervous system (NS)

1. Neurons: basic anatomical and functional units in nervous system (NS); each neuron has 3 parts:
   a. Cell body (major part of neuron)
   b. Axon, which carries stimulus away from cell body
      1) Axons extend a long way from cell body and do not branch until very end
      2) Axons in peripheral NS are covered with an insulating lipid layer called myelin sheath, which functions for rapid conduction of nerve impulses
      3) Each axon terminates at a synapse where neurotransmitters and other chemical substances are released
   c. Dendrites direct impulses toward cell body; they usually extend a short distance from cell body and branch copiously
   d. Nerve cells are separated by a synaptic cleft; neurotransmitters are secreted into cleft by 1 neuron to stimulate dendrites of another neuron
   e. Conduction of a nerve impulse is initiated when a stimulus is sufficient to create an action potential (summation of impulses from dendrites); it is then sent down axon by depolarization; in myelinated nerves the action potential hops from one node of Ranvier to the next for rapid conduction
2. Glial cells: supportive structures of NS that nourish, support, and protect brain neurons; because these cells divide by mitosis, they are a source of primary tumors of NS; there are 4 main types in brain and 1 in PNS:
   a. Astrocytes: star-like cells that provide nutrition to neurons, regulate synaptic connectivity, remove cellular debris, and control movement of molecules in blood–brain barrier

    b. Oligodendrocytes: produce myelin sheath within central nervous system (CNS) that insulates neurons allowing for fast transmission of impulses

    c. Ependymal cells: line ventricular system and choroid plexuses; they produce cerebral spinal fluid (CSF) and act as a barrier between fluid-filled ventricles and cerebral tissue

    d. Microglia: small phagocytic cells scattered in CNS that disintegrate and remove cellular debris and waste products

    e. Schwann cells: peripheral NS cells that produce insulating myelin sheaths, just as oligodendrocytes do in CNS, which facilitates rapid conduction of impulses

B. Central nervous system

    1. Consists of brain and spinal cord

    2. Brain is composed of divisions

        a. Cerebrum (largest division) composes top of brain and enables individuals to reason, function intellectually, express personality and mood, and interact with environment

            1) Includes 2 hemispheres; each has a frontal lobe, temporal lobe, parietal lobe, and occipital lobe; each lobe has specific functions

            2) Right hemisphere generally controls left side of body and left controls right; usually one hemisphere is considered dominant

            3) Frontal lobe performs high level cognitive function, has memory storage, influences somatic motor control, controls voluntary eye movements and controls motor aspect of speech in **Broca's area**, which is located in dominant hemisphere (usually left)

            4) Temporal lobe is located behind frontal and under parietal lobe and has primary auditory receptive areas and auditory association area (**Wernicke's area**), which is usually found on dominant side and is responsible for interpreting speech; another important area in temporal lobe is the interpretive area that integrates somatic, auditory, and visual data (this impacts perception, learning, memory, emotions, and intellectual abilities)

            5) Parietal lobe holds primary sensory cortex and sensory association areas; in these areas, sensations such as size, shape, weight, texture, and consistency are defined and localized; it also processes visual–spatial information and controls spatial orientation

            6) Occipital lobe is the visual center; it controls both eye reflexes and interpretation of sight

        b. Diencephalons and hypophysis are located at bottom of cerebrum near midbrain; this includes thalamus and related structures and pituitary gland; this area has many functions including temperature control, water metabolism, pituitary secretion, visceral and somatic activities, and visible physical expressions in response to emotions, sleep–wake cycle and hunger reflex

        c. Cerebellum is a double-lobed area posterior to pons that is responsible for muscle synergy and coordination, and maintains balance through feedback loops

        d. Brainstem is an integration system that also controls basic functions; there are 3 major divisions of brainstem (midbrain, pons, and medulla); reticular activating system (RAS) is responsible for alertness; substantia nigra is affected in Parkinson's disease; most cranial nerves originate in brainstem

    3. Spinal cord is an elongated mass of nerve tissue that runs most of length of vertebral column

        a. Spinal cord is divided into 4 areas: cervical area (C1–C7) transverses neck; thoracic area (T1–T12) goes through chest; lumbar area (L1–L5) goes through lower back; sacral area (S1–S4) is in sacrum

    b. Sensory tracts (dorsal roots) carry afferent impulses from periphery to dorsal root ganglia where cell bodies of sensory components are located; from this point they are then sent to brain by 2 types of sensory fibers:

        1) General somatic afferent fibers carry pain, temperature, touch, and proprioception from the musculoskeletal system, tendons, and joints

        2) General visceral fibers carry sensory input from organs of body

    c. Motor tracts (ventral roots) convey efferent impulses from spinal cord to body; there are 2 types of fibers:

        1) General somatic fibers that innervate voluntary striated muscles

        2) General visceral efferent fibers that innervate smooth and cardiac muscle and regulate glandular secretions

C. Peripheral nervous system

  1. Has 31 pairs of spinal nerves, 12 pairs of cranial nerves, and an autonomic system that is divided into sympathetic nervous system (SNS) and parasympathetic nervous system (PNS)

  2. Each pair of spinal nerves has dorsal and ganglion roots that exit spinal cord by way of an intervertebral foramina that corresponds with spinal level; these nerves carry input between specific areas called dermatomes and spine

  3. Cranial nerves (CN): 12 pairs of cranial nerves arise from brain; there are 3 pure sensory nerves, 5 pure motor nerves, and 4 mixed (sensory and motor) nerves; olfactory nerve (CN I) and optic nerve (CN II) arise from cerebrum; CN III and IV arise in midbrain; CN V through VIII arise in pons, while CN IX to XII arise in medulla (see Table 5-1 for overview of cranial nerves)

  4. Autonomic NS: a collection of motor nerves that regulate activities of viscera, smooth muscles, and glands to maintain a stable internal environment; there are 2 parts to system (SNS and PNS) that work antagonistically

    a. SNS is active during times of stress, such as fight or flight response; it increases heart rate and blood pressure and vasoconstricts peripheral blood vessels

    b. PNS is a conservation, restoration, and maintenance system; it decreases heart rate and increases gastrointestinal (GI) activity

Table 5-1   **Overview of Cranial Nerves**

Cranial Nerve Name	Type of Nerve	Physiological Functions
Olfactory (I)	Sensory	Ability to smell
Optic (II)	Sensory	Visual fields, visual acuity
Oculomotor (III)	Motor	Extraocular movements (EOM)
Trochlear (IV)	Motor	EOM
Trigeminal (V)	Mixed	Movement of eyelids, ability to clench jaw
Abducens (VI)	Motor	EOM
Facial (VII)	Mixed	Movement of eyelids, facial symmetry
Acoustic (VIII)	Sensory	Hearing ability
Glossopharyngeal (IX)	Mixed	Gag, swallow, and cough reflexes, voice quality
Vagus (X)	Mixed	Gag, swallow, and cough reflexes, voice quality
Spinal accessory (XI)	Motor	Neck strength and shoulder shrug
Hypoglossal (XII)	Motor	Tongue movement

D. Blood supply
1. Brain is unique in that it can only use glucose for its energy supply; a lack of glucose for 5 minutes results in irreversible brain damage; brain receives 750 mL/min of blood or 15–20% of resting cardiac output in adults; blood flow rates for specific sites correspond directly with rate of metabolism
2. Cerebral arteries are thinner, have more internal elasticity, and less smooth muscle than arteries in rest of body; brain is supplied with blood by 2 sets of arteries that divide it into anterior and posterior circulation
   a. Anterior circulation, fed by internal and external carotids, delivers blood to a central area at base of cerebrum named circle of Willis; from there it feeds anterior cerebrum via anterior cerebral artery, middle of cerebrum via middle cerebral artery, and posterior cerebrum via posterior cerebral artery; tissues that are at terminal areas fed by the 2 circulations are called watershed zones because they are subject to marginally adequate blood supply; during times of hypoperfusion, these may be first affected
   b. Posterior circulation, fed by vertebral arteries, delivers blood to posterior fossa; at bottom of posterior fossa, blood flows together into one basilar artery and delivers it to cerebellum, midbrain, pons, and medulla
   c. Meninges are supplied with blood from branches of external carotid arteries that ascend into brain at base of skull
3. Venous system of brain is unique
   a. Vessel walls are thinner than other veins of body
   b. They do not follow path of arteries but follow their own course
   c. There are no valves in brain's venous system, making drainage dependent on venous pressure and gravity
   d. Dural sinuses collect blood from brain and empty it into jugular veins

E. Blood–brain barrier
1. Is a descriptive term that refers to a network of endothelial cells in capillary walls and astrocyte projections in close proximity that do not have pores between them
2. This tight junction does not allow normal nonspecific filtering process that occurs in rest of body, so molecules must enter brain by active transport, endocytosis, and exocytosis, which creates a highly selective barrier that guards entrance to neurons
3. Movement of substances across this barrier depends on particle size, lipid solubility, chemical dissociation, and protein-binding potential
4. Barrier is very permeable to water, oxygen, carbon dioxide, other gases, glucose, and lipid-soluble compounds

F. Protective structures
1. Meninges: layer of tissue that covers brain and spinal cord to protect and support it; is divided into 3 layers from outer to inner (dura mater, arachnoid, and pia mater)
   a. Dura is a tough membranous tissue that surrounds and extends into brain tissue that provides important landmarks, such as falx cerebri and tentorium cerebelli; it is important to note whether an injury is supratentorial (above tentorium) or infratentorial (below tentorium) as nursing care will differ
   b. Arachnoid membrane lies below dura and is a network of delicate, elastic tissue that contains blood vessels of varying sizes
   c. Pia mater is a vascular membrane that covers entire brain with tiny vessels that extend into gray matter of brain
   d. Within meninges, there are important potential spaces (epidural, subdural, subarachnoid) where bleeding can occur
2. Skull: bony structure of head that includes 8 fused cranial bones and 14 facial bones; cranium encloses brain in a protective vault; many internal cranial surfaces are irregularly shaped; foramen magnum is a large hole at base of skull through which spinal cord runs

3. Spine: a flexible column that encloses spinal cord, formed from stacking of 33 bones called vertebrae; each vertebra has a body anteriorly and an arch that has 2 laminae and 2 pedicles that form 7 processes; this interlocking support structure provides protection and flexibility; spine is divided into 7 cervical, 12 thoracic, 5 lumbar, and 4 sacral vertebrae

4. Cerebrospinal fluid (CSF) and ventricular system

   a. CSF is a clear colorless, odorless solution that fills ventricular system and sub-arachnoid space of brain and spinal cord; it acts as a shock absorber to cushion brain from injuries caused by movement; it also has electrolytes, glucose, protein, oxygen, and carbon dioxide dissolved in solution

   b. Ventricular system is composed of 2 lateral ventricles (1 in each hemisphere of cerebrum), a third ventricle that lies midline in thalamic area, and a fourth that lies inferior to third ventricle and anterior to cerebellum and subarachnoid space

   c. Flow of CSF starts in choroid plexus in each lateral ventricle and travels to third ventricle via foramen of Monro; this landmark is used as a zero point in ventricular drainage systems; from third ventricle, CSF flows into fourth ventricle via aqueduct of Sylvius, through 2 lateral foramen of Luschka, midline through foramen of Magendie into subarachnoid space, down to spinal cord and up again to subarachnoid space on top of brain, where it is absorbed by arachnoid villi

II. DIAGNOSTIC TESTS AND ASSESSMENTS OF NERVOUS SYSTEM

A. Assessment of nervous system

1. Assess circumstances of injury and admission, pertinent family and social history
2. Assess chief complaint
   a. A—any associated symptoms with chief complaint
   b. P—what provokes (exacerbates or makes worse) or palliates (alleviates or makes better) symptoms
   c. Q—quality of symptom, description in client's own words
   d. R—region and radiation
   e. S—severity of symptom on a scale of 1–10
   f. T—timing—duration, when did it stop and start, note if intermittent or constant
3. Health information: including past medical or surgical history, current medications (prescribed, over the counter, herbal), other treatments or complementary therapies
4. Physical assessment of neurological functioning
   a. Mental status
      1) Assess mental status; include orientation to person, place, and time; note appearance, behavior, mood, speech pattern, thought and perception; include client's insight, thought, content, and judgment
      2) Obtain an accurate baseline by ensuring that client is fully awake, alert, and able to understand and respond to questions; note if client is impaired by drugs or alcohol (baseline would then be false)
      3) Assess level of consciousness (LOC); a client with an altered LOC may have a range of behaviors; terms used to describe this range vary from confused to comatose (see Table 5-2)
      4) Acute confusion or delirium should be recognized and treated by eliminating cause; try to avoid confusing delirium with dementia (the latter is a chronic problem)
   b. Cranial nerves: assessment of cranial nerves can be performed as described in Table 5-3; some methods of assessment test more than 1 cranial nerve at a time

Table 5-2	Terms Useful in Determining Level of Consciousness
Term	**Description**
Full consciousness	Alert; oriented to person, place, and time; and comprehends written and spoken words
Confusion	Disoriented to person, place, and/or time; misinterprets environment; has poor judgment; unable to think clearly
Lethargic	Oriented but slow and sluggish in speech, mental processes, and motor activity
Obtundation	Readily arousable to stimuli; responds with 1 or 2 words; can follow simple commands when asked, but quickly drifts back to sleep
Stupor	Lies quietly with minimal movement; responds with a groan or eye opening only to vigorous and repeated verbal with tactile stimuli; usually localizes painful stimuli
Coma	Unarousable to stimuli; nonverbal; may exhibit nonpurposeful response to stimuli
Light coma	Unarousable; withdraws nonpurposefully to pain; may decerebrate or decorticate; brainstem reflexes intact
Deep coma	Unarousable; unresponsive to painful stimuli; brainstem reflexes usually absent; decerebrate posturing usually noted
Delirium	Has rapid onset; brief impairment of cognition including a clouding of consciousness and difficulty sustaining and shifting attention
Dementia	A generalized, long-term decline in cognitive abilities such as memory, language, and clear consciousness

Source: Adapted from LeMone & Burke (2011). *Medical-surgical nursing: Critical thinking in patient care* (5th ed.). Upper Saddle River, NJ: Pearson Education, pp. 1431–1433.

c. Motor function
1) Inspect all body muscles for size, tone, movement, and strength
2) Compare left and right side for symmetry and equality
3) Assess for tremors (rhythmic movements) and fasciculations (twitching)
4) Criteria for grading muscle strength (see Box 5-1)
5) Common terms that are used when describing motor function are found in Table 5-4
d. Cerebellar examination: balance and coordination are under cerebellar control
1) To assess gait, have client walk normally and then on heels and toes and assess coordination; perform a Romberg's test and balance (have client stand with feet together and eyes closed for 20 seconds while the nurse stands close by to prevent falling); there should be minimal swaying

Box 5-1

Criteria for Grading Muscle Strength

0 = No contraction
1 = Trace of contraction
2 = Active movement with gravity
3 = Active movement against gravity
4 = Active movement against gravity and resistance
5 = Normal power

Note: Findings are recorded as a fraction with 5 (highest possible score) as the denominator; ex. normal finding is 5/5.

Table 5-3	Cranial Nerve Assessment Tests

Cranial Nerve	Assessment
Cranial nerve I (olfactory)	Assess ability to identify common odors
Cranial nerve II (optic)	Use Snellen chart to assess vision
Cranial nerves III, IV, and VI (oculomotor, trochlear, and abducens)	EOM: extraocular movements; have client follow finger through all visual fields Ptosis (III): droopy eyelid PEARLA: assess pupils equal and reactive to light and accommodation Nystagmus: pupil movement choppy, eye oscillates Doll's eyes: in a comatose client it is present when eyes stay center while moving head left and right; absent when eyes move with head
Cranial nerve V (trigeminal)	Jaw clench: palpate masseter and temporal muscles when client's jaw is clenched; note differences on left or right Compare light, dull, and sharp sensations on both sides of face Corneal reflex: on an unconscious client a wisp of cotton is touched to cornea; normal response is to blink Lids (V, VII): stroke each lid to elicit a blink response
Cranial nerve VII (facial)	Facial symmetry: note droopiness of nasal labia fold, lower eyelid or corner of mouth when asking client to grin, raise eyebrows and sniff; assess accuracy of tasting sweet, sour, and salty items on anterior two-thirds of tongue
Cranial nerve VIII (acoustic)	Assess hearing of each ear with a ticking watch or whispering Cold caloric testing: irrigating ear in cold or warm water causes a slow movement of eyes toward irrigated side with a rapid return to midline; this is called the oculovestibular reflex and indicates an intact brainstem
Cranial nerves IX and X (glossopharyngeal and vagus)	Swallow reflex: can client swallow water, or is there dysphagia (difficulty swallowing)? Gag reflex: assess gag by touching the back of both sides of throat; a unilateral loss may be noted Hoarseness: is client's voice hoarse? Cough reflex: is client's cough strong, weak, or absent? Assess sweet, salty, and sour taste on posterior third of tongue
Cranial nerve XI (spinal accessory)	Neck strength: have client turn head against resistance Shoulder shrug: have client shrug shoulders against resistance
Cranial nerve XII (hypoglossal)	Tongue deviation: have client stick out tongue and move it side to side against resistance; if there is a weakness, the tongue will go to stronger side

Table 5-4	Common Terms Associated with Motor Function

Term	Common Meaning
Strong	Normal strength
Weak	Not as strong as expected; moves against resistance but with little power
Unable to lift	Can't raise limb off the bed; can't move against gravity
Withdraws	Pulls back from pain source
Reflex	Involuntary contraction of muscle or groups of muscles in response to pain
Decorticate	To painful stimuli, flexes arms, wrists, and fingers with adduction of upper extremities and extension, internal rotation and plantar flexion of lower extremities
Decerebrate	To painful stimuli, extends, adducts, and hyperpronates arms and stiffly extends legs and plantar flexes feet
Flaccid	No response to pain; no muscle tone
Ataxia	Incoordination of voluntary muscle groups

2) Assess coordination, observe client's ability to touch own nose and then touch examiner fingers, then his or her nose again; next observe client's ability to touch each finger to thumb of same hand; finally, observe client's ability to run each heel down opposite shin while lying in supine position, note speed at which this can be performed without flaw to gain information about client's coordination

e. Sensory function

1) Have client close the eyes while examiner touches the client on all dermatomes with objects that are sharp, dull, light to touch, or vibrates (over bony prominence); client should be able to discriminate location and type of touch

2) To assess a client's sense of position (kinesthesia) have client close eyes and move client's finger or toe up or down and ask client to state how toe was moved

3) To assess for stereognosis, have client identify an object in his or her hand with eyes closed

4) To assess for graphesthesia have client identify a number or letter traced on palm of hand while eyes are closed

5) Test 2-point discrimination by touching a client with 2 simultaneous pinpricks and asking how many pinpricks there were; use dull edge object to perform this test

f. Reflexes

1) Deep tendon reflexes (patellar, biceps, brachioradialis, triceps, and Achilles) are assessed with a reflex hammer and scored; see Box 5-2 for criteria for scoring

2) Superficial abdominal reflex is assessed by lightly stroking abdomen from side to midline; normally side stroked will result in abdominal wall contraction

3) Cremasteric reflex is assessed by lightly stroking inside of thigh on a male client to raise testicle on that side

4) Babinski reflex is assessed by stroking lateral aspect of sole of foot from heel to ball, curving medially in ball; its presence is noted with dorsiflexion of big toe and fanning of other toes; is considered normal in infants but abnormal in adults; in adults, normal response is curling of toes (called a negative Babinski)

g. Speech: is usually described from interview

1) Clear: normal fluent speech

2) Dysarthria: ineffective articulation of speech; may be a motor deficit of tongue and/or speech muscles

3) Aphasia: a language disorder that is classified by type:

a) Expressive, motor, nonfluent or Broca's aphasia: an inability to express oneself using motor aspects of speech

b) Receptive, fluent, sensory or Wernicke's aphasia: an inability to comprehend spoken words

c) Global aphasia: a client can neither express nor comprehend language (mixed receptive and expressive)

Practice to Pass

A client newly admitted to a long-term care facility exhibits confusion. What client assessments would be necessary to determine whether the client is experiencing delirium (acute confusion) versus dementia (chronic confusion)?

Box 5-2

Standard Criteria for Grading Reflexes

0 = absent or no response
1 = hypoactive; weaker than normal (+)
2 = normal (++)
3 = stronger than normal (+++)
4 = hyperactive (++++)

B. Diagnostic studies of nervous system

1. CSF analysis: CSF is collected via lumbar puncture (LP); is studied for color, clarity, glucose, protein, blood, white blood cells (WBCs), and bacteria; normal CSF is colorless, clear, and without blood or bacteria (WBCs 0–5 cells/mm^3), glucose 40–80 mg/dL, and protein 16–45 mg/dL; position client side-lying with knees tucked toward chin for LP; assess site for CSF leakage and signs of infection postprocedure; following LP, position client with head elevated to low Fowler's with water-based contrast (to prevent spinal headaches) and flat with oil-based contrast

2. Radiological studies

   a. Cerebral angiography: used to view vascular structure of brain, detect arteriovenous malformation (AVM) and/or aneurysms; use standard nursing pre- and postprocedural care associated with use of contrast media (assess for allergy to iodine); increase fluids postprocedure to aid in excretion of contrast)

   b. Computed tomography (CT): scans brain in layers for density and digitally converts these to images; CT is painless and readily available; aids in detecting bleeding, hydrocephalus, and ischemic strokes older than 48 hours; may be done with or without contrast; see precautions noted above

   c. Magnetic resonance imaging (MRI): uses a magnet to line up hydrogen atoms and then converts findings of scan into images from various planes; detects soft tissue changes including necrotic tissue, tumors, edema, congenital disorders, and degenerative diseases; be sure to assess client for implanted metal that would contradict use of this diagnostic procedure

3. Electrographic studies

   a. Electroencephalography (EEG): measures brain waves with multiple scalp electrodes that is then interpreted by a neurologist; abnormal patterns of brain waves may suggest acute or neurodegenerative disorders, such as epilepsy, herpes simplex affecting the brain, encephalitis, or dementia; it is also an important criterion in determining brain death

      1) Teach client that test will not deliver electric shock

      2) Shampoo hair before procedure for cleanliness and postprocedure to remove residual electroconductive gel or paste

      3) Withhold antiepileptics and other medications as prescribed for 12–24 hours prior, if being done as emergency, note any drugs or medication taken within that time

      4) Have client eat regular meals to avoid hypoglycemia that could affect results

   b. Electromyography (EMG) and nerve conduction studies: are used to differentiate between peripheral nerve and muscle disorders; conduction velocity of muscles is measured between 2 points and recordings and measurements are taken at rest, with movement, and with electrical stimulation

4. Ultrasound (US)

   a. Carotid Doppler scan: a noninvasive US of carotids that detects occlusions and stenosis; US procedures cause minimal to no discomfort

   b. Transcranial Doppler ultrasonography (TCD): a portable noninvasive technique used to assess intracranial circulation by measuring blood flow velocity; it is used to assess vasospasm, transient ischemic attack (TIA), headache, subarachnoid hemorrhage (SAH), head injury, and AVM

III. ACUTE DISORDERS OF NERVOUS SYSTEM

A. Altered level of consciousness (LOC)

1. Description: a change in arousal or alertness and/or a change in cognition or solving complex problems (thought processes, memory, perception, problem solving, and emotion); is often first sign of a change in neurological status or may signal an underlying problem in older adult clients

2. Etiology and pathophysiology
   a. Causes for unconsciousness vary from primary CNS disorders (such as damage to RAS or cerebrum) to dysfunction of other organ systems
   b. In addition, metabolic disorders may alter cellular environment enough to inhibit neuronal activity
   c. The term *coma* is reserved for those who have long periods of unconsciousness, lasting from hours to months; neurological origin of coma results from damage to both hemispheres of the brain, damage to brainstem, or both
3. Assessment
   a. Clinical manifestations
      1) Except for cases where there is damage to brainstem, brain function deterioration and changes in LOC follow a predictable pattern from higher functions to primitive functions
      2) Confusion, forgetfulness, disorientation to time, then person, then place, agitation, poor problem-solving abilities, or any change in behavior may be an early change in cerebral function
      3) Changes to lethargy, obtundation, and stupor result from greater cerebral deterioration
      4) A change from purposeful movements to decorticate posturing (see Figure 5-1a) and small reactive pupils manifest midbrain deterioration
      5) Decerebrate posturing (see Figure 5-1b), fixed pupils, and positive cold caloric tests show deterioration at the level of the pons
      6) A positive vestibular-ocular reflex or doll's eyes (eyes move in opposite direction when head is turned), and positive cold caloric test (horizontal nystagmus when cold or warm water is used to irrigate ear canal) indicates brainstem is still intact
      7) Finally, flaccidity, fixed pupils, negative doll's eyes, and negative cold caloric tests indicate involvement at level of medulla
      8) Glasgow Coma Scale assessment includes components of eye opening (scored from 1–4), best verbal response (scored from 1–5), and best motor response (scored from 1–6); total score ranges from 3–15; a score of 8 or lower usually indicates coma (Teasdale G, Jennett B. *Assessment of Coma and Impaired Consciousness: A practical scale.* Lancet 1974, 2:81–84)
   b. Diagnostic and laboratory test findings
      1) CT and MRI may detect hemorrhage, tumor, cysts, edema, or brain atrophy
      2) EEGs evaluate unrecognized seizures as a cause for an altered LOC
      3) Cerebral angiography evaluates cerebral circulation for aneurysm and AVM
      4) Transcranial Doppler study is a less-invasive method to study blood flow
      5) A lumbar puncture with CSF analysis is done for infection
      6) Laboratory tests such as glucose, serum electrolytes, osmolarity, and creatinine, liver function, complete blood count (CBC), arterial blood gases (ABGs) may be done; toxicology screens may detect or rule out metabolic, toxic, or drug-induced disorders

Figure 5-1

Abnormal posturing.
A. Decorticate rigidity,
B. Decerebrate rigidity.

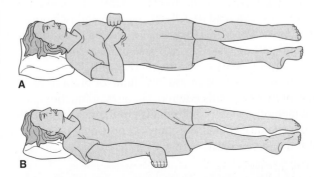

4. Therapeutic management: depends on cause of altered LOC; in addition to treating cause of problem, ongoing care focuses on airway maintenance, skin integrity, preventing contractures, and maintaining nutrition

5. Priority nursing problems: potential for ineffective cough and aspiration, potential for interrupted skin integrity, reduced mobility, risk for insufficient nutrients to meet bodily needs

6. Planning and implementation

    a. Assess for ability to clear secretions; assess breath sounds; maintain patent airway in unconscious client; maintain client with ineffective airway in side-lying position; provide tracheostomy care every 4 hours if client has one

    b. Assess swallow and gag reflex; use measures to prevent aspiration (side-lying, head of bed [HOB] at 30 degrees); monitor for and report possible aspiration

    c. Assess skin integrity every shift; reposition client every 2 hours; use measures to maintain intact skin; keep linens clean, dry, and wrinkle-free

    d. Provide proper support devices to maintain extremities in functional condition; perform passive range of motion (ROM) regularly

    e. Monitor nutritional status and assess daily weight; assess need for alternative methods of nutritional support

    f. DVT prophylaxis may include assessment, ROM exercises, antiembolism devices (elastic hose or sequential compression device), and antiplatelet agent

7. Medication therapy: depends on cause of altered LOC

8. Client education: client and family anxiety is common when clients have altered mental status, especially if prognosis is uncertain

    a. Reinforce information provided by health care provider

    b. Encourage family to talk to client (remember, hearing may remain even when client may be unable to respond)

    c. Provide information about client's care when family is ready

    d. Offer support services as needed

9. Evaluation: client maintains a clear and patent airway, remains aspiration free, has optimal motor and sensory functional capacity, has intact skin, and maintains adequate nutritional and elimination status

B. **Increased intracranial pressure (ICP)**

1. Description

    a. Increased ICP is defined as a prolonged pressure above 15 mmHg (normal 5–10 mmHg) measured in lateral ventricles

    b. Coughing, sneezing, straining, and bending forward cause a transient increase in ICP, this could be harmful in certain conditions

    c. Cushing's triad/response: involves 3 classic signs or responses to increased ICP: increased systolic blood pressure (while diastolic remains same), widening pulse pressure, and reflex bradycardia from stimulation of carotid bodies

    d. A prolonged increase in ICP causes tissue ischemia because cerebral blood flow and perfusion are compromised

    e. Autoregulation, a compensatory mechanism to maintain cerebral blood flow, if disrupted and can lead to cellular hypoxia and ischemia

    f. Untreated increased ICP leads to herniation and ultimately death

2. Etiology and pathophysiology: because brain is encased in a closed cavity, expansion of any contents of cavity can cause increased ICP

    a. Cerebral edema is an increase in volume of brain tissue due to increased capillary permeability (vasogenic edema), changes in functional or structural integrity of cell membrane (cytotoxic edema) or increased interstitial fluids (interstitial cerebral edema); edema is usually proportional to size of injury and may be localized or generalized

b. Hydrocephalus is an increase in volume of CSF within ventricular system; it may be "noncommunicating" where drainage from ventricular system is impaired (as when a mass blocks flow of CSF) or "communicating," such as when blood blocks arachnoid villi from absorbing CSF in a subarachnoid hemorrhage

3. Assessment

a. Clinical manifestations: earliest signs of increased ICP may be blurred vision, decreased visual acuity, and diplopia because of pressure on visual pathways; headache, papilledema, or swelling of optic disk and vomiting are next signs; most significant sign of increased ICP is a change in LOC; as pressure increases from front to back of brain, LOC deteriorates

b. Diagnostic and laboratory test findings are directed at identifying and treating underlying cause of increased ICP

1) CT or MRI scanning is generally the initial test

2) In general, a lumbar puncture is not performed because of risk of brain herniation caused by sudden release of pressure

3) Laboratory tests are performed to augment and monitor treatment approaches; serum osmolarity monitors hydration status and ABGs measure pH, oxygen, and carbon dioxide (hydrogen ions and carbon dioxide are vasodilators that can increase ICP)

4. Therapeutic management

a. Increased ICP is a medical emergency with little time for lengthy diagnostics; it centers on restoring normal pressure and can be accomplished through medications, surgery, and drainage of CSF from ventricular system

b. A drainage catheter can be inserted via ventriculostomy into lateral ventricle to monitor ICP and drain CSF to maintain normal pressure; if used, system is calibrated with transducer leveled 1 inch above ear (height of foramen of Munro); sterile technique is of utmost importance

5. Priority nursing problems: reduced perfusion to cerebral tissues, potential for infection, reduced mobility, potential for ineffective cough

6. Planning and implementation

a. Assess neurological status every 1–2 hours and report any deterioration; assess LOC, behavior, motor and sensory function, pupil size and reaction, and vital signs including temperature and pain

b. Maintain airway; elevate HOB 30 degrees or keep flat as prescribed; maintain head and neck in neutral position to promote venous drainage

c. Assess for bladder distention and bowel constipation; assist client when necessary to prevent Valsalva maneuver

d. Plan nursing care so it is not clustered because prolonged activity may increase ICP; provide for a quiet environment (lights kept low and limit stimuli such as radio, TV, and newspaper); avoid ingesting stimulants such as coffee, tea, cola drinks, and cigarette smoke

e. Maintain fluid restriction as prescribed

f. Keep dressings over catheter dry and change dressings as prescribed; monitor insertion site for CSF leakage or infection; use aseptic technique when in contact with ICP monitor

7. Medication therapy

a. Osmotic diuretics such as mannitol (Osmitrol) and loop diuretics such as furosemide (Lasix) are commonly used to decrease ICP; they work by moving water from edematous tissues to blood vessels; they can also disturb glucose and electrolytes so it is necessary to monitor these levels

b. Corticosteroids have been effective in decreasing ICP, especially with tumors, although mechanism of action is unclear

      c. Stool softeners are used to reduce constipation or need for Valsalva maneuver (bearing down or straining at stool)

  8. Client education

      a. Teach client at risk for increased ICP to avoid coughing, blowing nose, straining for bowel movements, pushing against bedside rails, or performing isometric exercises (or any other activity that closes glottis)

      b. Advise client to maintain neutral head and neck alignment

      c. Encourage family to maintain a quiet environment and minimize stimuli

      d. Educate family that upsetting client may increase ICP

  9. Evaluation: normal ICP (5–10 mmHg) is maintained; ischemia is minimized; airway patency and functional status are maintained

C. Head trauma: skull fractures

  1. Description: skull fracture is a break in skull that occurs with or without intracranial trauma; the force of impact significantly increases risk of hematoma formation; disruption of skull can lead to infection and cranial nerve injury

  2. Etiology and pathophysiology: skull fractures occur from trauma; they may be labeled as open or closed, depending on whether bone edges have lost contact; there are 4 classifications of fractures:

      a. *Linear* fractures are most common; risk of infection and CSF leakage is minimal because dura remains intact; hematoma formation is possible

      b. *Comminuted* and *depressed* skull fractures have a higher risk of brain tissue damage and infection especially if overlying skin and dura is torn or damaged; risk of secondary brain injury is reduced because impact injury causes bone fracture instead of being transferred to brain tissue

      c. *Basilar* skull fractures involve base of skull and are usually secondary injuries; most are uncomplicated, but those that disrupt sinuses and middle ear bones can lead to infection and CSF leakage

  3. Assessment

      a. Clinical manifestations may give clues to area of fracture; basilar skull fracture may produce these manifestations:

        1) Battle's sign: ecchymosis over mastoid process

        2) Hemotympanum: blood visible behind tympanic membrane

        3) Raccoon eyes: bilateral periorbital ecchymosis

        4) Rhinorrhea: fluid (CSF) leakage through nose

        5) Otorrhea: fluid (CSF) leakage through ear

      b. Diagnostic and laboratory test findings: x-rays and CT or MRI scans; basilar skull fractures may be difficult to identify on plain x-ray; extent of damage may be difficulty to determine if significant swelling present

  4. Therapeutic management: treatment depends on type and location of injury

      a. Linear skull fractures generally require bed rest and observation for underlying brain injury; no specific treatment is necessary

      b. Commuted and depressed skull fractures require surgery within 24 hours

      c. Basilar skull fractures do not require surgery unless there is persistent CSF leakage; regular neurological assessments and observations for meningitis are required

  5. Priority nursing problems: potential for infection, potential for injury

  6. Planning and implementation

      a. Observe client for otorrhea or rhinorrhea

      b. Test clear ear drainage and sinus drainage for glucose; only CSF has glucose; mucous secretions do not

      c. Observe blood tinged drainage for halo sign; CSF containing glucose dries in concentric rings on gauze or tissues

      d. Keep nasopharynx and external ear clean; use sterile technique and supplies when cleaning drainage from nose and/or ears

      e. Instruct client not to blow nose, cough, or inhibit sneeze, and to sneeze through an open mouth

      f. Use aseptic technique when changing head dressings

  7. Medication therapy

      a. Dexamethasone (Decadron), a potent corticosteroid, may reduce cerebral edema

      b. Antibiotics may be given when there is a risk of infection

  8. Client education: instruct client and family to go to emergency department if client experiences drowsiness or confusion, difficulty waking, vomiting, blurred vision, slurred speech, prolonged headache, blood or clear fluid leaking from ears or nose, weakness in an arm or leg, stiff neck, or seizures

  9. Evaluation: client recovers with minimal or no complications

D. Head trauma: intracranial hemorrhage

  1. Description: intracranial hemorrhage is an escape of blood into cranium, most commonly associated with blunt trauma; hemorrhage may cause a very slow to very rapid neurological deterioration

  2. Etiology and pathophysiology: results directly from trauma or from shearing forces on cerebral arteries and veins from acceleration–deceleration injuries; they are classified by location

      a. Epidural hematoma

          1) Develops between dura and skull; as hematoma forms, it strips dura away from skull

          2) Epidural hematomas usually develop from a tear in meningeal artery; because this is an arterial bleed, it rapidly expands, leading to a rapid deterioration in neurological status

      b. Subdural hematoma

          1) Forms between dura mater and arachnoid–pia mater layers of meninges; usually involves veins but may involve small arteries also

          2) As blood collects, pressure is applied to underlying brain tissue

          3) Subdural hematomas may be acute (developing within 48 hours after acute injury), subacute (developing 2 days to 3 weeks after lesser injury), or chronic (developing 3 weeks to months after a minor injury), or they may develop spontaneously

      c. Intracerebral hemorrhage

          1) Is bleeding into brain tissue

          2) Can occur anywhere in brain but is most common in frontal or temporal lobes

          3) May result from closed head trauma, where shearing forces are applied deep in brain; an example is a motor vehicle accident in which an individual hits head on the windshield, resulting in coup and contrecoup injury

  3. Assessment

      a. Clinical manifestations

          1) Epidural hematoma: client may initially lose consciousness then have a short period of lucidness, followed rapidly by deterioration from drowsiness to coma; other manifestations include headache, fixed dilated pupil on affected side, hemiparesis, hemiplegia, and possible seizures; this condition is a surgical emergency

          2) Subdural hematoma: manifestations may develop slowly and may be mistaken for dementia in older client; slow thinking, confusion, drowsiness, and lethargy are common; headaches, ipsilateral pupil dilation, sluggish pupillary response, and possible seizures are other signs

        3) Intracerebral hematomas vary in initial presentation depending on location; headache is common; as hematoma progresses, a decreased LOC, hemiplegia, and ipsilateral pupil dilation occurs; an expanding clot may lead to herniation

    b. Diagnostic and laboratory tests: may be diagnosed with CT and MRI scanning; laboratory values are of little use in establishing diagnosis, but may be used as baseline data for client's overall state of health

  4. Therapeutic management: small hematomas reabsorb spontaneously and may be treated conservatively; surgery is needed for epidural hematomas and larger subdural hematomas; surgery is less successful in intracerebral hematomas because of widespread tissue damage; supportive care and preventing complications are goals of therapy

  5. Priority nursing problems: alteration in respiratory pattern, potential for ineffective cough, potential for injury or reduced mobility, reduced perfusion to cerebral tissues

  6. Planning and implementation

    a. Assess neurological signs on a regular schedule; clear client's nose and mouth of secretions; (but avoid deep suctioning so as not to increase ICP)

    b. Monitor respirations for rate, depth, and rhythm if client is not ventilated; prepare for oxygen administration and endotracheal intubation for respiratory distress

    c. Prepare for cranial surgery for deteriorating neurological condition

    d. Provide appropriate preoperative and postoperative care as needed

    e. Provide previously discussed measures to manage increased intracranial pressure

  7. Medication therapy: none is specific to hematoma; medication such as antiepileptics and corticosteroids could be used as indicated to treat seizures and increased ICP if they occur as complications

  8. Client education: inform family of possibility of surgery to evacuate hematoma

  9. Evaluation: client maintains adequate respiratory rate and rhythm, adequate cerebral perfusion, and remains free of neurological complications

E. Inflammatory conditions: meningitis

  1. Description: an inflammation of meninges of brain and spinal cord; may be caused by infectious disease, basilar skull fracture, otitis media, sinusitis, mastoiditis systemic sepsis, impaired immune function, and neurosurgery or other invasive procedures

  2. Etiology and pathophysiology: most frequent cause is infection of meninges and CSF (rarely chemicals are the cause); infection (bacterial, viral, fungal, or parasitic) causes an inflammatory response in meninges; bacterial meningitis may be complicated by hydrocephalus, cerebral edema, arthritis, and cranial nerve damage; viral meningitis is usually less severe; with course of disease usually shorter and more benign

  3. Assessment

    a. Clinical manifestations

        1) Restlessness, agitation, and irritability

        2) Abdominal and back pain

        3) Nausea and vomiting

        4) Severe headaches

        5) Signs of meningeal irritation, nuchal rigidity (stiff neck), photophobia, positive Brudzinski's sign (pain, resistance, and hip and knee flexion occur when neck is flexed to chest while lying supine) and positive Kernig's sign (pain and/or resistance occurs with flexion of knee and hip and straightening of knee in supine position)

        6) Chills and high fever

        7) Confusion, altered LOC

        8) Seizures

        9) Signs and symptoms of increasing ICP

     b. Diagnostic and laboratory test findings: LP with CSF analysis including gram stain and cultures provides definitive diagnosis for meningitis; cultures of blood, urine, pharynx, and nose are collected to identify possible source of infection

  4. Therapeutic management: bacterial meningitis is a medical emergency that, if not treated, can be fatal within days; successful treatment depends on accurate diagnosis and aggressive treatment; treatment focuses on eradicating the infection with antibiotics, supportive treatment and managing symptoms; surgery may include placement of an Ommaya reservoir to allow **intrathecal** (into subarachnoid space) administration of antibiotics (rare)

  5. Priority nursing problems: risk for dehydration, potential for injury from seizures or loss of protective reflexes, potential for fever

  6. Planning and implementation

     a. Assess neurological status and vital signs (with temperature) regularly

     b. Assess and report changes in neurological status or presence of cranial nerve dysfunction

     c. Assess, prepare for, and report any seizure activity

     d. Assess for signs of increased ICP

     e. Administer prescribed medications and maintain fluid restrictions; a high-calorie, high-glucose diet may be prescribed

     f. Assess for fluid volume deficits, monitor intake and output and daily weights, skin turgor, laboratory values, and urine concentration

  7. Medication therapy: high-dose, broad-spectrum antibiotics initially (bacterial meningitis) to cross blood–brain barrier; when cultures are reported a more specific antibiotic may be used; antiepileptics (usually phenytoin [Dilantin]) are prescribed to prevent or control seizures; antipyretics, antiemetics, and analgesics are used for symptom relief; IV fluid replacement is continued until client can resume oral intake

  8. Client education

     a. Teach name and purpose of prescribed antibiotics (and other medications) and to take them as prescribed until they are finished

     b. Teach client and family to recognize and report signs and symptoms of ear, throat, and upper respiratory infections so they can be assessed for meningitis

  9. Evaluation: neurological status improves; symptoms of infection disappear; close contacts who develop symptoms receive proper and prompt medical care

F. Guillain–Barré syndrome

  1. Description: an acute, rapidly progressive inflammation of peripheral motor and sensory nerves characterized by motor weakness and paralysis that ascends from lower extremities in a majority of cases; outcome is generally excellent if care is appropriate

  2. Etiology and pathophysiology: occurs most often in clients 30–50 years; etiology is unknown, but autoimmune reaction is suspected (often develops after viral infection [especially GI or upper respiratory], immunizations, fever, injury, and sometimes surgery); antibody (IgM) formation targets peripheral nerve myelin, which damages myelin sheath and disrupts nerve conduction; remyelinization occurs in opposite direction of demyelination

  3. Assessment

     a. Clinical manifestations

        1) Weakness/paresis or partial paralysis progressing upward from lower extremities (paralysis in Guillain–Barré is "ground to brain") and then to total paralysis requiring ventilatory support

        2) Paresthesias (numbness and tingling) and pain

Practice to Pass

A college student visits health service complaining of a headache that does not ever go away. What other assessments would the nurse make to determine whether the client could be developing meningitis?

        3) Muscle aches, cramping, and nighttime pain

        4) Respiratory compromise and/or failure (dyspnea, diminished vital capacity, and breath sounds), decreasing O_2 saturation, abnormal ABGs

        5) Difficulty with extraocular eye movements, dysphagia, diplopia, difficulty speaking

        6) Autonomic dysfunction (orthostatic hypotension), hypertension, change in heart rate, bowel and bladder dysfunction, flushing, and diaphoresis

    b. Diagnostic and laboratory findings: nerve conduction test results are diminished, CSF examination shows elevated protein

  4. Therapeutic management

    a. Supportive care to maintain function of all body systems, including respiratory, cardiac, GI, renal, and skin; medications as discussed below

    b. Plasmapheresis (effective during first 2 weeks of disease): plasma is removed and separated from whole blood; blood cells are then returned without plasma to remove antibodies that cause disorder; monitor for complications of this therapy, which include bleeding from loss of clotting factors and fluid and electrolyte imbalance

  5. Priority nursing problems: alterations in respiratory pattern or gas exchange, insufficient nutrients to meet bodily requirements, potential for infection, potential loss of protective reflexes

  6. Planning and implementation

    a. Monitor respiratory status: rate, depth, breath sounds, vital capacity, note secretions, and check gag, cough, and swallowing reflexes

    b. Monitor cardiac status: heart rate, BP, dysrhythmias

    c. Administer chest physiotherapy and pulmonary hygiene measures

    d. Maintain adequate nutrition as appropriate: administer enteral or parenteral nutrition as needed; if client can swallow, assist with small frequent feedings of soft foods; weigh client weekly; check electrolyte status; provide mouth care every 2 hours

    e. Monitor bowel and bladder function: assess bowel sounds and frequency, amount, color and consistency of bowel movements; offer bedpan; check for distention and residual urine in a client who cannot void spontaneously; perform bladder scan to check for residual as needed and avoid intermittent catheterization when possible (this reduces nosocomial UTI); encourage fluid intake to 3,500 mL/day

    f. Prevent complications of immobility: encourage use of weak extremities; provide assistance with ROM and exercises prescribed by PT; protect immobile extremities with use of air mattress or special bed, and elbow and heel protectors; turn and reposition every 2 hours; elevate extremities to prevent dependent edema; use antiembolism compression devices or stockings

    g. Provide eye care for client who cannot close eyelids completely; instill artificial tears, cleanse eyes as needed, use eye shields and tape eyes closed if needed

    h. Provide therapeutic care and/or analgesics as needed

    i. Promote communication with client and family, using alternative means of communication if client is on ventilator or is unable to speak because of weak speech muscles

    j. Initiate discharge planning at time of admission

  7. Medication therapy: IV immunoglobulins (may result in low-grade fever, muscle aches, headache, or [rarely] acute renal failure or retinal necrosis); adrenocorticotropic hormone (ACTH) and corticosteroids or anti-inflammatory drugs; supportive medications that include stool softeners, antacids or H_2-receptor antagonists, analgesics, and antiplatelet agents or low molecular weight heparin such as enoxaparin (Lovenox)

  8. Client education: explain all care with rationales and provide information about progression of disease; encourage client and family to express feelings and participate in care as much as possible

9. Evaluation: client maintains satisfactory respiratory, cardiac, GI, and renal status; client resumes ability to move extremities and recovers from illness with no permanent loss of function

G. Cerebrovascular accident (CVA, brain attack, stroke)

1. Description: a CVA is a condition in which neurological deficits occur because of decreased blood flow to a localized area of brain; hypertension, diabetes mellitus, sickle cell disease, substance abuse, atrial fibrillation, and atherosclerosis are risk factors; onset may be rapid or gradual

2. Etiology and pathophysiology: ischemia followed by cell death results from severe and prolonged cerebral blood flow obstruction; deficits predict location of stroke; there are 4 types of brain attacks:

   a. Transient ischemic attack (TIA) is a brief period of neurological deficits that resolve within 24 hours; is a frequently precursor to a permanent CVA; causes of TIAs may be inflammatory arterial disorders, sickle cell anemia, atherosclerosis in cerebral vessels, thrombosis, and emboli

   b. Thrombotic CVA is caused by a thrombus (blood clot) occluding a cerebral vessel; thrombi tend to form on atherosclerotic plaque in larger arteries while blood pressure is lower (such as during sleep or rest); thrombosis occurs quickly but deficits progress slowly

   c. Embolic CVA is caused by a traveling blood clot; source of clot is elsewhere in body; has a sudden onset with immediate symptoms; if embolus is not absorbed, deficits will be persistent

   d. Hemorrhagic CVA or intracranial hemorrhage occurs when a blood vessel ruptures; this most often occurs with long-term, poorly controlled hypertension; other risk factors include a ruptured intracranial aneurysm, embolic CVA, tumor, AVM, anticoagulant therapy, liver disease, and blood disorders (such as disseminated intravascular coagulopathy [DIC], thrombocytopenia, or hypocoagulable state); this form of CVA is most often fatal because of rapidly increasing ICP; onset of symptoms is rapid; loss of consciousness occurs in about half the cases

3. Assessment

   a. Clinical manifestations: vary according to cerebral vessel involved

      1) Internal carotid: contralateral motor and sensory deficits of arm, leg and face; in dominant hemispheric CVA, **aphasia** (loss of ability to use language); in nondominant hemispheric CVA, **apraxia** (inability to perform known tasks), **agnosia** (inability to recognize) and unilateral neglect and homonymous **hemianopsia** (loss of one-half of visual field in each eye)

      2) Middle cerebral artery: drowsiness, stupor, coma, contralateral hemiplegia and sensory deficits of arm and face, aphasia, and homonymous hemianopsia

      3) Anterior cerebral artery: contralateral weakness or paralysis and sensory loss of foot and leg, loss of decision making and voluntary action abilities, and urinary incontinence

      4) Vertebral artery: pain in face, nose or eye, numbness or weakness of face on ipsilateral side, problems with gait, **dysphagia** (difficulty swallowing), and dysarthria (difficulty speaking)

   b. Diagnostic and laboratory test findings: a CT and MRI demonstrate hemorrhage, tumors, ischemia, edema, and tissue necrosis; cerebral angiography detects abnormal vessel structure, vasospasm, stenosis of carotid artery and loss of vessel wall integrity; ultrasound evaluates blood flow

4. Therapeutic management

   a. Drug therapy is most common treatment for CVAs; if it is a thrombotic stroke, medications could include thrombolytics and/or heparin

   b. It is imperative not to disrupt a clot that has formed after a hemorrhagic CVA

    c. Surgery is not usually indicated as a treatment modality

    d. Rehabilitation is crucial to improve deficits

5. Priority nursing problems: reduced mobility, insufficient ability to perform self-care, inadequate ability to communicate verbally

6. Planning and implementation

    a. Encourage active ROM on unaffected side and passive ROM on affected side

    b. Turn client every 2 hours

    c. Monitor lower extremities for thrombophlebitis

    d. Encourage use of unaffected arm for ADLs

    e. Teach client to put clothing on affected side first

    f. Resume diet orally only after successfully completing a swallowing evaluation; clients may need thickened liquids, foods with consistency of oatmeal or nectar, and to chew on unaffected side of mouth; this is sometimes referred to as a dysphagia diet; watch for pocketing of food in jaw, which may cause choking if inadvertently missed, similarly ensure medication is swallowed before leaving client's bedside

    g. Collaborate with occupational and physical therapy for rehabilitation

    h. Try alternate methods of communication with aphasic clients

    i. Help client to accept frustration and anger as common with this type of illness

    j. Teach client with homonymous hemianopsia to overcome deficit by turning head side to side to be able to fully scan visual field

7. Medication therapy

    a. Antiplatelet agents are used to treat TIAs and clients with previous CVA (except hemorrhagic CVAs)

Practice to Pass

What are the key differences in nursing management of a client who had a hemorrhagic stroke versus an ischemic stroke?

    b. During acute phase of thrombotic and embolic stroke, thrombolytic therapy may be administered within 3 hours to dissolve clot (note contraindication to thrombolytics)

    c. Anticipate anticoagulant therapy with heparin initially and then continued with an oral anticoagulant (sodium warfarin [Coumadin]) after acute phase

    d. In clients with cerebral edema, osmotic diuretics such as mannitol (Osmitrol) or loop diuretics such as furosemide (Lasix) may be given

    e. In clients with seizures, antiepileptics such as phenytoin (Dilantin), barbiturates, diazepam (Valium), and lorazepam (Ativan) may be given

8. Client and family education: CVA and CVA prevention (note client may extend a previous stroke), community resources, physical care and need for psychosocial support, medications, and injury prevention

9. Evaluation: client understands CVA and CVA prevention, and maximizes self-care and motor function

H. Spinal cord injury (SCI)

1. Description

    a. SCI is usually caused by trauma; young adults and adolescents are most commonly affected

    b. Injury affects motor and sensory function at level of and below injury

    c. SCIs are classified by amount of injury (complete or incomplete), cause of injury, and level of injury

    d. Perception, sexual function, and elimination are also affected

    e. Risk factors include age, gender, alcohol and drug abuse, and contact sports

2. Etiology and pathophysiology: spinal injuries usually result from excessive force applied to spinal cord and vertebral column; 4 types of injuries occur:

    a. Hyperflexion compresses vertebral bodies and disrupts ligaments and discs

    b. Hyperextension disrupts ligaments and causes vertebral fractures

    c. Axial loading is the application of excessive vertical force and may cause compression fractures

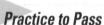

    d. Excessive rotation tears ligaments and fractures articular surfaces and causes compression fractures (see Figure 5-2)

  3. Assessment

    a. Clinical manifestations

      1) *Spinal shock* (temporary loss of reflex function), may occur after SCI: symptoms include bradycardia, hypotension, flaccid paralysis of skeletal muscles, loss of pain, touch, temperature, pressure, visceral and somatic sensations, bowel and bladder dysfunction, and loss of ability to perspire; spinal shock is resolved once spinal reflexes return

      2) Paraplegia is paralysis of lower portion of body; it occurs when injury level is in thoracic spine or lower

      3) Tetraplegia, formally quadriplegia, is paralysis of arms, trunk, legs, and pelvic portion; it occurs when level of injury is in cervical spine

      4) Autonomic hyperreflexia (also called autonomic dysreflexia) is an exaggerated sympathetic response that occurs in clients with injury at T6 or higher; this response is seen after spinal shock occurs when stimuli cannot ascend cord; a stimulus such as an urge to void or abdominal discomfort triggers massive vasoconstriction below injury, vasodilation above injury, and bradycardia

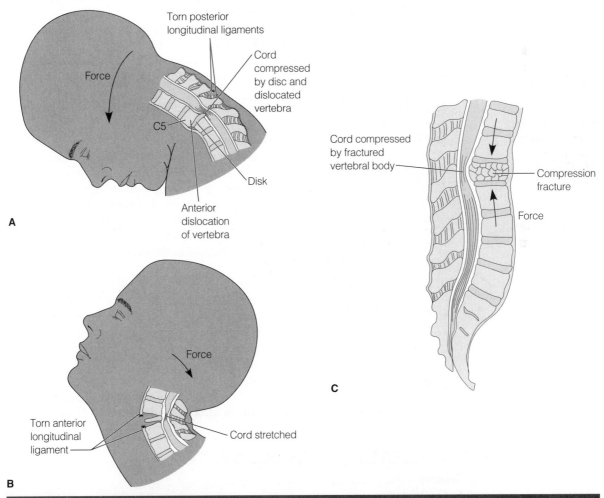

Figure 5-2

Spinal cord injury mechanisms. A. Hyperflexion, B. Hyperextension, C. Axial loading, a form of compression.

    b. Diagnostic and laboratory test findings: x-rays visualize fractures; CT and MRI scans show changes in vertebrae, spinal cord, and tissues surrounding cord; an EMG is done after acute injury to locate level of injury

4. Therapeutic management: acute management of SCI involves immobilizing injury and treating complications of respiratory distress, atonic bladder, paralytic ileus, and cardiovascular alterations; high-dose corticosteroid protocol is initiated to prevent secondary cord injury from edema and ischemia; stabilization with devices such as halo traction and Gardner–Wells tongs or surgery is done when indicated

5. Priority nursing problems: alterations in gas exchange, reduced mobility, potential for interrupted skin integrity or reduced self-esteem

6. Planning and implementation

    a. Monitor vital capacity and respiratory effectiveness; cervical cord injuries at C7 and higher may inhibit respiratory function and require mechanical ventilation

    b. Monitor for signs of ascending edema; may cause respiratory compromise

    c. Treat autonomic hyperreflexia immediately

      1) Elevate HOB and remove antiembolism stockings

      2) Assess BP every 2–3 minutes while assessing for causative stimulus; remove stimulus immediately when found (empty the bladder, remove fecal impaction or offending mechanical or thermal stimulus)

      3) If severe hypertension unresolved with removal of offending stimulus, notify provider and administer antihypertensives as prescribed per protocol

    d. Encourage client to verbalize feelings about loss of function and care

    e. Institute bowel and bladder training programs to restore a regular schedule for elimination

    f. Encourage self-care and independent decision making

    g. Include family and important others in discussions

    h. Clients with fracture or dislocation of cervical vertebrae may benefit from a halo brace; it is an external fixation device that allows earlier mobility because skeletal cervical traction by Gardner–Wells tongs or other apparatus is not needed

7. Medication therapy: corticosteroids (such as methylprednisolone, Solu-Medrol) to decrease or control edema of cord (monitor glucose levels); vasopressor to treat hypotension from spinal shock or antihypertensives for hypertension due to autonomic hyperreflexia; antispasmodics (baclofen [Lioresal] and diazepam [Valium] fort spasticity; analgesics and tricyclic antidepressants to treat pain

8. Client education

    a. Teach client and family to promote independence in self-care, such as self-catheterization technique, bowel evacuation, activities of daily living, etc.

    b. Educate client and family about variety of community resources that will be needed

    c. If client has a halo vest, teach that it raises center of gravity; avoid bending over to reduce risk of falls; neck is immobilized in midline so client needs to learn to turn entire body to scan environment; driving is prohibited; food is cut into small pieces and a straw is used for liquids to reduce risk for aspiration

9. Evaluation: autonomic hyperreflexia resolves; client maintains adequate respiratory status, makes satisfactory adjustments in lifestyle, and verbalizes feelings about loss of function

Practice to Pass

A client with recent spinal cord injury is beginning the rehabilitative phase of care. What ancillary services are needed to support the client's efforts to return to independent living?

IV. CHRONIC DISORDERS OF NERVOUS SYSTEM

A. Seizures

1. Description

    a. A seizure is an episode of excessive and abnormal electrical activity of all or part of brain that is manifested by disturbances in skeletal motor activity, sensation, behavior, consciousness, or autonomic dysfunction of viscera

    b. Seizures may result from an acute febrile state, head injury, infection, metabolic or endocrine disorders, or exposure to toxins

    c. Seizures are classified as partial or generalized; partial seizures begin in one area of cortex, and generalized involve both hemispheres and deeper brain structures

    d. If seizure activity is chronic (i.e., seizures recur within minutes, days, or even years), the diagnosis of epilepsy is given

2. Etiology and pathophysiology

    a. In some cases the exact initiating factor for seizures is unknown

    b. All people have a seizure threshold; when that threshold is exceeded, a seizure ensues

    c. Metabolic needs, oxygen requirements, metabolic by-products, and cerebral blood flow increase dramatically

    d. If cerebral blood flow can meet demands of a seizure, brain is protected from cellular exhaustion and destruction

    e. Epilepsy may be idiopathic (without identifiable cause) or secondary to a known cause such as birth trauma, infection, vascular abnormalities, trauma, or tumors

3. Assessment

    a. Clinical manifestations

       1) *Simple partial seizures* are limited to one hemisphere; manifestations include alterations in motor function, sensory signs, or autonomic or psychic symptoms

       2) *Complex partial seizures* originate in temporal lobe and may be preceded by an aura: an impaired LOC and repetitive nonpurposeful movements such as lip-smacking, picking, or aimless walking are noted; amnesia is common

       3) *Generalized partial seizure* is a partial seizure that has spread to both hemispheres and deeper structures of brain

       4) *Absence seizure* is a generalized seizure that lasts 5–30 seconds; there is a sudden brief cessation of motor activity and a blank stare; seizures may occur occasionally or up to 100 per day; they may be accompanied by eyelid fluttering or automatisms such as lip-smacking; more common in children than adults

       5) Tonic-clonic seizures (grand mal) are the most common type of seizure

          a) They may be preceded by an aura but are often without warning

          b) Typically, seizure starts with a loss of consciousness and sharp muscle contractions

          c) Client falls to floor and may have urinary and/or bowel incontinence

          d) Breathing ceases and cyanosis develops during tonic phase (about 15 sec to 1 min)

          e) Clonic phase (60–90 seconds) follows with alternating muscle contraction and relaxation in all extremities, hyperventilation, and eyes rolled back in head (see Figure 5-3)

          f) In next phase (postictal period), client is relaxed with quiet breathing, unconscious and unresponsive; client gradually regains consciousness and may have transient confusion and disorientation; clients often report head and muscle aches, fatigue, and may sleep several hours

          g) Clients will have amnesia of seizure and events just prior to seizure

       6) *Status epilepticus* is a life-threatening emergency that can occur during seizure activity; is characterized by continuous cycles of tonic-clonic activity with short periods of calm between them; this cumulative effect can interfere with respiration; client is in great danger of developing hypoxia, hyperthermia, hypoglycemia, and exhaustion if seizure activity is not stopped

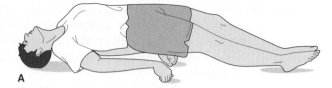

Figure 5-3

Tonic-clonic contractions in grand mal seizures. A. Tonic phase, B. Clonic phase.

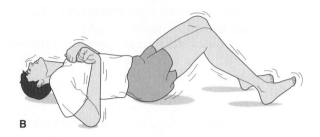

   b. Diagnostic and laboratory test findings: testing is done to confirm diagnosis and to determine treatable causes and precipitating factors; these include a complete neurological examination, EEG, skull x-ray series, CT scan, lumbar puncture with CSF analysis, blood studies, electrocardiogram and Wada procedure (neurological evaluation after injection of barbiturate into one hemisphere, then the other)

4. Therapeutic management: drug therapy is mainstay of controlling seizure activity; when all attempts fail, then surgery for excision of tissue involved in seizure activity may be safest alternative

5. Priority nursing problems: potential for ineffective cough, potential for injury, potential for anxiety

6. Planning and implementation

   a. During acute stay in hospital used padded side rails and keep call bell within reach

   b. Provide interventions during seizure to maintain airway patency; turn client to side if needed to maintain airway and promote drainage of secretions and prevent aspiration; keep oxygen and suction equipment at bedside for use after a seizure if needed; do not try to force an object, such as a tongue depressor or oral airway, into the mouth of a client who is seizing, as this may break teeth or cause other injury

   c. Provide interventions during a seizure to reduce risk of injury; do not restrain client but clear environment to prevent additional injury; teach family members how to protect client during seizures

   d. Document seizure activity promptly, include duration, preceding, accompanying, and post symptoms and report as appropriate

   e. During recovery (postictal) period, maintain a low-stimulus environment (low light, noise levels) to prevent recurrence of seizure activity

7. Medication therapy

   a. Antiepileptics that raise seizure threshold or limit spread of abnormal electrical activity are the mainstay of epilepsy treatment

   b. Some commonly used antiepileptics are phenytoin (Dilantin; be sure to monitor for therapeutic levels), divalproex sodium (Depakote), valproic acid (Depakene), carbamazepine (Tegretol), gabapentin (Neurontin), and lamotrigine (Lamictal)

   c. Diazepam (Valium), lorazepam (Ativan), and phenobarbital are also used intermittently to stop seizure activity during acute episodes

8. Client education

   a. Correct misconceptions, fears, and myths about epilepsy

   b. Encourage client and family to express feelings

    c. Provide information about community and national resources for epilepsy

    d. Stress importance of follow-up care

    e. Review any laws (such as driving a motor vehicle) that apply to people with epilepsy and risks of operating heavy equipment

    f. Provide support to client that concerns are normal; help client identify leisure activities that are safe; provide information about resources and support groups; provide accurate information about hiring practices; refer for employment or vocational counseling as needed

    g. Stress importance of wearing a medical alert band

    h. Emphasize aura alert

    i. Stress importance of continuing antiepileptic drug therapy

    j. Stress importance of avoiding physical and emotional stress

    k. Help client focus on positive aspects of life

    l. Teach to avoid alcohol and limit caffeine; and to take showers instead of baths to avoid drowning

    m. Discuss factors that may trigger seizure activity, such as increased stress, lack of sleep, emotional upset, alcohol use, overstimulation, flashlights, or loud noises

9. Evaluation: client has reduced or absent seizure activity, is protected from harm during seizures, verbalizes importance of continuing antiepileptic therapy, and obtains medical alert identification

B. Parkinson's disease (PD)

1. Description: a progressive, degenerative neurological disease characterized by bradykinesia, muscle rigidity, and nonintentional tremor; it affects older adults most often with a mean incidence of 60 years of age; it affects men more than women

2. Etiology and pathophysiology: in PD, atrophy occurs in substantia nigra that produces neurotransmitter dopamine; as dopamine decreases, acetylcholine is no longer inhibited; this imbalance in neurotransmitter is clinical basis for symptoms

3. Assessment

    a. Clinical manifestations: begin subtly; only fatigue and a slight resting tremor may be initial symptoms; in a small population of clients, dementia may be presenting symptom

        1) **Bradykinesia** is slow movement caused by muscle rigidity; also affects eyes, mouth, and voice; there is also a staring gaze

        2) Uncoordinated movements and postural disturbance (trunk tilted forward)

        3) Short-stepped, shuffling, and propulsive gait, which leads to increased risk of falls

        4) Slurred speech, soft voice tones, mask-like face, and dysphagia

        5) Excessive sweating of face and neck with absence of sweating on trunk and extremities

        6) Heat intolerance

        7) Constipation

        8) Anxiety and depression, with possible sleep disturbances

    b. Diagnostic and laboratory test findings

        1) CBC may show anemia of chronic disease

        2) Chemistry profile may show low albumin and protein

        3) Drug screens may be done to rule out toxic causes

        4) An EEG may show a slow pattern and disorganization

        5) An upper GI series may show delayed emptying, distention, and megacolon

        6) A video fluoroscopy may show a slowed response of cricopharyngeal muscles when swallowing

4. Therapeutic management: includes medications, surgery, and rehabilitation aimed at optimizing functional level; a team approach is essential to quality care of clients with PD

Practice to Pass

A client with seizure disorder is started on antiepileptic therapy with phenytoin (Dilantin). What are the key elements that should be included in a teaching plan about this medication?

   5. Priority nursing problems: reduced physical mobility, inadequate ability to communicate verbally, insufficient nutrients to meet bodily needs, potential for injury
   6. Planning and implementation
      a. Perform active ROM twice a day and ambulate at least 4 times a day
      b. Alternate rest periods with activity to avoid fatigue
      c. Use assistive devices when recommended; use clothing and shoes with Velcro closures to maintain self-care ability with loss of fine motor control
      d. Assess communication skills, speech, hearing, and writing
      e. Consult with a speech pathologist if necessary
      f. Assess nutritional status and self-feeding abilities
      g. Promote diet for foods high in bulk and fluids; limit protein (which may decrease effectiveness of medications)
   7. Medication therapy: monoamine oxidase (MAO) inhibitors, dopaminergics, dopamine agonists, and anticholinergics; eventually all these drugs lose effectiveness; a fluctuating response to drugs is called the on–off response; antidepressants, especially amitriptyline, are used to treat depression; propranolol may be used to treat tremors
   8. Client education
      a. Preventive measures for malnutrition, falls, and other environmental hazards, constipation, skin breakdown from incontinence, and joint contractures
      b. Gait training and exercises for improving ambulation, swallowing, speech, and self-care
      c. Discuss food to avoid when taking MAO inhibitors
   9. Evaluation: client maintains adequate mobility and nutritional status and remains free from falls; constipation is controlled

C. Multiple sclerosis
   1. Description: a chronic CNS disorder in which myelin and nerve axons in brain and spinal cord are destroyed; there are 4 forms based on rate of progression: benign, relapsing-remitting, primary progressive, and secondary progressive
   2. Etiology and pathophysiology
      a. Unknown etiology, possibly an autoimmune or genetic basis or may be caused by childhood viral infections
      b. Destruction of myelin and nerve axons causes a temporary, repetitive, or sustained interruption in conduction of nerve impulses, which causes symptoms of MS
      c. Plaque formation occurs throughout white matter of CNS, which also affects nerve impulses of optic nerves, cervical spinal cord, and thoracic and lumbar spine
      d. Inflammation occurs around plaques as well as normal tissue
      e. Astrocytes appear in lesions and scar tissue forms, replacing axons and leading to permanent disability
   3. Assessment
      a. Clinical manifestations: visual disturbances or blindness (retrobulbar neuritis); sudden, progressive weakness of one or more limbs; spasticity of muscles; nystagmus; tremors; gait instability; fatigue; bladder dysfunction (UTIs, incontinence); depression
      b. Diagnostic and laboratory findings: lumbar puncture for CSF (clonal IgG bands present); MRI, CT scans, muscle testing show characteristic changes
   4. Therapeutic management: no cure is available; supportive care is indicated
   5. Priority nursing problems: reduced physical mobility, possible loss of protective reflexes, body image alterations, potential for infection

6. Planning and implementation
    a. Overall goal of care is to maintain as much independent function as possible
    b. Include rest periods to prevent fatigue, which is an exacerbating factor
    c. Assist client to help set priorities for care on a daily basis whenever possible to maintain sense of control and independence
    d. Assist client with ADLs on an as-needed basis; provide adaptive utensils or other assistive devices as needed
    e. Maintain a fluid intake of at least 2,000 mL/day to maintain bowel and bladder function and prevent impaction and/or urinary tract infection
    f. Communicate with client about issues of concern, such as coping skills, sexuality, changing body image, or other issues perceived by client
    g. Avoid sources of infection; illness can act as a stressor and trigger an exacerbation
    h. Minimize extremes or large changes in environmental temperatures, which can trigger an exacerbation
7. Medication therapy: immunosuppressants, antivirals, corticosteroids, antibiotics for urinary tract infections, interferon-alpha, glatiramer (Copaxone), anticholinergics, and antispasmodics
8. Client education: medications, symptoms, bladder training, (may include intermittent self-catheterization), sexual functioning, complications, and possible triggers (fatigue, temperature extremes, illness)
9. Evaluation: client maintains maximum independence; is free of infection; verbalizes importance of preventing fatigue that would exacerbate disease process

D. **Myasthenia gravis**
1. Description: a chronic progressive disorder of peripheral NS affecting transmission of nerve impulses to voluntary muscles; causes muscle weakness and fatigue that increases with exertion and improves with rest; eventually leads to fatigue not relieved by rest
2. Etiology and pathophysiology
    a. Etiology unknown; thymus tumor (thymoma) and family history of autoimmune disorders are implicated
    b. An autoimmune process triggers formation of autoantibodies that decrease number of acetylcholine receptors and widen gap between axon ending and muscle fiber in neuromuscular (myoneural) junction
    c. Muscle contraction is hindered because IgG autoantibodies prevent acetylcholine from binding with receptors; destruction of receptors at neuromuscular junction occurs
    d. Is associated with continued production of autoantibodies by thymus gland in 75% of cases
    e. Onset is usually slow but can be precipitated by emotional stress, hormonal disturbance (pregnancy, menses, thyroid disorders), infections/vaccinations, trauma and surgery, temperature extremes, excessive exercise, and drugs that block or decrease neuromuscular transmission (opioids, sedatives, barbiturates, alcohol, quinidine, anesthetics), and thymus tumor
3. Assessment
    a. Clinical manifestations
        1) Mild diplopia (double vision) and unilateral ptosis (eyelid drooping) caused by weakness in extraocular muscles; weakness may also involve face, jaw, neck, and hip
        2) Complications arise when severe weakness affects muscles of swallowing, chewing, and respiration; respiratory distress is manifested by tachypnea, decreased depth, abnormal ABGs, O_2 sat less than 92%, and decreased breath sounds

3) Bowel and bladder incontinence, paresthesias and pain in weak muscles

4) Myasthenic crisis: sudden motor weakness; risk of respiratory failure and aspiration; most often caused by insufficient dose of medication or an infection

5) Cholinergic crisis: severe muscle weakness caused by overmedication; also cramps, diarrhea, bradycardia, and bronchial spasm with increased pulmonary secretions and risk of respiratory compromise

   b. Diagnostic and laboratory findings

1) ABGs and pulmonary function tests may show respiratory insufficiency

2) Electromyography (EMG) shows decreased amplitude when motor neurons are stimulated

3) Confirmation of clinical diagnosis can be made by IV administration of edrophonium chloride (Tensilon), which allows acetylcholine to bind with its receptors and temporarily improves symptoms; weakness returns after effects of Tensilon are discontinued; a positive Tensilon test confirms diagnosis of myasthenia gravis

   4. Therapeutic management: focuses on medication management with anticholinesterases: neostigmine (Prostigmin), pyridostigmine (Mestinon); immunosuppressants: corticosteroids, azathioprine (Imuran), and cyclosporine (Neoral); anti-inflammatory drugs; thymectomy (removal of thymus gland); plasmapheresis—removes IgG (antiacetylcholine) antibodies, atropine sulfate (Atropine) for cholinergic crisis

   5. Priority nursing problems: alterations in respiratory pattern, ineffective cough or swallowing ability, inability to endure activity or exercise, potential for injury or body image alterations

   6. Planning and implementation

   a. Maintain effective breathing pattern and airway clearance; thoroughly assess for respiratory distress

   b. Monitor meals and teach client to bend head slightly forward while eating and drinking to improve swallowing

   c. Teach client to avoid exposure to infections, especially respiratory

   d. Teach client effective coughing, use chest physiotherapy and incentive spirometry; have oral suction available, teach client how to use it; be prepared to intubate if needed

   e. Provide adequate nutrition: schedule meds 30–45 minutes before eating for peak muscle strength while eating; offer food frequently in small amounts that are easy to chew and swallow—soft or semisolid as needed; administer IV fluids and nasogastric tube feedings if client is unable to swallow

   f. Promote improved physical mobility with referrals to physical therapy and/or occupational therapy

   g. Provide eye care: instill artificial tears; use a patch over one eye for double vision; wear sunglasses to protect eyes from bright lights

   h. Promote positive body image and coping skills: encourage participation in treatment plan; plan time for active listening and encourage client to express feelings; reinforce progress and explain all care

   7. Medication therapy: anticholinesterases such as neostigmine (Prostigmin), pyridostigmine (Mestinon); immunosuppressants such as corticosteroids, azathioprine (Imuran), and cyclosporine (Neoral); anti-inflammatory drugs

   8. Client education

   a. Take medications on time and keep prescriptions filled ahead of time

   b. Plan rest periods and conserve energy; plan major activities early in day; schedule activities during peak medication effect

   c. Avoid extremes of hot and cold, exposure to infections, emotional stress and meds that may worsen or precipitate an exacerbation (alcohol, sedatives, and local anesthetics)

   d. Recognize and report signs of crisis

      e. Wear a medical identification bracelet or chain

      f. Use alternative methods of communication if needed: eye blink, finger wiggle for yes/no; flash cards or communication board; support lower jaw with hands to assist with speech

  9. Evaluation: client maintains patent airway and breathing without aspiration; maintains activities of daily living with assistance; demonstrates adequate coping skills for managing chronic and debilitating illness

E. Alzheimer's disease (AD)

  1. Description: a progressive dementia with irreversible deterioration of general intellectual function; it affects adults in middle to late life; incidence of AD increases with age

  2. Etiology and pathophysiology: cause is unknown; chemical changes in brain are found in hippocampus, and frontal and temporal lobes of cerebral cortex; clients lose nerve cells; perfusion to affected areas is decreased, and brain atrophies; amyloid a starchlike protein accumulates in brain tissue; as AD progresses more areas of brain are affected

  3. Assessment

      a. Clinical manifestations: AD is classified into 3 stages based on manifestations and abilities

        1) Early stage: lasts 2–4 years; client appears healthy and alert but may be restless or uncoordinated; cognitive impairment is not apparent; memory impairment, subtle changes in personality, and problems doing simple calculations may be first manifestations of AD

        2) Middle stage: lasts 2–12 years; memory impairment is more evident (recent memory is lost before remote memory); client is less able to behave spontaneously; client may wander or get lost; confusion and disorientation increases even though there are lucid periods; language deficits including paraphasia (using wrong word) and echolalia (repetition of words or phrases) are common; judgment is impaired; self-care is compromised because sequencing of tasks is lost; apraxia, astereognosis, and agraphia are common

        3) Late stage: lasts 2–4 years; this is characterized by increasing dependence, aphasia, incontinence, loss of motor skills, and gross loss of cognitive abilities

      b. Diagnostic and laboratory test findings: AD is a diagnosis of exclusion, meaning that other causes of symptoms are ruled out; CBC may reflect anemia; EEG may show slowing in later stages; CT and MRI may show atrophy; neurological evaluations reflect memory and cognitive impairment

  4. Therapeutic management: clients and their families require assessment of their support systems and extensive follow-up and support; because there is no cure for AD, the main objective of care is to match function with environment; safety and least restrictive environment are high priorities

  5. Priority nursing problems: alterations in thought processes, anxiety, loss of hope, potential for injury, potential for caregiver stress

  6. Planning and implementation

      a. Label room, drawers, or other items as needed

      b. Orient client to person, place, and time as needed

      c. Keep daily routine as consistent as possible

      d. Remove client from activities that increase anxiety

      e. Avoid criticizing or judging expressed feelings

      f. Provide realistic information about disease process

      g. Use therapeutic communication and listening skills to reduce agitation; listening to client's recollection of past events is helpful for client's psychosocial status

      h. Encourage family members to get involved in a support group

7. Medication therapy: reversible acetylcholinesterase inhibitors, such as tacrine (Cognex), donepezil (Aricept), and rivastigmine (Exelon) improve memory; antihistamines and tricyclic antidepressants are avoided because of high anticholinergic activity; occasionally tranquilizers are needed to treat agitation

8. Client education (focus is on client initially and in later stages centers on both client and support persons)
   a. Avoid stopping reversible acetylcholinesterase inhibitors suddenly because it can trigger behavior problems
   b. Teach caregivers about community resources
   c. Educate client and caregivers about expectations for disease process

9. Evaluation: safety is maintained, least restrictive environment is provided, and frequent follow-up care is provided

F. Cranial nerve (CN) disorders

1. Description: involve dysfunction of cranial nerves; most commonly affected are trigeminal nerve (CN V) and facial nerve (CN VII); trigeminal neuralgia and Bell's palsy are the respective disorders; trigeminal neuralgia is a chronic disease that causes severe facial pain; Bell's palsy is a unilateral paralysis of the facial muscles

2. Etiology and pathophysiology
   a. Trigeminal neuralgia has an unknown cause; it affects 1 or more of 3 divisions of trigeminal nerve (ophthalmic, maxillary, and mandibular); maxillary and mandibular divisions are affected most often
   b. Bell's palsy also has an unknown cause; inflammation of nerve and a viral cause has been suggested; 80% of clients recover completely within a few weeks to months; of those remaining 15% will recover some function but have permanent facial paralysis

3. Assessment
   a. Clinical manifestations
      1) Trigeminal neuralgia: characteristic symptom is brief, intense, superficial pain in face; episodes may occur as frequently as 100 times a day or as little as a few times each year; pain typically starts peripherally and advances centrally; motor or sensory deficits do not occur; some clients may have trigger zones that initiate onset of pain; in others, pain may be triggered by light touch, eating, swallowing, talking, shaving, sneezing, brushing teeth, or washing face
      2) Bell's palsy: manifestations include one-sided paralysis of facial muscles, paralysis of upper eyelid with loss of corneal reflex on affected side, loss or impairment of taste over anterior portion of tongue on affected side, and increased tearing from lacrimal gland on affected side
   b. Diagnostic and laboratory test findings: none specific; diagnosis is made by excluding other causes of symptoms

4. Therapeutic management
   a. Trigeminal neuralgia treatment is centered on controlling pain with antiepileptic medications such as carbamazepine (Tegretol); surgical procedures include microvascular decompression (removal of blood vessel from posterior trigeminal root), rhizotomy (surgical severing of nerve root), or Janetta procedure (sponge inserted at site of local nerve irritation as in arteriosclerosis)
   b. Bell's palsy: administration of corticosteroids (but their use has been questioned); antiviral medication is also currently very popular, as well as gentle massage, stimulation

5. Priority nursing problems: insufficient nutrients to meet bodily needs, pain, potential for injury, interrupted sleep

6. Planning and implementation
   a. Encourage client to chew on unaffected side
   b. Monitor dietary intake

     c. Assist with physiotherapy, including moist heat, gentle massage, and facial nerve stimulation

!   **d.** Protect cornea with artificial tears, sunglasses, eye patch at night, and gentle intermittent closure of eye

!   **7.** Medication therapy

     a. Trigeminal neuralgia: the most useful drug for controlling pain is carbamazepine (Tegretol); when this is not effective, phenytoin (Dilantin) is tried

     b. Bell's palsy: a corticosteroid such as prednisone (Deltasone) influences outcome by decreasing edema of nerve tissue; antivirals are also used

  8. Client education

     a. Wear an eye patch at night

     b. Wear protective glasses when outside

     c. Inspect inside of mouth on affected side for food that may collect between cheek and teeth

  9. Evaluation: eye is protected; pain is controlled

Case Study

A 24-year-old male is admitted to the neurology hospital unit following a motor vehicle incident in which he suffered a head injury after hitting the windshield while unrestrained in the front passenger seat. He is being evaluated for a possible intracranial hemorrhage secondary to the injury. You are the admitting nurse for this client.

1. What will you include in a focal neurological assessment of this client?

2. What diagnostic tests will confirm the presence of an intracranial hemorrhage?

3. What signs would indicate that the client is developing increased intracranial pressure?

4. How will the nurse plan care to minimize elevations in intracranial pressure?

5. What medications would the nurse anticipate being ordered for this client?

For suggested responses, see page 622.

POSTTEST

POSTTEST

① An unconscious client who is receiving continuous enteral feedings has a sudden onset of wheezes and rhonchi. The nurse identifies that which nursing problem is a priority for this client?

1. Risk for Aspiration
2. Risk for Excess Fluid Volume
3. Risk for Imbalanced Nutrition: Less than Body Requirements
4. Risk for Electrolyte Imbalance

② A client is admitted to the emergency department following a motor vehicle crash. While completing a neurological assessment, the client pulls his arms inward and upward while the nurse is eliciting a pain response. The nurse identifies that this positioning is significant for which of the following? Select all that apply.

1. Decerebrate posturing
2. Decorticate posturing
3. Injury to the brainstem
4. Injury to the pons
5. Injury to the midbrain

3 The nurse is admitting a client from the emergency department after a fall that resulted in increased intracranial pressure (ICP). The client opens his eyes when the nurse calls his name, and moans and pulls his hand away to a pain response. Using the chart provided, what is the client's Glasgow Coma Score?

Assessment	Response	Score
Eyes open	Spontaneously To speech To pain No response	4 3 2 1
Best motor response	Obeys commands Localizes pain Flexion-withdrawal Abnormal flexion Abnormal extension No response	6 5 4 3 2 1
Best verbal response	Oriented Confused Innapropriate words Incomprehensible sounds No response	5 4 3 2 1

4 The nurse is planning care for a client who experienced a cerebrovascular accident (CVA) with residual dysphagia. Which action will the nurse plan to avoid during meals?

1. Feed the client slowly.
2. Give the client thin liquids.
3. Give foods with the consistency of oatmeal.
4. Place food on the unaffected side of the mouth.

5 A client who experienced a spinal cord injury at the level of T5 rings the call bell for assistance. Upon entering the room, the nurse finds the client to have a flushed head and neck, is diaphoretic, and reports a severe headache. The client's pulse is 47 and BP is 220/114 mmHg. The nurse concludes that the client needs immediate treatment for which condition?

1. Malignant hypertension
2. Pulmonary embolism
3. Autonomic hyperreflexia
4. Spinal shock

6 A nurse is caring for a client who just experienced a seizure. While doing follow-up documentation, the nurse plans to include which items in the progress note? Select all that apply.

1. Reports of unusual sounds or smells prior to the seizure
2. What the client was doing prior to the seizure
3. Food and fluid intake prior to the seizure
4. The part of the body where the seizure started
5. The amount of lighting in the room when the seizure began

7 The home care nurse is doing an admission assessment on a client discharged from the hospital with a diagnosis of Parkinson's disease. When assessing the client's neurological status, the nurse anticipates which assessment finding?

1. Flaccidity of skeletal muscles
2. A shuffling and propulsive gait
3. An intention tremor
4. Droopy eyelids

8 A client with multiple sclerosis tells the nurse, "I am worried that this condition will make me too tired to do anything when I go home." Which response by the nurse most supports the goal of maintaining client independence?

1. "Maybe you can get a family member to help you out in the evenings."
2. "You are going to have to learn to be happy with doing less and taking more naps."
3. "You should go to the drugstore to get some assistive devices."
4. "Let's look at the things you do every day and figure out how to space the activities out through your day."

POSTTEST

9 The nurse reads in an admission note that the physical examination of a client revealed an impairment of cranial nerve II. The nurse gives ancillary caregivers which instructions when caring for this client? Select all that apply.

1. Whisper to the client.
2. Serve food at room temperature.
3. Clear the client's path of obstacles.
4. Report difficulty swallowing.
5. Ensure adequate lighting for tasks.

10 The nurse is providing a client with Bell's palsy with information about medications that might reduce nerve tissue edema. The nurse should explain the actions and side effects of which medication?

1. Acetaminophen (Tylenol)
2. Ibuprofen (Advil)
3. Dexamethasone (Decadron)
4. Prednisone (Deltasone)

➤ *See pages 177–178 for Answers and Rationales.*

ANSWERS & RATIONALES

Pretest

1 **Answer: 4** **Rationale:** Placing the client in a side-lying position allows saliva to run out of the mouth by gravity and reduces the risk of aspiration. Foam toothettes are appropriate to provide oral care on an unconscious client as a method to moisten the mouth. A soft bristle toothbrush may used to provide oral care as it is the best way to remove plaque from the mouth. Alcohol-based mouthwash should be avoided for oral hygiene as it is drying to the oral mucosa. **Cognitive Level:** Applying **Client Need:** Basic Care and Comfort **Integrated Process:** Nursing Process: Implementation **Content Area:** Fundamentals **Strategy:** The nurse should intervene when the student is observed performing a wrong action. As you read each option, ask yourself if this action is correct or incorrect. If an action is incorrect, then that is the correct response to this question. **Reference:** Berman, A., & Shirey, S.J. (2012). *Skills in clinical nursing* (7th ed.). Upper Saddle River, NJ: Pearson Education, pp. 193–199.

2 **Answer: 4** **Rationale:** Because the brain is enclosed in the rigid skull, it cannot accommodate the excessive increase in volume associated with tissue edema of head trauma. As the volume increases, pressure is exerted on the structures within the brain because there is no outlet for the edema fluid. Eventually, the pressure is exerted onto the brain structures and autoregulation is lost. Loss of autoregulation causes a late sign of increased intracranial pressure (ICP), the Cushing's reflex, which is manifested by rising systolic blood pressure accompanied by widening pulse pressure and bradycardia. Damage to the hypothalamus causes a temperature elevation and pressure on the medulla results in a decreased respiratory rate. **Cognitive Level:** Analyzing **Client Need:** Physiological Adaptation **Integrated Process:** Nursing Process: Assessment **Content Area:** Adult Health

Strategy: Pay attention to the critical words in the question *increasing intracranial pressure*. Review the autoregulatory responses in brain tissue and the result of a loss of the reflexes. **Reference:** LeMone, P., Burke, K., & Bauldoff, G. (2011). *Medical-surgical nursing: Critical thinking in patient care* (5th ed.). Upper Saddle River, NJ: Pearson Education, pp. 1438–1439.

3 **Answer: 2** **Rationale:** Clients with increased intracranial pressure (ICP) often require ventilation for airway support and respiratory management. Since carbon dioxide (CO_2) is a potent vasodilator, often clients with increasing ICP will be hyperventilated via a mechanical ventilator. Hyperventilation to achieve a $PaCO_2$ of 25 to 30 mmHg causes cerebral vasoconstriction that will lead to reduced intracranial blood volume and reduced ICP. **Cognitive Level:** Analyzing **Client Need:** Reduction of Risk Potential **Integrated Process:** Nursing Process: Evaluation **Content Area:** Adult Health **Strategy:** To answer this question, you need to understand the relationship between pCO_2 and cerebral circulation and the results of hyperventilation on cerebral circulation. This will enable you to draw the correct conclusion. **Reference:** LeMone, P., Burke, K., & Bauldoff, G. (2011). *Medical-surgical nursing: Critical thinking in patient care* (5th ed.). Upper Saddle River, NJ: Pearson Education, pp. 1441–1442.

4 **Answer: 2** **Rationale:** Because this client has hemiparesis on the right side, this indicates that the stroke is in the left cerebral hemisphere. It is not uncommon for a stroke in this area to cause loss of vision in the affected side. It is therefore best to place objects on the left side of the client so the client can see and reach them. If objects are placed on the right, the client will not see them because of visual field cuts. Placing objects far away from a client with hemiparesis will increase the risk of client injury because the client may attempt to reach for objects needed for self-care. **Cognitive Level:** Applying

Client need: Physiological Adaptation **Integrated Process:** Nursing Process: Implementation **Content Area:** Adult Health **Strategy:** Review the pathophysiology of cerebrovascular accident (CVA), and apply this to the symptoms that the client would experience. Then compare this information to the distracters and select the one that maximizes client independence. **Reference:** LeMone, P., Burke, K., & Bauldoff, G. (2011). *Medical-surgical nursing: Critical thinking in patient care* (5th ed.). Upper Saddle River, NJ: Pearson Education, pp. 1450–1457.

5 **Answer: 1, 2, 3** **Rationale:** Autonomic hyperreflexia, an exaggerated sympathetic response to noxious stimuli, is a risk for clients who sustain a spinal cord injury at the level of T6 or above. Massive vasoconstriction occurs below the level of the injury, causing hypertension and a severe pounding headache. Above the level of the injury, the heart responds to reflex vagal stimulation by slowing down. There is a baroreceptor-mediated vasodilation above the level of the injury, causing warm, flushed skin with sweating. **Cognitive Level:** Applying **Client Need:** Physiological Adaptation **Integrated Process:** Nursing Process: Assessment **Content Area:** Adult Health **Strategy:** Review the pathophysiology of the disease process and apply the expected signs and symptoms. Then treat each answer like a true-false question, marking the "true" responses as correct. **Reference:** LeMone, P., Burke, K., & Bauldoff, G. (2011). *Medical-surgical nursing: Critical thinking in patient care* (5th ed.). Upper Saddle River, NJ: Pearson Education, p. 1483.

6 **Answer: 1** **Rationale:** Decerebration frequently precedes brainstem herniation and is demonstrated by the client's extending the arms and internally rotating them. The feet may also be plantar flexed. Clients with injuries to the corticospinal tract will frequently exhibit decorticate posturing first characterized by flexion of the arms upward and toward the center of the body and then decerebrate posturing. Kernig's sign is an indicator of meningeal irritation and manifests as pain or resistance to flexing the knee at the hips and then straightening the leg. A positive Babinski reflex occurs when the toes of the foot dorsiflex and fan outward when the bottom of the foot is stroked and it is associated with upper motor neuron disease of the pyramidal tract. **Cognitive Level:** Applying **Client Need:** Physiological Adaptation **Integrated Process:** Communication and Documentation **Content Area:** Adult Health **Strategy:** Specific knowledge of abnormal neurological posturing is needed to answer the question. Review the positions that occur with deteriorating neurological status and the primary site of injury if this question was difficult. **Reference:** LeMone, P., Burke, K., & Bauldoff, G. (2011). *Medical-surgical nursing: Critical thinking in patient care* (5th ed.). Upper Saddle River, NJ: Pearson Education, pp. 1426–1427.

7 **Answer: 1, 2** **Rationale:** Parkinson's disease is characterized by tremors, rigidity, akinesia and postural instability. Rocking back and forth to initiate movement may help overcome akinesia and rigidity. Velcro fasteners assist clients with Parkinson's disease independence with dressing and grooming. Activities should be planned for immediately after taking medication when the client has the greatest range of motion. Clients with Parkinson's disease should sit in chairs that are high and firm, as it will help the client to rise from a sitting to a standing position. Buttons will be difficult to handle for clients with Parkinson's disease because of the hand tremors associated with this disorder. **Cognitive Level:** Applying **Client Need:** Physiological Adaptation **Integrated Process:** Teaching and Learning **Content Area:** Adult Health **Strategy:** Knowledge of the pathophysiology of Parkinson's disease and the pharmacologic management of the disease are required to answer this question correctly. Keep in mind the principle of promoting independence as long as possible to help make the correct selection. **Reference:** LeMone, P., Burke, K., & Bauldoff, G. (2011). *Medical-surgical nursing: Critical thinking in patient care* (5th ed.). Upper Saddle River, NJ: Pearson Education, p. 1531.

8 **Answer: 1** **Rationale:** Stage 2 Alzheimer's disease is characterized by mild memory lapses. Nursing interventions geared towards assisting these clients with memory impairments include ensuring a client is wearing an ID badge, using a calendar, and keeping lists of reminders. A quiet, calm environment may enhance the client's feelings of isolation and depression. Restraints are not indicated and violate the principle of "least restrictive measures." It is unnecessary to assess level of consciousness (LOC) hourly for a client in Stage 2 Alzheimer's disease as it is not affected at this stage. **Cognitive Level:** Applying **Client Need:** Management of Care **Integrated Process:** Nursing Process: Planning **Content Area:** Adult Health **Strategy:** Consider the stage of the disorder and the client presentation as well as the identified problem. Eliminate any option that is inconsistent with either the stage of the disease or the identified problem. **Reference:** LeMone, P., Burke, K., & Bauldoff, G. (2011). *Medical-surgical nursing: Critical thinking in patient care* (5th ed.). Upper Saddle River, NJ: Pearson Education, pp. 1511–1514.

9 **Answer: 1** **Rationale:** The pain of trigeminal neuralgia is triggered by stimulation of the sensory fibers of the trigeminal nerve, causing excessive firing to the irritated nerve. Minimal stimulation can evoke severe episodes of pain. Stimulation can be caused by pressure-related triggering events include shaving, toothbrushing, washing the face, and eating or drinking. Temperature-related triggers include environmental changes and hot or cold food and drink. Hypoglycemia, epinephrine, and the immune response are unrelated to trigeminal neuralgia. **Cognitive Level:** Applying **Client Need:** Physiological Adaptation **Integrated Process:** Nursing Process: Implementation **Content Area:** Adult Health **Strategy:** Focus on important syllables such as *neur-* involving a nerve and *-algia* involving pain. Apply this information to each answer option to select the correct response. **Reference:** LeMone, P., Burke, K., & Bauldoff, G. (2011). *Medical-surgical* *nursing: Critical thinking in patient care* (5th ed.). Upper Saddle River, NJ: Pearson Education, pp. 1545–1547.

10 **Answer: 2** **Rationale:** Antidepressants, tranquilizers, and antiepileptics (if ordered) are generally withheld for 24 to 48 hours before an EEG. The client does not have to be NPO because cellular activity is affected by insufficient amounts of glucose but stimulants such as coffee, tea, cola, alcohol, and cigarettes should be avoided. The client should be asked to shampoo the hair before the procedure to remove any gel or hairspray that may be in the hair. The test is not uncomfortable. **Cognitive Level:** Applying **Client Need:** Reduction of Risk Potential **Integrated Process:** Nursing Process: Implementation **Content Area:** Adult Health **Strategy:** Since an EEG assesses nerve transmission, eliminate any answer option that can influence this process. **Reference:** LeMone, P., Burke, K., & Bauldoff, G. (2011). *Medical-surgical nursing: Critical thinking in patient care* (5th ed.). Upper Saddle River, NJ: Pearson Education, p. 1416.

Posttest

1 **Answer: 1** **Rationale:** An unconscious client may have a decreased or absent gag reflex, making them unable to effectively protect the airway from aspiration. Enteral feedings place the client at even higher risk for aspiration and the development of aspiration pneumonia. While enteral feedings may place a client at risk for fluid volume overload, there is not enough data in the question to support that the client is at risk for fluid volume overload. An unconscious client is at risk for inadequate nutritional intake but it is not a priority for this client. Enteral feedings will provide an unconscious client with calories, nutrients and volume. Electrolyte imbalance as a collaborative problem is possible but it is not a priority for this client. **Cognitive Level:** Analyzing **Client Need:** Reduction of Risk Potential **Integrated Process:** Nursing Process: Diagnosis **Content Area:** Fundamentals **Strategy:** Read the information data provided in the questions and apply it to potential complications. Utilize the ABC's (airway, breathing, and circulation) as a method to eliminate the wrong answers. **Reference:** LeMone, P., Burke, K., & Bauldoff, G. (2011). *Medical-surgical nursing: Critical thinking in patient care* (5th ed.). Upper Saddle River, NJ: Pearson Education, p. 1436.

2 **Answer: 2, 5** **Rationale:** Decorticate posturing, a late sign of significant deterioration in neurologic status, is manifested by clients' rigidly flexing their elbows and wrists and it can be significant for injury to the midbrain. Clients with significant intracranial injury and edema will frequently exhibit decorticate posturing first and then decerebrate posturing. Decerebration frequently precedes brainstem herniation or injury to the pons. **Cognitive Level:** Applying **Client Need:** Physiological Adaptation **Integrated Process:** Nursing Process: Assessment **Content Area:** Adult Health **Strategy:** Read each answer carefully and use the process of elimination. Recall the positions that occur with deteriorating neurological

status and how they relate to the primary site of injury to make the correct selections. **Reference:** LeMone, P., Burke, K., & Bauldoff, G.(2011). *Medical-surgical nursing: Critical thinking in patient care* (5th ed.). Upper Saddle River, NJ: Pearson Education, p. 1427.

3 **Answer: 10** **Rationale:** The client opens his eyes to voice = 3. Withdrawing the hand to a pain response demonstrates that the client can localize pain = 5. The client is making incomprehensible sounds = 2. Then add the numbers: 3 + 5 + 2 = 10 **Cognitive Level:** Analyzing **Client Need:** Physiological Adaptation **Integrated Process:** Nursing Process: Assessment **Content Area:** Adult Health **Strategy:** Read the assessment data carefully and think about what the descriptions really mean. Apply the descriptions to the data given. **Reference:** LeMone, P., Burke, K., & Bauldoff, G. (2011). *Medical-surgical nursing: Critical thinking in patient care* (5th ed.). Upper Saddle River, NJ: Pearson Education, p. 1421.

4 **Answer: 2** **Rationale:** A client who experienced a cerebrovascular accident (CVA) may have involvement of the cranial nerves responsible for chewing and swallowing (dysphagia). The client with dysphagia may be started on a diet once the gag and swallow reflexes have returned. Feeding the client slowly will reduce the risk that the client will aspirate food due to impaired swallowing. Clients with impaired swallowing should have liquids the consistency of honey, not thin liquids. Oatmeal-consistency foods are easier for clients with dysphagia to swallow. Placing food on the unaffected side of the mouth helps prevent the food from collecting in the mouth and makes swallowing safer. **Cognitive Level:** Applying **Client Need:** Reduction of Risk Potential **Integrated Process:** Nursing Process: Implementation **Content Area:** Adult Health **Strategy:** The question is asking which action the nurse should avoid doing. Select the answer choice that is the wrong action based on the information given. **Reference:** LeMone, P., Burke, K., & Bauldoff, G. (2011). *Medical-surgical nursing: Critical thinking in patient care* (5th ed.). Upper Saddle River, NJ: Pearson Education, p. 1458.

5 **Answer: 3** **Rationale:** Above the level of T6, clients with spinal cord injury are at risk for autonomic hyperreflexia. It is a life-threatening syndrome triggered by a noxious stimulus below the level of the injury. This complication is characterized by severe, throbbing headache, flushing of the face and neck, bradycardia, and sudden severe hypertension. Given the presentation of the client's symptoms associated with a thoracic spinal cord injury, it is unlikely that the client is experiencing malignant hypertension. This symptom cluster is inconsistent with pulmonary emboli, which would include chest pain, anxiety, and hypoxia. Spinal shock occurs immediately after a spinal cord injury and is characterized by flaccidity and hypotension. **Cognitive Level:** Analyzing **Client Need:** Physiological Adaptation **Integrated Process:** Nursing Process: Diagnosis **Content Area:** Adult Health **Strategy:** This item is directly related to the spinal cord injury. Recall the possible complications of this type of injury and compare your list to the symptoms in the question. **Reference:** LeMone, P., Burke, K., & Bauldoff, G. (2011). *Medical-surgical nursing: Critical thinking in patient care* (5th ed.). Upper Saddle River, NJ: Pearson Education, p. 1483.

6 **Answer: 1, 2, 4** **Rationale:** The presence of an aura, unusual taste or smell prior to the seizure, should be included in documentation. The client's actions prior to the seizure may suggest precipitating factors for the seizure and should be documented. Documentation of food and fluid intake prior to the seizure is unnecessary. The part of the body where the seizure started may indicate the site of the seizure activity in the brain tissue. It is not necessary to document the amount of lighting in the room prior to the onset of the seizure. **Cognitive Level:** Applying **Client Need:** Physiological Adaptation **Integrated Process:** Nursing Process: Documentation **Content Area:** Adult Health **Strategy:** Treat each answer choice like a true-false question, applying your knowledge of seizure disorders. **Reference:** LeMone, P., Burke, K., & Bauldoff, G. (2011). *Medical-surgical nursing: Critical thinking in patient care* (5th ed.). Upper Saddle River, NJ: Pearson Education, pp. 1442–1448.

7 **Answer: 2** **Rationale:** Muscle rigidity, not flaccidity, occurs in Parkinson's disease as a result of involuntary contraction of skeletal muscles. Clients with Parkinson's disease walk with short, shuffling steps in order to try to maintain an upright position when walking. Intention tremors are common in multiple sclerosis, while clients with Parkinson's disease have resting tremors of the hands, feet, head, neck, and face. Droopy eyelids are a hallmark assessment finding in clients with myasthenia gravis, not Parkinson's disease. **Cognitive Level:** Analyzing **Client Need:** Reduction of Risk Potential **Integrated Process:** Nursing Process: Assessment **Content Area:** Adult Health **Strategy:** Review the answer choices and eliminate any answer choices not consistent with Parkinson's disease. **Reference:** LeMone, P., & Burke, K. (2011). *Medical-surgical nursing: Critical thinking in patient care* (5th ed.). Upper Saddle River, NJ: Pearson Education, pp. 1526–1528.

8 **Answer: 4** **Rationale:** Multiple sclerosis is an autoimmune disease that affects the myelin sheath and muscle innervations, characterized by remissions and exacerbations. Independence and self-control should be encouraged in clients with multiple sclerosis. Suggesting a family member help with activities is inconsistent with this goal. While naps and prioritizing activities may be necessary during some exacerbations of multiple sclerosis, telling the client to learn to be happy is not therapeutic. There is no indication that the client needs assistive devices at home. Arranging daily activities throughout the day and including rest periods are essential to manage feelings of fatigue and replenish energy reserves. **Cognitive Level:** Analyzing **Client Need:** Physiological Adaptation **Integrated Process:** Nursing Process: Implementation **Content Area:** Adult Health **Strategy:** Focus on the response that encourages the client to maintain as normal an existence as possible. **Reference:** LeMone, P., & Burke, K. (2011). *Medical-surgical nursing: Critical thinking in patient care* (5th ed.). Upper Saddle River, NJ: Pearson Education, pp. 1524–1525.

9 **Answer: 3, 5** **Rationale:** Cranial nerve II is the optic nerve, which controls visual acuity. It is appropriate to ensure adequate lighting for tasks and to clear obstacles out of the path of a client with impaired visual acuity. The ability to hear is controlled by cranial nerve VIII, not cranial nerve II. The trigeminal nerve (cranial nerve V) controls sensation on the tongue. Swallowing is managed by the glossopharyngeal nerve (cranial nerve IX). **Cognitive Level:** Analyzing **Client Need:** Management of Care **Integrated Process:** Nursing Process: Planning **Content Area:** Adult Health **Strategy:** This item requires you to know the names of the cranial nerves and the interventions that can compensate for the loss of function of that nerve. **Reference:** LeMone, P., & Burke, K. (2012). *Medical-surgical nursing: Critical thinking in patient care* (5th ed.). Upper Saddle River, NJ: Pearson Education, pp. 1422–1423.

10 **Answer: 4** **Rationale:** Bell's palsy is an inflammatory process of the fifth cranial nerve. It causes facial paralysis and can result in corneal abrasions because of an inability to close the eye on the affected side. Prednisone (Deltasone) is the treatment of choice because it reduces inflammation and edema and can help preserve a significant amount of function; it is also effective against pain when given early in the course of treatment. Ibuprofen (Advil) is classified as an anti-inflammatory medication but it is not the treatment of choice for Bell's palsy. Dexamethasone (Decadron) is the drug of choice in cerebral edema, not Bell's palsy. Acetaminophen (Tylenol) is an analgesic that works at the level of the peripheral nerves. **Cognitive Level:** Analyzing **Client Need:** Pharmacological and Parenteral Therapies **Integrated Process:** Nursing Process: Implementation **Content Area:** Adult Health **Strategy:** To select the best answer option, eliminate items that are not primarily related to the inflammatory process. Select the answer choice that is used for its broad anti-inflammatory properties. **Reference:** LeMone, P., & Burke, K. (2011). *Medical-surgical nursing: Critical thinking in patient care* (5th ed.). Upper Saddle River, NJ: Pearson Education, pp. 1547–1548.

References

Berman, A., & Snyder, S. (2012). *Kozier & Erb's fundamentals of nursing: Concepts, process, and practice* (9th ed.). Upper Saddle River, NJ: Pearson Education.

D'Amico, D., & Barbarito, C. (2012). *Health & physical assessment in nursing* (2nd ed.). Upper Saddle River, NJ: Pearson Education, Inc.

Ignatavicius, D. D., & Workman, M. L. (2013). *Medical-surgical nursing: Critical thinking for collaborative care* (7th ed.) Philadelphia: W. B. Saunders Company.

Kee, J. L. (2010). *Laboratory and diagnostic tests* (8th ed.). Upper Saddle River, NJ: Pearson Education.

Lehne, R. (2010). *Pharmacology for nursing care* (7th ed.). St. Louis, MO: Saunders.

LeMone, P., Burke, K., & Bauldoff, G. (2011). *Medical-surgical nursing: Critical thinking in patient care* (5th ed.). Upper Saddle River, NJ: Pearson Education.

Lewis, S., Dirksen, S., Heitkemper, M., Bucher, L., & Camera, I. (2011). *Medical surgical nursing: Assessment and management of clinical problems* (8th ed.). St. Louis, MO: Elsevier.

McCance, K. L., & Huether, S. E. (2010). *Pathophysiology: The biologic basis for disease in adults and children* (6th ed.). St. Louis, MO: Mosby, Inc.

Osborn, K. S., Wraa, C. E., & Watson, A. (2010). *Medical surgical nursing: Preparation for practice*. Upper Saddle River, NJ: Pearson Education.

Smith, S. F., Duell, D. J., & Martin, B. C. (2012). *Clinical nursing skills: Basic to advanced skills* (8th ed.). Upper Saddle River, NJ: Pearson Education.

6 Renal and Urinary Disorders

Chapter Outline

Overview of Anatomy and
Physiology of Renal and
Urinary Systems
Diagnostic Tests and Assessments
of Urinary System

Common Nursing Techniques
and Procedures
Nursing Management of
Clients Having Renal
or Bladder Surgery

Disorders of the Urinary
System

NCLEX-RN® Test Prep

Use the accompanying online resource,
NursingReviewsandRationales, to test
yourself with hundreds of NCLEX®-style
practice questions.

Objectives

➤ Identify basic structures and functions of the renal and urinary systems.
➤ Describe the pathophysiology and etiology of common renal and
urinary disorders.
➤ Discuss expected assessment data and diagnostic test findings for
selected renal and urinary disorders.
➤ Identify priority nursing problems for selected renal and urinary
disorders.
➤ Discuss therapeutic management of selected renal and urinary disorders.
➤ Discuss nursing management of a client experiencing a renal or
urinary disorder.
➤ Identify expected outcomes for a client experiencing a renal or
urinary disorder.

Review at a Glance

acute renal failure sudden interruption of renal function caused by obstruction, poor circulation, or kidney disease

anuria output of urine in quantities less than 100 mL in a 24-hour period

azotemia increased toxic levels of nitrogenous wastes in blood

chronic renal failure (CRF) slow, progressive loss of kidney function and glomerular filtration

cystectomy partial or total removal of urinary bladder and surrounding structures

cystitis inflammation of bladder

glomerulonephritis inflammation of renal glomerulus characterized by decreased urine production, blood and protein in urine, and edema

hematuria presence of blood in urine

hemodialysis procedure to remove wastes from blood by filtering client's blood through a machine

intravenous pyelography (IVP) a radiology technique that involves injecting a contrast medium into a vein and taking x-ray films of kidneys as medium is cleared from blood into urinary system

lithotripsy procedure that breaks up stones within urinary system

nephrotic syndrome renal disease characterized by massive edema and excess protein excretion

oliguria diminished urine production in relation to intake, usually less than 400 mL in 24 hours

peritoneal dialysis procedure during which blood is filtered through peritoneal membrane to remove waste products

polycystic kidney disease a disorder characterized by multiple cysts of kidney

polyuria excess production of urine

proteinuria presence of protein in urine

pyelonephritis a pus-forming infection of kidney that usually moves upward from lower urinary tract

pyuria pus in urine

urinary diversion procedure that provides an alternative route for urine excretion when normal channels are damaged or defective

vesicoureteral reflux backflow of urine from bladder into ureter

PRETEST

1 The nurse has admitted a client with uremia. The nurse questions the client about a history of which health problem?

1. Polycystic kidney disease
2. End-stage renal failure
3. Pyelonephritis
4. Cystitis

2 A client receiving peritoneal dialysis (PD) has outflow that is 200 mL less than the inflow for 2 consecutive exchanges. Which actions would be appropriate for the nurse to take at this time? Select all that apply.

1. Examine the abdominal dressing.
2. Change client's position.
3. Lower the drainage bag.
4. Continue to monitor the outflow in future exchanges.
5. Irrigate the peritoneal dialysis catheter.

3 The nurse is planning to teach the client with acute glomerulonephritis about necessary dietary restrictions. Which dietary changes should the nurse include in the plan?

1. Limit fluid intake to 500 mL per day.
2. Restrict protein intake by limiting meats and other high-protein foods.
3. Increase intake of high-fiber foods, such as bran cereal.
4. Increase intake of potassium-rich foods such as bananas or cantaloupe.

4 A client develops a renal disorder after taking an antibiotic that is known to have nephrotoxic effects. The nurse adds a standardized care plan to the client's medical record for which disorder?

1. Polycystic kidney disease
2. Glomerulonephritis
3. Acute renal failure
4. Chronic renal failure

5 A client with a chronic urinary tract infection (UTI) is scheduled for a number of laboratory tests. The nurse would note that which test result best evaluates whether the kidneys are being adversely affected?

1. Serum potassium 3.8 mEq/L
2. Urinalysis specific gravity 1.015
3. Serum creatinine 2.0 mg/dL
4. Urine culture negative

6 The nurse is teaching a female client with recurrent cystitis who is scheduled for cystoscopy in the morning. Which preprocedure instructions should the nurse include in the teaching?

1. Take acetaminophen (Tylenol) and diphenhydramine (Benadryl) the morning of the test to minimize allergic reaction.
2. Light breakfast may be eaten.
3. This test is only used to diagnose disorders.
4. Take a laxative the evening before procedure.

7 The nurse is teaching the client to perform peritoneal dialysis (PD). The nurse reviews which essential action that will help to prevent the major complication of peritoneal dialysis?

1. Monitor postvoid residuals.
2. Maintain strict aseptic technique during connection and disconnection.
3. Add heparin to dialysate at least once per day.
4. Change catheter site dressing twice daily.

8 A client is admitted to the emergency department with suspected urolithiasis. The nurse questions the client about the presence of which symptom that would be expected with urolithiasis?

1. Flank pain
2. Difficult urination
3. Absence of urine
4. Headache

PRETEST

9 The nurse is caring for a client immediately following a transurethral prostatectomy (TURP). The nurse places high priority on which nursing interventions in the immediate postoperative period for this client? Select all that apply.

1. Assess for signs of a urinary tract infection.
2. Prevent postoperative atelectasis.
3. Discontinue urinary catheter as soon as possible.
4. Adjust flow rate of the bladder irrigant to keep catheter patent.
5. Monitor the amount of blood in the urine.

10 The nurse is caring for a client following a renal transplant. The nurse places highest priority on which nursing diagnosis?

1. Anxiety related to postoperative pain
2. Disturbed Sleep Pattern related to frequent assessments
3. Disturbed Body Image related to fluid retention
4. Risk for Infection related to bone marrow suppression

➤ *See pages 212–214 for Answers & Rationales.*

I. OVERVIEW OF ANATOMY AND PHYSIOLOGY OF RENAL AND URINARY SYSTEMS

A. Renal structures (see Figure 6-1)

1. Adrenal glands: located on top each kidney; influence blood pressure (BP) and sodium (Na^+) and water retention; comprised of 2 parts: medulla and cortex
2. Kidneys: bean-shaped organs located on either side of spinal column behind peritoneal cavity; helps regulate fluid and acid–base balance
3. Renal cortex: outer region of kidneys; contains blood-filtering mechanisms
4. Renal medulla: middle region of kidneys; contains renal pyramids
5. Renal pyramids: triangular wedges containing tubular structures
   a. Apex: tapered section of each pyramid; empties into calyx (calyces)
   b. Calyx (calyces): channel urine from renal pyramids to renal pelvis
6. Renal pelvis: expansion of upper end of ureters, formed as calyces join together
7. Nephrons: basic functional units of kidneys; selectively secrete and reabsorb ions; perform mechanical filtration of fluid, wastes, electrolytes, acids, and bases
   a. Glomerular capsule (Bowman's capsule): surrounds glomeruli
   b. Glomerulus (glomeruli): tuft of capillaries within each nephron; filter large plasma proteins and blood cells
   c. Glomerular filtrate: fluid filtered by glomeruli; similar to plasma; made up of water, electrolytes, glucose, amino acids, and metabolic wastes
8. Proximal convoluted tubule: located in renal cortex; receives filtrate from glomerular capsules; reabsorbs water and electrolytes
9. Loop of Henle: forms renal pyramid in medulla; U-shaped portion of renal tubule
   a. Descending loop of Henle: removes water from filtrate
   b. Ascending loop of Henle: removes Na^+ and chloride from filtrate; helps maintain osmolality
10. Distal convoluted tubule: portion of tubule beyond loop of Henle; located in renal cortex; removes more Na^+ and water

B. Blood vessels of kidneys

1. Renal artery: large branch of abdominal aorta that delivers blood to each kidney
2. Interlobar arteries: branches of renal artery within each kidney
3. Peritubular capillaries: surround renal tubules
4. Renal vein: returns filtered blood to circulation; empties into inferior vena cava

C. Function of kidneys

1. Kidneys filter blood to remove waste products, byproducts of drugs, excess minerals and vitamins, excess electrolytes; this mechanism supports homeostasis and uses processes of filtration, absorption and osmosis

Figure 6-1

Urinary system of a female

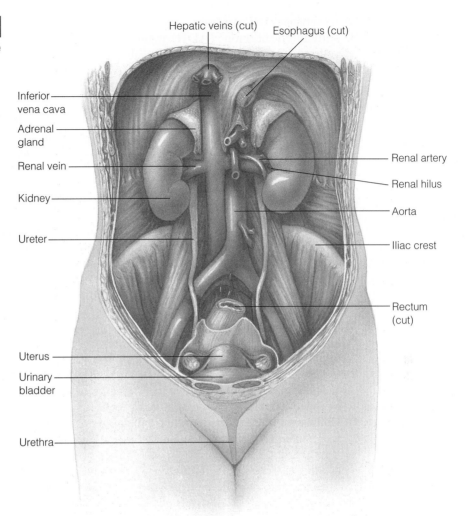

Hepatic veins (cut)

Esophagus (cut)

Inferior vena cava

Adrenal gland

Renal vein

Kidney

Ureter

Renal artery

Renal hilus

Aorta

Iliac crest

Rectum (cut)

Uterus

Urinary bladder

Urethra

2. Filtration: first step in blood processing; water and solutes move from plasma in glomerulus into Bowman's capsule; depends on pressure gradient between blood in glomeruli and filtrate in Bowman's capsule

3. Reabsorption: second step in urine formation; molecules move from tubules into blood; active and passive transport mechanisms are used in all parts of renal tubules
   a. Proximal tubules: reabsorb Na^+ and other major ions through active and passive transport
   b. Loop of Henle: reabsorbs through counter-current mechanism (passive); contents flow in opposite directions
   c. Distal tubules: reabsorb Na^+ by active and passive transport in smaller amounts than proximal tubules
   d. Collecting ducts: prevent water from leaving filtrate; use active and passive reabsorption

4. Tubular secretion: movement of substances out of blood into tubular fluid; tubule cells secrete certain substances in addition to performing reabsorption

5. Regulation of urine volume: hormones play a central part in urine regulation

6. Osmolality: osmotic pressure of a solution expressed as number of osmoles of pressure per kg of water; active transport and reabsorption mechanisms are based on osmolality of solutions

D. Renal hormones and enzymes

1. Antidiuretic hormone (ADH): regulates urine volume by acting on distal tubule and collecting ducts to increase water reabsorption and urine concentration
2. Atrial natriuretic hormone (ANH): secreted by muscle fibers in atrium of heart; promotes loss of Na^+ via urine
3. Aldosterone: secreted by adrenal cortex; increases Na^+ absorption in distal and collecting tubules and controls potassium (K^+) secretion, leading to osmotic imbalance that causes reabsorption of water; works in conjunction with ADH
   a. Increased serum K^+ levels lead to increased aldosterone secretion
   b. Increased aldosterone secretion increases Na^+ and water retention and depresses formation of renin
4. Renin: enzyme secreted by kidneys; helps regulate Na^+ retention and, therefore, BP and fluid volume
   a. Renin-angiotensin system: converts angiotensinogen to angiotensin I in liver
   b. Angiotensin II: formed in lungs from angiotensin I; vasoconstrictor that stimulates adrenal cortex to produce aldosterone
5. Erythropoietin: hormone produced by kidneys in response to low oxygen levels in arterial blood; travels to bone marrow and stimulates increased red blood cell (RBC) production

E. Urinary excretion

1. Ureters: extend from renal pelvis of kidney to urinary bladder; conduct urine to bladder
2. Bladder: elastic sac located behind symphysis pubis; stores and excretes urine
   a. Ruggae: ridges formed by mucous membrane on bladder wall
   b. Detrusor muscle: muscular layer of bladder
3. Urethra: tube that carries urine from bladder to exterior of body
   a. Female urethra: embedded in anterior wall of vagina; is approximately 23–26 cm in length
   b. Male urethra: passes through prostate gland, urogenital diaphragm (a ligament), and penis; passes both urine and semen and is approximately 40 to 44 cm in length
4. Urinary meatus: exterior opening of urethra
5. Urination: an involuntary or voluntary reflex allowing urine to leave body
   a. Micturition reflex: parasympathetic response that stimulates relaxation and contraction of external sphincter, allowing urine to pass
   b. Internal sphincter muscle: helps control urine passage into urethra; relaxes in response to parasympathetic nerve fibers in bladder wall
   c. External sphincter muscle: voluntary muscle that allows urine to pass into urethra; controlled by micturition reflex
6. Characteristics of normal urine
   a. Color: clear, pale amber
   b. Consistency: 95% water with many dissolved substances
   c. Output: 1,000–2,000 mL per 24-hour period
   d. Specific gravity: commonly 1.010–1.025
   e. Odor: faint ammonia

II. DIAGNOSTIC TESTS AND ASSESSMENTS OF URINARY SYSTEM

A. Urine studies

1. Urinalysis: evaluates specific gravity, color (light to dark yellow or amber, depending on concentration), pH (5–9, average 6), and substances that should be absent or negative (protein, glucose, ketone bodies, leukocytes); examines urine sediment for blood cells, casts, and crystals
2. Urine culture: checks urine for bacteria; urine is normally sterile

3. 24-hour urine specimen: urine is collected over 24 hours for these tests:
- **a.** Creatinine: nitrogenous waste product excreted by muscle tissue; normally found in urine (normal 15–25 mg/kg in 24 hours)
- **b.** Creatinine clearance: test to assess how well kidneys remove creatinine from blood (males 95–135 mL/min; females 85–125 mL/min)
- **c.** Protein: less than 150 mg/24 hours
- **d.** Urea nitrogen: end product of protein metabolism (normal 6–17 grams/24 hours)

4. Urine osmolality: osmotic pressure (concentration) of urine; average is 500–800 mOsm/kg water, with an extreme range of 50–1,400 mOsm/kg water

B. Renal scan: intravenous radioactive substance (radionuclide) is injected, then observed passing through kidneys; evaluates renal blood flow, nephrons, collecting system function, and renal structures

C. Radiographic studies

1. Kidney-ureter-bladder radiography (KUB): x-ray series that shows kidney size, position, and structure; provides limited diagnostic information
2. Renal angiography: x-ray images of renal blood vessels and tissues, obtained by injecting contrast medium via femoral artery; detects abnormalities such as cysts, renal artery stenosis, and renal infarction
3. Renal venography: x-ray images of renal veins, obtained by injecting contrast medium in a large vein; detects renal vein thrombosis
4. Retrograde cystography: contrast medium instilled into bladder, followed by x-ray examination; helps diagnose ruptured or neurogenic bladder and other conditions

D. Computerized tomography (CT) scan: generates a 3-dimensional, computerized image of kidneys; identifies masses and other lesions; contrast medium may be injected

E. Magnetic resonance imaging (MRI): passes magnetic energy through body to produce 3-dimensional images of renal tissue; also called nuclear magnetic resonance (NMR)

F. Ultrasonography: high-frequency sound waves are directed through body and reflect back to source; a computer evaluates reflection (echo) and records/displays it; useful for clients with renal failure and those allergic to contrast medium; evaluates kidney size, shape, and position

G. Blood studies

1. Blood urea nitrogen (BUN): measures nitrogenous urea in blood; urea is produced by protein metabolism; increases that are caused by reduced glomerular filtration rate (GFR) and insufficient excretion may indicate renal disease; also rises with dehydration and high-protein diet or other conditions where excess protein is metabolized
   - **a.** Normal: 8–22 mg/dL
   - **b.** BUN levels are best evaluated in conjunction with serum creatinine
2. Serum creatinine: a nitrogenous waste resulting from muscle metabolism of creatine; creatinine levels reflect GFR
   - **a.** Measures renal damage more reliably than BUN, because only severe renal damage causes significant elevation
   - **b.** Normal: 0.6–1.5 mg/dL for adult males; 0.6–1.1 mg/dL for adult females
3. Glomerular filtration rate
   - **a.** Is an estimate of how much blood passes through kidney per minute; is based on age, gender, height, race, weight, and creatinine clearance
   - **b.** Normal is 90–120 mL/min/1.73 m^2 and decreases with age

H. Hemodynamic studies

1. **Intravenous pyelography (IVP)**: x-ray of kidneys and urinary tract after IV injection of contrast medium; also called excretory urography
2. Cystoscopy or cystourethroscopy: insertion of a cystoscope with a fiberoptic light source and telescopic lens into urethra; procedures include biopsy of bladder and prostate, lesion resection, calculi collection, or passage of catheter to renal pelvis

3. Percutaneous renal biopsy: client is positioned on abdomen while needle is inserted into kidney to remove tissue; x-ray may be used to guide needle
    a. Tissue studies (histology) can reveal renal disease, malignant tumors, and other conditions
    b. Risks include bleeding, hematoma, AV fistula, and infection

III. COMMON NURSING TECHNIQUES AND PROCEDURES

A. **Urinary catheterization**: introduction of a catheter into urinary bladder
1. Indwelling urinary catheter: a retention (Foley) catheter with balloon is inserted and remains in place
    a. Explain procedure to client and ensure privacy
    b. *Female*: assist client to supine position, with knees flexed and thighs externally rotated; drape client
    c. Wearing disposable gloves, cleanse perineal area; remove gloves
    d. Prepare equipment and set up sterile field; don sterile gloves; drape client with sterile drape
    e. Moisten sterile cotton balls with antiseptic solution (agency policy may differ concerning use of antiseptic)
    f. Lubricate insertion tip of catheter
    g. Clean meatus with antiseptic (check agency policy)
    h. Use nondominant hand to separate labia minor and expose urinary meatus; assess meatus for trauma, swelling, discharge, or redness
    i. Grasp catheter near insertion end with sterile, gloved hand
    j. Gently insert catheter into meatus and advance catheter until urine flows; do not use forceful pressure; ask client to take deep breaths to relax external sphincter
    k. After urine begins to flow, advance catheter 1–2 cm more into bladder and inflate balloon by injecting contents of prefilled syringe; apply slight tension by pulling back on catheter until resistance is felt to confirm that balloon is in bladder
    l. Anchor catheter to client's thigh with nonallergenic tape or leg strap and secure drainage bag to bed frame in a dependent position
    m. *Male*: use same positioning except knees do not need to be flexed
    n. Wearing disposable gloves, wash penis, and dry it well
    o. Follow steps d, e, f, and g described above, but in uncircumcised male, retract foreskin to expose meatus before cleaning
    p. Grasp insertion end of catheter with sterile, gloved hand
    q. Lift penis to 90-degree angle with body and exert slight traction
    r. Insert catheter steadily until urine begins to flow; ask client to take deep breaths to relax external sphincter; rotate catheter during insertion if slight resistance is met because of curvature of urethra
    s. Advance catheter farther into bladder (1 to 2 cm) and follow steps k and l described above
    t. In uncircumcised male, return foreskin over glans of penis
2. Intermittent catheterization: used for clients with neurogenic bladder dysfunction; may be done by nurse or by client at home after proper instruction; teach client the following procedure:
    a. Catheterize as often as needed; may be every 2–3 hours at first, then every 4–6 hours; use a clean catheter for each insertion
    b. Encourage to void before procedure if appropriate; bladder scanning (noninvasive) may be used to determine residual quantities, use catheter to obtain residual urine if amount voided is less than 100 mL
    c. Procedure is similar to inserting indwelling catheter; assemble all supplies and use good lighting

       d. Wash hands and clean urinary meatus as previously described

       e. Assume comfortable position, such as standing with one foot elevated, semi-reclining in bed, or sitting on chair or toilet

       f. Apply lubricant to catheter tip

       g. Catheter insertion: for *females*: locate meatus using a mirror or touch, separate labia with dominant hand, and direct catheter through meatus, then forward and upward; for *males*: hold penis with slight upward tension to 90-degree angle and insert catheter

       h. Hold catheter in place until all urine is drained, then withdraw slowly

       i. Notify care provider of cloudy urine, sediment, bleeding, fever, or difficulty passing catheter

       j. Client should drink at least 2,000–2,500 mL of fluid daily; cranberry and prune juices help to acidify urine and possibly reduce bacterial growth

B. Urine collection

   1. 24-hour urine collection

       a. Obtain specimen container with preservative from laboratory

       b. Provide clean receptacle to collect urine (bedpan, urinal, commode, or collection device on toilet) unless client already has an indwelling urinary catheter

       c. Post signs in client's room, on chart, and in bathroom alerting personnel to save urine

       d. Have client void and discard this urine at beginning of collection period, if indwelling catheter used, empty the collection bag at start time

       e. During collection period, save all urine in container; place container on ice or refrigerate as indicated; don't contaminate urine with bathroom tissue or feces

       f. Instruct client to empty bladder at end of collection period and save this urine

       g. Send collected urine to laboratory with completed requisition

       h. Document collection of specimen, time started and completed, and any observations

   2. Clean catch (midstream)

       a. Many clients can obtain specimen themselves after instruction

       b. Male clients void directly into container, while females hold container between legs during voiding

       c. Ask client to wash genitals and perineal area with soap and water

       d. Instruct how to clean meatus with antiseptic towelettes

       e. Female clients: use 3 towelettes, clean perineal area from front to back; use each towelette only once

       f. Male clients: clean meatus and head of penis with circular motion; use each towelette only once

       g. For client who needs assistance: nurse may don gloves, clean perineal area, assist client to a comfortable position, and open clean-catch kit

       h. Instruct client to begin voiding, then place specimen container in stream of urine; collect 30–60 mL of urine

       i. Cap container, touching only outside

       j. Label container, place in biohazard bag along with requisition, and immediately send to laboratory

       k. Document pertinent data, such as difficulty voiding, strong odor to urine, or sediment

C. *Peritoneal dialysis*: removes toxins from blood of client with acute or chronic renal failure; uses peritoneal membrane as semipermeable dialyzing membrane

   1. Hypertonic dialyzing solution (dialysate) is instilled through a catheter in peritoneal cavity

   2. Excess concentrations of electrolytes and uremic toxins diffuse across peritoneal membrane into dialysis solution; excess water moves into solution by osmosis

   3. Dialysate is drained after appropriate dwelling time

   4. Procedure is performed manually or with a cycler machine; client may also perform continuous ambulatory peritoneal dialysis (CAPD)

   5. Possible complications

       a. Peritonitis from bacteria entering peritoneal cavity (use aseptic technique when handling catheter or tubing); this is critical to prevent because it could result in client's having to change therapy to hemodialysis

       b. Catheter obstruction from clots or kinking (keep all lines unobstructed; add heparin to dialysate per protocol)

       c. Insufficient outflow (reposition client as needed to bring fluid into contact with catheter; allow to ambulate if advisable due to condition)

       d. Hypotension and hypovolemia from excess fluid removal (carefully monitor intake and output (I & O) records; report accordingly)

       e. Hyperglycemia (from glucose in dialysate; monitor diabetic clients closely; do not allow fluid to dwell longer than ordered)

   6. Peritoneal dialysis procedure

       a. Explain procedure and check vital signs (VS) and weight

       b. Have client urinate if able to avoid bladder puncture or discomfort; perform catheterization if client unable to void

       c. Warm dialysate to body temperature in a warmer

       d. Use 1.5, 2.5, or 4.25% dextrose solution; heparin may be added to prevent catheter clotting; dialysate should be clear and colorless; add medication as prescribed

       e. Put on surgical mask and prepare dialysis administration set, maintaining strict sterile technique at all times

       f. Place drainage bag below client and connect outflow tubing

       g. Connect dialysis infusion line to dialysate bags and hang on IV pole

       h. Place client in supine or semi-recumbent position, prime tubing with solution, close clamps, and connect infusion line to abdominal catheter

       i. Test catheter by instilling 500 mL of dialysate into peritoneal cavity; clamp tubing; unclamp outflow line and drain fluid into collection bag; if outflow is brisk, catheter is patent

       j. Unclamp infusion lines and infuse prescribed amount of dialysate; close clamps when bag is empty

       k. Allow solution to dwell for prescribed time (usually up to 4 hours)

       l. Open outflow clamps and allow solution to drain

       m. Repeat cycle according to prescribed number of times; when completed, clamp peritoneal catheter and disconnect inflow line while wearing sterile gloves

       n. Apply sterile dressing to catheter site

       o. During procedure, monitor VS every 10 minutes until stable, then every 2–4 hours

       p. Observe for signs of peritonitis: fever, persistent abdominal pain, and cramping; slow or cloudy dialysate drainage; swelling, redness, or tenderness around catheter; increased WBC count

       q. Wear protective eyewear when draining or handling outflow solution

       r. Check outflow tubing periodically for clots or kinks; having client change position may increase flow

       s. Clients lose protein during peritoneal dialysis and require fewer or no dietary restrictions of protein

       t. Calculate fluid balance at end of each exchange (with manual dialysis) or at end of each session or every 8 hours, depending on protocol; include oral and IV intake, urine output (UO), and wound drainage in calculations; weigh dialysate bag before and after exchange if part of protocol

  D. Urinary diversion stoma care

   1. Collection device should fit snugly around stoma; allow no more than 1/8-inch margin of skin between stoma and faceplate

   2. Stoma should appear light or bright red; suspect a problem if it is deep red or bluish in color

3. Check peristomal skin for breakdown; main cause of irritation is urine leakage; change device and cleanse skin if leakage occurs
   a. Cleanse area with warm water and pat dry; apply light coating of karaya powder and thin layer of protective dressing
   b. Notify provider if severe skin excoriation occurs
4. Assess I & O; note changes in urine color, odor, or clarity
5. Home care by client
   a. Expect stoma shrinkage within 8 weeks after surgery; may require different pouch size
   b. Encourage client to change appliance as needed early in morning when urine production is less following sleep
   c. Appliance is often a one-piece unit (faceplate and collection bag), and needs to be emptied regularly and changed according to product directions
   d. Instruct client to report fever, chills, flank pain, abdominal pain, and pus in urine (**pyuria**) or blood in urine (**hematuria**)
   e. Refer client to support group, such as United Ostomy Association
   f. Encourage adequate oral fluid intake

E. **Care of an arteriovenous (AV) fistula**
   1. An AV fistula provides vascular access to a vein and an artery for hemodialysis; most common sites are radial or brachial artery and cephalic vein
   2. Assess circulation at access site by auscultating for bruits and palpating for thrills; lack of bruit may indicate blood clot and requires immediate surgical intervention
   3. Avoid using accessed arm for other procedures, such as IV insertion, BP monitoring, or venipuncture
   4. Monitor site for bleeding after completion of hemodialysis
   5. Home care instructions for client
      a. Keep fistula area clean and dry
      b. Notify health care provider of pain, swelling, redness, or drainage in accessed arm
      c. Exercise is beneficial and helps stimulate vein enlargement
      d. Don't allow any treatments or procedures on accessed arm
      e. Avoid excessive pressure to arm; don't sleep on it, wear constrictive clothing or jewelry, or lift heavy objects
      f. Avoid showering, bathing, or swimming for several hours after dialysis

F. *Hemodialysis*: a procedure to remove wastes from body by filtering blood using a machine; used primarily for clients with end stage renal disease; may also be used for emergency stabilization of clients, such as those with life-threatening electrolyte levels or poisoning or overdose with substances not eliminated with gastric lavage or activated charcoal
   1. Nurses who have undergone specialized instruction and training perform hemodialysis
   2. Before procedure, weigh client and take VS; check BP in lying and standing positions (orthostatic BPs); check orders to see what medication to withhold on morning of dialysis; may need to withhold antihypertensive(s) or any other vasoactive drugs until after dialysis; once daily medications that can be given after dialysis should be delayed until procedure is completed
   3. Wear protective eyewear, gown, and gloves for protection during procedure
   4. Dialysis is continued usually for 3–4 hours, depending on client's condition; monitor partial thromboplastin time or other standard laboratory studies according to protocol (heparin is used as an anticoagulant during procedure)
   5. At end of treatment, obtain blood samples as ordered, return blood remaining in dialyzer to client, and remove needles from vascular access device
   6. Monitor access device for bleeding and maintain pressure on site as needed
   7. Early in course of hemodialysis, assess for and report disequilibrium syndrome, a condition in which cerebral edema forms from slower excretion of wastes behind blood–brain barrier relative to rest of body and subsequent uptake of fluid by brain cells
      a. Assess client for headache, mental confusion, decreasing level of consciousness (LOC), nausea and vomiting (N/V), twitching, and possible seizure activity

    b. Call provider to obtain necessary orders for antiepileptic medication

    c. It is prevented by dialyzing for shorter times or at reduced blood flow rates early in the course of therapy

IV. NURSING MANAGEMENT OF CLIENT HAVING RENAL OR BLADDER SURGERY

A. ***Lithotripsy***: also called extracorporeal shock-wave lithotripsy (ESWL); uses high-energy shock waves to break up calculi, allowing normal passage of urine to resume

    1. Perform preoperative teaching about procedure and postoperative course and care

        a. Treatment takes 30 minutes to 1 hour

        b. Client will receive a general or epidural anesthetic

    2. Postprocedure care

        a. Perform baseline assessment and check VS following agency policy

        b. Maintain patency of indwelling urinary catheter and monitor I & O

        c. Strain urine for calculi fragments and send these to laboratory for analysis

        d. Slight hematuria is common, but report persistent bleeding

        e. Encourage ambulation to aid passage of calculi fragments

        f. Increase fluid intake as prescribed to aid passage of calculi fragments

        g. Give analgesics as needed; severe pain may indicate presence of new calculi—report such findings immediately

    3. Home care instructions for client

        a. Drink 3–4 L of fluid daily up to 1 month after treatment unless contraindicated

        b. Strain urine during first week and save any calculi fragments; bring these to first follow-up visit with health care provider

        c. Expect blood-tinged urine, mild GI upset, and pain in treated side as calculi fragments pass

        d. Report severe pain, persistent blood in urine, inability to void, fever and chills, or N/V

        e. Review prescribed medications or dietary regimen

        f. Ambulation assists in clearance of stone fragments

B. Ureterolithotomy, pyelolithotomy, nephrolithotomy: involve making an incision into ureter, renal pelvis, or renal calyx to remove urinary calculi

    1. Preoperative period

        a. Explain procedure to client

        b. Explain postoperative care, including presence of a urinary catheter

        c. Administer preanesthetic medications as ordered

    2. Postoperative period

        a. Perform baseline assessments as for all postoperative clients (VS, LOC, status of dressing)

        b. Monitor UO for amount, color, and clarity; urine may be bright red initially, but amount of bleeding should diminish; cloudy urine may indicate infection

        c. Maintain placement and patency of urinary catheters; irrigate gently as prescribed

        d. Assess for pain and administer analgesics as needed

        e. Increase client's fluid intake as prescribed to aid passage of calculi fragments

        f. Strain urine for calculi fragments and send these to laboratory for analysis

    3. Home care for client

        a. Follow agency policy for home incision care

        b. Drink 3–4 L of fluid daily up to a month after treatment

        c. Report bloody, cloudy, or foul-smelling urine

        d. Report inability to void, fever, chills, and redness, swelling, or purulent drainage from incision

        e. Strain urine during first week and save any calculi fragments; bring these to first follow-up visit with health care provider

      f. Avoid strenuous exercise, sexual activity, heavy lifting, or straining until advised otherwise by health care provider

      g. Mild activity aids passage of any retained calculi fragments

      h. Review prescribed medications or dietary regimen

      i. Outline catheter care if client is discharged with indwelling catheter

C. Cystectomy with urinary diversion

    1. Complete radical **cystectomy** involves surgical removal of bladder, plus adjacent muscles and tissues

      a. In men, prostate and seminal vesicles are removed, which results in impotence

      b. In women, uterus, uterine tubes, and ovaries are removed, resulting in sterility

      c. A urinary diversion is created to provide for urine collection and drainage

    2. Urinary diversion: a procedure that provides an alternative route for urine excretion when normal channels are damaged or defective

      a. Ileal conduit: also called ileal loop; reroutes urine from kidneys to pouch in abdominal wall created from a segment of the ileum; urine drains continuously from ileal pouch

      b. Nephrostomy: drains urine through a catheter placed directly into kidney; used when a ureter is blocked or damaged; may be temporary

    3. Preoperative period

      a. Reduce anxiety through preoperative teaching about procedure and postoperative course and care

      b. Client may awaken with nasogastric tube, IV, indwelling urinary catheter, Penrose drain, or other drains

      c. Assess client's support systems and ability to care for self after surgery

      d. Address concerns about changes in body image and loss of sexual or reproductive function

      e. Administer preanesthetic medications as prescribed

      f. Administer antibiotics (usually erythromycin and neomycin) for 24 hours before surgery, as prescribed

      g. Begin bowel preparations about 4 days prior to surgery

      h. Administer enema on night before surgery to clear fecal matter from bowel as prescribed or per protocol

    4. Postoperative period

      a. Perform baseline assessments as for all postoperative clients (VS, LOC, status of dressing, and patency of urinary catheter)

      b. Assess respiratory status frequently; encourage frequent position changes, coughing and deep breathing, and early ambulation, if appropriate

      c. Administer prescribed analgesic medications as needed

      d. Monitor amount and character of urine drainage every hour; report UO less than 30 mL/hour; irrigate catheter as ordered

      e. Observe for signs of hypovolemic shock, such as pallor, hypotension, and tachycardia

      f. Inspect stoma and incision for bleeding and observe urine for frank bleeding and clots; expect slight hematuria for several days; assess stoma color, expecting light or bright red (report deep red or bluish color)

      g. Observe incision for signs of infection (redness and purulent drainage); change dressing according to agency policy or surgeon's order

    5. Home care instructions for clients

      a. Report signs of infection, including fever, chills, cloudy urine, purulent drainage or redness of incision

      b. Report persistent blood in urine, inability to void, or painful urination

      c. Instruct in care of stoma and provide supplies as needed; refer client to support organization, such as the United Ostomy Association

      d. Weakness, incisional pain, and fatigue may persist for several weeks

    D. Ureteral stent: tube used to maintain patency and promote healing of ureter; may be temporary after surgery or used for long periods in clients with a damaged ureter

        1. Stent is positioned during surgery or cystoscopy

        2. Nursing care

            a. If stent has been brought to surface, secure it, and maintain its position

            b. Monitor UO, including color, consistency, and odor

            c. Observe for signs of infection, obstruction, or bleeding, including fever, tachycardia, cloudy urine, pain, hematuria

            d. Maintain fluid intake

            e. If stent is semi-permanent, instruct client and family in its care

    E. Nephrectomy: removal of kidney

        1. Preoperative period

            a. Reduce anxiety through preoperative teaching about procedure and postoperative course and care

            b. Client may awaken with nasogastric tube, IV, indwelling urinary catheter, Penrose drain, or other drains

            c. Assess client's support systems and ability to care for self after surgery

            d. Administer preanesthetic medications as prescribed

            e. Assess baseline urinary status

        2. Postoperative period

            a. Perform baseline assessments as for all postoperative clients (VS, LOC, status of dressing, and patency of urinary catheter)

            b. Assess client's fluid and electrolyte status, because significant amount of blood is lost during nephrectomy; monitor hemoglobin and hematocrit results and urine specific gravity

            c. Monitor amount and character of UO every hour; report UO less than 30 mL/hour; irrigate catheter as ordered

            d. Observe for signs of urinary infection: fever, redness at surgical site, cloudy urine, or discharge

            e. Assess patency of urinary or wound drainage tubes; reinforce or change dressing as needed

            f. Encourage frequent position changes, coughing and deep breathing, and early ambulation, if appropriate

            g. Assess respiratory status frequently

            h. Administer analgesic medications as needed

    F. Renal transplantation

        1. Preoperative period

            a. Reduce anxiety through preoperative teaching about procedure and postoperative course and care; encourage client to express feelings and ask questions

            b. Assess client's support systems and ability to care for self after surgery and follow medical regime

            c. Instruct client that rejection of donated organ by recipient's body is major obstacle in transplantation; reassure client that rejection usually isn't life-threatening and client can resume dialysis if needed (see Table 6-1 for types of rejection)

            d. Begin administering immunosuppressant drugs; explain their purpose and possible adverse effects; monitor for signs of anaphylaxis

            e. Plan for client to undergo dialysis on day before surgery, a cleansing enema, and many laboratory tests

        2. Postoperative period

            a. Perform baseline assessments as for all postoperative clients (VS, LOC, status of dressing)

Table 6-1	Renal Transplant Rejection	
Description	**Manifestations**	**Management**
Hyperacute		
Occurs within hours of surgery; results from antibody reaction to donor antigens; rare now due to better histocompatibility assessments	Urine output (UO) stops; examination of kidney shows a blue, flaccid appearance	Transplanted kidney must be removed; client must resume hemodialysis until (possibly) another kidney is available
Acute		
Occurs within days to months after surgery; body mounts an immune system defense against tissue in donor organ	UO drops sharply and BUN and creatinine rise; possible fever, graft tenderness, swelling	Increased dosage of immunosuppressant drugs, including steroids and monoclonal antibodies
Chronic		
Occurs from months to years after surgery; etiology is unclear, but may involve immune response to donor tissue	More gradual decline in kidney function, including UO, BUN, and creatinine; proteinuria may occur	No specific treatment; client must resume hemodialysis caused by loss of graft until or unless another donor kidney is transplanted

    b. Encourage frequent position changes, coughing and deep breathing, and early ambulation, if appropriate

    c. Use special infection control measures: strict aseptic technique when changing dressings or performing catheter care; limit client's contact with staff and visitors; wear a surgical mask when in client's room; monitor white blood cell (WBC) count and notify surgeon of significant drop

    d. Observe for signs of tissue rejection: flulike symptoms, decreasing UO, fever, weight gain, pain over site and fatigue; elevated WBC count, increased **proteinuria** (protein in urine); hypertension; elevated BUN and creatinine levels; mild cases can be treated with increased doses of immunosuppressant drugs

    e. Provide analgesic medications as needed; pain should decrease after 24 hours

    f. Monitor UO closely; report output less than 100 mL/hour; decreased urine may indicate thrombus formation at renal artery anastomosis site

    g. Expect blood-tinged urine for several days; irrigate catheter as ordered, using strict aseptic technique

    h. With a living donor transplant, urine flow should begin immediately after revascularization and connection of ureter to client's bladder; with a cadaver transplant, expect **anuria** for 2 days to 2 weeks (client will need dialysis during this period)

    i. Monitor daily renal function tests: serum creatinine, BUN, creatinine clearance, electrolytes, urine pH, and specific gravity

    j. Observe for signs of hyperkalemia (weakness, irregular pulse, tall peaked T waves on cardiac rhythm strip)

    k. Weigh client daily; rapid weight gain may indicate fluid retention

  3. Home care for client

    a. Carefully measure and record I & O; notify health care provider if UO falls below 600 mL for any 24-hour period

    b. Instruct client how to collect 24-hour urine samples

    c. Advise client to weigh self at least twice weekly

    d. Drink at least 1 liter of fluid daily, unless advised otherwise

e. Report signs of rejection: redness, warmth, tenderness, or swelling over the kidney; fever; decreased UO; elevated BP

f. Avoid crowds and persons with known infections for 3 months after surgery

g. Practice regular, moderate exercise, but avoid heavy lifting or contact sports for at least 3 months; beware of lap-style seat belts

h. Wait at least 6 weeks before engaging in sexual activity

V. DISORDERS OF URINARY SYSTEM

A. Urinary calculi

1. Description: presence of stones in urinary tract; a common urologic problem

2. Etiology and pathophysiology

a. Stones form when chemicals and other elements of urine become concentrated and form crystals; usually related to metabolic or dietary causes

b. Types of stones: calcium phosphate and/or oxalate (most common), struvite, uric acid, and cysteine (least common)

c. Most stones form in kidneys, but bladder stones are common in clients with indwelling urinary catheters or those unable to empty bladder completely (see Figure 6-2)

d. Stones may be single or multiple and vary in size; large calculi cause pressure necrosis and can also lead to obstruction

e. Risk factors

1) Dehydration: concentrates calculus-forming substances

2) Infection: damaged tissue and changing pH provide an environment for calculi to develop; bacteria may form nucleus of calculi

3) Obstruction: urine stasis allows solid materials to collect; also promotes infection, which worsens obstruction

4) Metabolic factors: hypoparathyroidism, renal tubular acidosis, elevated uric acid levels, defective oxalate metabolism, and excessive vitamin D or dietary calcium intake

Figure 6-2

Development and location of calculi within the urinary tract

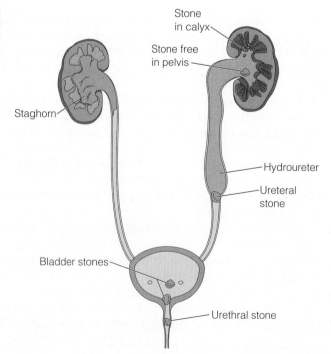

Stone in calyx

Stone free in pelvis

Staghorn

Hydroureter

Ureteral stone

Bladder stones

Urethral stone

3. Assessment
    a. Clinical manifestations
        1) Pain is most common symptom; renal calculi cause flank pain on side of affected kidney; may radiate to groin, called renal colic; pain fluctuates in intensity and may be severe; N/V sometimes accompany severe pain
        2) Other symptoms: abdominal distention, fever, and chills
    b. Diagnostic and laboratory test findings
        1) Urinalysis (may reveal hematuria, pyuria, and crystal fragments)
        2) 24-hour urine levels for calcium, uric acid, and oxalate
        3) Serum levels for calcium, phosphorus, and uric acid
        4) Chemical analysis of stones passed for content and type
        5) KUB, IVP, retrograde pyelography, renal ultrasound, CT scan, cystoscopy, and MRI
4. Therapeutic management
    a. Stones that are too large to be passed spontaneously (usually greater than 5 mm in diameter), multiple stones, and those that obstruct urinary tract usually require surgical intervention
        1) Extracorporeal shock-wave lithotripsy (ESWL) uses externally generated waves to pulverize or shatter urinary stones/calculi, which are then excreted in urine
        2) Ureterolithotomy, pyelolithotomy, or nephrolithotomy: utilize a surgical incision used to remove calculi from affected areas; requires a large flank incision and an extended recovery time
        3) Percutaneous nephrostomy: small incision in flank allows insertion of endoscope to visualize renal pelvis; stones are removed with forceps or a basket device, or lithotripsy is used to crush stones
        4) Transurethral uroscopy: a ureteral catheter is passed via a cystoscope to drain urine proximal to a stone and dilate ureter, allowing stone to pass; a basket catheter passed through cystoscope can also remove calculus
    b. Treatment for urinary stones
        1) Increase hydration (up to 3 liters daily) and exercise; excessive hydration is avoided in acute phase to avoid acute retention of urine proximal to blockage

Table 6-2	Dietary Alterations to Treat Renal and Urinary Stones	
Diet	**Dietary Alteration**	**Examples of Foods**
Acid ash	Increase intake of acid-ash foods	Acid-ash foods include cranberries, plums, grapes, and prunes; tomatoes; eggs and cheese; whole grains; meat and poultry
Alkaline ash	Increase intake of alkaline-ash foods	Alkaline ash foods include legumes, milk and milk products, green vegetables, rhubarb, fruits except those acid-ash fruits noted above
Calcium	May or may not be restricted	High-calcium foods include milk and other dairy products, beans and lentils, dried fruits, canned or smoked fish (except tuna), flour, chocolate, and cocoa
Low oxalate	Decrease intake of foods high in oxalates	Foods high in oxalate include dark green leafy vegetables, asparagus, beets, celery, cabbage, fruits, tomatoes, green beans, chocolate and cocoa, beer, cola beverages, nuts, and tea
Low purine	Decrease intake of foods high in purines	High-purine foods include organ meats, sardines and herring, venison, and goose; other meats also contain purines and should be limited in quantity

> **2)** Dietary measures (see Table 6-2 also)
>> **a)** Calcium phosphate and/or oxalate stones: acid-ash diet with limitations of foods high in oxalates and possibly calcium
>> **b)** Struvite stones: acid-ash diet
>> **c)** Uric acid stones: alkaline-ash and low-purine diet
>> **d)** Cysteine stones: alkaline-ash diet

5. Priority nursing problems: pain, alterations in urinary elimination, potential for infection, inadequate knowledge

6. Planning and implementation
  a. Treatment is aimed at symptom relief, removal or destruction of calculi, and prevention of future stones
  b. 90% of calculi pass out of urinary system without invasive treatment
  c. Treatments are carried out as described in section 4 above on therapeutic management
  d. Provide pain relief measures and treat other symptoms as they occur
  e. Assess urinary function and monitor I & O
  f. Strain all urine and save solid material for analysis
  g. Encourage ambulation and high fluid intake to help client pass calculi
  h. Record daily weights to assess fluid status and renal function

7. Medication therapy: antimicrobials for infection; analgesics for pain; and diuretics to prevent urine stasis

8. Client education
  a. Proper diet is essential to prevent recurrence of stones; teach dietary needs related to type of calculus (see Table 6-2 again)
  b. Increase fluid intake to 2,500–3,000 mL/day
  c. Maintain activity at level that will prevent urinary stasis and resorption of calcium from bone
  d. If discharged prior to stone passage, collect and strain all urine and bring stones to follow-up visit; observe amount and character of urine and report to health care provider at follow-up visit also
  e. Report increased pain, persistent blood in urine, inability to void, significant decrease in UO
  f. Report signs of infection: burning with urination, cloudy urine, or fever
  g. Review specific drug information and how to self-administer

9. Evaluation: client states understanding of medications and correctly demonstrates use; has recovered stone; identifies dietary and lifestyle measures to prevent calculi; has relief of pain; and exhibits no sign of complications

B. Urinary retention

1. Description: inability to empty bladder that leads to bladder distention, poor contractility of detrusor muscle, and further inability to urinate

2. Etiology and pathophysiology
  a. Mechanical obstruction of bladder outlet is most often caused by benign prostatic hyperplasia or acute inflammation
  b. Functional problems
    1) Surgery may disrupt function of detrusor muscle, leading to retention of urine
    2) Many medications can interfere with detrusor muscle function, including anticholinergics, antidepressant and antipsychotic agents, anti-Parkinson drugs, antihistamines, and some antihypertensives

3. Assessment
  a. Clinical manifestations
    1) Firm, distended bladder that may be displaced to one side of midline
    2) Overflow voiding or incontinence may occur, with 25–50 mL of urine eliminated at frequent intervals

     b. Diagnostic and laboratory test findings

       1) Residual urine (postvoiding catheterization) in amounts over 50 mL obtained from bladder catheterization

       2) Positive urine culture indicates presence of urinary tract infection (UTI)

       3) Elevated serum creatinine and BUN levels indicate disturbances in renal function

       4) Elevated blood glucose may indicate diabetes

       5) Cystometrography evaluates muscle function

4. Therapeutic management: surgical correction of any condition causing mechanical obstruction of urine flow, including benign prostatic hyperplasia (BPH) and calculi

5. Priority nursing problems: retention of urine, possible infection, inadequate knowledge

6. Planning and implementation

     a. Palpate bladder for distention at regular intervals

     b. Monitor I & O and observe urine

     c. Attempt to stimulate relaxation of urethral sphincter by running water, providing warm water in which client could place fingers, pour warm water over perineum, or provide warm sitz bath

     d. Perform intermittent straight catheterization as ordered

     e. Evaluate client's medication regime for drugs that cause urinary retention

     f. Clients with mechanical obstruction need surgery to remove or repair obstruction; men with BPH may require resection of prostate gland

7. Medication therapy: cholinergic medications to promote detrusor muscle contraction and bladder emptying; anticholinesterase drugs to increase detrusor muscle tone

8. Client education

     a. How to perform straight catheterization at home, if needed

     b. Recognize and report signs of urinary tract infection: burning with urination, cloudy urine, pelvic pain, fever, and strong urine odor

     c. Maintain moderate to high fluid intake and a diet that acidifies urine; cranberry juice and ascorbic acid (vitamin C) help maintain acidity

     d. Review specific drug information and procedures for self-administration

9. Evaluation: client maintains a normal voiding pattern or is able to self-catheterize at home; has normal UO; and verbalizes signs and symptoms of infection

C. Urinary incontinence

1. Description: involuntary urination

     a. Urinary incontinence can be subdivided for classification according to its various causes

       1) Loss of urine with increased abdominal pressure

       2) Involuntary loss of urine at somewhat predictable intervals when a specific bladder volume is reached

       3) Involuntary passage of urine soon after a strong urge to void

       4) Involuntary, unpredictable passage of urine

       5) Frequent small involuntary voidings after inability to empty bladder

     b. Incontinence is a symptom of other problems, not a disease in itself, although it has a significant impact on client's life

2. Etiology and pathophysiology

     a. May be acute or chronic, and the cause may be congenital or acquired

     b. Occurs when pressure within bladder exceeds urethral resistance, allowing urine to escape; any condition causing increased bladder pressure or reduced urethral resistance may lead to incontinence

     c. Common causes: pelvic muscle relaxation, disruption of cerebral and nervous system control, and disturbances of bladder musculature

Practice to Pass

A female client who voids 50 mL of urine at a time states, "This is normal for me." How should you respond?

      d. Risk factors for incontinence in older clients: decreased bladder capacity, laxity of pelvic muscles in females, immobility, chronic degenerative diseases, low fluid intake, diabetes, stroke, and other brain disorder

  3. Assessment

      a. Clinical manifestations: involuntary passage of urine

      b. Diagnostic and laboratory test findings

         1) Weak abdominal and pelvic muscle tone in women

         2) Enlarged prostate in men

         3) Postvoiding residual urine greater than 50 mL

         4) Cystometrography: reduced muscle function and tone

         5) Ultrasonography and cystoscopy identify possible causes of the incontinence

  4. Therapeutic management

      a. Surgical suspension of bladder neck to treat stress incontinence associated with urethrocele

      b. Prostatectomy to treat overflow incontinence due to enlarged prostate

      c. Implantation of an artificial sphincter to treat clients with neurogenic bladder

  5. Priority nursing problems: alterations in urinary elimination, incontinence (of various types), potential for alteration in body image, potential for interrupted skin integrity, insufficient ability to adequately care for self

  6. Planning and implementation

      a. Goal is to identify and correct underlying cause; if unable, client may learn techniques to manage UO

      b. Monitor diagnostic tests to evaluate cause of incontinence

      c. Employ behavioral techniques, such as bladder training, for clients who are cognitively and functionally intact

      d. Insert urinary catheter as ordered and monitor client's UO

  7. Medication therapy: anticholinergics for stress incontinence to increase bladder capacity and inhibit detrusor muscle contractions; antihistamines to enhance contraction of smooth muscles of bladder neck; estrogen therapy for incontinence associated with postmenopausal atrophic vaginitis

  8. Client education

      a. How to care for indwelling urinary catheter at home

      b. Recognize and report signs of urinary tract infection: burning with urination, cloudy urine, pelvic pain, fever, and strong urine odor

      c. Maintain moderate to high fluid intake and a diet that acidifies urine; cranberry juice and ascorbic acid (vitamin C) help maintain acidity

      d. Avoid foods and fluids that may be implicated in urge incontinence, such as chocolate or caffeine

      e. Perform Kegel exercises to strengthen pelvic floor muscles (see Box 6-1)

      f. Modify diet and fluid intake to reduce stress and urge incontinence; consume most fluids during times of day client is most able to remain continent

      g. Wear clothing that is easily removed for ease in toileting

---

Box 6-1 **Teaching Kegel Exercises**	• First, sit or stand with the legs apart. • Tense your muscles to pull your rectum, urethra, and vagina up inside, and hold for a count of 3 to 5 seconds. The pull should be felt at the cleft of your buttocks. • Try to stop and start your stream of urine. • Develop a schedule that will help remind you to do these exercises. • To control episodes of stress incontinence, brace the muscles and use the Kegel maneuver when doing any activity that increases intra-abdominal pressure, such as coughing, laughing, sneezing, or lifting.

Practice to Pass

A female client reports dribbling of urine when she laughs, sneezes, or coughs. What advice should you give this client based on the type of incontinence she describes?

    h. Use assistive devices, such as raised toilet seats, bedside commode, and urinal or bedpan, as needed

    i. Review specific drug information and procedures for self-administration

    j. Some clients may be asked to keep a voiding diary to help diagnose the cause(s) of incontinence

9. Evaluation: client states understanding of medications and demonstrates their use; uses safety measures; reports fewer incontinent episodes; monitors UO; verbalizes a state of dryness that is personally satisfactory; states diet and fluid modifications, and demonstrates care of indwelling urinary catheter

D. Urinary tract infections (UTIs)

  1. Description: presence of microorganisms in urinary tract leading to inflammation

  2. Etiology and pathophysiology

    a. UTIs are classified according to region and primary site affected

    b. Urinary tract is sterile above urethra; pathogens enter by ascending from perineal area (most common) or from bloodstream

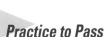

    c. *Escherichia coli* is most frequent infective organism (80% of all cases); 5–15% are caused by *staphylococcus*

    d. Free urine flow, large UO, and pH are antibacterial defenses

    e. Microscopic urine examination identifies organism (especially important for clients acquiring infection while institutionalized)

    f. Females are prone to UTIs because urethra is shorter than male urethra

  3. Assessment

    a. Clinical manifestations: burning, frequency, fever, cloudy urine, strong odor to urine, and pain in pelvic area

    b. Diagnostic and laboratory findings

      1) Urine cultures and gram stain determine presence and number of bacteria; check for resistant strains in clients with repeated UTI

      2) WBCs are elevated with an increase in neutrophils

      3) Blood or urine tests are also performed to rule out sexually transmitted infections (STIs), which produce similar symptoms especially in young males

Practice to Pass

How would you respond to a female client who asks you why she seems to have more urinary tract infections as compared to her husband?

  4. Therapeutic management

    a. Surgical intervention may be needed if recurrent UTI is caused by structural abnormalities

    b. These procedures may include:

      1) Ureteroplasty (surgical repair of ureter) for stricture

      2) Ureteral stent (catheter in ureter to provide free flow of urine)

  5. Priority nursing problems: pain, altered urinary elimination, inadequate knowledge

  6. Planning and implementation

    a. Increase fluid intake to 3,000 mL per day

    b. Encourage client to void every 2–3 hours and to completely empty bladder to reduce urinary stasis

    c. Monitor I & O and observe urine characteristics

  7. Medication therapy

    a. Antimicrobials (sulfonamides and urinary antiseptics frequently)

    b. Antispasmodics and analgesics to relieve pain, frequency, and burning

  8. Client education

    a. Avoid beverages that irritate bladder: carbonated or caffeinated drinks and alcohol

    b. Females should use hygiene measures to prevent reoccurrence: wipe from front to back, keep perineum clean and dry, do not douche, avoid tight-fitting pants, use cotton-lined underwear, void after sexual intercourse

    c. Finish complete course of antibiotics, even if symptoms subside

    d. Correct use, purpose, and effects of medication

       e. Phenazopyridine (Pyridium), a urinary analgesic, turns urine and other body fluids (such as tears) reddish orange; protect clothing, be aware of discoloration of contact lenses, and do not mistake urine discoloration for bleeding (hematuria)

       f. Recognize signs of infection: frequency, burning, cloudy urine, fever, and malodorous urine

       g. Maintain acidic urine by drinking cranberry juice daily or take ascorbic acid (helps prevent bacteria from clinging to bladder wall)

       h. Maintain fluid intake of at least 8–10 eight ounce glasses per day

  9. Evaluation: client states understanding of medications and demonstrates their use; identifies measures to prevent infection; identifies signs of infection; normal voiding pattern is restored

E. *Cystitis*

  1. Description: inflammation (infection) of bladder

  2. Etiology and pathophysiology

       a. Infection or obstruction of urethra is most common cause

       b. Noninfectious cystitis results from exposure to radiation, chemical agents, or a metabolic disorder

       c. Gram-negative bacteria from lower GI tract usually cause infectious cystitis

       d. Females are more prone to cystitis because:

          1) Urethra is short and straight

          2) Urinary meatus is close to the vagina and anus

          3) Tissue trauma and potential contamination occurs during sexual intercourse

          4) In some cases, poor personal hygiene and voluntary urinary retention contribute to risk

       e. Males are more likely to develop urinary infection with aging because of prostatic hyperplasia, which impedes urine flow leading to incomplete bladder emptying and urinary stasis

  3. Assessment

       a. Clinical manifestations

          1) Older clients may have nonspecific symptoms, such as nocturia, incontinence, confusion, lethargy, or anorexia

          2) See previous section on UTI

       b. Diagnostic and laboratory test findings: see previous section on UTI

  4. Therapeutic management: see previous section on UTI

  5. Priority nursing problems: pain, altered urinary elimination, inadequate knowledge

  6. Planning and implementation

       a. Assist in identifying and removing cause of condition (infection, obstruction, etc.)

       b. Administer antimicrobial medications as ordered

       c. Collect uncontaminated urine specimens as needed

       d. Maintain acid urine (pH 5.5)

       e. Encourage bedrest or decreased activity during acute stage

       f. Increase fluid intake to 3,000 mL/day

  7. Medication therapy

       a. Antimicrobials to eradicate bacteria if that is the cause

       b. Antispasmodics and analgesics to relieve pain, frequency, and burning

  8. Client education

       a. See previous section on UTI

       b. Practice frequent voiding (every 2–4 hours) to flush bacteria from urethra

       c. Avoid bubble bath, powder, or sprays in perineal area; use mild soap

       d. Take showers rather than baths if recurrent infection is a problem

  9. Evaluation: client states medication instruction and demonstrates its use; states measures to prevent infection and signs of infection; normal voiding pattern is restored; verbalizes 3 methods to prevent recurrence of infection

F. *Pyelonephritis*

1. Description: infection of one or both kidneys that usually begins in renal pelvis; may be acute or chronic
2. Etiology and pathophysiology
   a. Affects renal pelvis and parenchyma (functional portion of kidney)
   b. Infection develops in scattered areas and spreads from renal pelvis to cortex; kidney becomes edematous and abscesses may develop; tissue destruction primarily affects tubules; with healing, scar tissue replaces normal tissue and affected tubules atrophy
   c. *E. coli* causes 85% of cases; *Proteus* and *Klebsiella* bacteria are examples of less common causes
   d. Acute form is a bacterial infection, usually caused by bacteria that ascend from lower urinary tract
   e. Risk factors: pregnancy, urinary tract obstruction, congenital malformation, urinary tract trauma, calculi, and diabetes
   f. Asymptomatic bacteriuria or cystitis may lead to acute pyelonephritis
   g. Chronic form is associated with nonbacterial infections and noninfectious processes caused by metabolic, chemical, or immunologic disorders
      1) Often results from an autoimmune process leading to inflammation
      2) Acute episodes may contribute to inflammation and scarring associated with chronic form
      3) Fibrosis and scarring lead to dilation of renal pelvis and gradual destruction of tubules
      4) May lead to chronic renal failure and end-stage renal disease
   h. **Vesicoureteral reflux** (urine moves from bladder back toward kidneys) is a common risk factor in children who develop pyelonephritis; it is also seen in adults when bladder outflow is obstructed
3. Assessment
   a. Clinical manifestations: urinary frequency, dysuria, flank pain, costovertebral tenderness, tachypnea, GI symptoms, muscle tenderness, fever, chills, malaise
   b. Diagnostic and laboratory findings: hematuria, pyuria, bacteriuria, leukocyte casts in urine, and leukocytosis
4. Therapeutic management: same as for UTI
5. Priority nursing problems: pain, alterations in urinary elimination, inadequate knowledge
6. Planning and implementation
   a. Administer and monitor drug therapy
   b. Maintain bed rest until symptoms subside
   c. Encourage increased fluids to maintain UO of 1,500 mL/day
   d. Continue monitoring for presence of bacteria
   e. Monitor urinalysis: concentration and electrolytes
   f. If oliguria present, maintain diet low in protein and high in calories and vitamins
   g. Observe for edema and signs of renal failure
7. Medication therapy: antimicrobial therapy; urinary antiseptics; and analgesics for pain
8. Client education
   a. Monitor UO and notify care provider if less than 1,500 mL/day
   b. Instruct in methods to prevent chronic renal insufficiency
   c. Eat a high-calorie, low-protein diet if oliguria present
   d. Use proper hygiene to prevent further infections
   e. Maintain bed rest during acute stage
   f. Finish complete course of antibiotics, even if symptoms resolve
   g. Correct use, purpose, and effects of medication

9. Evaluation: client states understanding of medications and demonstrates proper use; identifies measure to prevent further infection; identifies signs of infection; normal voiding pattern is restored; and verbalizes methods to prevent recurrence of infection

G. **Glomerulonephritis**

1. Definition: a group of kidney diseases caused by inflammation of capillary loops in glomeruli of kidneys
2. Etiology and pathophysiology
   a. Caused by an immunologic reaction to an antigen
   b. Endogenous antigens are already present in glomerulus or other body tissues
   c. Exogenous antigens come from infections occurring in body
   d. Antigen–antibody complexes trapped within glomeruli produce an inflammatory response that damages glomeruli
   e. Most often follows infections with group A beta-hemolytic streptococcus
   f. Upper respiratory infection, skin infection, and autoimmune processes (systemic lupus erythematosus) predispose to glomerulonephritis
   g. Symptoms appear 2–3 weeks after original infection
   h. Has higher incidence in men than women; may occur at any age
3. Assessment
   a. Clinical manifestations
      1) Early symptoms may be mild: pharyngitis, fever, and malaise
      2) Recent upper respiratory or skin infections, pericarditis, or lower UTI
      3) Weakness and fatigue
      4) Anorexia, N/V
      5) Cocoa-colored urine
      6) Peripheral edema
      7) Hypertension
   b. Diagnostic and laboratory test findings
      1) Hematuria, proteinuria (most important indicator of glomerular injury), hypoalbuminemia
      2) Pulmonary infiltrates
      3) Positive antibody response tests for streptococcal exoenzymes
      4) Elevated erythrocyte sedimentation rate (ESR)
      5) Elevated BUN and creatinine; decreased creatinine clearance
      6) Decreased serum Na^+, elevated K^+, and decreased phosphate
      7) Delayed uptake and excretion of radioactive dye in renal scan
      8) Positive renal biopsy findings
4. Therapeutic management
   a. Plasmapheresis: removal of harmful components in plasma
   b. Sodium restriction
   c. Dialysis if disease progresses to renal failure
5. Priority nursing problems: alterations in urinary elimination, inability to endure exercise or activity, fluid overload
6. Planning and implementation
   a. Administer penicillin as prescribed for residual infection
   b. Provide appropriate diet: protein restriction if oliguria is severe; high carbohydrate to provide energy; K^+ usually restricted; Na^+ restriction for hypertension and edema
   c. Maintain fluid restriction as needed
   d. Encourage complete bedrest during acute stage
   e. Monitor VS frequently; observe for hypertension
   f. Monitor I & O and daily weight
   g. Evaluate for signs of renal failure: oliguria, **azotemia**, and acidosis

Practice to Pass

During a routine assessment, a client tells you, "I've been noticing blood in my urine." What would be your appropriate nursing action?

7. Medication therapy: antimicrobials for infection; analgesics for pain relief; and vitamin and electrolyte replacement as needed
8. Client education
   a. Maintain strict bed rest during acute phase
   b. Dietary changes and importance of maintaining diet
   c. Importance of fluid restriction if oliguria present
   d. Purpose of laboratory tests and other procedures
   e. Monitor daily UO and daily weight
9. Evaluation: client is able to resume usual activities of daily living, demonstrates knowledge of diet and fluid restrictions, and maintains desired weight; signs of fluid overload and N/V are absent

H. *Nephrotic syndrome*
   1. Description: renal disease characterized by massive edema and albuminuria
   2. Etiology and pathophysiology
      a. Seen with any renal condition that damages glomerular capillary membrane: glomerulonephritis, lipoid nephrosis, syphilitic nephritis, amyloidosis, or systemic lupus erythematosus
      b. Allows plasma proteins to escape into urine, resulting in hypoalbuminemia, with decreased oncotic pressure in plasma and fluid shifts from intravascular to interstitial spaces; this leads to edema
      c. Salt and water retention contribute to edema, which may be severe
      d. Kimmelstiel-Wilson syndrome, a specific form of intercapillary glomerulosclerosis, is associated with diabetes mellitus
      e. Thromboemboli (mobilized blood clots) are a common complication and may occlude peripheral veins and arteries, pulmonary arteries, and renal veins
      f. Prognosis is poor for adults with this syndrome; less than 50% experience complete remission; at least 30% develop end-stage renal failure
   3. Assessment
      a. Clinical manifestations
         1) Severe generalized edema
         2) Symptoms of renal failure
         3) Loss of appetite and fatigue
         4) Amenorrhea
      b. Diagnostic and laboratory test findings
         1) Pronounced proteinuria, hypoalbuminemia, and hyperlipidemia
         2) Positive renal biopsy finding
   4. Therapeutic management
      a. No specific treatment
      b. Since 30% of adults progress to end-stage renal failure, see section on therapeutic management of renal failure
   5. Priority nursing problems: fluid overload, fatigue, insufficient ability to perform usual roles
   6. Planning and implementation
      a. Provide nursing care to control edema
         1) Sodium-restricted diet
         2) Avoid Na^+-containing drugs (such as several OTC products)
         3) Diuretics that block aldosterone formation (Lasix and Edecrin)
         4) Administer salt-poor albumin to reduce fluid retention
      b. Provide high-protein diet to restore body proteins, high-calorie diet, and a restricted Na^+ diet if edema is present
      c. Administer drug therapy as prescribed
      d. Maintain bed rest until edema begins to subside

   e. Monitor laboratory and diagnostic test results, including BUN, creatinine, serum electrolytes, urinalysis, hemoglobin, and hematocrit
   f. Observe for signs of pulmonary edema: tachypnea, dyspnea, crackles in the lungs
   g. Tally I & O records every 4–8 hours and weigh client daily
   h. Maintain fluid restriction; offer ice chips and provide frequent mouth care
   i. Provide for adequate rest and energy conservation
   j. Be aware that immune system depression increases risk of infection
      1) Assess for signs of infection, such as purulent wound drainage and signs of UTI
      2) Monitor CBC, with close attention to WBC and differential
      3) Use good hand hygiene and infection control techniques
      4) Avoid or minimize invasive procedures
7. Medication therapy: immunosuppressives for clients with autoimmune disorders; angiotensin converting enzyme (ACE) inhibitors to reduce protein loss; NSAIDs to reduce proteinuria; penicillin or other broad-spectrum antibiotics to eradicate bacteria; and antihypertensives to maintain normal BP if needed
8. Client education
   a. Take measures to maintain general health, as disorder may persist for months or years
   b. Avoid sources of infection such as people with upper respiratory infections
   c. Nutritious diet (low Na^+, high protein)
   d. Activity as tolerated
   e. Use and potential effects of medications
   f. Signs, symptoms, and implications of improving or declining renal function
9. Evaluation: client maintains BP within normal limits; returns to usual weight with no evidence of edema; consumes adequate calories while following dietary limitations; and demonstrates understanding of disease and prescribed management regimen

I. Neoplastic disease

1. Description
   a. Neoplastic disease is a pathologic tissue overgrowth that may be benign or malignant
   b. Other classifications: solid, cystic, superficial, invasive, primary, or metastatic
2. Etiology and pathophysiology
   a. Most urinary tract tumors arise from epithelial tissue that lines entire urinary tract
   b. Even nonmalignant tumors may lead to obstruction, renal failure, hemorrhage, and invasion and inflammation of surrounding tissues
   c. Tissue destruction may cause fistulas, which can allow urine to leak into the pelvis, vagina, or bowel
   d. Renal cancer accounts for only 2% of adult cancers
   e. Bladder cancer occurs most often after age 50, and is more common in men than women
      1) Major factors in bladder cancer are presence of carcinogens in the urine (highly associated with smoking), and chronic inflammation or infection of bladder mucosa
      2) Other risk factors: exposure to industrial chemicals and dyes, chronic use of phenacetin-containing analgesics; carcinogenic agents from these materials are excreted in urine and stored in bladder between voidings, leading to abnormal cell development
3. Assessment of bladder cancer
   a. Clinical manifestations
      1) Observe for painless hematuria (presenting symptom in 75% of cases); hematuria may be gross or microscopic, and is often intermittent
      2) Inflammation surrounding tumor may cause signs of urinary tract infection, such as frequency, urgency, and dysuria

Table 6-3	Renal Cell Cancer Staging
Stage of Tumor	**Extent of Tissue Involvement**
I	Kidney capsule only
II	Kidney capsule with invasion through capsule into local fascia only
III	Kidney, regional lymph node, ipsilateral renal vein, and possibly inferior vena cava
IV	Kidney, as well as local invasion or distant metastases

   3) With ureteral tumors, observe for colicky pain from obstruction
   4) Neoplasms cause few outward symptoms and may not be discovered until urinary obstruction occurs or a fistula develops
 b. Diagnostic and laboratory test findings
   1) Urinalysis shows gross or microscopic hematuria
   2) Urine cytology shows abnormal tumor or pre-tumor cells; see Table 6-3 for information about renal cell cancer staging
   3) Visualization of tumors via intravenous pyelography, ultrasound, CT scan, cystoscopy, or ureteroscopy
4. Therapeutic management of renal cancer: is treated primarily with radical nephrectomy (removal of kidney, adrenal gland, upper ureter, and fat and fascia around kidney); see discussion of care of client undergoing nephrectomy earlier in chapter
5. Therapeutic management of bladder cancer
 a. Radiation therapy
 b. Surgical intervention for bladder tumors includes tumor resection, partial cystectomy, or radical cystectomy (removal of bladder and adjacent structures)
 c. Urinary diversion may also be created
   1) Cutaneous ureterostomy: one or both ureters are excised from bladder and brought to a stoma
   2) Ileal conduit: portion of ileum is isolated from small intestine that is formed into a pouch; ureters are attached to pouch; pouch has open stoma
   3) Colon conduit: same as ileal conduit but a portion of sigmoid colon is used
   4) Kock pouch: same as ileal conduit but nipple valves are formed preventing leakage and reflux (see Figure 6-3)

Figure 6-3

A continent urinary diversion. A segment of ileum is separated from the small intestine and formed into a pouch. Nipple valves are formed at each end of the pouch by intussuscepting tissue backward into the reservoir to prevent leakage.

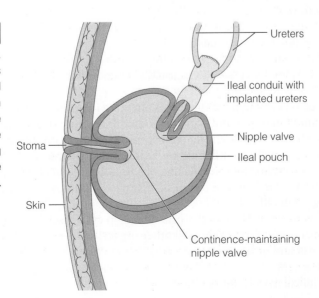

         5) Indiana continent urinary reservoir: reservoir is formed from colon and cecum and portion of ileum is brought to surface

         6) Ileocystoplasty: section of ileum is used; this procedure is ideal for men because it allows client to void

6. Priority nursing problems: alterations in urinary elimination, inadequate knowledge, anxiety, body image alterations, potential for infection

7. Planning and implementation

  a. Monitor urinary status, including I & O, signs of infection, hematuria, and BUN and creatinine levels

  b. Monitor UO from all catheters, stents, and tubes for amount, color, and clarity

  c. Prepare client for invasive tests to confirm location and size of neoplasm

  d. Follow guidelines for care before and after surgery, chemotherapy, and radiation treatments

  e. Encourage increased fluid intake, unless contraindicated

  f. Provide analgesics as needed for pain

  g. Encourage client to express feelings about potentially life-threatening illness and ask questions

8. Medication therapy for bladder cancer: chemotherapeutic agents may be given IV or administered by intravesical instillation (into bladder)

9. Client education

  a. Explain all nursing and medical interventions, including benefits and possible adverse effects

  b. Provide information about diagnosis and client's specific neoplasm

  c. Stress importance of compliance with long-term treatment plan and follow-up care

  d. Instruct client in methods to prevent infection

  e. For clients with a stoma or indwelling catheter, teach home care procedures and when to consult health care provider

  f. For clients with a continent ileostomy, teach how to catheterize pouch (approximately every 4 hours) and wear a small dressing to protect stoma and clothing

  g. Teach relaxation techniques and other coping mechanisms

10. Evaluation: client states understanding of disorder and proposed treatment plan; client's fluid I & O is balanced; client communicates fears and concerns about diagnosis; and client demonstrates appropriate care of stoma or catheter

J. Polycystic kidney disease

1. Description

  a. Hereditary disease characterized by cyst formation and massive kidney enlargement, affecting both children and adults

  b. Autosomal dominant form affects adults

  c. Autosomal recessive form usually diagnosed in childhood

2. Etiology and pathophysiology

  a. Renal cysts are fluid-filled sacs affecting nephron; they develop in tubular epithelium of nephron and fill with glomerular filtrate or secreted solutes and fluid

  b. Cysts range in size from microscopic to several centimeters

  c. As cysts enlarge and multiply, kidneys also enlarge; renal blood vessels and nephrons are compressed and obstructed, and functional tissue is destroyed

  d. Disorder is slow and progressive; adult symptoms usually manifest themselves by age 30 to 40

  e. Clients with this disorder often develop cysts elsewhere in body, including liver, spleen, pancreas, brain, and other organs; some clients also have aneurysms in aorta and/or brain

3. Assessment

  a. Clinical manifestations

    1) Flank pain

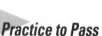

Practice to Pass

The nurse is preparing a client with glomerulonephritis for discharge. What dietary instructions should be included in the teaching plan?

          2) Polyuria and nocturia

          3) Signs of UTI and possibly renal calculi

          4) Hypertension

          5) Palpable, enlarged, and knobby kidney

          6) Signs of chronic renal failure as client approaches 50–60 years of age

      b. Diagnostic and laboratory test findings

          1) Gross hematuria, proteinuria

          2) Positive findings in renal ultrasonography, IVP, and CT scan

   4. Therapeutic management

      a. Largely consists of symptom management

      b. Eventually will require dialysis or transplantation

   5. Priority nursing problems: fluid overload, inadequate knowledge, anticipatory grief, potential for inadequate coping

   6. Planning and implementation

      a. Provide supportive care to help client cope with symptoms; no effective treatment is available

      b. Encourage fluid intake of 2,000–2,500 mL/day to help prevent UTI and calculi

      c. Administer antihypertensive agents as prescribed

      d. Discuss that hemodialysis and possibly renal transplant will be indicated as disease progresses

      e. Provide nursing care directed toward edema control

          1) Sodium restriction in diet

          2) Diuretics that block aldosterone formation

   7. Medication therapy: ACE inhibitors to control hypertension; diuretics to control edema; and antibiotics if infection develops

   8. Client education

      a. Maintenance of general health status, as disorder is chronic and progressive

      b. How to avoid UTI and to recognize early signs of infection

      c. Avoid nephrotoxic medications and check with provider before taking any new drug

      d. Genetic counseling and screening of family members for evidence of disease

      e. Maintain fluid intake of at least 2,500 mL/day

      f. Referral to support groups such as American Kidney Foundation

   9. Evaluation: client can state measures to prevent UTI; recognizes early signs of infection; verbalizes need to avoid nephrotoxic medications; maintains fluid intake of 2,500 mL/day; and states knowledge of disease and sequelae

K. *Acute renal failure*

   1. Description: a sudden loss of kidney function caused by failure of renal circulation or damage to tubules or glomeruli

   2. Etiology and pathophysiology

      a. Usually reversible, with spontaneous recovery in a few days to weeks

      b. Ischemia is primary cause; when allowed to continue for more than 2 hours, it produces irreversible damage to tubules

      c. Etiologic categories

          1) Prerenal: accounts for 55% of cases; caused by decreased blood flow to kidneys; readily reversible when recognized and treated early; may be caused by severe dehydration, diuretic therapy, circulatory collapse, hypovolemia, or shock

          2) Intrarenal: caused by a disease process, ischemia, or toxic conditions such as acute glomerulonephritis, vascular disorders, toxic agents, or severe infection; iatrogenic causes include such items as antibiotics and contrast dyes

          3) Postrenal: caused by any condition that obstructs urine flow such as in benign prostatic hyperplasia, renal or urinary tract calculi, or tumors

3. Assessment
   a. Clinical manifestations follow 3 phases: initiation, maintenance, and recovery; initiation stage has very few manifestations; maintenance phase is characterized by **oliguria** (UO less than 400 mL/24 hours); signs of improving renal function characterize recovery stage
     1) Muscle weakness, N/V, and diarrhea may occur
     2) Neurologic symptoms such as confusion, agitation, disorientation, seizures, and coma may also be present
   b. Diagnostic and laboratory test findings
     1) Hyperkalemia, hyperphosphatemia, and hypocalcemia
     2) Metabolic acidosis
     3) Anemia
     4) Elevated creatinine and BUN levels; azotemia
     5) Urinalysis shows specific gravity (SG) equal to SG of plasma; proteinuria; presence of casts, RBC, WBC, and renal tubular epithelial cells
     6) Positive renal biopsy findings
4. Therapeutic management: fluid and electrolyte management and supportive therapy with dialysis
5. Priority nursing problems: fluid overload, insufficient nutrients to meet bodily needs, inadequate knowledge, potential for infection
6. Planning and implementation
   a. Monitor intake and UO
   b. Observe for oliguria followed by **polyuria** (excess UO from diuresis)
   c. Weigh daily and observe for edema
   d. Monitor for complications of electrolyte imbalances, such as acidosis and hyperkalemia
   e. Allow client to verbalize concerns regarding disorder
   f. Encourage prescribed diet: moderate protein restriction, high in carbohydrates, restricted K^+
   g. Once diuresis phase begins, evaluate slow return of BUN, creatinine, phosphorus, and K^+ to normal
7. Medication therapy
   a. Avoid nephrotoxic drugs: aminoglycoside antibiotics, platinoid chemotherapy agents, NSAIDs, contrast media
   b. Use volume expanders as prescribed to restore renal perfusion in hypotensive clients and dopamine (Intropin) IV to increase renal blood flow
   c. Use loop diuretic to reduce toxic concentration in nephrons and establish urine flow
   d. Use ACE inhibitors to control hypertension
   e. Use antacids or histamine H_2-receptor antagonists to prevent gastric ulcers
   f. Use sodium polystyrene sulfate (Kayexalate) to reduce serum K^+ levels and sodium bicarbonate to treat acidosis
8. Client education
   a. Dietary and fluid restrictions, including those that may be continued after discharge
   b. Signs of complications, such as fluid volume excess, CHF, and hyperkalemia
   c. Monitor weight, BP, pulse, and UO
   d. Avoid nephrotoxic drugs and substances: NSAIDs, some antibiotics, radiologic contrast media, and heavy metals; consult provider before taking any OTC drugs
   e. Recovery of renal function requires up to 1 year; during this period, nephrons are vulnerable to damage from nephrotoxins
9. Evaluation: client states understanding of dietary and fluid restrictions, need to avoid nephrotoxic substances, signs of infection and when to notify provider; demonstrates ability to monitor BP, pulse, and UO; maintains weight; VS are within normal range

L. End-stage renal disease (ESRD)
 1. Definition
  a. Loss of renal function characterized by a GFR less than 20% of normal
  b. Final stage of **chronic renal failure (CRF)** (slow, progressive loss of kidney function and glomerular filtration); ends fatally with uremia
 2. Etiology and pathophysiology
  a. Most common causes of CRF are diabetic neuropathy, hypertension, glomerulonephritis, systemic lupus erythematosus, and cystic kidney disease
  b. Progressive loss of renal function occurs in 4 stages; fourth stage ends with ESRD (uremia)
  c. As 90% or more of nephrons are destroyed, BUN and creatinine clearance rise, and urine SG is fixed at 1.010 (normal up to 1.025)
  d. Uremia: "urine in blood"; term used for symptoms associated with ESRD
  e. Loss of erythropoietin leads to chronic anemia and subsequent fatigue
  f. There is inadequate clearance of fluid and electrolytes, leading to fluid and Na^+ retention, as well as hyperkalemia, hypermagnesemia, hyperphosphatemia, azotemia, and hypocalcemia; hypocalcemia leads to increased parathyroid secretion and calcium loss from bones (renal osteodystrophy); metabolic acidosis occurs because of impaired hydrogen ion excretion
 3. Assessment
  a. Clinical manifestations
   1) Early: nausea, apathy, weakness, and fatigue
   2) Late: possible frequent vomiting, increasing weakness, lethargy, and confusion
   3) Client may report "restless leg syndrome," paresthesia, and sensory loss
   4) Personality changes, such as anxiety, irritability, and hallucinations; seizures and coma may occur in late stages
   5) Respirations may change to Kussmaul pattern, with deep coma following
   6) Skin becomes pale and dry, with yellowish hue; metabolic wastes cause itching and uremic frost (crystallized deposits of urea on the skin)
  b. Diagnostic and laboratory test findings
   1) Urinalysis shows fixed SG approximately 1.010, equivalent to plasma; abnormal proteins, blood cells, and casts are present
   2) Elevated creatinine and BUN; decreased creatinine clearance
   3) Abnormal electrolyte values as noted above
   4) Moderate anemia
   5) Decreased platelets
   6) Decreased renal size by ultrasonography
   7) Positive renal biopsy if damage caused by cancer
 4. Priority nursing problems: reduced kidney tissue perfusion, fluid overload, insufficient nutrients to meet bodily needs, potential for infection, alterations in body image, reduced endurance for exercise or activity
 5. Planning and implementation
  a. Provide low-protein diet supplemented amino acids; restrict fluids as prescribed
  b. Provide electrolyte replacement or restriction
   1) Sodium and potassium restriction
   2) Replacement of calcium
   3) Replacement of bicarbonate stores to treat acidosis
  c. Monitor and plan nursing care for hypertension and heart failure
  d. Prepare client for dialysis or kidney transplant
  e. Administer medications with caution because of inability to excrete efficiently, check for toxicity
  f. Monitor I & O and VS

g. Monitor results of BUN and serum creatinine, pH, electrolytes, and CBC
h. Provide symptomatic relief for N/V
i. Observe for signs of infection
j. Provide rest periods to combat fatigue, which is chronic in nature
k. Help client learn about and adjust to diagnosis; support coping strategies and work with client to develop realistic goals
6. Medication therapy: limited by kidneys' inability to excrete; diuretics to reduce volume of extracellular fluid; ACE inhibitors to maintain normal BP; electrolyte replacement; phosphate binding agents; sodium polystyrene sulfonate (Kayexalate) to reduce serum K^+ levels; folic acid, iron supplement, and perhaps epoetin alfa (Epogen) to combat anemia; and multivitamins
7. Client education
a. Monitor weight, VS, and UO at home
b. Fluid and dietary restrictions (low Na^+, low K^+, low phosphorus, low protein) need to be followed carefully
c. Monitor symptoms of uremia
d. Avoid nephrotoxic drugs and substances: NSAIDs, some antibiotics, radiologic contrast media, and heavy metals
e. Teach strategies to avoid thirst, yet continue fluid restrictions, such as frequent mouth care, sugarless hard candy, using ice chips instead of liquids, or using a spray bottle instead of a cup to limit fluids ingested
f. Discuss hemodialysis or renal transplant therapies as indicated
g. Recommend methods to combat nausea: antiemetics; mouth care; small, frequent meals
h. Provide referral to mental health counseling or support group
8. Evaluation: client states understanding of dietary and fluid restrictions, need to avoid nephrotoxic substances, and signs of infection; takes medications as prescribed

Case Study

C. S., a 60-year-old truck driver, has been diabetic and has required insulin therapy for the past twenty years. Diabetic neuropathy has led to several complications, including end-stage renal disease, which he developed two years ago. He now receives hemodialysis three times a week and has an AV fistula in his left forearm. Yesterday, C. S. presented in the Emergency Department with a respiratory infection and was hospitalized with pneumonia, hypertension, and fluid overload. He will receive dialysis while on your nursing unit.

1. Is it appropriate to administer an aminoglycoside antibiotic for his respiratory infection? Why or why not?

2. What changes would you expect to see in this client's blood glucose levels during and after hemodialysis?

3. C. S. missed his dialysis treatment on the day of admission. How might this be evidenced in his respiratory status?

4. His wife comments on the fruity odor of his breath. What complication would cause this sign?

5. C. S. reports dry, itching skin. How would you explain this symptom to him? What nursing measures for skin care would you provide?

For suggested responses, see page 622.

POSTTEST

1 The nurse is reviewing health care provider prescriptions for a client diagnosed with end-stage renal failure. Which diet should the nurse expect the provider to prescribe for this client?

1. Increased protein, decreased carbohydrates
2. Restricted protein, increased carbohydrates
3. Increased potassium and sodium
4. Increased phosphorus and magnesium

2 The client diagnosed with cystitis asks the nurse about the purpose of the prescribed phenazopyridine (Pyridium). What is the nurse's best explanation?

1. Eases discomfort of the bladder mucosa
2. Eliminates urinary bacteria
3. Eases urinary tract spasms
4. Should be taken after sexual intercourse

3 The nurse is assessing cognitive status on a client who has developed urinary incontinence. When questioned by the family, the nurse explains that this assessment will help to determine which condition?

1. Stress incontinence
2. Overflow incontinence
3. Functional incontinence
4. Mixed incontinence

4 An older adult male reports to the nurse that he has difficulty starting urination and is voiding several times during the night. The nurse suspects that this client has which condition?

1. Benign prostatic hyperplasia (BPH)
2. Urinary tract infection
3. Urethral strictures
4. Urethritis

5 A client diagnosed with acute renal failure after surgical repair of a ruptured diverticulum is now receiving peritoneal dialysis (PD). From 7:00 to 11:00 a.m. the client has received IV fluids at a rate of 125 mL/hr and urine output was 150 mL total; Salem sump drainage was 250 mL; and peritoneal dialysis balance is −475. In calculating the client's 4-hour intake and output (I & O) totals, what is the client's total net fluid loss in mL considering all forms of I & O? Provide a numerical response.

_____ mL

6 Which nursing action is most appropriate when caring for a client with a nursing diagnosis of Excess Fluid Volume related to renal insufficiency?

1. Teaching clients about sodium content of foods
2. Administering vitamin D supplements
3. Assessing and documenting client's energy level
4. Observing for signs of hypocalcemia

7 The nurse is caring for a client with recurrent cystitis. Which instruction should be included prior to discharge?

1. Limit fluid daily intake to decrease the urge to void.
2. There is no relationship between sexual intercourse and cystitis.
3. Void at least every 4 hours even if the urge is absent.
4. Daily cranberry juice has been proven to decrease the number of UTIs.

POSTTEST

8 A client has undergone creation of an ileal conduit. Which instruction to the client about urostomy care would be appropriate to include in the teaching plan?

1. Cut the faceplate of the appliance so that the opening is slightly smaller than the stoma.
2. Plan to do appliance changes just before bedtime.
3. Limit fluids to minimize odor from urine breakdown to ammonia.
4. Cleanse the skin around the stoma using gentle soap and water, rinse and dry well.

9 The nurse is reviewing the past medical history of a client diagnosed with chronic renal failure. Which conditions in the client's history most likely contributed to the client's renal failure? Select all that apply.

1. Type 1 diabetes
2. Hypertension
3. Systemic lupus erythematosus
4. Hypothyroidism
5. Hiatal hernia

10 The nurse is conducting discharge teaching with a client following insertion of a new arteriovenous fistula in the left arm for hemodialysis. The nurse will be sure to include which topics in discussions with this client? Select all that apply.

1. Avoid carrying items with the left arm.
2. Assess the fistula site daily for redness or drainage.
3. Blood pressures should be taken in the right arm only.
4. Sleep on the left side.
5. It is expected to have some bleeding at the access site after a dialysis treatment.

➤ *See pages 214–215 for Answers and Rationales.*

ANSWERS & RATIONALES

Pretest

1 **Answer: 2** **Rationale:** Uremia is a manifestation of renal failure characterized by an elevated BUN and creatinine. Pyelonephritis, an inflammation of the kidney and renal pelvis, may be acute or chronic. If acute, it is manifested as an acute febrile process. Chronic pyelonephritis causes an inability to concentrate urine. Cystitis is an inflammation of the urinary bladder and has symptoms of a urinary tract infection. Polycystic kidney disease is a hereditary disease characterized by kidney enlargement and cyst formation rather than renal failure. **Cognitive Level:** Analyzing **Client Need:** Physiological Adaptation **Integrated Process:** Nursing Process: Planning **Content Area:** Adult Health **Strategy:** Define uremia. Compare the definition of uremia with each of the answer choices. Eliminate every answer choice that is inconsistent with the definition. This also requires an understanding of the various renal diseases listed. Anything ending in *-itis* means there is an inflammatory process involved. **Reference:** LeMone, P., Burke, K., & Bauldoff, G. (2011). *Medical-surgical nursing: Critical thinking in patient care* (5th ed.). Upper Saddle River, NJ: Pearson Education, p. 848.

2 **Answer: 1, 2, 3** **Rationale:** Checking the abdominal dressing allows the nurse to examine whether the dialysis tubing is kinked or obstructed at the site of insertion. To facilitate drainage, the client's position should be changed to move the dialysate solution into contact with the tip of the catheter. Dialysate drains from the abdomen by gravity. Lowering the drainage bag may increase the gravitational pull of drainage. The catheter would only need to be irrigated if there is a cessation of drainage and the nurse suspects that the catheter is completely obstructed. Continuing to monitor does not correct the current problem. **Cognitive Level:** Applying **Client Need:** Physiological Adaptation **Integrated Process:** Nursing Process: Implementation **Content Area:** Adult Health **Strategy:** Treat each answer choice as an individual true or false option as it relates to the question. The key to answering the question is to understanding the peritoneal dialysis process and the nurse's role in troubleshooting problems with peritoneal dialysis. **Reference:** LeMone, P., Burke, K., & Bauldoff, G. (2011). *Medical-surgical nursing: Critical thinking in patient care* (5th ed.). Upper Saddle River, NJ: Pearson Education, p. 845.

3 **Answer: 2** **Rationale:** The primary function of the kidneys is to clear nitrogenous waste from the body. Ingested protein breaks down into a nitrogenous waste and increases the workload of the kidney. By limiting the protein intake, protein catabolism is decreased, and the kidneys are allowed to rest and heal. Fluid replacement in glomerulonephritis is usually the urinary output plus 500 mL. Bran is more relevant in preventing colon cancer and is irrelevant in renal disease. Clients with glomerulonephritis are likely to have hyperkalemia so potassium-rich foods are contraindicated. **Cognitive Level:** Applying **Client Need:** Physiological Adaptation **Integrated Process:** Nursing Process: Implementation **Content Area:** Adult Health **Strategy:** To answer this question, you must know the normal functioning of the kidney as well as have an understanding of glomerulonephritis. Integrating both concepts helps to determine the correct response. **Reference:** LeMone, P., Burke, K., & Bauldoff, G. (2011). *Medical-surgical nursing: Critical thinking in patient care* (5th ed.). Upper Saddle River, NJ: Pearson Education, pp. 822–827.

4 **Answer: 3** **Rationale:** Acute renal failure is a condition that may be caused by nephrotoxic drugs such as aminoglycoside antibiotics. Acute renal failure has a rapid onset and is potentially reversible. Polycystic kidney disease is a genetic disorder and it is not related to ingestion of nephrotoxic substances. Glomerulonephritis is frequently caused by infectious organisms. Chronic renal failure develops over time, usually secondary to other disorders like hypertension and diabetes. **Cognitive Level:** Applying **Client Need:** Pharmacological and Parenteral Therapies **Integrated Process:** Nursing Process: Planning **Content Area:** Pharmacology **Strategy:** Recall the definition of nephrotoxicity. Comparing this definition to the answer choices helps eliminate the wrong ones and select the correct one. **Reference:** LeMone, P., Burke, K., & Bauldoff, G. (2011). *Medical-surgical nursing: Critical thinking in patient care* (5th ed.). Upper Saddle River, NJ: Pearson Education, p. 837.

5 **Answer: 3** **Rationale:** Serum creatinine measures the amount of creatinine and indicates renal function (normal 0.8–1.6 mg/dL). An elevation suggests that the kidneys are not functioning correctly. Urinalysis is a gross and microscopic view of the urine that can indicate such disorders as urinary tract infection and dehydration. The specific gravity of 1.015 is within normal limits (1.010–1.025). Urine culture specifically examines the type and amount of microscopic organisms present in the urine and should be negative. Serum potassium may be increased in renal failure as well as other disorders, so it is not a definitive diagnostic test for renal function; this value is normal (range 3.5–5.1 mEq/L). **Cognitive Level:** Applying **Client Need:** Reduction of Risk Potential **Integrated Process:** Nursing Process: Assessment **Content Area:** Adult Health **Strategy:** The question is asking what diagnostic test is an indicator of renal function. Only the answer choice that directly answers this question is correct. **Reference:** LeMone, P., Burke, K., & Bauldoff, G. (2011). *Medical-surgical nursing: Critical thinking in patient care* (5th ed.). Upper Saddle River, NJ: Pearson Education, pp. 774–775.

6 **Answer: 4** **Rationale:** Because general anesthesia may be used for cystoscopy, the client is instructed to remain NPO after midnight. Because radiopaque dye is not

used, allergic reactions are not of concern. Visualization of the bladder is enhanced when the colon is empty. A cystoscopy is used as a diagnostic test to visualize obstructions, tumors, or trauma but it is also can be used to remove bladder tumors and enlarged prostate glands. **Cognitive Level:** Applying **Client Need:** Reduction of Risk Potential **Integrated Process:** Nursing Process: Implementation **Content Area:** Adult Health **Strategy:** Any *-oscopy* involves direct visualization, in this case, visualization of the bladder using an endoscope. Review each answer choice and select the option that applies best to this test. **Reference:** LeMone, P., Burke, K., & Bauldoff, G. (2011). *Medical-surgical nursing: Critical thinking in patient care* (5th ed.). Upper Saddle River, NJ: Pearson Education, p. 775.

7 **Answer: 2** **Rationale:** Peritonitis is the major complication of peritoneal dialysis (PD). The nurse should use strict aseptic technique and should teach the client to use it whenever accessing the catheter. The client does not need postvoid residuals as it is irrelevant to the question of PD complications. Heparin is added to dialysate as ordered to prevent clot formation and clogging of the catheter. It would be added to each bag, not to one bag per day. The catheter site dressing is changed daily and when wet. **Cognitive Level:** Analyzing **Client Need:** Safety and Infection Control **Integrated Process:** Nursing Process: Implementation **Content Area:** Adult Health **Strategy:** It is important to understand the process of peritoneal dialysis and related complications to correctly answer the questions. Select the answer choice that best applies to your knowledge of peritoneal dialysis. **Reference:** LeMone, P., Burke, K., & Bauldoff, G. (2011). *Medical-surgical nursing: Critical thinking in patient care* (5th ed.). Upper Saddle River, NJ: Pearson Education, pp. 843–845.

8 **Answer: 1** **Rationale:** Urolithiasis is the development of renal calculi that cause an acute, severe pain in the flank and upper abdominal quadrant on the affected side. It is sudden in onset and may be accompanied by nausea, diaphoresis, and vomiting. Difficult or painful urination is usually associated with an infectious process in the urinary tract. Absence of urine or anuria is associated with renal failure or complete urinary obstruction. Headache may result from disequilibrium syndrome following hemodialysis or other problems not related to the renal system. **Cognitive Level:** Applying **Client Need:** Physiological Adaptation **Integrated Process:** Nursing Process: Assessment **Content Area:** Adult Health **Strategy:** Define urolithiasis. Compare this definition to each answer choice. **Reference:** LeMone, P., Burke, K., & Bauldoff, G. (2011). *Medical-surgical nursing: Critical thinking in patient care* (5th ed.). Upper Saddle River, NJ: Pearson Education, p. 794.

9 **Answer: 2, 4, 5** **Rationale:** Following a transurethral prostatectomy (TURP), the client has a 3-way urinary catheter with continuous bladder irrigation to remove blood from the bladder and prevent occlusion of the urethra and meatus with a blood clot. Priorities during the immediate postoperative period are to maintain irrigation and urinary drainage to prevent clots that could cause obstruction and lead to possible disruption of the surgical site. This is done by adjusting the flow rate of the irrigant according to the amount of blood in the urine. Preventing atelectasis postoperatively is a general priority to prevent respiratory complications. Postoperative infection would not be evident immediately after surgery so this is a lesser priority. While discontinuing a urinary catheter is also a general priority, it is not the focus immediately after this surgery, since the catheter is needed to facilitate clearance of blood and possible clots. **Cognitive Level:** Analyzing **Client Need:** Reduction of Risk Potential **Integrated Process:** Nursing Process: Planning **Content Area:** Adult Health **Strategy:** Note the critical words *immediate postoperative period*. View each answer choice in relation to the surgical procedure performed. **Reference:** LeMone, P., Burke, K., & Bauldoff, G. (2011). *Medical-surgical nursing: Critical thinking in patient care* (5th ed.). Upper Saddle River, NJ: Pearson Education, p. 1663.

10 **Answer: 4** **Rationale:** Transplant clients receive immunosuppressant drugs to prevent organ rejection, and these drugs suppress the bone marrow, making the client at risk for infection. Anxiety is a concern but is not the priority in the postoperative period. Ensuring continued functioning of the transplanted kidney is of greater priority than sleep disturbance. Body image disturbance is not the highest priority for this client. **Cognitive Level:** Analyzing **Client Need:** Physiological Adaptation **Integrated Process:** Nursing Process: Diagnosis **Content Area:** Adult Health **Strategy:** Use Maslow's hierarchy of needs to prioritize nursing diagnoses. Physical needs take priority over psychosocial needs. **Reference:** LeMone, P., Burke, K., & Bauldoff, G. (2011). *Medical-surgical nursing: Critical thinking in patient care* (5th ed.). Upper Saddle River, NJ: Pearson Education, p. 856.

Posttest

1 **Answer: 2** **Rationale:** Kidneys are not able to excrete the by-products of protein metabolism in end-stage renal disease so protein should be restricted to 0.6 gram/kg/day. Carbohydrate intake should be increased to maintain energy requirements. In end-stage renal failure, protein should be restricted and carbohydrates should be increased. Clients with end-stage renal disease should be on a potassium-restricted diet. Due to hyperphosphatemia and hypermagnesemia in chronic renal failure, intake of phosphorus and magnesium is restricted. **Cognitive Level:** Applying **Client Need:** Physiological Adaptation **Integrated Process:** Nursing Process: Implementation **Content Area:** Foundational Sciences **Strategy:** Apply the pathophysiology of renal failure to dietary implications. **Reference:** LeMone, P., Burke, K., & Bauldoff, G. (2011). *Medical-surgical nursing: Critical

thinking in patient care (5th ed.). Upper Saddle River, NJ: Pearson Education, pp. 850–853.

2 **Answer: 1** **Rationale:** Phenazopyridine (Pyridium) is a urinary tract analgesic for relief of the symptoms of urinary tract infections. Phenazopyridine does not eliminate bacteria. Antibiotic therapy is needed to eliminate urinary bacteria. The mechanism of action of phenazopyridine does not include easing urinary tract spasms. Clients with chronic cystitis are usually prescribed a dose of antibiotic or antiseptic to be taken immediately after intercourse. **Cognitive Level:** Applying **Client Need:** Pharmacological and Parenteral Therapies **Integrated Process:** Teaching and Learning **Content Area:** Pharmacology **Strategy:** Recall what cystitis is and the mechanism of action of phenazopyridine. Note that the drug in the question does not have any of the typical prefixes or suffixes found in the various classes of antibiotics, suggesting this drug is not an antimicrobial. Use nursing knowledge and the process of elimination to make a selection. **Reference:** LeMone, P., Burke, K., & Bauldoff, G. (2011). *Medical-surgical nursing: Critical thinking in patient care* (5th ed.). Upper Saddle River, NJ: Pearson Education, p. 788.

3 **Answer: 3** **Rationale:** Functional incontinence is usually associated with impaired cognitive functioning as that seen with dementia. Stress incontinence is usually associated with coughing or sneezing, or loss of estrogen postmenopause. Overflow incontinence occurs when the bladder becomes overdistended and urine leaks out to prevent rupture of the bladder. Mixed incontinence is a combination of stress and urge incontinence. **Cognitive Level:** Applying **Client Need:** Physiological Adaptation **Integrated Process:** Nursing Process: Assessment **Content Area:** Adult Health **Strategy:** Identify the types of urinary incontinence and compare them to the scenario identified in the question. **Reference:** LeMone, P., Burke, K., & Bauldoff, G. (2011). *Medical-surgical nursing: Critical thinking in patient care* (5th ed.). Upper Saddle River, NJ: Pearson Education, p. 811.

4 **Answer: 1** **Rationale:** Benign prostatic hyperplasia (BPH) partially obstructs the neck of the bladder, making voiding difficult. Clients with BPH have difficulty starting the urinary stream and frequently feel an urge to void because of incomplete bladder emptying. A urinary tract infection presents with urgency and frequency but does not affect the ability to start a urinary stream. Urethral strictures are usually related to trauma or sexually transmitted diseases. Urethritis is similar to a urinary tract infection with symptoms of burning or difficulty with urination or discharge from the meatus. **Cognitive Level:** Analyzing **Client Need:** Physiological Adaptation **Integrated Process:** Nursing Process: Assessment **Content Area:** Adult Health **Strategy:** The client's age and gender help focus the selection of the correct response. Eliminate the distracters that are not gender and age related. **Reference:** LeMone, P., Burke, K., & Bauldoff, G. (2011).

Medical-surgical nursing: Critical thinking in patient care (5th ed.). Upper Saddle River, NJ: Pearson Education, p. 1661.

5 Answer: 375 **Rationale:** Nondialysis intake includes all IV and oral fluids (although this client has only IV fluids ordered); this total is 500 mL. Nondialysis output includes urine and Salem sump drainage, which totals 400 mL. The dialysis fluid loss is 475 mL. The total output (400 + 475) is 875 mL. After subtracting total intake (500 mL), the client's net fluid loss for the 4-hour period is 375 mL. **Cognitive Level:** Analyzing **Client Need:** Basic Care and Comfort **Integrated Process:** Nursing Process: Implementation **Content Area:** Adult Health **Strategy:** Calculate the intake and output separately. Then to obtain the total fluid balance, subtract the total intake from the total output. **Reference:** Berman, A., Snyder, S., Kozier, B., & Erb, G. (2008). *Fundamentals of nursing: Concepts, process, and practice* (9th ed.). Upper Saddle River, NJ: Pearson Education, pp. 1473–1473.

6 Answer: 1 **Rationale:** Clients with excess fluid volume need to have restrictions in sodium intake because of the relationship of water and sodium. Elevated serum sodium will cause water to be retained. The client should avoid foods that are high in sodium such as cured meats, preserved foods, and canned goods. Vitamin D and hypocalcemia bear no relationship with fluid volume overload. Clients with an excess fluid volume may have decreased energy levels, but this is not directly related to decreasing the amount of fluid retention. **Cognitive Level:** Applying **Client Need:** Physiological Adaptation **Integrated Process:** Nursing Process: Implementation **Content Area:** Adult Health **Strategy:** The relationship between fluid balance and sodium is fundamental to answering this item. Recall that "water wants to follow salt" to help you choose correctly. **Reference:** LeMone, P., Burke, K., & Bauldoff, G. (2011). *Medical-surgical nursing: Critical thinking in patient care* (5th ed.). Upper Saddle River, NJ: Pearson Education, p. 850.

7 Answer: 3 **Rationale:** A client with frequent cystitis must void whenever the urge occurs and at least every 4 hours. Cranberry juice is used to decrease the incidence of urinary tract infections (UTIs) but its effectiveness has not been empirically proven. There is a direct relationship between the development of a UTI and sexual intercourse in many women. Increasing the fluid intake to 2 to 3 L per day helps to flush the bladder, while limiting fluids should be avoided. **Cognitive Level:** Applying **Client Need:** Physiological Adaptation **Integrated Process:** Nursing Process: Implementation **Content Area:** Adult Health **Strategy:** The possible mechanisms for bacterial migration up the urethra are explored in this item as well as interventions to flush the bacteria out. Select the answer choice that meets both criteria. **Reference:** LeMone, P., Burke, K., & Bauldoff, G. (2011). *Medical-surgical nursing: Critical thinking in*

patient care (5th ed.). Upper Saddle River, NJ: Pearson Education, pp. 785–791.

8 Answer: 4 **Rationale:** Peristomal skin should be cleansed with each appliance change using a gentle soap and water, and then should be rinsed and dried thoroughly. The client should change the appliance early in the morning, when urine production is slowest from lack of fluid intake during sleep. The opening of the appliance should be cut no larger than 3 mm greater than the opening of the stoma. An opening smaller than the stoma could decrease circulation to the stoma, causing ischemia. Fluids should be encouraged to maintain proper fluid and electrolyte balance and to dilute the urine and decrease the odor. **Cognitive Level:** Applying **Client Need:** Basic Care and Comfort **Integrated Process:** Nursing Process: Planning **Content Area:** Adult Health **Strategy:** This item is related to the selection of the appropriate interventions. Select the answer choice that does not pose a risk to the skin or the stoma. **Reference:** LeMone, P., Burke, K., & Bauldoff, G. (2011). *Medical-surgical nursing: Critical thinking in patient care* (5th ed.). Upper Saddle River, NJ: Pearson Education, pp. 802–803.

9 Answer: 1, 2, 3 **Rationale:** Diabetes is the leading cause of chronic kidney disease due to glomerular scarring. Clients with a history of hypertension are at risk for developing chronic renal disease. Clients with lupus are at high risk for developing lupus nephritis, which can lead to chronic renal disease. Hypothyroidism is not known to contribute directly to chronic renal failure. There is no relationship between a history of hiatal hernia and renal disease. **Cognitive Level:** Applying **Client Need:** Physiological Adaptation **Integrated Process:** Nursing Process: Assessment **Content Area:** Adult Health **Strategy:** The question is asking for the risk factors for chronic renal disease. Select the answer choices that are risk factors for chronic renal disease. **Reference:** LeMone, P., Burke, K., & Bauldoff, G. (2011). *Medical-surgical nursing: Critical thinking in patient care* (5th ed.). Upper Saddle River, NJ: Pearson Education, pp. 848–849.

10 Answer: 1, 2, 3 **Rationale:** To avoid the risk of clotting, the client should avoid carrying things with the affected arm. Infection is one of the leading complications of vascular access for hemodialysis. Blood pressures and venipunctures should be avoided on the arm on the fistula side. Sleeping on the affected side should be avoided. The client should alert the provider if any bleeding is experienced from the vascular access site. **Cognitive Level:** Applying **Client Need:** Safety and Infection Control **Integrated Process:** Teaching and Learning **Content Area:** Adult Health **Strategy:** Pay attention to the side of the affected extremity and apply your knowledge of dialysis care to the question. **Reference:** LeMone, P., Burke, K., & Bauldoff, G. (2011). *Medical-surgical nursing: Critical thinking in patient care* (5th ed.). Upper Saddle River, NJ: Pearson Education, pp. 844–845.

ANSWERS & RATIONALES

References

Berman, A. J., & Snyder, S. (2011). *Kozier and Erb's fundamentals of nursing: Concepts, process, and practice* (9th ed.). Upper Saddle River, NJ: Pearson Education.

D'Amico, D., & Barbarito, C. (2012). *Health & physical assessment in nursing* (2nd ed.). Upper Saddle River, NJ: Pearson Education.

Ignatavicius, D. D., & Workman, M. L. (2010). *Medical-surgical nursing: Patient-centered collaborative care* (6th ed.). St. Louis, MO: Elsevier.

Kee, J. F. (2010). *Laboratory and diagnostic tests with nursing implications* (8th ed.). Upper Saddle River, NJ: Pearson Education.

Lehne, R. (2010). *Pharmacology for nursing care* (7th ed.). St. Louis, MO: Elsevier.

LeMone, P., Burke, K., & Bauldoff, G. (2011). *Medical-surgical nursing: Critical thinking in patient care* (5th ed.). Upper Saddle River, NJ: Pearson Education.

Lewis, S., Dirksen, S., Heitkemper, M. Bucher, L., & Camera, I. (2011). *Medical surgical nursing: Assessment and management of clinical problems* (8th ed.). St. Louis, MO: Elsevier.

McCance, K., & Huether, S. (2010). *Pathophysiology: The biologic basis for disease in adults and children* (6th ed.). St. Louis, MO: Elsevier.

Smith, S.F., Duell, D.J., & Martin, B.C. (2012). *Clinical nursing skills: basic to advanced skills* (8th ed.). Upper Saddle River, NJ: Pearson Education.

Hepatobiliary and Pancreatic Disorders

7

Chapter Outline

Overview of Anatomy and Physiology of Hepatobiliary System

Diagnostic Tests and Assessments of Hepatobiliary System

Disorders of the Liver
Disorders of the Gallbladder
Disorders of the Pancreas

Objectives

➤ Identify basic structures and functions of the hepatobiliary and pancreatic systems.
➤ Describe the pathophysiology and etiology of common hepatobiliary and pancreatic disorders.
➤ Discuss expected assessment data and diagnostic test findings for selected hepatobiliary and pancreatic disorders.
➤ Identify priority nursing problems for selected hepatobiliary and pancreatic disorders.
➤ Discuss therapeutic management of selected hepatobiliary and pancreatic disorders.
➤ Discuss nursing management of a client experiencing a hepatobiliary or pancreatic disorder.
➤ Identify expected outcomes for the client experiencing a hepatobiliary or pancreatic disorder.

NCLEX-RN® Test Prep

Use the accompanying online resource, NursingReviewsandRationales, to test yourself with hundreds of NCLEX®-style practice questions.

Review at a Glance

ascites accumulation of fluid that is rich in proteins in abdominal (peritoneal) cavity
asterixis flapping tremor of hands from an increased serum ammonia level
cholecystectomy surgical removal of gallbladder either through a laparoscope or an abdominal incision
cholecystitis acute or chronic inflammation of gallbladder
cholelithiasis gallstones in biliary tree most commonly formed from cholesterol
cirrhosis fibrosis of liver from chronic inflammation
esophageal tamponade direct pressure applied to bleeding esophageal varices using a special nasogastric tube with esophageal and gastric balloons that are inflated to apply pressure
esophageal varices distended tortuous veins in esophagus that are prone to rupture

hepatic encephalopathy accumulation of ammonia in blood from chronic liver disease that results in neurological symptoms of confusion, irritability, coma, and asterixis
hepatitis inflammation of liver caused by numerous viruses, bacteria, alcohol, toxic chemicals, and drugs
hepatorenal syndrome renal failure caused by alterations in circulation resulting from chronic liver disease without primary renal disease
hyperbilirubinemia elevated serum bilirubin, both indirect and direct bilirubin
hypoalbuminemia low serum albumin resulting from chronic liver disease
icteric second phase of acute viral hepatitis marked by jaundice and lasting from 2 to 6 weeks
jaundice yellow-orange discoloration of skin and mucous membranes caused

by disrupted metabolism and excretion of bilirubin, which allows it to accumulate in and stain tissues
lithotripsy a procedure in which sound waves are passed through calculi to disintegrate stones
pancreatitis acute or chronic inflammation of pancreas
paracentesis a procedure used to remove excess fluid from peritoneal cavity
portal hypertension abnormally high blood pressure in portal venous circulation contributing to ascites formation and esophageal varices
sclerotherapy treatment for esophageal varices in which a sclerosing agent is injected into a bleeding vessel causing it to thrombose
steatorrhea fatty, frothy, foul-smelling stools caused by a decrease in pancreatic enzyme secretion

PRETEST

1 A female client who needs a cholecystectomy asks the nurse how she can live without her gallbladder. Which response by the nurse is most appropriate?

1. "Bile produced by the liver will go directly to your intestinal system."
2. "Your doctor will prescribe bile replacement therapy."
3. "Try not to be concerned; all the gallbladder does is store bile."
4. "You will have to permanently reduce your fat intake and take extra fat-soluble vitamins."

2 The nurse reviews a client's laboratory tests and notices that the total serum bilirubin is 2.5 mg/dL. Which clinical manifestation would the nurse identify as most likely to be present?

1. Ascites
2. Diarrhea
3. Scleral icterus
4. Hypertension

3 A client is diagnosed with obstructive jaundice. The nurse should ask the client about which of the following manifestations?

1. Clear, pale urine
2. Clay-colored stools
3. Lactose intolerance
4. Ankle edema

4 A client with cirrhosis who is receiving lactulose (Cephulac) is currently having 6 diarrhea stools per day. Which of the following prescriptions does the nurse anticipate from the health care provider?

1. Take Neomycin sulfate (Neo Tabs) orally 4 times daily.
2. Repeat serum ammonia level now.
3. Decrease the frequency of the lactulose dose.
4. Restrict fluids to 1,500 mL/day.

5 The nurse is assessing a client admitted to the emergency room with severe abdominal pain and possible cholelithiasis. The client states, "Right before you came in the pain just completely stopped!" What action should the nurse take next? Select all that apply.

1. Document effectiveness of the pain medication just administered.
2. Teach the client how to prevent future problems.
3. Notify the health care provider immediately of the change in condition.
4. Prepare client for the prescribed gallbladder study.
5. Reassess the client's pulse and blood pressure.

6 The client newly diagnosed with cirrhosis of the liver asks the nurse why he has edema. The nurse would make which response to explain how edema results from pathophysiologic changes in cirrhosis?

1. "The edema occurs because your liver produces fewer proteins that help draw fluid into the bloodstream."
2. "The high osmotic pressure of proteins in your blood pushes fluid into body tissues."
3. "Because of the liver disease, the kidneys are able to filter less fluid, so the body cannot excrete it as urine very easily."
4. "Your body is metabolizing sex hormones more quickly, leading to fluid retention."

7 The client has just had a liver biopsy. Which of the following nursing actions is the highest priority after the biopsy?

1. Monitor vital signs every 15 minutes the first hour, every 30 minutes the second hour, and then hourly.
2. Assess prothrombin times (PT), partial thromboplastin time (PTT), and platelet counts hourly.
3. Check bowel sounds every 2 hours and report an absence of or decrease in frequency.
4. Maintain NPO status for 4 hours post-biopsy or until the gag reflex returns.

8 The visiting nurse is caring for a client with a diagnosis of hepatitis A. The nurse is developing a teaching plan for the client and the family. What should the nurse include in this plan? Select all that apply.

1. Client should sleep in a single room away from spouse.
2. Sexual intimacy between client and significant other is prohibited.
3. Everyone should wash his or her hands frequently to prevent transmission.
4. Plan for frequent periods of rest during recovery stage.
5. Eat small frequent meals to minimize nausea.

9 The nurse teaches a client about the pathophysiological processes of acute pancreatitis. The nurse should explain that the pathophysiological events occur in what sequence? Place the following choices in the correct order.

1. Proteolysis, edema, hemorrhage, and necrosis occurred
2. Activated pancreatic enzymes released into pancreas tissue
3. Elastic tissue of blood vessel walls digested
4. Precipitating event
5. Enzymes digested pancreatic tissue and activate other enzymes

10 The client is diagnosed with chronic pancreatitis and nonenteric coated pancrelipase (Lipancreatin) is prescribed. Which of the following instructions should the nurse give to this client about this medication?

1. "Take the drug with your ranitidine (Zantac) at mealtimes."
2. "You should have bulkier stools while taking this medication."
3. "This drug is a natural product so it does not have side effects."
4. "Take this medication whenever you notice excess fat in your stools."

➤ *See pages 245–247 for Answers and Rationales.*

I. OVERVIEW OF ANATOMY AND PHYSIOLOGY OF HEPATOBILIARY SYSTEM

A. Basic structures of the hepatobiliary system (see Figure 7-1)

1. Liver: located in right upper quadrant (RUQ) of abdomen, beneath the diaphragm and weighing 1,200–1,600 grams
   a. Composed of two lobes; right is larger than left
   b. Lobes are separated by a mesenteric ligament, which suspends liver from diaphragm and anterior abdominal wall

Figure 7-1

Anatomy of hepatobiliary-pancreatic system

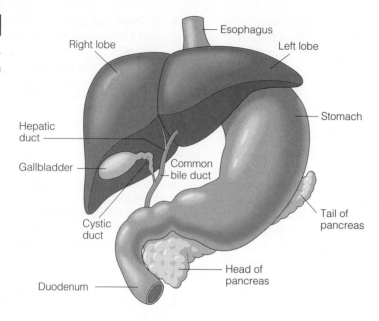

    c. Covered with a fibroelastic capsule (Glisson capsule) that contains blood vessels, lymphatics, and nerves

    d. Hepatic artery receives 400–500 mL/min of oxygenated blood from abdominal aorta; hepatic portal vein receives about 1,000–1,200 mL/min of deoxygenated blood from superior and inferior mesenteric veins and splenic vein, and sends blood on to vena cava and heart

2. Biliary tract: composed of gallbladder and associated ducts; cystic, hepatic, and common bile ducts

    a. Bile is synthesized in liver and transported to bile ducts via bile canaliculi that surround each hepatic cell

    b. Bile canaliculi drain into right or left hepatic bile ducts, which come together to form the common hepatic duct

    c. Sphincter of Oddi is at distal end of common hepatic duct and controls flow of bile into duodenum

    d. Cystic duct connects gallbladder with hepatic duct and they merge to form the common bile duct

    e. Common bile duct opens into duodenum allowing secretion of bile necessary for digestion

3. Gallbladder: saclike organ located on inferior surface of liver

    a. Mucosa of gallbladder wall absorbs water and electrolytes resulting in a high concentration of bile salts, bile pigments, and cholesterol

    b. Primary purpose of gallbladder is to store and concentrate bile; about 90 mL

4. Pancreas: primary enzyme-producing gland of digestive system with both exocrine and endocrine functions; is located along upper quadrants of abdomen; head is located within curve of duodenum; tail touches spleen; body lies behind stomach

B. Basic functions of hepatobiliary system

  1. Liver

    a. Produces 700-1,200 mL per day of bile per day, a bitter-tasting, alkaline, yellow-green fluid necessary for fat emulsification and absorption; bile is formed by hepatocytes and secreted into biliary canaliculi; bile contains bile salts (conjugated bile acids), cholesterol, bilirubin, electrolytes, phospholipids, lecithin, and water

      b. Stores fat-soluble vitamins (A, D, E, and K)

      c. Metabolizes bilirubin, a by-product of destruction of old red blood cells (RBCs)

      d. Stores and releases blood during hemorrhage

      e. Synthesizes plasma proteins to maintain plasma oncotic pressure

      f. Synthesizes prothrombin, fibrinogen, and clotting factors I, II, VII, IX, and X

      g. Synthesizes fats from carbohydrates and proteins to be either used for energy or stored as adipose tissue

      h. Synthesizes phospholipids and cholesterol necessary for production of bile salts, steroid hormones, and plasma membranes

      i. Converts amino acids to carbohydrates through deamination

      j. Stores glucose as glycogen during times of hyperglycemia or converts it to fat

      k. Releases glucose during times of hypoglycemia

      l. Stores and releases copper

      m. Stores iron as ferritin and releases it as needed for the production of RBCs

      n. Alters alcohol, certain drugs, chemicals, foreign molecules, and hormones to make them less toxic

      o. Phagocytosis

   2. Biliary tract: functions to transport bile formed in liver to bile ducts and eventually to duodenum

   3. Gallbladder: stores and concentrates bile; stores about 90 mL of bile

      a. Contracts and releases bile into cystic duct that joins hepatic duct and together form the common bile duct, which terminates in the duodenum

      b. Sphincter of Oddi controls release of bile into duodenum; gallbladder contraction is regulated by hormones secreted by duodenal mucosa in presence of fat, which acts to relax sphincter of Oddi and allow flow of bile into duodenum

   4. Pancreas: produces enzymes (exocrine) and hormones (endocrine) that assist in digestive process

      a. The endocrine pancreas secretes insulin and glucagon hormones from islets of Langerhans directly into circulation

         1) Insulin: protein hormone that promotes storage and utilization of food, primarily glucose and fats

         2) Glucagon: stimulates glycogenolysis in liver

      b. Exocrine pancreas is composed of secretory units called *acini* that secrete 1–1.5 L of enzymes and alkaline fluids per day into pancreatic ducts, which empty into common bile duct at ampulla of Vater; secretion of these enzymes and fluids is controlled by the vagus nerve and the intestinal hormones secretin and cholecystokinin

         1) Lipase promotes fat breakdown and absorption

         2) Amylase promotes carbohydrate breakdown

         3) Trypsin, chymotrypsin, and carboxypeptidase break down proteins

         4) Nucleases break down nucleic acids

         5) Alkaline-rich fluid neutralizes acidic chyme from stomach and prepares it for further enzymatic digestion

II. DIAGNOSTIC TESTS AND ASSESSMENTS OF HEPATOBILIARY SYSTEM

A. Laboratory tests

   1. Alanine aminotransferase (ALT): normal 5–35 units/L; enzyme found within liver cells and released with liver cell damage; helps eliminate hemolysis as a cause of jaundice; higher elevations result from drug- or chemical-induced liver damage;

more significant elevations with acute **hepatitis** (inflammation of liver from a variety of causes) than with **cirrhosis** (fibrosis of liver from chronic inflammation)

2. Albumin: normal 3.5 to 5.0 grams/dL; synthesized by liver and makes up more than half of plasma proteins; levels decrease with diminished liver function, resulting in reduced osmotic (oncotic) pressure and fluid shifts from within blood vessels to tissues, with resulting edema and/or **ascites** (accumulation of fluid in peritoneal cavity)

3. Alkaline phosphatase (ALP): normal 30–85 units/mL (adult); found mainly in liver and bone; increases with biliary obstruction; more significant elevations with acute hepatitis than with cirrhosis

4. Alpha-fetoprotein (AFP): high elevations in 70% of those with hepatocellular cancer but may also increase with cirrhosis or hepatitis

5. ALT/AST ratio: ALT is more elevated than AST in acute hepatitis and liver necrosis from drug or chemical toxicity; in cirrhosis, AST is more elevated than ALT in liver cancer and chronic hepatitis

6. Ammonia: normal 15–45 mcg/dL; end product of protein digestion (nitrogenous waste) synthesized by liver to urea for excretion by kidneys; elevations seen with liver cell damage

7. Amylase
   a. Serum amylase: enzyme from pancreas that changes starch to sugar; increases early in **pancreatitis** and may return to normal levels within 48 hours
   b. Urine amylase: increases in acute pancreatitis

8. Aspartate aminotransferase (AST): normal 5–40 units/L (adults); enzyme found primarily in heart and liver cells; severe liver damage may cause elevations of 20–100 times normal; stays elevated for longer periods than ALT; more significant elevations with acute hepatitis than with cirrhosis; also increases with acute pancreatitis

9. Bilirubin

   a. Total bilirubin (serum)—normal 0.1–1.2 mg/dL; includes both indirect (unconjugated) and direct (conjugated) forms
      1) Indirect (unconjugated) bilirubin: normal less than 1.0 mg/dL; increases with hemolytic jaundice and may increase with hepatic jaundice
      2) Direct (conjugated) bilirubin: normal 0.1–0.3 mg/dL; increases with obstructive jaundice and may increase with hepatic jaundice
   b. Urine bilirubin: normal 0–0.2 mg/dL; increases are always due to high levels of direct (conjugated) bilirubin because direct bilirubin is water-soluble and indirect bilirubin is not

10. C-reactive protein; produced in liver in response to tissue injury and acute inflammation anywhere in body; elevations seen with pancreatitis

11. Electrolyte abnormalities
    a. Hypocalcemia seen with severe pancreatitis
    b. Hypomagnesemia seen with alcohol abuse and cirrhosis
    c. Hypokalemia may be seen secondary to vomiting or diuretic therapy
    d. Hyperkalemia if renal failure
    e. Hyponatremia if excess free water (hemodilution)

12. Erythrocyte sedimentation rate (ESR): nonspecific; elevations occur with inflammation of liver and other inflammatory disorders

13. Gamma-glutamyl transferase (GGT): enzyme found primarily in liver and kidney; acutely elevated with alcohol consumption use of and hepatotoxic drugs, remains elevated as long as cellular damage persists

14. Glucose: normal 60–100 mg/dL; stored in liver as glycogen, requires insulin produced by pancreas to be used by cells; elevations may be seen with liver damage, pancreatitis

15. Lipase: an enzyme secreted by pancreas to aid in digesting fats; increases with pancreatitis and pancreatic pseudocyst, elevations may persist for up to 14 days

Box 7-1	• Vital signs q 15 min × 4; q 30 min × 2; q 4 hr × 4; then q 6 hr
Nursing Care after Liver Biopsy	• Observe dressing for oozing on same schedule as vital signs
	• Monitor for signs and symptoms of bleeding
	• Apply direct pressure to biopsy site immediately after procedure
	• Position on right side for compression over biopsy site
	• Maintain NPO for 2 hr postprocedure
	• Bed rest for 24 hr
	• Avoid activities that increase intra-abdominal pressure (coughing, lifting, straining) for 1–2 weeks

16. Platelet count: decreases with platelet destruction by spleen seen with cirrhosis
17. Prothrombin time (PT): prolonged if liver is injured to the point that it can no longer produce proteins necessary for blood coagulation
18. Hemoglobin, hematocrit, and RBC count: decrease with anemia secondary to bleeding; cirrhosis may also cause bone marrow suppression, increased RBC destruction, and deficiencies of folic acid and vitamin B_{12} needed for RBC production
19. Specific serological tests to detect either viral antigens, antibodies or the virus itself
20. White blood cells: elevations seen with infections frequently present with **cholecystitis** (inflammation of gallbladder) or pancreatitis; decreases secondary to splenomegaly seen with cirrhosis

B. **Radiologic procedures**
1. Abdominal ultrasound: identifies gallstones, pancreatic mass or pseudocyst, liver changes
2. Abdominal x-ray: identifies ascites, some gallstones (most are not radiopaque)
3. Chest x-ray: identifies pleural effusion resulting from enzymatic irritation from leaking pancreatic fluid
4. Computed tomography (CT, CAT) scans: visualize size of organs, identify fluid collections, abscesses, masses, lesions and areas of hemorrhage or necrosis; contrast may be used to enhance visualization; can be used to guide needle biopsies
5. Nuclear scan: radioisotope administered intravenously; abnormal tissue absorbs more radioisotope than normal tissue; injected radionuclide is safe and should not affect others
   a) Hepatobiliary iminodiacetic acid (HIDA) scan: evaluates for acute cholecystitis
   b) Liver imaging: detection of hepatic metastases and hepatocellular diseases
6. Liver biopsy: removal and examination of liver tissue; provides definitive diagnosis for liver cancer, cirrhosis; there is risk for postprocedure bleeding, especially if abnormal coagulation studies are present; apply pressure dressing and position client on right side after procedure to decrease risk of hemorrhage; see Box 7-1 for nursing care after liver biopsy
7. Magnetic resonance imaging (MRI): may reveal focal lesions, more sensitive than CT scan; magnet can damage metal so is contraindicated if client has a pacemaker, internal metal clips or other metal within body; external metal (including piercings, jewelry, cosmetics with metallic fragments) should be removed; closed MRI may require sedation if client is claustrophobic, open MRIs are available but result in a decrease in image quality

III. DISORDERS OF THE LIVER

A. *Jaundice*: also referred to as icterus
1. Description
   a. Yellow-orange discoloration of skin and mucous membranes; caused by a disturbance of bilirubin metabolism or excretion causing **hyperbilirubinemia**

(serum bilirubin level greater than 2.5–3.0 mg/dL); is frequently seen first in sclera of eyes and then skin

   b. Associated with diffuse hepatocellular disorders or present in newborns because of impaired bilirubin uptake and conjugation

  2. Etiology and pathophysiology

   a. RBCs are destroyed because of cell aging or disease, leading to release and breakup of hemoglobin molecule

    1) Biliverdin, later converted to fat-soluble bilirubin (unconjugated or indirect bilirubin), is released

    2) Unconjugated bilirubin is transported to liver

    3) Liver converts bilirubin to a water-soluble form (conjugated or direct bilirubin) to be excreted in bile

   b. Hyperbilirubinemia and jaundice result from accumulation of bilirubin pigments; jaundice is classified as hepatic, obstructive, or hemolytic

   c. Hepatic jaundice

    1) Disturbance of hepatocyte function caused by impairment of liver cells (hepatocytes), leading to increases in both conjugated and unconjugated forms of bilirubin

    2) Common causes are drug reactions (phenothiazines) or hepatitis

    3) Stools may appear normal or clay-colored, and urine is dark because conjugated bilirubin is excreted by kidneys

   d. Obstructive jaundice

    1) Common bile duct is occluded by gallstones or a tumor, preventing transport of bile into duodenum

    2) Bile accumulates within liver and overflows into blood, causing hyperbilirubinemia and elevated conjugated bilirubin level

    3) Stools are light or clay-colored from lack of bile pigment; urine is dark because kidneys excrete bilirubin

   e. Hemolytic jaundice is caused by excessive breakdown of RBCs

    1) Amount of bilirubin produced exceeds liver's ability to conjugate it, leading to increase in unconjugated or indirect serum bilirubin

    2) Unconjugated bilirubin is insoluble in water and will not be found in urine

    3) Causes include blood transfusion reactions, sickle cell disease, membrane defects of erythrocytes, severe infection, or toxic substances

  3. Assessment

   a. General assessments

    1) Vital signs and full physical examination focused on skin, mucous membranes, and eyes assessing for yellowish discoloration

    2) Abdominal swelling, pain in right upper quadrant, and presence of hepatomegaly

    3) Questions regarding appetite and color of urine and stool

   b. Clinical manifestations

    1) Yellowish discoloration of skin and mucous membranes caused by deposition of bilirubin

    2) Scleral icterus (yellowish discoloration of sclera) may be present before discoloration of skin

    3) Pruritus (severe itching) secondary to accumulation of bilirubin in skin

    4) Elevation of conjugated bilirubin that causes urine to be dark (tea- or cola-colored); may be present before jaundice appears

    5) Complete obstruction of flow of bile into duodenum causes light or clay-colored stools

6) Jaundice caused by an infectious process may be accompanied by fever and chills

7) Any client with liver dysfunction or injury may complain of nausea, anorexia, and/or fatigue

8) Abdominal pain may be present because of liver inflammation or pressure from obstructed bile flow

4. Therapeutic management is aimed at treating cause of jaundice

5. Priority nursing diagnosis: Altered Comfort: Itching

6. Planning and implementation

a. Cool or tepid/warm (but not hot) baths containing colloidal substances (oatmeal, cornstarch, soybean powder); limit duration, pat dry, do not rub skin

b. Cool room (68 to 70°F) with 30 to 40% humidity

c. Use an emollient lotion rather than one containing alcohol, which is too drying

d. Wear loose cotton garments that allow moisture to evaporate from skin

e. Keep fingernails short, and wear cotton mittens or gloves as needed to prevent scratching during sleep

7. Medication therapy: there is no specific medication therapy for jaundice

a. Topical corticosteroids may provide some relief of itching

b. Bile-sequestering agents, such as cholestyramine (Questran), bind bile acids in intestine and may remove excess bile from fat deposits under skin, decreasing pruritus

8. Client education

a. Diagnostic tests required to determine cause of jaundice and once diagnosed, the disease process and future management

b. The causes of jaundice are usually correctable

c. Avoid alcohol and acetaminophen with liver damage, since both can cause further liver damage

9. Evaluation: client verbalizes the disease process; identifies appropriate dietary adjustments as indicated; identifies ways to reduce itching

B. Hepatitis

1. Description

a. Inflammation of liver, usually caused by a virus (hepatitis A, hepatitis B, hepatitis C, hepatitis D or hepatitis E) but may result from other pathogens, exposure to alcohol, drugs (acetaminophen overdose is the leading cause of acute liver failure) and toxins, or autoimmune processes

b. Chronic hepatitis is caused by hepatitis B virus, hepatitis C virus, and hepatitis D virus; may cause few symptoms but is primary cause of liver damage leading to cirrhosis, liver cancer, and liver transplantation

c. Cirrhosis, discussed in the next section, is a potential consequence

2. Etiology and pathophysiology

a. Causative agent triggers inflammatory process with edema within liver

b. Cell-mediated immune responses damage hepatocytes and Kupffer cells, leading to hyperplasia, necrosis, and cellular regeneration

c. Flow of bile may be impaired, leading to jaundice

d. Damage may be mild to severe

e. Metabolism of nutrients, drugs, alcohol, and toxins may be disrupted as well as the process of bile elimination

f. Toxic substances, such as alcohol or drugs, directly damage liver cells; degree of damage depends on age and extent of exposure to hepatotoxin

g. Viruses replicate in liver, provoking an immune response that causes inflammation and necrosis of hepatocytes; see Table 7-1 for comparison of types of viral hepatitis

Practice to Pass

A client with jaundice is complaining of severe itching. What instructions can the nurse give to help relieve the itching?

Practice to Pass

What information should the nurse give to a client with viral hepatitis about its transmission?

Table 7-1 **Comparison of Types of Viral Hepatitis**

Virus	Hepatitis A (HAV)	Hepatitis B (HBV)	Hepatitis C (HCV)	Hepatitis D (HDV)	Hepatitis E (HEV)
Mode of transmission	Fecal–oral	Blood and body fluids; perinatal	Blood and body fluids	Blood and body fluids; perinatal	Fecal–oral
Incubation (in weeks)	2–6	6–24	5–12	3–13	3–6
Onset	Abrupt	Slow	Slow	Abrupt	Abrupt
Carrier state	No	Yes	Yes	Yes	Yes
Possible complications	Rare	Chronic hepatitis	Cirrhosis	Liver cancer	Chronic hepatitis
Cirrhosis	Liver cancer	Chronic hepatitis	Cirrhosis	Fulminant hepatitis	May be severe in pregnant women
Laboratory findings	Anti-HAV antibodies present	Positive HBsAg (HBV surface antigen); anti-HBV antibodies present	Anti-HCV antibodies present	Positive HDVAg (delta antigen) early; anti-HDV antibodies later	Anti-HEV antibodies present

Source: LeMone, Priscilla; Burke, Karen M.; Bauldoff, Gerene, *Medical-Surgical Nursing: Critical Thinking in Patient Care* 5th Ed., © 2011. Reprinted and Electronically reproduced by permission of Pearson Education, Inc., Upper Saddle River, New Jersey.

3. Assessment

   a. Acute viral hepatitis is divided into 3 phases
      1) Prodromal (preicteric) phase (most contagious) occurs before jaundice appears, about 2 weeks after exposure to virus; no manifestations are present during incubation period; manifestations begin abruptly or insidiously and include flulike symptoms (general malaise, gastrointestinal [GI] complaints, nausea or vomiting [N/V], diarrhea, and anorexia), headache, fatigue, myalgia, joint pain, chills, and low-grade fever; food odors, smoking, or alcohol may cause nausea
      2) **Icteric** phase is marked by onset of jaundice; may not occur with hepatitis C but is common with acute hepatitis A or B; occurs about 5–10 days after onset of symptoms and lasts 2–6 weeks; includes dark-colored urine and clay-colored stools prior to appearance of jaundice and pruritis; decrease in preicteric phase symptoms; liver remains enlarged and may be tender to touch
      3) Recovery (posticteric) phase begins with resolution of jaundice and lasts several weeks; during this phase symptoms improve, energy level increases, and serum enzymes normalize
   b. Chronic hepatitis may have few symptoms; liver enzymes (especially serum aminotransferase), are typically elevated
   c. Toxic hepatitis; symptoms vary depending on degree of damage to liver cells
   d. Specific assessments
      1) Vital signs, including weight and reported weight loss
      2) Skin assessment for jaundice, pruritis, signs of bleeding, petechiae or ecchymotic areas, dehydration, and scleral icterus
      3) Lymphadenopathy
      4) Abdominal assessment for pain (location, type), hepatomegaly, and swelling of abdomen (may indicate ascites)
      5) Edema
      6) Current nutritional state (adequate intake, anorexia, N/V) and elimination pattern (diarrhea)
      7) Activity level, fatigue, ability to perform ADLs
      8) Risk factors: IV drug use, homosexual or bisexual lifestyle, unprotected sexual contact, blood transfusion, tattoos

4. Therapeutic management: consists primarily of medication therapy

    a. Vaccines are available for hepatitis A and hepatitis B

    b. Postexposure prophylaxis

        1) Hepatitis A: a single dose of immune globulin (IG) within 2 weeks of exposure; not necessary if exposed person is known to be immune or has been vaccinated

        2) Hepatitis B: administration of hepatitis B immune globulin (HBIG); may give HBV vaccine concurrently

    c. Disease treatment

        1) Most recover fully without pharmacologic treatment

        2) Anti-retroviral, such as lamivudine (Epivir) may be given for severe cases of acute hepatitis B

        3) Interferon alpha, an antiviral agent, may be given to reduce risk of chronic hepatitis C

        4) Milk thistle (active ingredient silymarin) has been demonstrated to promote quality of life and reduce symptoms in clients with hepatitis C and other types of liver damage

        5) Antiemetics, antihistamines and analgesics may be provided for symptom relief; most analgesics are metabolized in liver so their use must be limited; acetaminophen is contraindicated

        6) IV fluids may be necessary if client is unable to tolerate oral fluids

        7) Vitamin K is indicated if prothrombin time is prolonged

5. Priority nursing problems

    a. Potential for infection related to transmission of viral hepatitis

    b. Fatigue or inability to endure exercise or activity (as appropriate to client) related to inadequate liver function

    c. Insufficient nutrients to meet bodily needs related to N/V, anorexia, and diarrhea

    d. Altered comfort related to pain and pruritis

    e. Potential for interrupted skin integrity related to jaundice and pruritus

6. Planning and implementation

    a. Use of standard precautions (including use of goggles, gown, and gloves when splattering of blood or body fluids is likely) and meticulous hand hygiene by client, family, and staff is imperative

    b. Clients should have a private bathroom

    c. Proper bagging, labeling, cleansing, and disposal of contaminated items is needed

    d. Provide anti-emetic medications as prescribed and encourage a diet high in carbohydrates and low in fat

    e. Abstinence from alcohol is essential

    f. If liver function is compromised, protein and salt should be restricted

    g. Encourage a good breakfast; clients tend to be more nauseous later in day

    h. Initiate intravenous (IV) fluids as prescribed

    i. Assess for signs of dehydration and monitor electrolyte status

    j. Encourage gradual increase of activity as tolerated

    k. Plan nursing activities to allow for adequate rest

    l. Inform clients they may never donate blood

    m. Observe for blood in stool or urine, multiple ecchymosis, or petechiae, or oozing of blood from gums or minor cuts, which may indicate a complication

7. Client education

    a. Since most clients with acute viral hepatitis are not hospitalized, provide detailed education about the disease and prevention of transmission (such as meticulous hand hygiene; avoid sharing eating utensils, bath towels, and other personal care items that are in contact with body fluids)

            b. Avoid alcohol and drugs that may be hepatotoxic (such as acetaminophen)

            c. Use safe sex practices as a general health measure

            d. Importance of rest and good nutrition for liver repair

            e. Reinforce possibility of chronic disease and importance of maintaining medication therapy if prescribed

     8. Evaluation

            a. Client demonstrates understanding of disease process and necessary steps to avoid transmitting infection both in hospital and after discharge

            b. Resumes normal bowel elimination pattern

            c. Activity progressively increases to a level normal for client

            d. Client is able to meet daily caloric intake and maintain a stable weight

            e. Practices safe sex

            f. Obtains vaccinations (if appropriate)

C. Cirrhosis

     1. Description

            a. Chronic liver disease characterized by diffuse inflammation and fibrosis of liver tissue

            b. Previously believed irreversible; not recognized that fibrosis might be reversed to some degree if underlying cause is eliminated

            c. Structural changes lead to loss of liver function because of scarring and obstruction of hepatic blood flow

     2. Etiology and pathophysiology (see Figure 7-2)

            a. Three classifications: Laënnec's (also called alcoholic), biliary, and postnecrotic

                1) Laënnec's (alcoholic) cirrhosis is most prevalent type in United States, and is highest among middle-aged men

                    a) Caused by prolonged, excessive alcohol intake with or without malnutrition; is directly related to toxic effects of alcohol on liver

                    b) Alcohol is metabolized to acetaldehyde and causes metabolic changes in liver with increased triglyceride and fatty acid synthesis, decreased formation and release of lipoproteins and leads to fatty infiltration of liver, causing a large firm liver (reversible at this stage if alcohol intake is stopped)

                    c) With continued alcohol abuse inflammatory cells infiltrate liver, causing necrosis, fibrosis, and destruction of functional liver tissue (irreversible)

                    d) In final stage regenerative nodules form, liver becomes smaller and develops a nodular appearance (irreversible)

                2) Biliary cirrhosis is caused by obstruction of bile canaliculi and ducts and results in necrosis and fibrosis; the cause can be autoimmune in nature or from tumors, gallstones, or chronic pancreatitis

                3) Posthepatic (also called postnecrotic) cirrhosis results from a chronic, severe liver disease such as hepatitis B or C, autoimmune hepatitis, or from nonalcoholic fatty liver disease (from obesity); as with other types the liver becomes shrunken and nodular, with extensive liver cell loss and fibrosis

            b. Regardless of cause, cirrhosis develops slowly; severity and rate of progression depend on cause and repeated injury to hepatocytes

            c. Disruption of portal blood flow secondary to structural changes in liver results in edema, ascites, splenomegaly (caused by splanchnic venous congestion), portal hypertension (see section that follows), hemorrhoids, varicose veins, and **esophageal varices** (see section that follows)

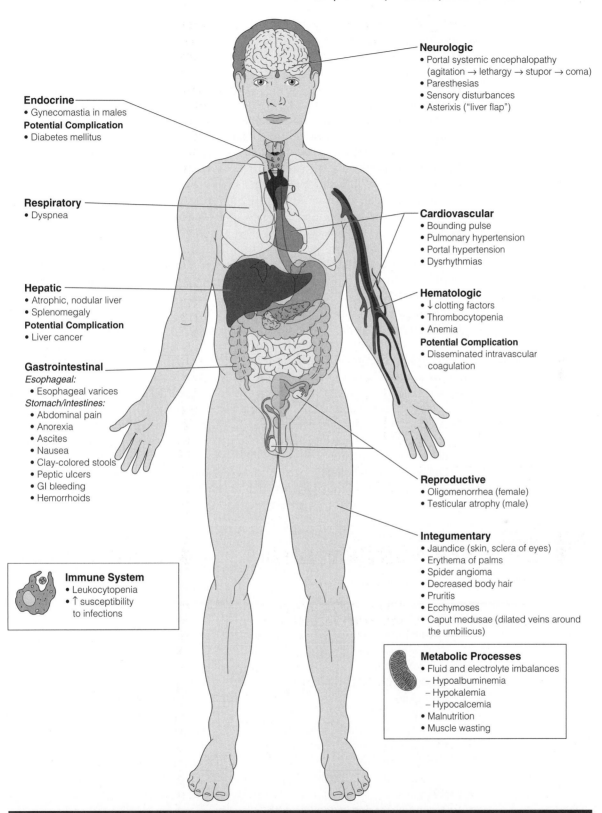

Neurologic
- Portal systemic encephalopathy (agitation → lethargy → stupor → coma)
- Paresthesias
- Sensory disturbances
- Asterixis ("liver flap")

Endocrine
- Gynecomastia in males
Potential Complication
- Diabetes mellitus

Respiratory
- Dyspnea

Cardiovascular
- Bounding pulse
- Pulmonary hypertension
- Portal hypertension
- Dysrhythmias

Hepatic
- Atrophic, nodular liver
- Splenomegaly
Potential Complication
- Liver cancer

Hematologic
- ↓ clotting factors
- Thrombocytopenia
- Anemia
Potential Complication
- Disseminated intravascular coagulation

Gastrointestinal
Esophageal:
- Esophageal varices
Stomach/intestines:
- Abdominal pain
- Anorexia
- Ascites
- Nausea
- Clay-colored stools
- Peptic ulcers
- GI bleeding
- Hemorrhoids

Reproductive
- Oligomenorrhea (female)
- Testicular atrophy (male)

Integumentary
- Jaundice (skin, sclera of eyes)
- Erythema of palms
- Spider angioma
- Decreased body hair
- Pruritis
- Ecchymoses
- Caput medusae (dilated veins around the umbilicus)

Immune System
- Leukocytopenia
- ↑ susceptibility to infections

Metabolic Processes
- Fluid and electrolyte imbalances
  – Hypoalbuminemia
  – Hypokalemia
  – Hypocalcemia
- Malnutrition
- Muscle wasting

Figure 7-2

Multisystem effects of cirrhosis

3. Assessment
    a. Specific assessments
        1) Vital signs: orthostatic measurement of blood pressure and pulse, temperature, and weight
        2) Skin: signs of jaundice and scleral icterus, bruises, hematomas, petechiae, evidence of pruritus, spider angiomata, telangiectasia, hair loss, palmar erythema, caput medusa, and edema
        3) Pulmonary: decreased breath sounds in bases (may indicate pleural effusion), crackles (may indicate development of heart failure), or lower oxygen saturation (with ascites and upward pressure on diaphragm)
        4) Abdomen: swelling, shifting dullness, fluid wave, or increasing abdominal girth that are indicative of ascites; change in bowel sounds, pain or tenderness in the right upper quadrant, hepatomegaly, splenomegaly
        5) Nutritional status: muscle atrophy and wasting; check color and character of urine (dark) and stool (possibly clay-colored)
        6) Neurological: decreased level of consciousness, disorientation, tremor, **asterixis** (flapping tremor of hand from increased ammonia levels), and decreased deep tendon reflexes (DTRs)
    b. Clinical manifestations (see Box 7-2)
        1) GI symptoms include N/V, anorexia, constipation, weight loss
        2) Decreased ability to metabolize carbohydrates (CHOs) leads to hypoglycemia, decreased energy, and alterations in glycogenolysis, gluconeogenesis, and glycogenesis
        3) Alteration in fat metabolism causes increased synthesis of fatty acids and triglycerides leading to fatty liver and hepatomegaly
        4) Altered protein metabolism leads to low albumin levels and with decrease in osmotic pressure, development of edema and ascites; decreased protein also decreases production of clotting factors that increases risk of bleeding
        5) Decreased metabolism of sex steroids (estrogen, progesterone, and testosterone) leads to gynecomastia, loss of body hair, development of palmar erythema and spider angiomata, erectile dysfunction, and menstrual disorders

| **Box 7-2**

Signs and Symptoms
of Cirrhosis | • General malaise
• Skin
  Pruritis
  Spider angiomata
  Ecchymosis
  Propensity for bleeding
  Edema
  Palmar erythema
• Gastrointestinal
  Nausea and vomiting
  Anorexia
  Pyrosis
  Malnutrition and weight loss
  Constipation and flatulence
  Possible clay color stools
  Hemorrhoids
• Abdomen
  Ascites (increasing abdominal girth)
  Abdominal pain (RUQ) | Positive fluid wave
Shifting dullness
Caput medusa
• Neurological
  Fatigue
  Encephalopathy
  Asterixis
• Miscellaneous
  Gynecomastia
  Loss of body hair
  Testicular atrophy
  Erectile dysfunction
  Menstrual irregularities
  Anemia
  Dark urine |

      6) Decreased metabolism of aldosterone results in sodium and water retention and adds to development of edema and ascites

      7) Decreased metabolism of ammonia leads to increased serum ammonia levels and **hepatic encephalopathy** (manifests as lack of coordination, decreased memory, lack of orientation, and coma)

      8) Decreased stores of vitamins (especially fat-soluble A, D, E, and K) and minerals lead to malnutrition, fatigue, and anemia

      9) Obstruction of bile flow leads to hyperbilirubinemia and jaundice, clay-colored stools, dark-colored urine

      10) Splenomegaly leads to pancytopenia

      11) Fibrosis and scarring continue, resulting in increased portal pressure that causes ascites, hemorrhoids, esophageal varices, caput medusa (superficial abdominal veins)

      12) Involuntary tremor or flapping of hands is called liver flap or asterixis

      13) Malnutrition: leads to muscle atrophy and bitemporal wasting

4. Therapeutic management

  a. Abdominal **paracentesis** is performed with severe ascites to reduce respiratory distress; it is an invasive procedure that is accomplished by draining fluid from abdomen via a needle; fluid is often sent for culture

  b. Surgical intervention (to prevent reaccumulation of ascitic fluid and relieve portal hypertension) includes insertion of a transjugular intrahepatic portosystemic shunt (TIPS); shunt allows blood to flow from portal to hepatic vein, therefore bypassing liver and reducing portal pressure; stenosis and occlusion are frequent complications and it increases risk of developing hepatic encephalopathy; TIPS is generally a short-term measure until liver transplant is performed

  c. Liver transplantation may be indicated for a decline in functional status, increased bilirubin levels, decreased albumin levels and increasing complications that respond poorly to treatment; contraindications include malignancy, active alcohol or drug abuse, and poor surgical risk

5. Priority nursing problems

  a. Fluid overload related to **hypoalbuminemia** (low serum albumin levels) and hyperaldosteronism

  b. Insufficient nutrients to meet bodily needs related to anorexia, liver failure, dietary restrictions, and inability to store or metabolize vitamins and other nutrients

  c. Potential for injury related to bleeding, fatigue, and activity intolerance

  d. Potential for alterations in respiratory pattern related to ascites

  e. Potential for interrupted skin integrity related to jaundice, malnutrition, edema, and prolonged bleeding time, pruritis

  f. Potential for reduced coping related to health crisis (and for those with cirrhosis related to alcohol, inability to cope with life pressures)

  g. Potential for confusion related to effects of high ammonia

  h. Potential for bleeding related to fewer platelets and portal hypertension

6. Planning and implementation

  a. Clients with ascites are fluid restricted to prevent further accumulation of ascitic fluid

  b. Diet restrictions include low sodium (1,500–2,000 mg) intake to prevent further ascitic fluid accumulation; damaged liver struggles to process protein but protein malnutrition causes more problems than maintaining normal protein levels in diet; decrease protein intake if impending encephalopathy

  c. Provide small, frequent meals with between meal snacks

  d. Administer antiemetics and diuretics as prescribed

    e. Weigh daily, and monitor intake and output (I&O)

    f. Monitor for signs of impaired renal function such as oliguria, a fixed specific gravity, central (around the eyes and face) edema, and increasing serum creatinine and blood urea nitrogen (BUN) levels

    g. Measure abdominal girth to assess progression of ascites

    h. For respiratory support, use high-Fowler's position and use supplemental O_2 as prescribed; encourage deep breathing; allow activity as tolerated; measure oxygen saturation, and arterial blood gases as prescribed

    i. Maintain skin integrity; remove moist linens promptly; keep client's skin clean and moistened with emollient; administer antihistamines cautiously (decreased liver function increases risk for altered drug responses) as prescribed; encourage activity as tolerated or reposition every 2 hours

    j. Institute bleeding precautions: prevent constipation, avoid injections, observe for signs and symptoms of bleeding, encourage use of soft toothbrush, monitor labs (CBC, PT); if bleeding occurs monitor closely for encephalopathy as blood in intestinal tract is digested as a protein

    k. Assess understanding of illness; identify support system; assess coping skills; offer clergy support; encourage Alcoholics Anonymous for those with cirrhosis secondary to alcohol dependence; provide substance abuse consultation as indicated

7. Medication therapy

    a. Diuretics: these are given cautiously to promote excretion of excess fluid to decrease ascites; most commonly used drugs are spironolactone (Aldactone) to lowers aldosterone level, a potassium-sparing diuretic, and furosemide (Lasix), a loop diuretic

    b. Lactulose (Cephulac); a disaccharide laxative that is not absorbed by GI tract; it reduces ammonia producing bacteria and lowers pH in colon (which decreases absorption of ammonia); dosage is adjusted to average 2–4 stools per day

    c. Oxazepam (Serax): a benzodiazepine antianxiety and sedative drug that is not metabolized by liver

    d. Other medications include vitamin K to treat prolonged PT, an antiinfective such as neomycin to reduce intestinal bacteria, beta blockers to reduce portal hypertension, antihistamines, and antiemetics

8. Client education

    a. Lifestyle changes include dietary restrictions, abstinence from alcohol, fluid restrictions; suggest nutrition consultation to optimize client's nutritional state

    b. Reduce intake of foods that are high in sodium; avoid canned foods, highly processed cheeses, potato chips, etc.

    c. If impending encephalopathy, limit intake of foods high in protein: eggs, cheese, milk, and meats

    d. Avoid taking any over-the-counter medications without checking with health care provider first since many medications are hepatotoxic (such as acetaminophen)

    e. Be aware of signs and symptoms that require medical attention after discharge: weight gain, increased abdominal girth, respiratory distress, changes in handwriting, bleeding gums, blood in stool or urine, fever, abdominal pain

    f. Adjust dose of lactulose according to number of loose stools per day (average of 2–4 per day)

    g. Involve family and other support persons in client's care; refer as appropriate to Alcoholics Anonymous, Narcotics Anonymous

9. Evaluation

    a. Client demonstrates understanding of illness and importance of making lifestyle changes after discharge from hospital

    b. Client participates in care while hospitalized such as monitoring I & O, daily weights

      c. Client demonstrates understanding of dietary restrictions by verbalizing foods high in protein and sodium

      d. Client contacts Alcoholics Anonymous if appropriate

      e. Client verbalizes understanding of bleeding precautions

      f. Client demonstrates good skin care

D. Complications of cirrhosis (see Box 7-3)

    1. Portal hypertension: an abnormally high blood pressure (BP) in portal venous system; most commonly caused by cirrhosis but can be caused by anything that impedes blood flow through portal veins or through vena cava, such as fibrosis or inflammation of liver tissue secondary to cirrhosis, hepatitis or infection, hepatic vein thrombus, tumor, or right-sided heart failure

      a. Assessment

        1) Clinical manifestations include all findings described with cirrhosis

        2) Other potentially fatal conditions that can develop as a result of portal hypertension are esophageal varices, ascites, hepatic encephalopathy leading to coma, and hepatorenal syndrome; each of these is discussed in more detail below

        3) Most common clinical manifestation is vomiting of blood secondary to rupture of esophageal varices; clients with oozing varices may present with anemia and melanotic stools

        4) Splenomegaly can result from increased pressure within splenic vein, which branches from portal vein

        5) Clients may report irritation from hemorrhoids or have bright red rectal bleeding from hemorrhoids

      b. Therapeutic management: parallels treatment for cirrhosis and is based on symptomatic treatment of varices, ascites, encephalopathy, and hepatorenal syndrome, which are discussed in sections to follow

      c. Planning and implementation: nursing care is similar to care given for esophageal varices, ascites, encephalopathy, and hepatorenal syndrome

      d. Medication therapy: is aimed at decreasing portal venous pressure without precipitating hypotensive crisis; diuretics and fluid restriction are treatments of choice; propranolol (Inderal), a beta blocker, has also been used to decrease portal venous pressures

    2. Esophageal varices: develop as a result of increased portal pressure; are distended and tortuous vessels that can rupture secondary to coughing, sneezing, vomiting, or ingestion of foods high in roughage; bleeding can be abrupt and painless with mortality reaching 50%; ruptured esophageal varices are considered a medical emergency

      a. Assessment: if bleeding is slow, melena and decreasing hemoglobin and hematocrit are present, but if bleeding is abrupt, severe hematemesis and signs of hypovolemic shock (tachycardia, hypotension) can occur

      b. Therapeutic management: includes stopping bleeding either by **sclerotherapy** (drug therapy to sclerose bleeding vessel) or **esophageal tamponade** (direct pressure by use of a special nasogastric tube with esophageal and gastric balloons)

Practice to Pass

The client with hepatic encephalopathy is prescribed to receive lactulose. What is the purpose of this medication?

Box 7-3	• Portal hypertension
	• Right-sided heart failure
Complications of Cirrhosis	• Esophageal varices
	• Varicose veins
	• Ascites
	• Encephalopathy/coma
	• Hepatorenal syndrome

    c. Planning and implementation

        1) Maintain airway, breathing, and circulation and measure VS

        2) Start 2 large-bore IVs with infusion of normal saline (NS) as ordered

        3) Draw serum laboratory tests (CBC, type and cross-match, chemistries)

        4) Begin gastric lavage if prescribed

        5) Esophageal tamponade/balloon tamponade applies direct pressure to varices and is done via placement of Sengstaken-Blakemore or Minnesota tubes, which are multi-lumen gastric tubes, placed nasally and extend into stomach; there are 2 balloons, 1 in esophageal area that, when inflated, tamponades bleeding varices in esophagus and a gastric balloon, which serves as an anchor (see Chapter 8)

        6) Sclerotherapy and banding are accomplished via endoscopy; with sclerotherapy, bleeding vessel is located via endoscope and a sclerosing agent is injected (causes thrombosis and hemostasis) and may be done emergently or as an elective procedure; banding involves placing a rubber band–like ligature around a varice to slow and stop bleeding

        7) Keep clients NPO for either of the above procedures (if elective); reinforce explanation of procedure as needed, and give a mild sedative as prescribed before procedure

        8) Prepare client for transfer to a setting with cardiac monitoring capability

    d. Medication therapy

        1) Sandostatin (Octreotide); given intravenously to decrease splanchnic blood flow, constricts blood vessel in gut and reduces bleeding from esophageal varices

        2) Propranolol (Inderal); beta blocker that reduces portal pressure, not effective in all clients; given in low doses such as 10 mg qid

3. Ascites: an accumulation of plasma-rich fluid in peritoneal cavity secondary to portal hypertension, increased aldosterone, and decreased oncotic pressure (hypoalbuminemia); cirrhosis is the most common cause; kidneys retain sodium and thus water, further increasing third-spaced fluid and anasarca (severe, generalized edema)

    a. Assessment: abdominal distention, weight gain, increased abdominal girth, dilated abdominal veins (caput medusa), generalized edema, and respiratory distress if accumulation of ascitic fluid is large

    b. Therapeutic management

        1) Diuretics; shunting devices (to treat portal hypertension); paracentesis to remove fluid if fluid impinges on diaphragm

        2) Diagnostic testing to identify liver disease: abdominal ultrasound, paracentesis with fluid examination, liver biopsy

        3) Comfort measures

    c. Planning and implementation

        1) Monitor fluid and electrolyte status

        2) Give fluids as prescribed

        3) Monitor daily weights and measure abdominal girth every 8–24 hrs

        4) Restrict sodium intake; if impending encephalopathy, restrict intake of dietary protein

        5) Provide education about disease process and diagnostic tests

        6) Assess for respiratory distress, monitor vital signs for hypotension and/or tachycardia

        7) Administer albumin intravenously if needed to maintain intravascular volume

    d. Medication therapy: there are no specific medications for treatment of ascites; management is aimed at treating cause; beta blockers may help to decrease portal hypertension

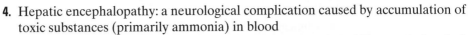

Practice to Pass

The client with cirrhosis has just had a liver biopsy. What does the usual postbiopsy care include?

4. Hepatic encephalopathy: a neurological complication caused by accumulation of toxic substances (primarily ammonia) in blood
   a. Assessment: change in handwriting, loss of memory, irritability, confusion, lethargy, sleep disturbances, stupor, coma, and asterixis
   b. Therapeutic management: aimed at reducing production of nitrogenous wastes (urea) and ammonia, correcting fluid and electrolyte imbalances, and eliminating use of sedating drugs and drugs metabolized by liver
   c. Planning and implementation
      1) Perform frequent neurologic assessment to note progression of lethargy
      2) Administer medications to reduce ammonia levels (lactulose) and intestinal bacteria as prescribed (neomycin)
      3) Restrict dietary protein
      4) Avoid sedating medications
      5) Monitor for fluid and electrolyte imbalances and implement corrective measures as prescribed
      6) Treat cause of liver disease by implementing prescribed therapies
   d. Medication therapy: lactulose (Cephulac) and neomycin as previously discussed

5. **Hepatorenal syndrome**: renal failure associated with advanced liver failure and caused by alterations in circulation without primary renal disease; results in sudden renal failure possibly from imbalanced blood flow leading to constriction of vessels leading to and within the kidneys; may be precipitated by GI bleeding, diuretics or by an unknown cause; is associated with a poor prognosis
   a. Assessment: decreased urine output, hypotension, increased BUN and creatinine levels
   b. Therapeutic management
      1) Fluid and electrolyte imbalances and encephalopathy are treated with aim of restoring renal and liver function
      2) Nephrotoxic or hepatotoxic drugs are eliminated (such as neomycin sulfate)
      3) Hemodialysis is used to treat hyperkalemia and fluid overload
   c. Planning and implementation involves carefully assessing I & O, daily weights, monitoring electrolyte status, and educating client about hemodialysis
   d. Medication therapy includes stopping use of all nephrotoxic and hepatotoxic medications

E. **Cancer of the liver**
   1. Description
      a. Most common types are metastases from colon, lung, breast, kidney, and other forms of GI cancers
      b. Primary liver cancer (hepatoma) is uncommon in United States, but is more prominent in areas with increased chronic liver disease (Africa, Asia)
      c. Prognosis is poor; there is less than 20% survival rate for those with primary liver cancer
   2. Etiology and pathophysiology
      a. Tumors arise in liver cells (hepatocellular) or bile duct (cholangiocellular)
      b. Primary liver cancer is more common in the presence of chronic liver disease
      c. Tumors can be diffuse, nodular, or single nodule
      d. Tumor compresses surrounding cells and can invade blood supply causing necrosis or hemorrhage
      e. Most primary hepatic cancers in United States result from chronic alcohol consumption, cirrhosis, HBV or HCV; other etiologic agents are nitrosamines, prolonged androgen therapy, pesticides, and contraceptive steroids

3. Assessment
   a. Clinical manifestations: RUQ pain or mass, epigastric fullness, fatigue, general malaise, anorexia and weight loss; later signs can include ascites, fever, jaundice, bleeding varices, liver failure, and splenomegaly
   b. Diagnostic and laboratory test findings: degree of abnormal findings depends on degree of liver damage (see earlier section for specific diagnostic studies)
4. Therapeutic management
   a. Partial hepatectomy for clients with solitary lesions and without extrahepatic manifestations; serial AFPs are done following procedure to assess effects of intervention
   b. Liver transplantation may be done for those meeting established criteria (stage 1 or 2 tumors with no lymph node involvement or distant metastasis) for procedure
   c. Radiation therapy may be a palliative measure employed to shrink tumor or reduce pain or pressure on surrounding structures
   d. Chemotherapy as a primary therapy has limited response; direct continuous hepatic arterial administration prolongs survival
   e. Pain control is important
   f. Follow principles of therapeutic management of other liver disorders when other manifestations of liver failure are present
5. Priority nursing problems
   a. Potential for grief response related to loss, poor prognosis
   b. Potential for infection related to altered immune response and malnutrition
   c. Potential for injury related to weakness, prolonged bleeding, and malnutrition (see other sections related to liver failure)
6. Planning and implementation
   a. Provide care as outlined for other complications of liver failure or liver disorders
   b. Provide education regarding liver cancer and chemotherapy
   c. Refer to other sections for measures related to liver failure complications
7. Medication therapy
   a. Chemotherapy can include 5-fluorouracil, methotrexate, and doxorubicin
   b. Other medications may be used, as discussed in prior sections related to liver failure or liver complications
8. Client education
   a. Disease process, expected outcomes, and chemotherapy
   b. Etiologic agents that cause or contribute to development of hepatic cancer
   c. Refer to prior sections on liver disorders and complications for other teaching points related to liver disease
9. Evaluation
   a. Demonstrates effective coping skills
   b. Has stable or decreasing serial AFP levels
   c. Demonstrates appropriate knowledge regarding complications of liver failure

IV. DISORDERS OF THE GALLBLADDER

A. Description

1. **Cholelithiasis**: gallstones that can occur anywhere in biliary tree, although stones within gallbladder are most common; 80% are composed of cholesterol, while 20% are pigmented; 20 to 25 million adults have gallstones and most are asymptomatic; they affect 10% of males and 15% of females over age 55

2. Cholecystitis: an acute or chronic inflammation of gallbladder, most often caused by gallstones obstructing cystic duct resulting in distention and inflammation of gallbladder; pain is similar to that of gallstones; approximately 5% of clients develop

Practice to Pass

What dietary instructions should the nurse give to the client with cholelithiasis?

acalculous cholecystitis precipitated by trauma, prolonged total parenteral nutrition (TPN), fasting, or surgery

B. Etiology and pathophysiology

1. Cholesterol gallstone (80%); formation is enhanced by production of mucin glycoprotein, which traps cholesterol leading to stasis of bile, and contributes to stone formation; cholesterol stones (usually several) develop slowly, are hard, white, or yellow-brown, radiolucent, and can be up to 4 centimeters in size

2. Pigmented stones form because of an increase in unconjugated bilirubin and calcium with a concurrent decrease in bile salts; usually develop within the intra- and extra-hepatic ducts and are preceded by bacterial invasion

3. Increased bile concentration, bile stasis, and hypercholesterolemia contribute to stone formation

4. Most stones are formed within gallbladder and migrate out through ducts of biliary tree; symptoms are consistent with location of stone; many clients are asymptomatic

5. Risk factors associated with formation of gallstones are listed in Box 7-4

C. Assessment

1. Clinical manifestations
   a. Depend on location of the stones and whether or not cholecystitis is present
   b. Classic manifestations include severe and steady (RUQ) pain that may radiate to back, right scapula or shoulder; sudden onset, lasting up to 5 hours
   c. May occur after a high-fat meal
   d. Other symptoms include N/V, heartburn, and flatulence
   e. Fever and chills occur with development of acute cholecystitis
   f. Biliary colic or cramping-type pain occur when stone is lodged in cystic or common bile duct; if stone blocks duct, edema and inflammation of gallbladder (cholecystitis) occur and may be associated with jaundice
   g. Physical exam findings include positive Murphy's sign—palpation of RUQ causes severe pain with inspiratory arrest; bowel sounds may be absent; abdominal guarding, rigidity, and rebound tenderness suggest peritoneal involvement
   h. Jaundice is not usually seen unless common bile duct is blocked

2. Diagnostic and laboratory test findings: see previous section of this chapter

D. Therapeutic management

1. Oral dissolution therapy using ursodiol (Actigall) for clients who are poor surgical risks or refuse surgery; given orally to dissolve cholesterol stones; effective for small stones less than 2 cm in diameter, full treatment can take 2 or more years and 50% of clients experience reoccurrence of stones within 5 years

Box 7-4	
Risk Factors for Gallstones	• Female gender • Caucasian race • Aging • Obesity (and possible sedentary lifestyle) • Family history (may relate to familial hyperlipidemia or high fat diet) • Pregnancy • Type 1 diabetes mellitus • Very low calorie diet with rapid weight loss • Use of estrogen-containing medications (oral contraceptives or hormone replacement therapy) • Other gastrointestinal problems such as cirrhosis, Crohn's disease, or jejunal bypass surgery

2. Extracorporeal shock wave **lithotripsy** uses shock waves to disintegrate stones; oral dissolution therapy is used postprocedure to dissolve stone fragments; clients may experience biliary colic postprocedure when gallbladder is contracting to pass stone fragments

3. Endoscopic retrograde cholangiopancreatography (ERCP) is used for both diagnostic and treatment purposes; involves use of fiberoptic endoscope to visualize biliary tree, remove stones, drain bile sludge, and collect biopsies

4. Laparoscopic **cholecystectomy** is less invasive and involves shorter hospital stay; abdomen is insufflated with CO_2; laparoscope is introduced through a small incision, and gallbladder is deflated and removed through small abdominal incision

5. Cholecystectomy (open, traditional): surgical removal of gallbladder through an abdominal incision in right upper quadrant; T-tube placement may accompany surgery, in which a T-tube is placed in common bile duct to assist passage of bile until edema has decreased; bile collects in a bag by gravity drainage

E. **Priority nursing problems**
1. Pain related to pathophysiological effects
2. Possible altered gas exchange related to pain and ineffective inspiratory effort
3. Potential for infection from bile duct obstruction or postoperative complications
4. Insufficient nutrients to meet bodily needs related to N/V and anorexia
5. Potential for dehydration
6. Anxiety related to lack of knowledge about disease process and treatment measures

F. **Planning and implementation**
1. Implement comfort measures including analgesics and antiemetics as prescribed
2. Provide education regarding diagnostic tests, disease process, and postoperative course if surgery indicated
3. Maintain NPO status preprocedure as prescribed; institute IV fluids as prescribed
4. Provide diet instruction regarding low-fat diet, frequent small meals
5. Encourage obese individuals to lose weight
6. Monitor fluid and electrolyte balance
7. Postoperative nursing care
   a. Prevent infection: administer IV antibiotics as prescribed, keep incision clean and dry; assess abdomen for signs of peritonitis q 4 hr; monitor vital signs, report any temperature greater than 100°F
   b. Prevent pain: administer pain medication as prescribed; instruct client to request pain medication before pain becomes intense; medicate for pain prior to postoperative activity; keep client comfortable to promote deep breathing, turning, and coughing
   c. Prevent pulmonary infection: promote q 2 hr turning, coughing, deep breathing; reinforce importance of incentive spirometry q 1 hr postoperatively
   d. Maintain clients who have had T-tube placement in a Fowler's position to promote gravity drainage of bile
      1) Keep collection container below level of incision
      2) Assess bile drainage and record amount (expect up to 500 mL in first 24 hours, with decrease to less than 200 mL in 2–3 days); report bile drainage in excess of 500 mL per day after 2 days to surgeon
      3) Assess skin for inflammation secondary to bile leakage
      4) Instruct client about proper handling of tube for turning and ambulating
      5) Instruct client that T-tube is removed when bile drainage has subsided and stools have returned to a normal brown color
   e. Maintain NPO status as prescribed; advance diet as tolerated
   f. Monitor bowel sounds and encourage ambulation to promote peristalsis

Practice to Pass

The client has just returned from surgery following a cholecystectomy. What should be included in the postoperative care?

       g. Prevent deep vein thrombosis with leg exercises and frequent ambulation; question client about pain when foot is dorsiflexed (Homan's sign)

       h. Provide general postoperative instruction before discharge about wound care, analgesia, diet, and signs of infection

G. Medication therapy

  1. Symptomatic treatment of pain and nausea with analgesics and antiemetics as prescribed

  2. Opioid analgesics such as morphine (generic) or fentanyl (Sublimaze) are used for severe pain; research has indicated that morphine is no more likely to cause spasms of sphincter of Oddi than meperidine (Demerol)

  3. Cholestyramine (Questran) is used for severe cases of pruritus; binds bile salts to hasten excretion through feces

  4. Oral dissolution medications

       a. Chenodeoxycholic acid (CDCA): a bile acid, taken orally for dissolving cholesterol stones

       b. Ursodeoxycholic acid (UDCA): similar to CDCA—less hepatotoxic and does not cause fatty diarrhea as does CDCA

H. Client education

  1. Disease process and gallstone formation

  2. Diagnostic procedures, therapeutic management, and expected outcomes

  3. Dietary management, particularly to avoid foods high in fat

I. Evaluation

  1. Client is pain free

  2. Client verbalizes disease process and dietary restrictions

IV. DISORDERS OF THE PANCREAS

A. Acute pancreatitis

  1. Description

       a. Occurs when there is obstruction to flow of pancreatic enzymes resulting in inflammation of pancreas

       b. Types

          1) Acute interstitial pancreatitis: diffuse inflammation and edema of pancreas is present but pancreas maintains anatomical features; there is no necrosis or hemorrhage within gland; it is less severe than hemorrhagic

          2) Acute hemorrhagic pancreatitis: a more severe form of interstitial pancreatitis with inflammation, hemorrhage, and necrosis of pancreatic tissue

          3) Biliary pancreatitis: more common in females 55–65 years of age caused by transient obstruction of ampulla of Vater by a gallstone or biliary sludge

          4) Alcoholic pancreatitis: more common in younger males, cause is not understood but is most likely toxic in nature

          5) Chronic pancreatitis: a chronic irreversible process of inflammation, fibrosis, and gradual destruction of functional pancreatic tissue

  2. Etiology and pathophysiology

       a. Inflammatory process can be associated with alcoholism, obstructive biliary disease, peptic ulcer disease (PUD), medications (thiazide diuretics, NSAIDs, estrogens, steroids, salicylates), malnutrition, hyperlipidemia or idiopathic (no identified cause)

       b. Alcohol abuse and gallbladder disease constitute 80% of acute pancreatitis cases in United States

          1) Obstructive cholelithiasis that causes reflux of bile into pancreas can precipitate acute pancreatitis

        2) Alcohol causes duodenal edema, and may increase pressure and spasms of sphincter of Oddi and ampulla of Vater, which can also obstruct flow of pancreatic enzymes; alcohol also stimulates pancreatic enzyme production

    c. Exact pathophysiologic mechanism is unknown; most likely it results from a combination of factors

        1) Activated pancreatic enzymes released into pancreatic tissue

        2) Activated proteolytic enzymes digest pancreatic tissue and activate other enzymes that digest cell membrane phospholipids and elastic tissue of blood vessel walls

        3) Proteolysis, edema, vascular damage and hemorrhage, and necrosis of parenchymal cells occur

        4) Cellular damage and necrosis release activated enzymes and vasoactive substances that produce vasodilation, increase vascular permeability, and cause edema

        5) Large volume of fluid may shift from circulating blood into retroperitoneal space, peripancreatic spaces, and peritoneal cavity

    d. Systemic complications, which can result in death, include intravascular volume depletion with shock, acute tubular necrosis and renal failure, and acute respiratory distress syndrome (ARDS)

    e. Local complications include pancreatic abscesses, pseudocysts (encapsulated collections of fluid), and pancreatic ascites

3. Assessment

    a. Clinical manifestations vary with severity of attack

        1) Acute epigastric pain, steady and severe, can occur in umbilical area and radiate into back; it may be temporally associated with ingestion of alcohol or a fatty meal

        2) Pain is greater when lying supine and improves with sitting up and leaning forward, flexion of the knee, or fetal positioning

        3) Nausea and vomiting is common and worsens with any oral intake and does not relieve abdominal pain

        4) Vital signs: fever (rarely above 102°C), hypotension, and tachycardia

        5) Leukocytosis, hyperglycemia, and elevated amylase and lipase

        6) Abdominal tenderness, rigidity, progressive distention, and decreased bowel sounds

        7) Mild jaundice may appear within 24 hours

        8) Grey Turner sign is a bluish discoloration over flank area and represents accumulation of blood in that area

        9) Cullen sign is a bluish discoloration around umbilicus that is a sign of bleeding

    b. Diagnostic and laboratory test findings: see discussion earlier in chapter

4. Therapeutic management: treatment is aimed at supportive care, preventing further autodigestion of pancreatic tissue, and preventing systemic complications

    a. NPO status with nasogastric tube if ileus or protracted vomiting

    b. IV hydration to prevent hypotension and shock

    c. TPN as needed for prolonged episodes; reverses catabolic state

    d. Possible peritoneal lavage to remove toxic exudates from abdominal cavity

    e. Endoscopic transduodenal sphincterotomy to remove retained obstructing gallstones

    f. Surgical removal of gallbladder for gallstones after acute pancreatitis is resolved

    g. Surgical removal/drainage of pseudocyst or abscess may be necessary for recovery

5. Priority nursing problems

    a. Pain related to pancreatic edema, stretching, and chemical irritation

    b. Insufficient nutrients to meet bodily needs related to poor oral intake and malabsorption

        c. Potential for dehydration related to fluid shifts into abdominal cavity (third spacing) and decreased intake

        d. Potential for infection related to adverse effects of malnutrition

    6. Planning and implementation

        a. Administer pain medications as prescribed and on regular schedule

        b. Keep NPO with nasogastric suction to decrease gastric secretions that stimulate pancreatic secretions; teach family and visitors to avoid bringing food into room because sight or smell of food may stimulate pancreatic enzyme secretion

        c. Monitor lab results for increase leukocytosis, signs of increased catabolism, malnutrition

        d. Monitor vital signs, daily weights, hourly urine outputs, bowel sounds, and stool chart (frequency, color, odor, and consistency)

        e. Assess respiratory function; provide pulmonary hygiene measures to prevent pneumonia

        f. Educate client regarding disease process and therapeutic procedures

        g. Provide diet instruction when oral feeding is resumed (usually when amylase level returns to normal and abdominal pain subsides)

        h. Maintain bed rest during acute phase and increase activity as tolerated

        i. Monitor renal function, neurologic function, and cardiovascular status

    7. Medication therapy

        a. Opioid analgesics such as morphine sulfate (generic) or hydromorphone (Dilaudid)

        b. Antiemetics

        c. Gastric protection with IV H_2 blocker such as famotidine (Pepcid) and proton-pump inhibitor such as omeprazole (Prilosec)

        d. Antispasmodics such as dicyclomine (Bentyl)

        e. Electrolyte replenishment as indicated by laboratory tests

        f. Insulin as required to regulate serum glucose levels

        g. Antibiotics as prescribed for infection

        h. Pancreatic enzyme replacement with pancrelipase (Viokase) to manage abdominal pain and reduce **steatorrhea**; clients with chronic pancreatitis may require therapy for life

        i. Octreotide (Sandostatin), a synthetic hormone, to suppress pancreatic enzyme secretion; may be used to ease pain in chronic pancreatitis

    8. Client education

        a. Disease process and expected outcomes

        b. Nutrition: explain necessity for NPO status during acute phase and once oral feeding resumes, provide several small meals with no alcohol allowed; a low-fat diet is recommended

        c. Importance of taking enzyme replacement to prevent malnutrition and weight loss

        d. Smoking and stress stimulate pancreas and should be avoided

    9. Evaluation

        a. Client verbalizes understanding of disease process and necessary steps to prevent future attacks

        b. Follows dietary restrictions in accordance with etiologic factors, no alcohol and low cholesterol

B. Cancer of the pancreas

    1. Description: most involve cancer of ductal epithelium and are adenocarcinomas; comprises 3–4% of all cancers and can occur at any age but most often after age 50; survival rate at 5 years is approximately 5%

2. Etiology and pathophysiology
   a. Is associated with cigarette smoking and in women with long history of diabetes
   b. Other risk factors include exposure to industrial chemicals, environmental toxins, high-fat diet, and pancreatitis
   c. Incidence is 30% higher in men than in women, 65% greater in African Americans than Caucasians
   d. Is usually located in head of pancreas, deep within tissue, often causing obstruction of common duct
   e. Metastasis almost always occurs prior to symptoms with invasion of tumor into posterior wall of stomach, duodenal wall, colon, and common bile duct
3. Assessment
   a. Clinical manifestations
      1) Early manifestations are nonspecific and include anorexia, nausea, weight loss, flatulence, and dull epigastric pain
      2) Later pain is severe and may be worse when lying down or eating because of pressure on celiac ganglion
      3) Jaundice, pruritis, clay-colored stools, and dark urine occur when there is involvement of bile ducts
      4) Late manifestations include a palpable abdominal mass or ascites
   b. Diagnostic and laboratory test findings
      1) Similar to those for pancreatitis, jaundice, and cholelithiasis
      2) CT scan will reveal a mass and a histological diagnosis can be made via CT-guided needle biopsy
4. Therapeutic management
   a. Most clients do not present for treatment until cancer is too advanced, and thus treatment is in most cases aimed at supportive or palliative care
   b. Pancreatic cancer is usually fatal within 6 months regardless of treatment
   c. ERCP may be performed to place stents within ductal system to facilitate bile drainage
   d. Surgical management
      1) Gastrojejunostomy: bypasses duodenum
      2) Choledochojejunostomy: relieves biliary obstruction
      3) Pancreatoduodenectomy (Whipple's procedure): surgical removal of head of pancreas, entire duodenum, distal third of stomach, a portion of jejunum, and lower half of common bile duct
   e. Chemotherapy and radiation therapy are usually adjuncts to surgical intervention
5. Priority nursing problems
   a. Inadequate knowledge of disease process and treatment options
   b. Insufficient nutrients to meet bodily needs related to decreased intake and disease process
   c. Pain related to disease process
   d. Anxiety or fear about diagnosis
   e. Loss of hope related to diagnosis
6. Planning and implementation
   a. Provide supportive care and education regarding treatment options and assistance with educated decision making
   b. Pain management is integral to quality of life; administer analgesics as prescribed and assess effectiveness for appropriate discharge regimen
   c. Provide preoperative teaching if client opts for surgical intervention
   d. Provide information about support groups in geographical area

7. Medication therapy
   a. No specific medications for treatment of pancreatic cancers
   b. All medications are aimed at controlling symptoms: pain, N/V
   c. Chemotherapy is rarely effective and is used most often for palliative treatment; gemcitabine (Gemzar) and 5-fluorouracil (5-FU) are drugs of choice
8. Client education
   a. Disease process and poor prognosis
   b. Importance of pain control and symptom relief
   c. Importance of abstinence from smoking and alcohol
9. Evaluation
   a. Client verbalizes understanding of potential for developing tolerance and physical dependence to opioid analgesics
   b. Client has support system in place prior to discharge
   c. Client verbalizes importance of ample rest and proper nutrition
   d. Client is comfortable with decisions regarding treatment choices
   e. Client has adequate control of pain allowing for optimal amount of activity

POSTTEST

Case Study

S. D., a 60-year-old male, is admitted to the hospital with cirrhosis. He has a history of alcoholism and hepatitis B.

1. What should the nurse expect to find on his initial laboratory results?

2. S. D. is scheduled for a liver biopsy. What are the priorities of care for this procedure?

3. What are the complications of cirrhosis and hepatitis B, and what assessments should the nurse make to determine the presence of complications?

4. What instructions about diet modifications should the nurse give to S. D.?

5. If S. D. asks the nurse about the long-term outcome of cirrhosis, what should be included in the response?

For suggested responses, see pages 622–623.

POSTTEST

1 A client with cirrhosis is admitted to the hospital. Which assessment finding by the nurse is consistent with development of portal hypertension?

1. Hematemesis
2. Asterixis
3. Elevated blood pressure
4. Confusion

2 The nurse should teach the client with liver disease to avoid which over-the-counter medication after discharge?

1. Ferrous sulfate (Feosol)
2. Psyllium (Metamucil)
3. Folic acid (Folate)
4. Acetaminophen (Tylenol)

3 The nurse is doing discharge teaching for a client who has cirrhosis and ascites. Which of the following foods used by the client as snacks should the nurse instruct the client to avoid?

1. Whole wheat bread
2. Cookies
3. Potato chips
4. Hard candy

4 The client who has liver disease asks the nurse why he bruises so easily. What information should the nurse include in a response to the client?

1. "Your liver is unable to make the proteins that are needed to make clotting factors."
2. "Your liver can no longer metabolize drugs and render them inactive."
3. "Your liver is breaking down blood cells too rapidly."
4. "Your liver can't store vitamin C any longer."

5 The nurse is caring for a client who had a liver biopsy approximately 15 minutes ago. The client is lying supine in bed with the head elevated 30 degrees. The nurse notes that the client's skin is pale and cool, and he reports lightheadedness. The nurse's immediate response is to carry out which interventions? Select all that apply.

1. Place client on his right side.
2. Lower the head of the bed.
3. Obtain vital signs.
4. Check urine output.
5. Call emergency response team.

6 The client who has esophageal varices is started on propranolol (Inderal). What explanation does the nurse provide to the client about the purpose for this medication?

1. "This drug will help prevent esophageal bleeding."
2. "You need this drug to prevent getting high blood pressure from your liver disease."
3. "This medication helps to decrease the number of ammonia-forming organisms in your bowel and prevent encephalopathy."
4. "Your heart's extra workload is causing your esophageal varices; this medication helps decrease that workload."

7 The client who had a cholecystectomy asks why a T-tube has been inserted. What is the best response by the nurse?

1. "T-tubes drain edema fluid and bile to keep the duct patent."
2. "T-tubes drain small gallstones."
3. "T-tubes are always inserted following gallbladder surgery."
4. "T-tubes help us monitor for infection."

8 A client with a possible exposure to hepatitis B asks what type of symptoms will occur if they acquire the disease. What is the typical manner in which acute hepatitis progresses that will guide the nurse's response? Place the following choices in the correct order.

1. No manifestations
2. Yellowing of the sclera
3. Flulike symptoms
4. Serum bilirubin and liver enzymes decrease

9 The client is admitted to the hospital with acute pancreatitis. The nurse taking a history should question the client about which of these risks for developing pancreatitis?

1. Inflammatory bowel disease
2. Alcoholism
3. Diabetes mellitus
4. High-fiber diet

10 The nurse administers the first dose of hepatitis A vaccine to a client on 1/10. When is the earliest the client should return for the second dose? Put a check mark in the box below the correct date on the image shown.

Date (Month and day of month)															
1/10	1/17	1/24	1/31	2/7	3/10	4/10	5/10	6/10	7/10	8/10	9/10	10/10	11/10	12/10	1/10
Dose 1															

➤ *See pages 247–248 for Answers and Rationales.*

ANSWERS & RATIONALES

Pretest

1 **Answer: 1** **Rationale:** The nurse should respond in a manner that is factually correct and that addresses the client's concerns. After the gallbladder is removed the bile produced by the liver flows directly through the common bile duct to the small intestine. Although the gallbladder stores and concentrates bile, it is not a necessary organ. Once the flow of bile into the intestines is restored, the bile will help absorb fat-soluble vitamins. **Cognitive Level:** Applying **Client Need:** Physiological Adaptation **Integrated Process:** Communication and Documentation **Content Area:** Adult Health **Strategy:** Be sure to address the client's concern, which is how the body adapts to the removal of the gallbladder. Compare the normal function of the gallbladder with the remainder of the gastrointestinal (GI) system. Understanding how the normal GI system functions will enable you to answer this question. **Reference:** LeMone, P., Burke, K., & Bauldoff, G. (2011). *Medical-surgical nursing: Critical thinking in patient care* (5th ed.). Upper Saddle River, NJ: Pearson Education, pp. 721–726.

2 **Answer: 3** **Rationale:** The normal total bilirubin is 0.3–1.2 mg/dL. Hyperbilirubinemia manifests as jaundice, a yellow discoloration of the body tissues and sclera. Ascites is associated with low serum albumin and may accompany liver disease in later stages but would not be the clinical manifestation to be most likely seen. Hypertension and diarrhea are unlikely to be present with elevations in bilirubin. **Cognitive Level:** Applying **Client Need:** Reduction of Risk Potential **Integrated Process:** Nursing Process: Assessment **Content Area:** Adult Health **Strategy:** First recall concepts related to both the function of bile and elimination of bilirubin. Then note (even if only because of the wording of the question) that the client's serum bilirubin is elevated. Next evaluate each of the options against this knowledge base to enable you to eliminate choices that are unrelated to the question. **Reference:** LeMone, P., Burke, K., & Bauldoff, G. (2011). *Medical-surgical nursing: Critical thinking in patient care* (5th ed.). Upper Saddle River, NJ: Pearson Education, pp. 723, 728.

3 **Answer: 2** **Rationale:** Obstructive jaundice is caused by an obstruction of bile flow within the biliary system. Clay-colored stools indicate that no bile is reaching the intestine and is consistent with the diagnosis of obstructive jaundice. Clear, pale urine is normal and in obstructive jaundice, the urine is dark because of the presence of bile. Lactose intolerance is unrelated to obstructive jaundice. Ankle edema is more likely to be present in cardiovascular disease or as an indirect consequence of portal hypertension. **Cognitive Level:** Applying **Client Need:** Physiological Adaptation **Integrated Process:** Nursing Process: Assessment **Content Area:** Adult Health **Strategy:** Recall the pathophysiology behind the development of obstructive jaundice. If you can explain why obstructive jaundice occurs, the unrelated choices become evident. It will also help you select the correct answer. **Reference:** LeMone, P., Burke, K., & Bauldoff, G. (2011). *Medical-surgical nursing: Critical thinking in patient care* (5th ed.). Upper Saddle River, NJ: Pearson Education, p. 728.

4 **Answer: 3** **Rationale:** The frequency of the dose of lactulose should be decreased if the client is having more than 2–4 diarrhea stools per day. Should the diarrhea continue, the client may require additional fluids, not restriction. Lactulose is given to reduce the ammonia levels in a person with hepatic encephalopathy. The presence of diarrhea indicates it is having the expected results and is not an indication for a repeat serum ammonia level. Neomycin is also administered to reduce serum ammonia levels; there is no indication that it is needed. **Cognitive Level:** Analyzing **Client Need:** Pharmacological and Parenteral Therapies **Integrated Process:** Nursing Process: Implementation **Content Area:** Adult Health **Strategy:** To select the correct response, you need to know the indication for lactulose in cirrhosis and the intended effect. The question is not asking why it is used. **Reference:** LeMone, P., Burke, K., & Bauldoff, G. (2011). *Medical-surgical nursing: Critical thinking in patient care* (5th ed.). Upper Saddle River, NJ: Pearson Education, p. 742.

5 **Answer: 3, 5 Rationale:** Rupture of an acutely inflamed gallbladder may be heralded by abrupt pain relief as contents are released from the distended gallbladder into the abdomen. The nurse should first notify the health care provider of the client's change in condition. The nurse should also reassess the vital signs to determine the stability of the client's condition. Pain medication causes a gradual reduction in pain, not an abrupt discontinuation of pain. A gallbladder scan may be prescribed to confirm the diagnosis of cholelithiasis but the change in condition may result in the client's orders may be modified. Teaching methods to prevent future problems should not be done until the cause of the problem is confirmed. **Cognitive Level:** Analyzing **Client Need:** Physiological Adaptation **Integrated Process:** Nursing Process: Implementation **Content Area:** Adult Health **Strategy:** When clinical manifestations abruptly disappear consider whether this may indicate a complication rather than an improvement in the client's condition. **Reference:** LeMone, P., Burke, K., & Bauldoff, G. (2011). *Medical-surgical nursing: Critical thinking in patient care* (5th ed.). Upper Saddle River, NJ: Pearson Education, pp. 722–723.

6 **Answer: 1 Rationale:** The liver is responsible for the production of albumin, which in turn is responsible for maintaining colloidal osmotic pressure. With less production of albumin, osmotic pressure decreases and edema develops. The loss of protein production does not increase osmotic pressure. The edema is unlikely to be related to renal function in a client with a new diagnosis of cirrhosis and is unrelated to sex hormones. **Cognitive Level:** Applying **Client Need:** Physiological Adaptation **Integrated Process:** Nursing Process: Implementation **Content Area:** Adult Health **Strategy:** Recall the principles of fluid transmission across body compartments, the role of albumin in the body, as well as the pathophysiology of cirrhosis to enable you to answer this question. **Reference:** LeMone, P., Burke, K., & Bauldoff, G. (2011). *Medical-surgical nursing: Critical thinking in patient care* (5th ed.). Upper Saddle River, NJ: Pearson Education, pp. 728, 736–737, 740–741.

7 **Answer: 1 Rationale:** The liver is the most vascular organ in the body. Therefore, a liver biopsy may cause hemorrhage. The nurse should assess for signs of hemorrhage (increased pulse, decreased blood pressure). Laboratory tests that reflect clotting function, including prothrombin times (PT), partial thromboplastin time (PTT), and platelet counts are assessed prior to a liver biopsy, not after. Bowel sounds and gastrointestinal status are monitored after a liver biopsy but are not the highest

priority. The client should be NPO for 4–6 hours prior to the procedure but does not need to be NPO after the procedure. Medications that interfere with the gag reflex are not given for a liver biopsy. **Cognitive Level:** Applying **Client Need:** Reduction of Risk Potential **Integrated Process:** Nursing Process: Implementation **Content Area:** Adult Health **Strategy:** Consider the risks associated with an invasive procedure of a vascular surface. The goal of initial management is to allow time for a clot to form so homeostasis can be achieved. **Reference:** Kee, J. L. (2010). *Laboratory and diagnostic tests* (8th ed.). Upper Saddle River, NJ: Prentice Hall, pp. 457–460.

8 **Answer: 3, 4, 5 Rationale:** Hepatitis A is transmitted via the fecal–oral route so hand hygiene is essential to prevent transmission to others. Additional isolation measures are not needed. Rest is important to allow the liver time to heal. Nausea frequently accompanies hepatitis, and eating small frequent meals aids in digestion and prevents nausea. **Cognitive Level:** Applying **Client Need:** Safety and Infection Control **Integrated Process:** Nursing Process: Planning **Content Area:** Adult Health **Strategy:** The correct answers are related to the route of transmission and symptoms. Select answers that would alleviate symptoms or prevent transmission of the hepatitis A virus to others by the fecal–oral route. **Reference:** LeMone, P., Burke, K., & Bauldoff, G. (2011). *Medical-surgical nursing: Critical thinking in patient care* (5th ed.). Upper Saddle River, NJ: Pearson Education, pp. 729–735.

9 **Answer: 4, 2, 5, 3, 1 Rationale:** Exact causes are not known but some event such as gallstones or alcohol intake causes the process to begin. The result is the release of activated pancreatic enzymes into pancreas tissue. The activated enzymes digest pancreatic tissue and progress to destruction of blood vessel walls. This destruction leads to proteolysis, edema, hemorrhage, and necrosis. **Cognitive Level:** Applying **Client Need:** Physiological Adaptation **Integrated Process:** Teaching and Learning **Content Area:** Adult Health **Strategy:** Remember that pancreatitis is an acute inflammatory disorder. Apply principles of inflammation. **Reference:** LeMone, P., Burke, K., & Bauldoff, G. (2011). *Medical-surgical nursing: Critical thinking in patient care* (5th ed.). Upper Saddle River, NJ: Pearson Education, pp. 751–753.

10 **Answer: 1 Rationale:** Pancrelipase (Lipancreatin) is a pancreatic enzyme replacement of porcine (pig) origin that aids in the digestion of starches and fats. The nonenteric coated version is most effective; it should be taken with meals. Concurrent administration of H_2 antagonists or antacids helps prevent destruction of the enzyme by hydrochloric acid. Allergic reactions and other side effects can occur. The client should see a decrease in steatorrhea (fatty, frothy, foul-smelling stools), decreased bulk of stools, and increase or maintenance of weight. The client should take the medication with each meal and with any foods eaten between meals. The medication should be continued unless advised by the health care provider that it is no longer necessary. **Cognitive Level:** Applying **Client Need:** Pharmacological and Parenteral Therapies **Integrated Process:** Nursing Process: Implementation **Content Area:** Adult Health **Strategy:** Apply the principles of the inflammatory process to the pancreas as well as the functions of the gallbladder. This information will enable you to select the response that indicates that the pancrelipase is replacing normal pancreatic function. **Reference:** LeMone, P., Burke, K., & Bauldoff, G. (2011). *Medical-surgical nursing: Critical thinking in patient care* (5th ed.). Upper Saddle River, NJ: Pearson Education, pp. 753–754. Wilson, B. A., Shannon, M. T., & Shields, K. M. (2012). *Pearson nurse's drug guide 2012*. Upper Saddle River, NJ: Prentice Hall, pp. 1144–1145.

Posttest

1 **Answer: 1** **Rationale:** In cirrhosis, the liver becomes fibrotic, which obstructs the venous blood flow through the liver. This increases the vascular pressure in the portal system and causes congestion in the spleen and development of varicosities in the esophagus. Bleeding esophageal varices are a complication of portal hypertension and result in vomiting of blood and possible hemorrhage and death. Asterixis is flapping of the hands when they are held up and indicates encephalopathy. The client with cirrhosis is more inclined to hypotension because of the loss of circulating blood volume. Confusion indicates the onset of encephalopathy. **Cognitive Level:** Analyzing **Client Need:** Physiological Adaptation **Integrated Process:** Nursing Process: Assessment **Content Area:** Adult Health **Strategy:** For each choice identify which complication is directly related to it. Select the answer that is vascular in nature. **Reference:** LeMone, P., Burke, K., & Bauldoff, G. (2011). *Medical-surgical nursing: Critical thinking in patient care* (5th ed.). Upper Saddle River, NJ: Pearson Education, pp. 736–738.

2 **Answer: 4** **Rationale:** Any medication that is metabolized by the liver and has not been prescribed by the health care provider should be avoided, such as acetaminophen, sedatives, and barbiturates. Iron and folic acid supplementation is used to treat anemia. Psyllium is a bulk laxative and may be prescribed to prevent the occurrence of constipation and subsequent encephalopathy **Cognitive Level:** Applying **Client Need:** Pharmacological and Parenteral Therapies **Integrated Process:** Nursing Process: Implementation **Content Area:** Adult Health **Strategy:** The core issue of the question is knowledge of drugs that are metabolized or biotransformed by the liver. Review each choice to determine whether that drug has side effects or adverse effects that could increase the severity of the liver disease, and choose the one that is most harmful. Recall that acetaminophen is a prime drug that is commonly used and harmful to the liver. **Reference:** LeMone, P., Burke, K., & Bauldoff, G. (2011).

Medical-surgical nursing: Critical thinking in patient care (5th ed.). Upper Saddle River, NJ: Pearson Education, pp. 742–743.

3 **Answer: 3** **Rationale:** A low-sodium diet is recommended for clients who have cirrhosis and ascites. Potato chips are high in sodium. Cookies and hard candy are high in sugar. While they provide no nutrient value, they do increase the calorie intake, which is important for tissue metabolism. Whole wheat bread is high in complex carbohydrates and fiber and is a good nutrient source for fiber and carbohydrates. **Cognitive Level:** Applying **Client Need:** Physiological Adaptation **Integrated Process:** Teaching and Learning **Content Area:** Adult Health **Strategy:** The critical words in the question are *cirrhosis* and *ascites*. Consider the relationship between ascites, fluid retention, and sodium and choose the item that is highest overall in sodium, such as salty snacks. **Reference:** LeMone, P., Burke, K., & Bauldoff, G. (2011). *Medical-surgical nursing: Critical thinking in patient care* (5th ed.). Upper Saddle River, NJ: Pearson Education, p. 743.

4 **Answer: 1** **Rationale:** The liver synthesizes clotting factors I, II, VII, IX, and X as well as prothrombin and fibrinogen. These proteins are needed for adequate clotting, so their reduction leads to increased risk of bleeding. The inability of the liver to detoxify drugs actually raises the serum level of the drug. The spleen is responsible for breaking down blood cells, while the liver processes the bilirubin that results from RBC destruction. The liver stores the fat-soluble vitamins A, D, E, and K. **Cognitive Level:** Applying **Client Need:** Physiological Adaptation **Integrated Process:** Nursing Process: Implementation **Content Area:** Adult Health **Strategy:** The question is focused on the normal function of the liver directly related to clotting. Eliminate any choices that are unrelated to the clotting. **Reference:** LeMone, P., Burke, K., & Bauldoff, G. (2011). *Medical-surgical nursing: Critical thinking in patient care* (5th ed.). Upper Saddle River, NJ: Pearson Education, pp. 728, 741.

5 **Answer: 1, 3** **Rationale:** The liver is highly vascular and is therefore prone to bleeding following a biopsy. Following a biopsy, the best position for the client is to lie on his right side to apply pressure to the vessels of the liver and prevent bleeding. Because this client could be experiencing early signs of shock, the nurse should quickly check vital signs. This would provide additional data to report to the health care provider. Lowering the head of the bed will not help control possible bleeding and is not called for at this time. Decreased urine output can be seen with bleeding but not in the 15 minutes since the liver biopsy was performed. This would not be an appropriate immediate response. The nurse needs to gather further data before activating the emergency response team. **Cognitive Level:** Analyzing **Client Need:** Reduction of Risk Potential **Integrated Process:** Nursing Process: Implementation **Content Area:** Adult Health **Strategy:** Correlate the anatomy of the liver with the clinical signs of the client. Select first an option that will provide compression to the vascular liver and increase homeostasis. Then choose an option that will provide quick information about hypovolemia from bleeding, such as vital signs. Recall that nurses do not report a single piece of data when a client's situation is deteriorating; rather, the nurse quickly gathers data that are directly relevant to the suspected problem. **Reference:** LeMone, P., Burke, K., & Bauldoff, G. (2011). *Medical-surgical nursing: Critical thinking in patient care* (5th ed.). Upper Saddle River, NJ: Pearson Education, p. 575.

6 **Answer: 1** **Rationale:** Beta-blockers such as propranolol (Inderal) may be given to reduce portal hypertension and prevent bleeding of esophageal varices. Liver disease is associated with portal hypertension, but not with elevated systemic blood pressure. Medications given to decrease ammonia-forming organisms include lactulose (Cephulac) and antibiotics such as neomycin (generic), metronidazole (Flagyl), or rifaximin (Xifaxan). While propranolol does decrease cardiac workload, cardiac workload is not the cause of esophageal varices. **Cognitive Level:** Analyzing **Client Need:** Pharmacological and Parenteral Therapies **Integrated Process:** Nursing Process: Implementation **Content Area:** Adult Health **Strategy:** The mechanism of action of propranolol is directly related to its effectiveness in the treatment of esophageal varices. Correlate these two content areas. **Reference:** LeMone, P., Burke, K., & Bauldoff, G. (2011). *Medical-surgical nursing: Critical thinking in patient care* (5th ed.). Upper Saddle River, NJ: Pearson Education, pp. 737–743.

7 **Answer: 1** **Rationale:** Manipulation of the common bile duct causes inflammation that may occlude the duct, preventing bile excretion. Insertion of the T-tube prevents the inflammation from occluding the common bile duct. While it may drain some small stones that were not removed during the procedure, this is not the purpose for the tube. Not all clients have a T-tube after a cholecystectomy, only those with significant risk for edema. The T-tube actually can increase the risk of infection because it provides a direct opening into the abdomen. **Cognitive Level:** Applying **Client Need:** Reduction of Risk Potential **Integrated Process:** Nursing Process: Implementation **Content Area:** Adult Health **Strategy:** Remember that tissue edema follows surgical manipulation of a body part. The T-tube is intended to prevent the edema from occluding the duct. **Reference:** LeMone, P., Burke, K., & Bauldoff, G. (2011). *Medical-surgical nursing: Critical thinking in patient care* (5th ed.). Upper Saddle River, NJ: Pearson Education, p. 724.

8 **Answer: 1, 3, 2, 4** **Rationale:** There is an incubation period after exposure to the hepatitis virus where no manifestations are present but the virus is replicating. The prodromal or preicteric (before jaundice stage) occurs after the incubation period with general malaise, anorexia, fatigue, and muscle and body aches. Chills, fever, nausea, vomiting, diarrhea, or constipation may develop, as well as mild RUQ abdominal pain. The icteric (jaundiced) phase usually begins 5 to 10 days after the onset of symptoms. Besides jaundice (yellowing of the skin and mucous membranes) common manifestations include pruritus, light brown or clay-colored stools, and brown urine. The convalescent phase follows jaundice and lasts several weeks. Manifestations gradually improve with a decrease in bilirubin and liver enzymes, an increase in energy, a decrease in liver pain and minimal to absent gastrointestinal symptoms. **Cognitive Level:** Applying **Client Need:** Physiological Adaptation **Integrated Process:** Teaching and Learning **Content Area:** Adult Health **Strategy:** Apply common principles of progression of infection and inflammatory response to select the correct order. **Reference:** LeMone, P., Burke, K., & Bauldoff, G. (2011). *Medical-surgical nursing: Critical thinking in patient care* (5th ed.). Upper Saddle River, NJ: Pearson Education, pp. 729–730.

9 **Answer: 2** **Rationale:** Pancreatitis is typically associated with alcoholism and gallstones. Inflammatory bowel disease is unrelated to the pancreas. Diabetes is caused by an inability of the pancreas to secrete insulin, but this is unrelated to pancreatitis. A high-fiber diet is believed to decrease the risk of colon cancer but has no association with pancreatitis. **Cognitive Level:** Applying **Client Need:** Physiological Adaptation **Integrated Process:** Nursing Process: Assessment **Content Area:** Adult Health **Strategy:** Eliminate any choices that are directly related to other GI diseases. Then select the answer that has a direct link with pancreatitis. **Reference:** LeMone, P., Burke, K., & Bauldoff, G. (2011). *Medical-surgical nursing: Critical thinking in patient care* (5th ed.). Upper Saddle River, NJ: Pearson Education, pp. 751–752.

10 **Answer: 7/10** **Rationale:** The hepatitis A vaccine is given in 2 doses with at least 6 months between doses. Thus, a dose that is given on January 10 can be followed up by a second dose no earlier than July 10. **Cognitive Level:** Applying **Client Need:** Pharmacological and Parenteral Therapies **Integrated Process:** Nursing Process: Planning **Content Area:** Adult Health **Strategy:** Specific knowledge of the immunization schedule for hepatitis A vaccine is needed to answer the question. Recall the schedule to choose correctly. **Reference:** LeMone, P., & Burke, K. M. (2011). *Medical-surgical nursing: Critical thinking in patient care* (5th ed., Vol. Single). Upper Saddle River, NJ: Pearson Education, pp. 731–732.

References

Berman, A., & Snyder, S. (2012). *Kozier & Erb's fundamentals of nursing: Concepts, process, and practice* (9th ed.). Upper Saddle River, NJ: Pearson Education.

Black, J., & Hawks, J. (2009). *Medical surgical nursing: Clinical management for positive outcomes* (8th ed.). St. Louis, MO: Elsevier.

D'Amico, D. & Barbarito, C. (2012). *Health & physical assessment in nursing* (2nd ed.). Upper Saddle River, NJ: Pearson Education, Inc.

Ignatavicius, D. D., & Workman, M. L. (2013). *Medical-surgical nursing: Critical thinking for collaborative care* (7th ed.) Philadelphia: W. B. Saunders Company.

Kee, J. L. (2010). *Laboratory and diagnostic tests* (8th ed.). Upper Saddle River, NJ: Pearson Education.

Lehne, R. (2010). *Pharmacology for nursing care* (7th ed.). St. Louis, MO: Saunders.

LeMone, P., Burke, K., & Bauldoff, G. (2011). *Medical surgical nursing: Critical thinking in patient care* (5th ed.). Upper Saddle River, NJ: Pearson Education.

Lewis, S., Dirksen, S. Heitkemper, M., Bucher, L., & Camera, I. (2011). *Medical surgical nursing: Assessment and management of clinical problems* (8th ed.). St. Louis, MO: Elsevier.

McCance, K. L., & Huether, S. E. (2010). *Pathophysiology: The biologic basis for disease in adults and children* (6th ed.). St. Louis, MO: Mosby, Inc.

Osborn, K. S., Wraa, C. E., & Watson, A. (2010). *Medical surgical nursing: Preparation for practice*. Upper Saddle River, NJ: Pearson Education.

Smith, S. F., Duell, D. J., & Martin, B. C. (2012). *Clinical nursing skills: Basic to advanced skills* (8th ed.). Upper Saddle River, NJ: Pearson Education.

8 Gastrointestinal Disorders

Chapter Outline

NCLEX-RN® Test Prep

Use the accompanying online resource, NursingReviewsandRationales, to test yourself with hundreds of NCLEX®-style practice questions.

Objectives

➤ Identify basic structures and functions of the gastrointesinal system.
➤ Describe the pathophysiology and etiology of common gastrointestinal disorders.
➤ Discuss expected assessment data and diagnostic test findings for selected gastrointestinal disorders.
➤ Identify priority nursing problems for selected gastrointestinal disorders.
➤ Discuss therapeutic management of selected gastrointestinal disorders.
➤ Discuss nursing management of a client experiencing a gastrointestinal disorder.
➤ Identify expected outcomes for a client experiencing a gastrointestinal disorder.

Review at a Glance

Barrett's epithelium esophageal epithelial tissue that has undergone change as a result of repeated exposure to gastric juice and is more resistant to erosion, but is premalignant

body mass index (BMI) estimates total body fat stores in relation to height and weight

bulk-forming agents high-fiber supplements that increase fecal bulk

chyme stomach contents consisting of partially digested food mixed with gastric juice

colostomy surgical diversion of large intestine fecal contents to an external collection device

diarrhea increase in frequency, amount, or liquidity of stool that is a change from normal pattern

dumping syndrome complication of gastric resections where there is rapid emptying of stomach contents into jejunum causing physiologic manifestations

esophagogastroduodenos-copy (EGD) direct visualization of esophagus, stomach, and duodenum through a fiberoptic endoscope and used to diagnose disorders of these structures

esophagogastric tube also known as a Sengstaken-Blakemore or Minnesota tube, consisting of a tube with several lumens used to inflate a gastric

balloon, esophageal balloon, and drain stomach contents

fistula abnormal pathway between structures or from an internal organ to an outside surface

gastroesophageal reflux the backward flow of gastric contents into lower portion of esophagus

gavage referring to intermittent feeding through a tube in stomach or jejunum

hernia referring to a protrusion of an organ through a weakness in muscle

ileostomy surgical diversion of fecal contents at level of ileum to an external collection device

lavage irrigation of stomach using a tube inserted into stomach

lower esophageal sphincter (LES) sphincter located at esophageal gastric junction

nasogastric (NG) tube a tube inserted through nose and into stomach

and used to drain contents or for feeding

nonsteroidal anti-inflammatory drugs (NSAIDs) medications usually used for analgesia and to reduce inflammation

Zollinger-Ellison syndrome disorder in which a pancreatic tumor secretes gastrin, which then stimulates secretion of acid and pepsin

PRETEST

1 Which of the following assessments is essential for the nurse to make when caring for a client who has just had an esophagogastroduodenoscopy (EGD)?

1. Auscultate bowel sounds.
2. Check gag reflex.
3. Monitor gastric pH.
4. Measure abdominal girth.

2 A client has a nasogastric (NG) tube in place for gastric decompression and complains of increasing nausea. Which action should the nurse take first?

1. Advance the tube 2 cm.
2. Place client in a recumbent position.
3. Irrigate with 20 mL of saline.
4. Obtain abdominal x-ray to assess placement.

3 A client with a subtotal gastrectomy is scheduled for discharge. Which instruction should the nurse give the client to reduce the possibility of dumping syndrome?

1. "Be sure to eat foods high in complex carbohydrates."
2. "It is helpful to take a walk after eating."
3. "Avoid drinking fluids with your meal."
4. "Don't lie down for at least 2 hours after eating."

4 An obese client is considering having a gastric banding procedure. Which diagram does the nurse use to illustrate the surgical procedure?

1.   2.   3.   4.

5 The nurse teaches the client with gastroesophageal reflux disease (GERD) about ways to minimize symptoms. Which client statement indicates that more teaching is needed?

1. "I will be sure to drink tea instead of coffee."
2. "I will take a walk after I eat."
3. "I will try to eat smaller meals more frequently."
4. "I will sleep with the head of the bed elevated about 12 inches."

6 The client with a gastric ulcer is admitted to the hospital. The nurse should assess the client for intake of which substance that increases the risk of developing a gastric ulcer?

1. Aspirin
2. Chili
3. Acetaminophen (Tylenol)
4. Coffee

7 The nurse is caring for a client who is receiving enteral feedings via a nasoduodenal tube. Upon entering the client's room, what should the nurse assess to determine that the client's airway is protected? Select all that apply.

1. Bowel sounds
2. Breath sounds
3. Gag reflex
4. Client's position
5. Rate of the feeding

8 The client is admitted to the hospital with ulcerative colitis. The nurse should assess the client for which sign that indicates a complication of the disease?

1. Low hemoglobin and hematocrit
2. Low platelet count
3. Epigastric or right-sided pain following a high-fat meal
4. Presence of fat in the stools

9 The nurse is developing a health promotion program for intestinal health. Which of the following pieces of information should the nurse include in the program?

1. The addition of dietary fiber can reduce the risk of diverticulosis.
2. A diet high in fat increases the risk of developing Crohn's disease.
3. Irritable bowel syndrome is caused by a deficiency in soluble fiber.
4. Laxatives can improve motility and bowel health.

10 A client is admitted to the hospital with a bowel obstruction. Which finding by the nurse would indicate that the obstruction is in the early stages?

1. High-pitched tinkling bowel sounds
2. Soft rumbling bowel sounds
3. No bowel sounds auscultated
4. Normal bowel sounds heard in all four quadrants

➤ *See pages 278–279 for Answers and Rationales.*

I. OVERVIEW OF ANATOMY AND PHYSIOLOGY

A. Oral cavity/pharynx

1. Mouth, also referred to as oral or buccal cavity
   a. Lined with mucous membranes
   b. Bordered by lips, cheeks, hard and soft palate, and tongue
      1) Lips and cheeks: keep food in mouth during chewing
      2) Hard palate: hard surface at roof of mouth against which tongue pushes food during chewing and swallowing
      3) Soft palate: distal to hard palate and rises during swallowing (reflex) to close oropharynx
      4) Tongue: mostly skeletal muscle and contains mucous and serous glands, papillae and taste buds; mixes food and saliva to form bolus and initiates swallowing
   c. Salivary glands: drain into mouth; secrete saliva to moisten food and provide amylase to initially break down carbohydrates (CHOs)
   d. Teeth: 32 permanent in adults; tear and grind food into smaller pieces providing more surface area for action of saliva
2. Pharynx: composed of oropharynx and laryngopharynx
   a. Passageway for food, fluids, and air; moves food into esophagus by peristalsis
   b. Lined with mucous membranes and mucous-secreting glands to ease passage of food

B. Esophagus: muscular tube 10 in. (25 cm) extending from pharynx to stomach

1. Lined with squamous epithelium, except where it joins stomach, where it is lined with columnar epithelium
2. Enters stomach through cardiac orifice that is surrounded by gastroesophageal sphincter (also called **lower esophageal sphincter or LES**), which keeps orifice closed when no food is swallowed; keeps gastric contents (acid) out of esophagus

C. Stomach: distensible food reservoir located high on left side of abdomen; can hold as much as 4 L of food and fluid; empty it is about 10 in (25 cm) in size; continues mechanical breakdown of food and mixes food with gastric juice forming a mixture called **chyme**

Figure 8-1

Regions of the stomach

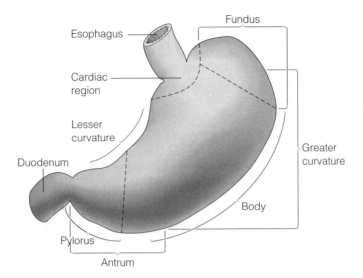

1. Divided into 4 regions (see Figure 8-1)
   a. Cardiac region: surrounds cardiac orifice
   b. Fundus: upper portion (high concentration of gastric glands)
   c. Body: includes greater and lesser curvatures (high concentration of gastric glands)
   d. Pyloric region: surrounds pyloric sphincter
2. Lined with columnar epithelial cells that contain secretory cells
   a. Mucous cells: secrete alkaline mucus to protect stomach lining from acidic gastric juice
   b. Zymogenic cells: produce pepsinogen, a precursor to pepsin, which digests proteins
   c. Parietal cells: produce hydrochloric (HCl) acid and intrinsic factor
      1) HCl acid: converts pepsinogen to pepsin for protein digestion and acts as a bactericidal agent
      2) Intrinsic factor: needed for absorption of vitamin B_{12} in small intestine
   d. Enteroendocrine cells: secrete hormones gastrin, histamine, endorphins, serotonin, and somatostatin
3. Gastric secretion is under neural (sympathetic, parasympathetic) and hormonal control and is divided into 3 phases
   a. Cephalic phase: preparation for digestion; stimulated by sight, odor, taste, or thought of food
   b. Gastric phase: starts when food enters stomach and is initiated by stimulation of gastric stretch receptors and chemically by partially digested proteins; gastrin is secreted and stimulates production of more gastric juice
   c. Intestinal phase: initiated when chyme enters small intestine
4. Mechanical churning of gastric contents via peristalsis aids digestion and is influenced by gastric distention and gastrin; normal gastric emptying takes 4 to 6 hours (but is shorter with larger volumes of fluids and takes longer with solids and fats)

D. **Small intestine**: begins at pyloric sphincter and ends at ileocecal valve; is about 20 ft (6 m) long and 1 in. (2.5 cm) in diameter
   1. Divided into 3 regions
      a. Duodenum: begins at pyloric sphincter near head of pancreas; pancreatic enzymes (trypsin, chymotrypsin, lipase, and amylase) and bile enter in response to secretin and cholecystokinin (produced by intestinal mucosa cells in response to presence of chyme)

      b. Jejunum: middle section

      c. Ileum: terminal section

  2. Digestion is completed and most absorption occurs in small intestine through microvilli, villi, and circular folds that increas absorptive surface area

E. Large intestine: also known as colon; is 5 ft (1.5 m) long and extends from ileocecal valve to anus

  1. Divided into 5 areas

      a. Cecum

      b. Appendix: small outpouching attached to cecum where bacteria accumulate and may cause inflammation

      c. Colon: ascending, transverse, and descending segments

      d. Rectum: mucosa-lined reservoir for feces; 12 cm in length

      e. Anus: terminal end of digestive tract with internal and external sphincters that control defecation through defecation reflex (spinal cord reflex)

  2. Major function is to absorb water, salts, and vitamins formed by bacteria in large intestine and eliminate undigestible food and residue from body

F. Digestion: breakdown of food into molecules that can be absorbed and used by body cells

  1. Begins in mouth by action of chewing and addition of salivary amylase from salivary glands, which initiates CHO digestion

  2. Continues in stomach where food is mixed by muscular action of stomach and gastric juice is added; gastric juice contains acid, enzymes, hormones, intrinsic factor, and mucus

      a. HCl acid is secreted by parietal cells in gastric mucosa; acts to dissolve food fibers

      b. Pepsinogen, enzyme precursor to pepsin, is secreted by zymogenic (chief) cells; converted to pepsin in an acid environment; breaks down protein

      c. Hormones: gastrin to stimulate HCl acid and pepsinogen secretion

      d. Intrinsic factor: necessary for absorption of vitamin B_{12}

      e. Mucus: protects gastric mucosa from digestive action of acid and enzymes

  3. Digestion continues in proximal portion of small intestine; pancreatic enzymes, intestinal enzymes, and bile salts are added

      a. Pancreatic enzymes: trypsin, chymotrypsin, and carboxypeptidase break down proteins; pancreatic lipase breaks down fats

      b. Intestinal enzymes: lactase, maltase, and sucrase break down CHOs; aminopeptidases and dipeptidase break down proteins

      c. Bile salts: emulsify fats and make them ready for action by pancreatic lipase

  4. Absorption of nutrients takes place in capillaries in villae of small intestine; nutrients are then transported to liver via portal vein

G. Elimination: end process of digestion where food residue, unabsorbed GI secretions, shed epithelial cells, and bacteria are removed from body

  1. Accomplished by segmental contractions in colon that propel fecal material toward rectum

  2. Once in rectum, defecation reflex is triggered by stretch receptors in rectal wall; evacuation is accomplished by Valsalva maneuver

II. DIAGNOSTIC TESTS AND ASSESSMENTS

A. Upper GI series: series of x-rays using contrast medium (barium sulfate or Gastrografin)

  1. Lower esophagus, stomach, and duodenum are examined for tumors, ulcerations, inflammation, varices, obstruction, and/or anatomic abnormalities (hiatal **hernia**)

  2. After client drinks barium, a series of x-rays document progression of contrast as client is placed in different positions

  3. Gastroesophageal reflux (reflux from stomach into esophagus) can be assessed during procedure with client in a flat or head-down position

    4. Contraindications: complete bowel obstruction, esophageal or gastric perforation (may use Gastrografin), or unstable vital signs

    5. Possible complications: aspiration of contrast medium, constipation (if barium used), or partial bowel obstruction; if Gastrografin is used, there may be significant **diarrhea** (increase in frequency, amount, or liquidity of stool that is a change from normal pattern)

    6. Increase fluids and take a laxative after the test if barium was used; stools may be white until barium is eliminated

B. Lower GI series: series of x-rays using contrast medium (barium enema) and often followed with air contrast

    1. Colon, including appendix, is visualized for anatomic abnormalities, polyps, ulcers, tumors, Crohn's disease, **fistulas** (abnormal pathway between structures or from an internal organ to an outside surface) and diverticula

    2. Barium enema can also stop bleeding from diverticula

    3. Contraindications: perforated colon or uncooperative clients

    4. Possible complications: colonic perforation or barium impaction

    5. Scheduling considerations: should be performed before an upper GI study to prevent residual barium from being in colon, and colon should also be empty

        a. Clear liquid diet day before test

        b. Magnesium citrate or other bowel prep night before test

        c. NPO after midnight and continue until test is complete

        d. Cleansing enemas may be prescribed before test

    6. Client should increase fluids and take a laxative after test; stools may be white until barium is eliminated

C. Upper GI endoscopy: *esophagogastroduodenoscopy (EGD),* gastroscopy

    1. Direct visualization of esophagus, stomach, and duodenum through lighted endoscope; detects mucosal inflammations (gastritis, gastroesophageal reflux), tumors, varices, hiatal hernias, polyps, ulcers, and obstruction

    2. Endoscopy can also be used to directly sample tissues and fluids, stop areas of active GI bleeding by injection of sclerosing agents or cautery, and to perform GI surgery using laser beams

    3. Contraindications: uncooperative clients, esophageal diverticula, suspected perforation, recent upper GI surgery, and severe upper GI hemorrhage

    4. Possible complications: pulmonary aspiration of GI contents; perforation of esophagus, stomach or duodenum; bleeding from biopsy site; and reactions to sedative medication given during test

    5. Special nursing considerations postprocedure: NPO until client is completely alert and swallowing/gag reflexes have returned (2–4 hours); general safety precautions because of sedation; monitor for signs of bleeding, dyspnea, or dysphagia

D. Colonoscopy: fiberoptic direct visualization of colon from anus to cecum

    1. Detects tumors (benign or malignant), polyps, inflammation, ulcerations, and bleeding; may biopsy any suspicious tissue

    2. Contraindications: uncooperative or medically unstable clients, rectal hemorrhage, suspected colon perforation

    3. Possible complications: perforation of colon, bleeding from biopsy sites, oversedation

    4. Special nursing considerations: requires complete bowel prep similar to prep for lower GI series; general safety precautions because of sedation; monitor vital signs postprocedure for signs of bleeding and colon perforation

E. Sigmoidoscopy: direct visualization of anus, rectum, and sigmoid colon with either a rigid or flexible sigmoidoscope; similar to colonoscopy in procedure, contraindications, complications, and nursing considerations, but is a less extensive study

F. **Ultrasonography**: visualization of abdominal organs using high-frequency sound waves that penetrate organ and are bounced back to a transducer where sound waves are converted to an electronic pictorial image
   1. Can detect organ size, cyst formation, tumors, and filling defects
   2. No contrast medium or radiation is involved so there are no contraindications
   3. Possible complications: none

G. **CT (computed tomography) scan**: radiologic procedure (with or without contrast medium) used to diagnose conditions such as tumors, cysts, abscesses, perforation, bleeding, inflammation, aneurysms, and obstruction
   1. X-rays are passed through abdominal organs at many angles because of differing organ densities, penetration of x-rays varies, producing an image after digital computation into shades of gray
   2. Contraindications: allergy to iodine or iodinated contrast media, pregnancy, unstable vital signs, morbid obesity, and claustrophobia
   3. Possible complications: allergic reaction to contrast media (iodinated), and renal failure from contrast
   4. Special nursing considerations: instruct client to drink fluids to aid elimination of contrast; monitor for delayed reaction to contrast medium

H. **Gastric analysis**: stomach contents are aspirated with an NG tube and pH is measured at a basal rate (BAO–basal acid output) and also during a stimulated state (MAO–maximal acid output); or tubeless gastric analysis where a resin dye (Diagnex Blue) is ingested and gastric acid displaces dye from resin and dye is absorbed by bowel and excreted by kidneys
   1. Used to differentiate causes of hypergastrinemia including **Zollinger-Ellison syndrome** (elevated levels of gastrin from pancreatic tumor), chronic antacid ingestion or atrophic gastritis
   2. May be used to assess effect of antiulcer therapy (surgical or medical)
   3. Precautions: anyone with heart failure, carcinoid syndrome, or hypertension may have an exacerbation of symptoms with this test since histamine is used to stimulate gastric acid

I. **Stool examination**: fecal specimen is examined for obvious and occult blood, and fat, as well as assayed for clostridial toxin, and cultured for infective and parasitic pathogens
   1. Stool culture: common bacterial pathogens include *Salmonella, Shigella, Campylobacter, Yersinia*, pathogenic *Escherichia coli, Clostridium,* and *Staphylococcus*; parasitic pathogens include *Ascaris* (hookworm), *Strongyloides* (tapeworm), and *Giardia* (protozoans)
   2. Stool for occult blood: stool is tested with a reagent to detect blood that is not visible; causes of occult blood include: benign and malignant GI tumors, ulcers, inflammatory bowel disease, diverticulosis, and hemorrhoids; see Box 8-1 for substances that cause a false-positive test for blood
   3. Fecal fat: measures fat content of stool over a 24-hour period
      a. Conditions causing fat in stool: cystic fibrosis, celiac disease, sprue, Crohn's disease (regional enteritis), Whipple's disease, and maldigestion from pancreato-biliary tree obstruction
      b. Nursing considerations: instruct client to eat a diet that contains 100 grams of fat per day for 3 days before and during stool collection
   4. Stool for Clostridial toxin: *Clostridium difficile* bacteria release a toxin that causes necrosis of bowel epithelium; infection occurs in people who are immunocompromised or after taking broad-spectrum antibiotics

Practice to Pass

A client is scheduled for a CT scan of the abdomen. What questions should the nurse ask before the test can be done?

Box 8-1	**Common Substances Causing False-Positive Results**

Stool for Occult Blood

Common Substances Causing False-Positive Results
- Red meat or red liquids (rule of "no reds")
- Fish
- Oral iron supplements
- Iodine
- Boric acid
- Colchicine
- Drugs irritating to gastric mucosa
  - Aspirin
  - NSAIDs
  - Corticosteroids

Common Substances Causing False-Negative Results
- Vitamin C
- Turnips
- Horseradish
- Beets
- Melons

III. COMMON NURSING TECHNIQUES AND PROCEDURES

A. ***Nasogastric (NG) tube***: pliable plastic tube inserted through nose and advanced to stomach

    1. Types of tubes include: double lumen gastric sump tube (most common), single lumen tube, nasogastric feeding tubes

        a. Gastric sump tube: two-lumen tube in various sizes (14 to 18 Fr) and 120 cm (48 in.) long; the large lumen is used for suction and drainage of stomach contents while the small lumen (blue vent) acts as an air vent preventing tube from being sucked up against gastric mucosa when attached to a suction device; tube can also be used for short-term gastric feeding and medication administration

        b. Single lumen gastric tube: larger lumen tube used to quickly drain stomach contents in cases of poisoning

        c. Feeding tubes: smaller diameter tubes (6 to 12 Fr) that often have a weighted tip and are placed using a stylet

    2. Purpose: NG tubes are used for gastric decompression (drainage), gastric **lavage** (gastric irrigation), or gastric feeding (**gavage**)

    3. Nursing interventions

        a. Insertion

            1) Measure tube from tip of nose to ear and then to xyphoid process; place adhesive tape at this measurement (approximate length of esophagus from nose to stomach)

            2) Insert tube in nares with client in a high-Fowler's position and with head hyperextended (to reduce curvature of nasopharyngeal junction)

            3) Once tube is in posterior pharynx, ask client to tilt head forward and sip water through a straw to facilitate passage into esophagus (rather than trachea) if able

        b. Check placement

            1) Tube placement is checked immediately after insertion and each time before placing anything into tube; initial placement of feeding tubes should be verified by x-ray; after initial verification mark tube position with indelible marker

2) Prior to each feeding (or every 4–6 hours if continuous feedings are being administered) check pH of aspirated secretions (should be less than 5.0); small bore tubes may collapse with aspiration; use a 60 mL syringe to insert 20–30 mL of air, then aspirate a small amount secretions for testing

3) Do not administer a feeding or insert fluid if client is having difficulty speaking or is coughing

    c. Maintain suction when NG tube is used for gastric decompression and assess every 1–4 hours

    d. Tube patency: assess every 4 hours or according to agency policy; thick secretions and/or particles may obstruct holes in tube and drainage ceases; tube can be irrigated with 20 mL of saline or water to keep tube clear as per agency policy

    e. Oral and nasal care is important (presence of tube is irritating to mucosa)

B. Enteral feedings

  1. Types

    a. Feeding can be given through an NG tube or gastrostomy tube either continuously or intermittently; can be given through a jejunostomy tube or nasojejunal tube continuously but is controlled by an enteral feeding pump

    b. Numerous formulas are commercially available and vary in proportions of nutrients, calories, and osmolarity; health care provider usually prescribes formula and rate of administration

  2. Purpose: enteral feedings bypass mouth to deliver a balance of nutrients directly to GI system; are indicated for clients who are unable to eat for a variety of reasons (including coma, oropharyngeal surgery/cancer, anatomical abnormalities, inability to swallow, esophageal obstruction) and to clients who are able to eat but cannot ingest an adequate number of calories

  3. Nursing interventions

    a. Assess proper placement of feeding tube by checking pH before beginning enteral feedings; if tube is placed in stomach assess residual feeding contents before each intermittent feeding (or every 4–6 hours if on continuous feeding); if tube is in small intestine residual contents cannot be aspirated

    b. Place the client in Fowler's position if client can tolerate it to decrease risk of aspiration

    c. Administer feeding formula at room temperature to prevent abdominal cramping, but do not leave at room temperature (continuous feeding) for more than 8–12 hours (or less according to product directions) to limit bacterial growth; change equipment every 24 hours

    d. If the feeding is intermittent, clamp feeding tube before gavage bag or syringe is attached to prevent air from entering stomach

    e. Give intermittent feeding slowly (over 10–15 min) to prevent nausea, vomiting, flatus, and abdominal cramps

    f. When an intermittent feeding is finished, clamp tube and flush with water to prevent blockage

    g. Recheck placement and residual every 4 hours (or according to agency policy) when giving continuous feedings

    h. Ensure that head of bed remains elevated to at least 30 degrees at all times while continuous NG tube feedings are given

C. Esophageal and gastric tubes (*esophagogastric tube*): tubes with multiple lumens and two balloons; a large esophageal balloon to provide tamponade to bleeding in esophagus and a smaller gastric balloon that provides tamponade to cardiac region and distal esophagus (see Figure 8-2)

Practice to Pass

The client is to have an NG tube inserted. How should the nurse explain the procedure to the client?

Figure 8-2

Sengstaken-Blakemore tube

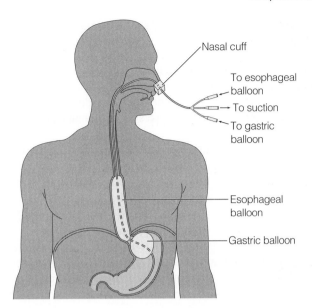

1. Types
   a. Sengstaken-Blakemore tube: triple lumen tube; esophageal balloon lumen, gastric balloon lumen, and a distal lumen to tip that drains stomach contents
   b. Minnesota tube: similar to Sengstaken-Blakemore tube but has 4 lumens; additional lumen opens proximal to esophageal balloon and drains esophageal secretions
2. Purpose: classic method to treat bleeding esophageal varices by applying direct pressure (tamponade) via inflated balloons
3. Nursing interventions
   a. Maintain pressure of esophageal balloon at 20–25 mmHg and monitor for loss of pressure or overinflation, which can cause tissue ischemia, necrosis and/or rupture of esophagus
   b. Apply traction to tube so gastric balloon is tight against lower esophageal (cardiac) sphincter to keep tube in place
    c. Monitor for sudden respiratory distress caused by upward displacement of esophageal balloon; always deflate esophageal balloon before gastric balloon (prevents esophageal balloon displacement and airway occlusion); if respiratory distress occurs, use an appropriate syringe to deflate esophageal balloon; if necessary cut tube to deflate both balloons and remove tube; keep appropriate syringe and scissors at bedside for emergency use

D. **Gastric lavage**: irrigation of stomach
   1. Purpose: remove toxic substances from stomach or slow bleeding
      a. Lavage is performed in cases of accidental poisoning or drug overdose; a large diameter tube (30–36 Fr) is used for rapid removal of stomach contents and irrigation is done to dilute toxins
      b. Lavage (with cool saline or sometimes with iced saline) and aspiration are performed in cases of upper GI bleeding to remove blood and slow bleeding; an 18-Fr tube is used for removing blood; use of iced saline poses risk of ischemia to hypothermic tissue and is controversial
   2. Nursing interventions
      a. Assess placement of gastric tube before instilling any fluid into stomach
      b. Strictly measure fluid instilled and removed to assess quantity of bleeding
      c. In cases of poisoning, fluid removed from stomach may be sent to laboratory for examination

IV. NURSING MANAGEMENT OF CLIENT HAVING GASTROINTESTINAL SURGERY

A. Bowel resection: ranges from endoscopic excision for small tumors to abdominal incision with removal of sigmoid colon, rectum, and anus

B. *Colostomy*: fecal diversion to an external collection device; named for portion of colon from which they are formed: ascending, transverse, descending, or sigmoid colostomy

1. Preoperative period

   a. Provide teaching about procedure and what to expect in postoperative period, including pain relief, breathing exercises, and appearance of stoma; this will reduce client anxiety and promote postoperative participation in care

   b. Allow client to verbalize fears and concerns about surgery and lifestyle changes and provide appropriate referrals and support (United Ostomy Association, enterostomal therapy nurse referral as examples)

   c. Carry out bowel preparation orders, which usually include bowel cleansing with cathartics and enemas as well as oral or parenteral antibiotics

   d. Ensure that usual preoperative activities are completed, consent for procedure is signed, and preanesthetic medications are given as prescribed

2. Postoperative period

   a. Routine care for surgical client: monitor vital signs and bowel sounds; assess intake and output including wound drainage and drainage from tubes (NG, urinary drainage, etc.); evaluate incision(s) and perianal area; assess level of consciousness, and encourage deep breathing, use of incentive spirometer, and splinting of incision

   b. Assess appearance and drainage from stoma; identify changes and notify surgeon if stoma becomes pale or cyanotic or if bleeding increases

   c. Apply ostomy appliance (pouch) over stoma and teach client and family about procedure and nature of effluent (initially dark green, more liquid, but will thicken over time and become yellow-brown)

   d. Use a skin barrier to protect skin around stoma from irritating effects of effluent (contains digestive enzymes and bile salts)

   e. Monitor pain control and take appropriate actions if pain is not controlled (check patency of IV access, notify surgeon, provide comfort measures)

   f. Maintain intravenous fluid and electrolyte replacement during nasogastric suction

   g. If abdominal perineal resection is done, avoid rectal temperatures, suppositories, or other rectal procedures (may disrupt anal suture line)

   h. Encourage ambulation as ordered to stimulate peristalsis

   i. Resume oral intake as ordered (often progress from clear liquids to full liquids, then frequent small feedings of regular foods) and monitor for nausea, abdominal distention, and adequacy of bowel sounds

   j. Begin discharge teaching: possible postoperative complications and preventive measures (infection, bowel obstruction, abdominal abscess); colostomy care (irrigation depending on location of stoma, pouch management, skin care)

C. *Ileostomy*: large intestine is removed and permanent fecal diversion is created at level of ileum; may be required for clients with extensive chronic ulcerative colitis

1. Preoperative and postoperative care as per bowel resection previously noted

2. Ileostomy will have liquid drainage because contents of small intestine are liquid

3. Emphasize importance of good nutrition, need for adequate fluid and electrolyte intake, and signs and symptoms of an imbalance (excess fluid and electrolytes are lost through ileostomy drainage); water intake should be sufficient to maintain pale urine and an output of at least 1 quart per day

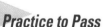

Practice to Pass

The client returns from the operating room following a colostomy. What should the nurse include in the initial assessment?

D. Continent ileostomy: an intra-abdominal reservoir is constructed and a nipple formed from terminal ileum; stool collects in internal pouch; nipple valve prevents it from leaking through stoma; a catheter is inserted into pouch intermittently to drain stool

E. Gastrectomy: removal of stomach with anastomosis of esophagus to jejunum (esophagojejunostomy); rarely performed, usually only for extensive gastric cancer or Zollinger-Ellison syndrome unresponsive to medical treatment

1. Preoperative period
   a. Clarify procedure with client and family so they understand risks and benefits and obtain a signed consent form as per hospital policy
   b. Prepare client and family about what to expect postoperatively, including pain relief, breathing exercises, expected tubes (NG, drains, jejunostomy feeding tube), and ambulation

2. Postoperative period
   a. Assess vital signs, lung and bowel sounds, intake and output including drainage from nasogastric tube, wound drainage (amount and character), effectiveness of pain control measures
   b. Do not reposition, irrigate, or check NG tube for placement because of risk of disrupting esophagojejunostomy sutures (depending on surgeon's orders)
   c. Implement standard postoperative care (intravenous fluid and electrolyte replacement, pain management, progressive activity to ambulation)
   d. Discuss limitations in oral intake and alternative methods to maintain nutrition; may require jejunostomy tube with an elemental (requires no digestion) enteral feeding
   e. Teach client about postoperative complications, including pernicious anemia, abdominal abscess or infection, and decreased nutrition

F. Gastric resection: portion of stomach is removed for diseases such as cancer and peptic ulcer disease refractory to medical management; in this case, the antrum, which contains most of gastrin-producing cells, is removed

1. Preoperative period: insert NG tube if ordered and connect to suction (may be inserted in operating room); provide standard preoperative care as for any abdominal surgery

2. Postoperative period
   a. Assess vital signs, lung and bowel sounds, intake and output including drainage from NG tube, wound drainage (amount and character), effectiveness of pain control measures
   b. Do *not* reposition, irrigate, or check NG tube for placement (unless the surgeon's orders specifically indicate to do so) because of risk of disrupting sutures inside stomach
   c. Implement standard postoperative care for clients with abdominal surgery as previously described
   d. Be alert for development of acute gastric dilation as a postoperative complication; signs and symptoms include epigastric pain, fullness, hiccups, tachycardia, and hypotension; results from a malfunctioning NG tube and rapidly improves after flushing tube (surgeon order) or placement of a new one

3. **Dumping syndrome** is a common complication of gastric resection when pylorus is bypassed and is a postprandial problem of rapid dumping of food into jejunum without proper mixing and duodenal digestion
   a. Early manifestations: occur 5–30 minutes after eating and include nausea with possible vomiting, epigastric pain with cramping and borborygmi (loud, hyperactive bowel sounds) and diarrhea; systemic symptoms include vertigo, tachycardia, orthostatic hypotension, sweating, and flushing; believed to result from a rapid shift of extracellular fluid into bowel to dilute hypertonic chyme, which causes decreased blood volume

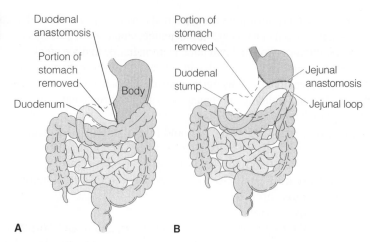

Figure 8-3

Partial gastrectomy.
A. Billroth I, B. Billroth II

    b. Late manifestations occur 2–3 hours postprandial and include hypoglycemic symptoms such as pale, cool skin with anxiety, shakiness, irritability and hunger; these symptoms are caused by excessive release of insulin in response to a rapid rise in blood glucose due to high-CHO bolus entering jejunum

    c. Dumping syndrome can be minimized by measures that delay gastric emptying and allow smaller boluses of undigested food to enter intestine, including a low-CHO, high-protein, high-fat diet; avoiding drinking fluids with meals; lying down for 30–60 minutes after eating and use of anticholinergics, antispasmodics or sedatives if prescribed

G. Billroth I (gastroduodenostomy): a partial gastrectomy where distal portion of stomach (including antrum) is removed and remainder is anastomosed to duodenum (see Figure 8-3a); gastrin-producing cells in antrum are removed as well as some parietal cells (acid-pepsinogen secreting cells)

    1. Preoperative and postoperative care is same as for any client having gastric surgery

    2. Dumping syndrome is a common complication of this procedure

H. Billroth II (gastrojejunostomy): a partial gastrectomy where lower portion of stomach is removed and proximal remnant is anastomosed to jejunum (see Figure 8-3b); used to treat gastric and duodenal ulcers

    1. Preoperative and postoperative care is same as for any client having gastric surgery

    2. Dumping syndrome is a common complication of this procedure

I. Roux-en-Y gastric bypass: a small stomach pouch is created to restrict food intake; a Y-shaped section of jejunum is attached to pouch to allow food to bypass lower stomach and duodenum; used to treat obesity; nutrient deficiencies are common

    1. Preoperative and postoperative care is same as for any client having gastric surgery but includes special needs related to obesity (expanded-capacity equipment, extra caregivers for movement and transfers, continuous positive airway pressure, cardiac monitoring)

    2. Dumping syndrome is a common complication of this procedure

J. Restrictive procedures: adjustable gastric banding; safer but less effective in the long term; few nutritional deficiencies; vomiting is a common postoperative risk

V. MALNUTRITION

    A. Description

        1. Dietary intake of nutrients does not meet body's energy needs

        2. Less than 90% ideal body weight and or body mass index below 18.5 kg/m^2

B. Etiology and pathophysiology

1. When more energy is expended by body than is consumed in food, body uses stored forms of energy in a certain order: first are CHOs stored as glycogen, then fat stores and finally protein stores in form of muscle tissue
2. Malnutrition can result from a variety of conditions and diseases
   a. Insufficient nutrients: liver failure (liver normally synthesizes proteins), starvation, anorexia nervosa/bulimia, severe illness/trauma (increases protein and calorie requirements)
   b. Improper proportions: fad dieting, unavailability of a variety of foods, maldigestion of certain foods because of a loss of enzymes, acid, or hormones
   c. Malabsorption: rapid GI transit time, gastric resection, partial gastrectomy, intestinal infections, absence of some enzymes as in celiac disease, decreased production or release of bile
   d. Improper distribution: in the absence of insulin glucose cannot enter cell to be used for energy
   e. Loss of nutrients: vomiting and severe diarrhea
   f. Increased metabolic needs: infection or physiologic stressors

C. Assessment

1. Ideal body weight (IBW): compare actual weight to body weight (as indicated for height on a standardized table)
   a. A weight 10–20% less than IBW indicates malnutrition
   b. A weight 10% above IBW is considered overweight
   c. A weight 20% above IBW is considered obese
2. **Body mass index (BMI)** estimates total body fat stores in relation to height and weight (weight in kg divided by height in meters^2); is less accurate for clients who are highly muscular or who have lost muscle mass (see Box 8-2)
3. Clinical manifestations
   a. Integumentary: brittle, dry and dull hair; decreased hair pigmentation; nails fragile, brittle and spoon-shaped; dry scaling skin,
   b. GI: cheilosis (painful lesions at corners of mouth), glossitis (smooth, bright-red tongue), stomatitis (dry and reddened oral mucosa), spongy bleeding gums
   c. Musculoskeletal: muscle wasting, subcutaneous fat loss, impaired strength
   d. Neurologic: confusion, disorientation, paresthesia
   e. Respiratory and cardiovascular: anemia, dysrhythmias, decreased respiratory rate, decreased vital capacity, decreased heart rate, decreased blood pressure, enlarged heart with possible heart failure
   f. Reproductive: amenorrhea
   g. Immune system: increased susceptibility to infections
   h. Metabolic processes: decreased weight, decreased core body temperature, edema
4. Laboratory studies
   a. Serum albumin: reflects long term changes in nutritional status; less than 3.0 grams/dL indicative of chronic malnutrition
   b. Prealbumin: reflects acute changes in nutritional status; less than 10 mg/dL indicates severe nutritional deficiency; less than 5 mg/dL indicates severe protein depletion

Box 8-2 **Interpretation of Body Mass Index Values**	Malnutrition = less than 18.5 kg/m^2 Normal = 18.5–24.9 kg/m^2 Overweight = 25–29.9 kg/m^2 Obese = greater than 30 kg/m^2 Extreme obesity = greater than 40 kg/m^2

Source: Centers for Disease Control http://www.cdc.gov/healthyweight/assessing/bmi/adult_bmi/index.html

      c. Total lymphocyte count: reduced in protein-calorie malnutrition

      d. Serum electrolytes, potassium levels are low in severe malnutrition

D. Priority nursing problems

  1. Insufficient nutrients to meet bodily needs

  2. Potential for interrupted skin integrity related to depleted protein

  3. Potential for infection related to suppressed immune system

  4. Potential for dehydration related to difficulty swallowing or administration of hyper-osmolar nutritional solutions

E. Planning and implementation

  1. Ensure that proper prescribed diet (high-calorie, high-protein) is delivered to client; provide a pleasant eating environment by removing sources of unpleasant odors (such as bedpans, urinals)

  2. Encourage client to eat in a slow relaxed manner, offer oral hygiene before and after meals, offer smaller and more frequent meals including preferred foods

  3. Provide enteral nutrition following guidelines previously discussed and as prescribed by health care provider

  4. Provide skin care and encourage activity to prevent skin breakdown

  5. Assess for signs of infection and instruct client about signs and symptoms of infection and to report them to health care provider if they occur

  6. Weigh daily and monitor intake and output

F. Medications

  1. Indicated for treatment of malnutrition as a result of enzyme deficiency, diarrhea, vomiting, vitamin and mineral deficiency, and when GI tract must be bypassed

  2. Generally includes pancreatic enzymes, vitamins, minerals, antiemetics, antidiarrheals, antibiotics (for infectious diarrhea), insulin, and last, total parenteral nutrition (TPN)

G. Client education

  1. Reinforce diet teaching provided by dietitian and importance of adhering to diet prescription; safe weight gain is 1 to 2 lbs/wk

  2. Help client choose high-calorie, high-protein foods

  3. Teach client about use of medications for digestion, vomiting, diarrhea, or intestinal infections if ordered

  4. Teach client about proper administration of enteral or parenteral feedings if prescribed

H. Expected outcomes: client gains weight; experiences no further weight loss, symptoms of vitamin or mineral deficiency decrease, and ingests a diet with proper proportions of nutrients

VI. OBESITY

A. Description: a state of being more than 20% above ideal body weight; obesity is more accurately defined by BMI

B. Etiology and pathophysiology

  1. Caused by excess of body fat; can be present with normal weight

    a. Men: greater than 22% body fat in young men and greater than 25% body fat in older men

    b. Women: greater than 35% body fat

  2. Genetic factors may contribute to up to 40% of risk for obesity with several genes contributing to appetite and fat deposition; obesity as a purely genetic condition is rare

  3. Neuroendocrine causes of obesity include Cushing syndrome, polycystic ovarian syndrome, hypogonadism, insulinoma, and growth hormone insufficiency

  4. Physical inactivity combined with excessive caloric intake is probably the most important factor contributing to obesity

  5. Some drugs promote obesity, such as estrogens, corticosteroids, antidepressants, antiepileptics, antihypertensives, **nonsteroidal anti-inflammatory drugs (NSAIDs)**, and phenothiazines

6. Psychological factors, such as loneliness, stress, depression, guilt, boredom, and low self-esteem may precipitate unhealthy eating behaviors

7. Cultures that view obesity as desirable and a sign of prosperity along with environmental influences contribute to increased food intake leading to obesity

8. Nearly two-thirds of adult Americans are overweight and more than 30 % are obese

9. Complications of obesity include the following:
   a. Cardiovascular disease (hypertension, hyperlipidemia, coronary artery disease, metabolic syndrome, heart failure, venous thrombosis, stroke)
   b. Endocrine and reproductive disorders: diabetes mellitus, breast and endometrial cancers, polycystic ovarian syndrome, complications of pregnancy
   c. Respiratory disorders: asthma, sleep apnea
   d. Other disorders (hiatal hernia, cholelithiasis, osteoarthritis, back pain, and increased susceptibility to infection)

C. **Assessment**
   1. Compare the client's actual weight to ideal body weight (see section on malnutrition)
   2. Diagnose by calculating BMI (see section on malnutrition), percent of body fat as measured by skinfold thickness, underwater weight, or bioimpedance
   3. Phsyiological causes of obesity, complications of obesity or comorbid conditions are determined by measuring thyroid profile, serum glucose, serum cholesterol, lipid profile, and electrocardiogram (ECG)
   4. Obtain history of eating habits, duration of obesity, medications, culture, 24-hour food recall, usual physical activity, situations that trigger eating and eating behavior
   5. Assess methods used for previous attempts at weight loss

D. **Priority nursing problems**: excess nutrients above bodily needs, inability to endure exercise or activity, reduced self esteem, inability to self-manage treatment regimen

E. **Planning and implementation**
   1. Assist client in decision making about weight loss options appropriate for client's situation
      a. Diet therapy is developed collaboratively among client, health care provider, and dietitian; plan to create a daily 500- to 1,000-kcal deficit; adherence to diet and participation in group sessions is more important than type of diet
      b. Exercise is a critical element in weight loss and maintenance, as it increases energy consumption while preserving lean body mass, decreasing appetite, improving self-esteem, increasing BMR, and improving physical fitness
      c. Behavioral therapy is aimed at ways to assist client to change daily eating habits and includes keeping a food diary, establishing exercise patterns, controlling external cues to eating behavior, and switching focus from physical appearance to health
      d. Surgery is limited to extremely obese patients (BMI over 40 kg/m^2) or those who have additional health risks; operative procedures include gastroplasty (most common), intestinal bypass, maxillomandibular fixation, and esophageal banding; pre- and postoperative care is similar to that described earlier for gastric surgery
   2. Reinforce explanations about various weight loss methods and importance of maintaining calorie expenditure greater than intake; exercise recommendations for a healthy lifestyle include at least 30 minutes per day; walking is recommended; plan with client an activity that is appropriate considering physical and environmental limitations
   3. Provide information about support groups for obese individuals such as Overeaters Anonymous and Weight Watchers

F. **Medications**
   1. Drug treatment is controversial and is usually only suggested for clients with a BMI greater than 30 (or greater than 27 with comorbidities) and in conjunction with diet and exercise modifications

2. Anorexic medications are commonly used to suppress appetite so client eats less and loses weight slowly over time; these drugs are contraindicated in pregnant or lactating clients or those who have cardiac, hepatic, or renal disease
   a. Sibutramine (Meridia) acts on central nervous system to increase metabolic rate; increases pulse rate and blood pressure, use caution in clients with hypertension, coronary heart disease, or heart failure
   b. Amphetamines and antidepressants also suppress appetite but are controversial because of reported cases of toxicity and dependency
3. Orlistat (Xenical) is a lipase inhibitor that reduces fat absorption from GI tract; adverse effects (oily stools, flatulence, and fecal urgency) diminish when dietary fat intake is limited

G. Client education
   1. Reinforce information about prescribed diet therapy and exercise
   2. Provide information about portion sizes, for example, a serving of meat is 3 oz and is about the size of a deck of cards; a serving of dry breakfast cereal is 1 oz or 1 cup
   3. Clients taking medications to assist in weight loss should be instructed about symptoms of possible side effects, such as chest pain, shortness of breath, insomnia, and nervousness
   4. Have client establish strategies for dealing with "stress" eating or interruptions in therapeutic regimen

H. Expected outcomes: client identifies importance of healthful lifestyle change to affect long-term weight loss and establishes a sustained pattern of change

VII. GASTROESOPHAGEAL REFLUX DISEASE (GERD)

A. Description: backward movement of stomach contents into esophagus

B. Etiology and pathophysiology
   1. Caused by relaxation of lower esophageal sphincter (LES), decreased LES tone, increased intra-abdominal pressure, increased gastric volume, or a combination (see Box 8-3 for factors influencing LES tone)
   2. Reflux of gastric contents is irritating to esophagus and causes breakdown of mucosal barrier leading to inflammation; erosion may develop
   3. Healing of lower esophageal erosion involves substitution of columnar epithelium (**Barrett's epithelium**) for normal squamous epithelium
   4. Barrett's epithelium resists acid (and thus supports healing) but is a premalignant tissue associated with an increased risk of esophageal cancer
   5. Occurs at any age, but increases in clients over age 50; availability of H_2 receptor antagonists over-the-counter (OTC) have decreased reported mild cases

C. Assessment
   1. Heartburn or substernal burning pain is the most common symptom and is exacerbated by bending over, recumbent position, or straining
   2. Other clinical manifestations include regurgitation not associated with vomiting or nausea; bad or sour taste upon awakening; coughing, hoarseness, or wheezing at night; belching; and flatulence
   3. Chronic GERD may cause dysphagia indicating possible stricture or cancer
   4. Diagnosis is most accurate through 24-hour pH monitoring
   5. Other studies include barium swallow, endoscopy, Bernstein test, and esophageal manometry

D. Priority nursing problems: pain related to pyrosis; inability to self-manage treatment regimen

E. Planning and implementation
   1. Avoid factors that reduce LES tone (see Box 8-3)

Box 8-3	• Nicotine

Factors Decreasing Lower Esophageal Sphincter (LES) Tone

- Nicotine
- Caffeine (coffee, tea, cola)
- Chocolate
- Fatty foods
- Alcohol
- Peppermint, spearmint
- High levels of estrogen and progesterone
- Anticholinergic drugs
- Beta-adrenergic blockers
- Calcium channel blockers
- Nitrates
- Theophylline
- Diazepam (Valium)
- Tight, restrictive clothing
- Bending, straining
- Hiatal hernia

2. Do not eat within 3 hours of bedtime or assume a recumbent position after eating
3. Avoid restrictive clothing that increases intra-abdominal pressure
4. Avoid large meals; eat smaller meals more frequently
5. Elevate head of bed for sleeping
6. Stop smoking
7. Surgery may be used for clients who do not respond to medication and lifestyle management; treatment of choice is laparoscopic fundoplication where gastric fundus is wrapped around distal esophagus; provide preoperative and postoperative care as discussed previously for client undergoing gastric surgery

F. Medications
1. Antacids such as Mylanta or Maalox neutralize stomach acid and are used to treat mild to moderate symptoms
2. Histamine$_2$ receptor antagonists such as ranitidine (Zantac), famotidine (Pepcid), nizatidine (Axid), and cimetidine (Tagamet) reduce gastric acid production, are available OTC and are widely advertised for treatment of symptoms associated with GERD
3. Proton pump inhibitors (PPIs): omeprazole (Prilosec) and lansoprazole (Prevacid) reduce gastric secretions and are FDA-approved for long-term treatment (8 weeks to 6 months); they promote healing of erosive esophagitis but interfere with absorption of calcium and vitamin B, placing clients on PPI therapy for a year or longer at increased risk of hip fracture; some PPIs are available OTC
4. Promotility agent such as metoclopramide (Reglan) is used short term to enhance esophageal clearance and gastric emptying
5. Antiulcer agent such as sucralfate (Carafate) reacts with gastric acid to form a thick paste that adheres to damaged mucosal tissue

G. Client education
1. Reinforce importance of smoking cessation and avoidance of caffeine
2. Avoid bending over, especially after eating
3. Take medications as prescribed
4. Lose weight if overweight to decrease intra-abdominal pressure
5. Raise head of bed by using 6- to 8-inch concrete or wooden blocks (or wedge) to reduce nighttime reflux

H. Expected outcomes: identifies ways to reduce symptoms of reflux and incorporates them into lifestyle; experiences no GERD symptoms

Practice to Pass

The client with GERD is diagnosed with Barrett's epithelium. How should the nurse explain this condition?

VIII. HIATAL HERNIA

A. **Description**
1. Diaphragmatic weakness through which a portion of stomach protrudes into thoracic cavity
2. Affects women more than men and incidence increases with age

B. **Etiology and pathophysiology**
1. Caused by congenital weakness of diaphragm, trauma, obesity, aging, increased intra-abdominal pressure, or a combination of these factors
2. Two major types (see Figure 8-4)
   a. Sliding hernia: gastroesophageal junction and portion of fundus move into thorax through esophageal hiatus
   b. Rolling hernia (paraesophageal): only fundus and (less frequently) part of greater curvature roll into thorax

C. **Assessment**
1. Most cases are asymptomatic
2. Symptoms include heartburn (pyrosis), substernal burning or pain, feeling of fullness, dysphagia, belching; these are usually worse when reclining
3. Diagnosed by upper GI series or an upper endoscopy and symptom history

D. **Priority nursing diagnosis**: Acute Pain related to heartburn (pyrosis)

E. **Planning and implementation**
1. Conservative treatment: diet therapy and lifestyle modifications (same as discussed for GERD) and surgical procedures (same as discussed for GERD)
2. Assist client in decision making about surgical procedure (only used when conservative treatment has failed)

F. **Medications**
1. Part of conservative treatment regimen
2. Generally includes antacids and histamine H_2 receptor antagonists (see treatment for GERD)

G. **Client education**
1. Report any increase in symptoms
2. Do not take antacids within 2 hours of other medications
3. Avoid alcohol, caffeine, NSAIDs, and any medication that contains aspirin (such as Alka-Seltzer™)
4. Reinforce diet and lifestyle modifications

H. **Expected outcomes**: identifies and maintains diet, lifestyle, and medication regimen and experiences a decrease in symptoms

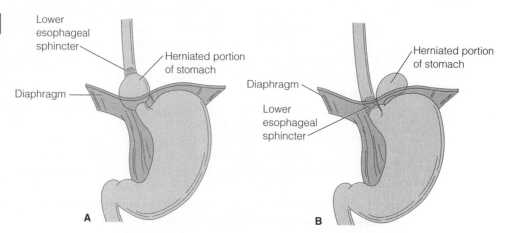

Figure 8-4

Hiatal hernias.
A. Sliding hernia,
B. Rolling hernia

Lower esophageal sphincter

Herniated portion of stomach

Diaphragm

A

Diaphragm

Herniated portion of stomach

Lower esophageal sphincter

B

IX. PEPTIC ULCER DISEASE (PUD)

    A. Description: generic term for ulcers or breaks in mucosal lining in GI tract that come in contact with gastric juice; can occur in stomach (gastric ulcers), duodenum (duodenal ulcers), or rarely lower esophagus (esophageal ulcers)

    B. Gastric ulcer

        1. Occurs most often on lesser curvature near pylorus

        2. Results from a disruption in normal protective mechanism that keeps gastric epithelial pH normal, including chronic *H. pylori* infection

        3. Prostaglandins in gastric mucosa increase resistance to acid, so substances (medications) that reduce prostaglandins (such as aspirin, NSAIDs, alcohol) will decrease gastric mucosal resistance

        4. Gastric ulcers are associated with gastritis and an increased incidence of gastric cancer

    C. Duodenal ulcer

        1. A chronic break in duodenal mucosa to muscularis mucosae layer; is the most common type of ulcer

        2. Results from increased gastric acid from increased number of parietal cells, increased vagal activity, increased secretion of gastrin, or chronic *H. pylori* infection

        3. Not associated with an increase in gastric cancer

    D. Peptic ulcer disease (PUD)

        1. Description (see previous descriptions for gastric and duodenal ulcers)

        2. Etiology and pathophysiology

            a. 10–15% of clients infected with *H. pylori* will develop PUD

            b. Chronic NSAID use (aspirin is worst) is associated with a fourfold increased risk for gastric ulcers

            c. Factors that increase risk for PUD include cigarette smoking, family history, blood group O (duodenal ulcer), alcohol use

            d. Incidence of ulcers increases steadily with age and peaks in sixth decade

            e. Men and women are affected equally

            f. Zollinger-Ellison syndrome is PUD caused by a gastrinoma, or gastrin-secreting tumor of pancreas, stomach or intestine; gastric analysis is performed when it is suspected

        3. Assessment

            a. Pain: gnawing, burning, aching, hunger-like, in the epigastrium, sometimes radiating to back

            b. Duodenal ulcers: pain relieved by eating

            c. Gastric ulcers: pain exacerbated by food

            d. Diagnosis is made most conclusively by EGD (see previous section for discussion)

            e. Upper GI series often done initially (less expensive and less invasive)

            f. Tests for *H. pylori* usually positive (includes biopsy specimen–most accurate–fecal tests, or urea breath tests)

            g. Observe for complications: perforation (signaled by pain, signs of peritonitis, shock), hemorrhage (noted by hematemesis, tarry stool, stool positive for occult blood), or pyloric obstruction (noted by vomiting, feeling of fullness)

        4. Priority nursing diagnosis: Pain related to mucosal injury

        5. Planning and implementation

            a. Reinforce importance of following treatment plan in reducing symptoms

            b. Prepare client for upper GI or EGD diagnostic test (discussed earlier)

            c. Refer client to smoking cessation program as smoking slows rate of healing and increases frequency of relapses

Practice to Pass

A client with peptic ulcer disease asks the nurse what the difference is between a gastric ulcer and a duodenal ulcer. How should the nurse respond?

      6. Medications

        a. Antacids, H$_2$ receptor antagonists, PPIs (antiulcer agents as discussed for GERD)

        b. Prostaglandin analogs: misoprostol (Cytotec) contributes to mucosal barrier preventing NSAID-induced ulcers

        c. Treatment for *H. pylori* changes frequently but generally includes antibiotics, antisecretory agents, and bismuth subsalicylate (Pepto-Bismol™)

      7. Client education

        a. Take medications as prescribed

        b. Report signs of complications: persistent anorexia, nausea or vomiting, blood (often black or tarry) in stool, increased pain, light-headedness or fainting

        c. Consume balanced meals at regular intervals; bland or restrictive diets are unnecessary

        d. Limit food intake after evening meal to decrease production of gastric acid and decrease likelihood of nighttime pain

      8. Expected outcomes: reduction or relief of pain following treatment

X. IRRITABLE BOWEL SYNDROME (IBS)

A. Description

    1. Common noninflammatory functional bowel disorder also known as spastic bowel, functional colitis, and mucous colitis

    2. Motility disorder of lower GI tract

B. Etiology and pathophysiology

    1. Cause is unknown, but aggravating factors are stress, anxiety, depression, certain foods and food additives in some clients, drugs, toxins, and hormones

    2. There is no change in physical characteristics of intestinal mucosa

    3. Usually manifests in three patterns: predominantly diarrhea, predominantly constipation, or combination of diarrhea and constipation; each pattern may or may not include abdominal pain

C. Assessment

    1. Abdominal pain

      a. Often relieved by defecation

      b. Intermittent and colicky or continuous and dull

    2. Change in bowel motility and character

      a. Diarrhea or constipation, or alternating with each

      b. Presence of mucus

      c. Altered stool passage (feeling of incomplete evacuation, straining, or urgency)

      d. Bloating and flatulence

    3. Diagnosis

      a. Exclude organic causes of clinical manifestations

      b. Abdominal pain or discomfort at least 3 days per month in previous 3 months with at least 2 of these characteristics:

        1) Improved with defecation

        2) Associated with a change in frequency of elimination

        3) Associated with a change in stool form

    4. Sigmoidoscopy may demonstrate spastic contractions that may be painful; mucosa is normal in appearance

D. Priority nursing problems: constipation; diarrhea

E. Planning and implementation

    1. No specific treatment

    2. Dietary fiber 30-40 grams may help in predominantly constipation type, while soluble fibers such as bran may help as well with diarrheal type

3. Assist client to identify and eliminate foods that exacerbate problem, including fruit, berries, lettuce, lactose, caffeinated drinks, preservatives (sodium sulfite), alcohol

4. Probiotic therapies (such as yogurt with active bacterial cultures) have been shown to benefit some clients with IBS

5. Encourage a program of relaxation and stress reduction; hypnosis has been shown to be beneficial

6. Regular exercise may help control symptoms

F. **Medications**

1. No standard pharmacologic treatment

2. **Bulk-forming agents** (Metamucil, Fibercon) may help reduce bowel spasm and normalize the number and form of bowel movements

3. Antidiarrheal agents (Imodium, Lomotil) may be used for predominantly diarrhea-type IBS

4. Antidepressants, anxiolytics, antispasmodics, or anticholinergics may be used

5. Herbal preparations with an antispasmodic effect (anise, chamomile, peppermint, sage) may reduce some manifestations of IBS while ginger root may reduce gas, bloaoting, and diarrhea

G. **Client education**

1. Fiber content of various foods

2. Follow prescribed regimen

3. Ensure bathroom privacy and a regular time for defecation

4. Information about programs of relaxation or support groups

H. **Expected outcomes**: client identifies triggers for IBS symptoms and follows prescribed treatment plan

XI. CHRONIC INFLAMMATORY BOWEL DISEASE

A. **Ulcerative colitis**

1. Description

   a. Area of chronic inflammation of mucosa and submucosa in colon and rectum

   b. Peak incidence is at 15–30 years of age with a second peak in people aged 60–80 years

   c. Characterized by periods of exacerbation and remission

2. Etiology and pathophysiology

   a. Cause is unknown

   b. May have relationship to stress, genetics, infection, dietary factors (low fiber intake), or antibody formation

   c. Inflammation (at base of crypts of Lieberkuhn usually in rectum) develops into abscesses that penetrate mucosa and spread laterally

   d. Begins in rectum and can progress proximally, but is usually limited to sigmoid colon and rectum

   e. Can range in severity from mild to severe

3. Assessment

   a. Diarrhea; 5–30 liquid stools per day often containing blood and sometimes mucus; nocturnal diarrhea is common

   b. May report fatigue resulting from blood loss, lack of sleep, and/or fluid imbalance

   c. May affect quality of life; client may be afraid to leave house because of severe diarrhea

   d. Complications include hemorrhage, abscess formation, toxic megacolon, malabsorption, bowel obstruction, bowel perforation, increased risk of colon cancer, and extraintestinal symptoms (arthritis, uveitis)

      e. Diagnosed conclusively by sigmoidoscopy (characteristic edematous, friable mucosa with a granular appearance with evident crypt abscesses), laboratory tests to identify effects and complications of disease, and stool examination and cultures to rule out infectious causes

   4. Priority nursing problems: diarrhea related to bowel inflammation; pain related to bowel mucosal inflammation

   5. Planning and implementation

      a. Provide pre- and postsigmoidoscopy care as outlined earlier in this chapter

      b. Rest is required to decrease intestinal activity

      c. Diet therapy: a low-residue diet or in severe cases nothing by mouth to rest bowel; TPN may be used in severe cases

      d. Surgery may be necessary if disease cannot be controlled by medical means; ranges from resection of affected portions of bowel to total colectomy with ileostomy (see section earlier in this chapter)

      e. Provide an atmosphere in which client feels free to talk about concerns related to disease process and its effect on lifestyle

   6. Medications

      a. Corticosteroids during exacerbations to decrease bowel inflammation

      b. Salicylate compounds (sulfasalazine [Azulfidine], mesalamine [Asocol]) are used to decrease prostaglandin formation in bowel thus reducing inflammation

      c. Antidiarrheal drugs are used to provide symptom management with mild, chronic manifestations but are not given during acute attacks as they may precipitate toxic dilation of colon

      d. Immunosuppressive agents such as azathioprine (Imuran), methotrexate, and cyclosporine (Sandimmune) may allow withdrawal from corticosteroids, maintain remission, and facilitate healing

      e. Immune response modifiers such as monoclonal antibody infliximab (Remicade) may suppress tumor necrosis factor (an inflammatory mediator substance) in clients who have not responded to standard therapies

   7. Client education

      a. Take medications as ordered

      b. Avoid foods that exacerbate symptoms: raw vegetables, raw fruits, whole-grain breads and cereals, seeds, nuts, popcorn, and any highly spiced or flavorful food; some clients benefit from eliminating all milk and milk products

      c. Notify health care provider if symptoms increase or there is blood in stool

      d. If surgery is required instruct client in postoperative care of stoma and incision as described in earlier section

      e. Provide information about ulcerative colitis support groups in the area

      f. Teach client importance of good perianal skin care to prevent complications

      g. Educate client about exacerbation and remission nature of disease and symptom management

   8. Expected outcomes/evaluation: identifies measures to decrease diarrhea and pain; has less diarrhea and pain; identifies signs and symptoms of complications and notifies healthcare provider of these if they occur

B. Crohn's disease (regional enteritis)

   1. Description

      a. Chronic inflammation of GI mucosa occurring anywhere from mouth to anus but occurring most often in terminal ileum

      b. Characterized by exacerbations and remissions

      c. Peak onset is ages 15–30

   2. Etiology and pathophysiology

      a. Cause is unknown

      b. Possible factors are autoimmune, genetics, infectious agents, and environmental (stress)

      c. Lesions extend to all thicknesses of bowel wall and are prone to fistula formation

      d. Lesions have a "cobblestone appearance" with sections of normal mucosa between lesions called "skip" lesions

      e. Over time chronic inflammation causes fibrotic changes in bowel wall leading to obstruction

      f. Depending on severity and location of lesions, malabsorption may occur as well as losses of protein from lesions themselves

3. Assessment

      a. Diarrhea (5-6 liquid to semiformed stools/day) is most common symptom (usually without mucous or blood); depending on location, steatorrhea (fatty stool) may occur

      b. Abdominal pain in RLQ that is relieved by defecation

      c. Systemic manifestations include fever, fatigue, malaise, weight loss, anemia, multiple vitamin and mineral deficits

      d. Complications include abscess and fistula formation, intestinal obstruction (common due to strictures), and malnutrition; bowel perforation and hemorrhage are uncommon

      e. Barium enema and upper GI series are often diagnostic showing areas of ulceration, narrowing, strictures, and fistulas

      f. Diagnosed by colonoscopy; characteristic aphthoid ulcers, strictures, and segmental involvement is visualized; biopsy of lesion is done

      g. Other tests are ordered to assess for complications and to rule out other causes of diarrhea (serum albumin, folic acid, hemoglobin, and hematocrit)

4. Priority nursing problems: diarrhea related to bowel inflammation; pain related to bowel inflammation; insufficient nutrients to meet bodily needs from malnutrition and protein losses

5. Planning and implementation

      a. Provide prescribed diet: usually high calorie, high protein, low fat; involve client in making appropriate menu choices

      b. Encourage intake of prescribed nutritional supplements

      c. Weigh daily, maintain calorie count, and monitor intake and output

      d. Allow client to express fears and anxiety about course of illness and possibility of surgical intervention (not as common as for ulcerative colitis because it is not necessarily curative)

6. Medications

      a. Are the same as those used for ulcerative colitis (antidiarrheals, salicylate-containing compounds, corticosteroids)

      b. Metronidazole (Flagyl), a broad-spectrum antimicrobial, is also given

      c. Antispasmotics decrease abdominal cramping following eating

      d. TPN may be prescribed during severe exacerbations to totally rest bowel

7. Client education

      a. Reinforce information about disease process, prescribed medication regimen, and dietary needs

      b. Teach client and family signs and symptoms of complications: increased pain, rectal bleeding, fever, chills, lethargy

      c. If TPN is ordered, teach client and family about proper catheter care and feeding techniques

      d. Encourage intake of nutritional supplements, such as Ensure™, which provide optimal elemental nutrition while providing for bowel rest

8. Expected outcomes: client has fewer episodes of diarrhea and associated abdominal pain; identifies foods high in protein, low in fat, and high in nutritional value, and follows prescribed nutrition regimen

XII. DIVERTICULITIS

A. Description

1. Inflammation of diverticula, which are outpouchings in wall of intestine (diverticulosis is presence of diverticula)
2. Majority of diverticula occur in sigmoid colon (90–95%)
3. Incidence increases with age
4. Diverticular disease is unknown in countries where people eat a high-fiber, unrefined diet

B. Etiology and pathophysiology

1. Caused by increased pressure in intestinal lumen and herniation of mucosa through defects in bowel wall; decreased fecal bulk (low-fiber diet) contribute to bowel wall hypertrophy and resultant narrowing of bowel with increased intraluminal pressure
2. Diverticula become inflamed when undigested food or bacteria are trapped; abscess formation contributes to disease and diverticulum may rupture

C. Assessment

1. Pain, usually left-sided, ranging in severity from mild to severe and can be constant or cramping; if perforation occurs, abdominal pain is generalized
2. Most cases of diverticular disease are asymptomatic, but nausea, vomiting, and a low-grade fever (less than 100°F) may occur; abdomen may be distended with tenderness and a palpable mass in left lower quadrant
3. May note constipation alternating with increased frequency bowel elimination pattern
4. Fever, chills, and tachycardia along with generalized abdominal pain may indicate perforation of diverticulum and onset of peritonitis
5. Diverticular disease is diagnosed with barium enema; however, this is contraindicated when diverticulitis is present because of risk of rupturing diverticulum with instillation of barium
6. CT scan or ultrasonography can be used to diagnose acute diverticulitis

D. Priority nursing problems: pain related to inflamed diverticula; interrupted gastrointestinal tissue integrity; inadequate knowledge related to dietary management

E. Planning and implementation

1. Reinforce dietary modifications to reduce complications of diverticulosis
   a. High-fiber diet after acute phase
   b. Bowel rest: NPO or low-residue diet during initial acute phase
   c. Addition of bran to everyday foods
   d. Avoid intake of seeds and foods with small seeds such as berries and figs
2. Assess for signs of bleeding: check stool for occult blood
3. Prepare for possible surgical intervention related to generalized peritonitis, abscess or hemorrhage; colon resection is done in 25% of cases of diverticulitis; may have a temporary colostomy

F. Medications

1. Antibiotics decrease bowel flora and reduce infection
2. Opioid analgesics relieve pain
3. Stool softeners may be used but laxatives and enemas are contraindicated (cause further increases in intraluminal pressure in colon)

G. Client education

1. Fiber content of various foods
2. Self-administration and side effects of medications ordered
3. Signs and symptoms of complications of diverticulitis

H. Expected outcomes: client identifies ways to increase dietary fiber; demonstrates understanding of disease process and symptoms of complications; follows therapeutic regimen

XIII. INTESTINAL OBSTRUCTION

A. Description
1. Failure of bowel contents to be moved forward
2. Can be partial or complete

B. Etiology and pathophysiology
1. Mechanical obstruction results from forces outside of intestines (adhesions, hernia, fibrosis); or blockage in lumen (fecal impaction, edema, stricture, volvulus, intussusception); or problems within intestine (tumors or inflammatory bowel disease)
2. Nonmechanical (functional) obstruction or paralytic ileus results from impairment of muscle tone or nervous system innervation preventing forward movement of intestinal contents (anesthesia, abdominal surgery, spinal injuries, peritonitis, vascular insufficiency)
3. Obstructions occur most often in ileum where the intestinal diameter is the smallest
4. Peristalsis increases in the intestine above the blockage, leading to increased secretions, edema, and increased capillary permeability and resulting in fluid and electrolyte imbalances and hypovolemia

C. Assessment
1. Early in bowel obstruction, bowel sounds may be high pitched and tinkling proximal to obstruction and silent distal to obstruction
2. Late in bowel obstruction bowel sounds become absent
3. Abdominal pain can be colicky and increase in intensity as obstruction progresses
4. Vomiting is common with a small-bowel obstruction and may have a fecal odor; vomiting is a late sign with a large-bowel obstruction, if it occurs at all
5. Abdominal distention is minimal with proximal obstructions but may be pronounced with distal obstruction and paralytic ileus
6. Vital signs may be normal in early obstruction but client can demonstrate signs of shock as dehydration and hypovolemia develop (tachycardia, fever, tachypnea, hypotension)
7. Diagnosed by history, physical findings, and abdominal x-ray; dilated loops of bowel can be seen (barium studies are contraindicated but gastrografin can be used); free air under diaphragm indicates a perforation

D. Priority nursing problems: interrupted gastrointestinal tissue perfusion, potential for dehydration, pain

E. Planning and implementation
1. Prepare client for possibility of surgery: laprascopic, exploratory laparotomy, colon resection, colostomy (see earlier section)
2. Prepare client for insertion of NGT (see earlier section)
3. Provide mouth care to minimize the fecal nature of secretions
4. Provide IV therapy as prescribed to restore fluid and electrolyte balance
5. Maintain NPO status until peristalsis returns
6. Provide comfort measures such as frequent position changes
7. Monitor vital signs including intake and output; early detection of hypovolemic shock can prevent complications (bowel ischemia and necrosis, multisystem organ failure); urine output of less than 30 mL per hour often indicates hypovolemia and an increased risk for shock and acute renal failure
8. Monitor level of pain: sudden change in the nature of pain may indicate complications (ischemia and necrosis)
9. Measure abdominal girth every 4–8 hours; mark level of measurement on abdomen to allow consistent, accurate measurements

F. Medications
1. Analgesic medication is generally limited because opioid analgesics decrease GI motility, which will further compromise bowel

! ▸ **2.** IV fluid with appropriate electrolyte replacement will be prescribed to prevent hypovolemia and shock; calculate urinary and nasogastric drainage losses every 2–4 hours to help determine fluid replacement needs

G. Client education

1. Instruct client about insertion and maintenance of NG tube
2. Reinforce instructions for postoperative use of incentive spirometer, coughing and deep-breathing exercises, ambulation, activity, and wound care
3. Provide support to client and family in dealing with possibility of a colostomy
4. Stress importance of maintaining a healthy lifestyle on discharge

H. Expected outcomes: client identifies understanding of disease process and treatment options; verbalizes ways to prevent future bowel obstructions

Case Study

M. W., a 47-year-old female, is admitted to the hospital to rule out chronic gastroesophageal reflux disease (GERD) versus peptic ulcer disease (PUD). You are the nurse assigned to care for this client.

1. What diagnostic tests should you anticipate being ordered to differentiate her diagnoses?

2. What are the priorities of care after these tests?

3. What instructions about lifestyle changes should you give M. W. if she has gastroesophageal reflux disease (GERD)?

4. What instructions about signs and symptoms of complications of GERD and PUD should you provide to M. W.?

5. If M. W. asks you about the possibility of developing cancer, how would you respond?

For suggested responses, see page 623.

For suggested responses, see page 623.

POSTTEST

POSTTEST

❶ A client is to receive gavage feeding through a nasogastric (NG) tube. Which action should the nurse take to prevent complications?

1. Flush with 20 mL of air.
2. Place client in high-Fowler's position.
3. Advance tube 1 cm.
4. Plug the air vent during feeding.

❷ The nurse is preparing to insert a small-bore nasogastric feeding tube. Which actions are appropriate for the nurse to take? Select all that apply.

1. Measure the tube from the tip of the nose to the xiphoid process.
2. Insert the tube into the nares with the client's head hyperextended.
3. Use a 3 mL syringe to aspirate stomach contents.
4. Check the pH of stomach contents.
5. Place the client in a Fowler's position during administration of the feeding.

3 The nurse is caring for a client with a Sengstaken-Blakemore tube. What action should the nurse take first if the client suddenly experiences difficulty breathing?

1. Elevate head of the bed.
2. Apply oxygen with a nasal cannula.
3. Listen to the client's lungs.
4. Deflate balloons and remove tube.

4 The client returns to the nursing unit postoperatively after a colostomy. Which of the following assessments would require immediate action by the nurse?

1. Stoma is bright red.
2. Stoma is bluish.
3. Stoma is draining serous fluid.
4. Stoma is draining no fluid.

5 The nurse assesses a client admitted 4 hours ago with a diagnosis of diverticulitis. Which assessment findings must be reported immediately to the health care provider? Select all that apply.

1. Left-sided abdominal pain
2. Temperature 101.6°F
3. Palpable mass in the left lower quadrant
4. Abdominal girth distended to same level as upon admission
5. Bowel sounds change from normoactive to hypoactive

6 A client is admitted to the hospital in a malnourished state. The nurse understands the client is at a high risk for which health problem as a result of decreased nutrition?

1. Infection
2. Diarrhea
3. Ulcerative colitis
4. Tumor formation

7 The client with gastroesophageal reflux disease (GERD) is prescribed famotidine (Pepcid). In order to provide effective teaching, the nurse must include which information about the action of the drug?

1. It improves gastric motility.
2. It coats the distal portion of the esophagus.
3. It increases the gastric pH.
4. It decreases the secretion of gastric acid.

8 The nurse should question the client with gastroesophageal reflux disease (GERD) about the use of which type of medication that decreases lower esophageal sphincter (LES) tone?

1. Antidepressant
2. Calcium channel blocker
3. Antiestrogen agent
4. Alpha-adrenergic blocking agent

9 The client with irritable bowel syndrome (IBS) asks the nurse what causes the disease. Which response by the nurse would be most appropriate?

1. "This is an inflammation of the bowel caused by eating too much roughage."
2. "IBS is caused by a stressful lifestyle."
3. "The cause of this condition is unknown."
4. "There is thinning of the intestinal mucosa caused by ingestion of gluten."

10 A client with Crohn's disease (regional enteritis) who is taking sulfasalazine (Azulfidine) asks the nurse why this medication is necessary. Which information should the nurse include in the response?

1. The drug decreases abdominal cramping by slowing peristalsis.
2. The drug decreases prostaglandin production in the bowel so it decreases inflammation.
3. The drug inhibits neurotransmission of pain impulses.
4. The drug stimulates the release of endorphins so pain is relieved.

➤ *See pages 279–281 for Answers and Rationales.*

ANSWERS & RATIONALES

Pretest

1 **Answer: 2** **Rationale:** The posterior pharynx is anesthetized for easy passage of the endoscope into the esophagus. The return of the gag reflex indicates that normal function is returning and the client is able to swallow. Bowel sounds and abdominal girth are more associated with caring for a client with a nasogastric tube in place. Gastric pH is related to the client with peptic ulcer disease. **Cognitive Level:** Applying **Client Need:** Reduction of Risk Potential **Integrated Process:** Nursing Process: Assessment **Content Area:** Adult Health **Strategy:** Apply the principle of ABCs (airway, breathing, and circulation) in priority setting to select the correct response. **Reference:** LeMone, P., Burke, K., & Bauldoff, G. (2011). *Medical-surgical nursing: Critical thinking in patient care* (5th ed.). Upper Saddle River, NJ: Pearson Education, p. 572.

2 **Answer: 3** **Rationale:** Thick secretions and particulate matter may obstruct the tube, causing drainage to cease, and the client may experience nausea and vomiting. The tube should be gently flushed to ensure patency and rule out obstruction as the cause of the client's symptoms. Manipulating or advancing the position of the tube would be a later choice. Repositioning the client may help increase drainage but will not affect drainage if the tube is occluded. If placement has been confirmed and the tube secured, a second chest x-ray is unnecessary. **Cognitive Level:** Applying **Client Need:** Reduction of Risk Potential **Integrated Process:** Nursing Process: Implementation **Content Area:** Fundamentals **Strategy:** Apply the principles for care and management of a client with a nasogastric tube in place. **Reference:** Berman, A. J., & Snyder, S. (2011). *Kozier and Erb's fundamentals of nursing: Concepts, process, and practice* (9th ed.). Upper Saddle River, NJ: Prentice Hall, pp. 985–986.

3 **Answer: 3** **Rationale:** Dumping syndrome is the rapid dumping of food into the jejunum without proper mixing and digestion. Interventions that help to minimize dumping syndrome are drinking fluids in between meals instead of with meals, which will help to prevent dilution and rapid propulsion into the small intestines. Other helpful interventions are lying down after eating to slow passage of food into the small intestines and eating a diet high in fat and protein and low in carbohydrates so the food stays in the stomach longer. **Cognitive Level:** Applying **Client Need:** Physiological Adaptation **Integrated Process:** Nursing Process: Implementation **Content Area:** Adult Health **Strategy:** Review the cause of dumping syndrome and then choose the interventions that will offset or counteract these effects. Those are the items the client can implement to prevent its occurrence. **Reference:** LeMone, P., Burke, K., & Bauldoff, G.

(2011). *Medical-surgical nursing: Critical thinking in patient care* (5th ed.). Upper Saddle River, NJ: Pearson Education, pp. 647–648.

4 **Answer: 3** **Rationale:** A gastric banding procedure involves the placement of a hollow band of silicone rubber around the upper portion of the stomach. No surgical resection is performed. **Cognitive Level:** Applying **Client Need:** Physiological Adaptation **Integrated Process:** Teaching and Learning **Content Area:** Adult Health **Strategy:** Differentiate between bypass procedures and banding procedures. **Reference:** LeMone, P., Burke, K., & Bauldoff, G. (2011). *Medical-surgical nursing: Critical thinking in patient care* (5th ed.). Upper Saddle River, NJ: Pearson Education, pp. 594–595.

5 **Answer: 1** **Rationale:** The client with GERD is encouraged to eat smaller, more frequent, low-fat meals and to avoid lying down after eating. Clients are instructed to not eat for at least 2 hours before bedtime and sleep with the head of the bed elevated. They should also avoid foods that decrease lower esophageal sphincter pressure such as caffeine-containing coffee, tea, cola, and chocolate. **Cognitive Level:** Analyzing **Client Need:** Physiological Adaptation **Integrated Process:** Teaching and Learning **Content Area:** Adult Health **Strategy:** Recall the pathophysiology of GERD and its causes. The actions that will counteract the triggers are correct items of client teaching. Because this question has the critical words *more teaching*, choose the item that reflects misinformation on the part of the client. **Reference:** LeMone, P., Burke, K., & Bauldoff, G. (2011). *Medical-surgical nursing: Critical thinking in patient care* (5th ed.). Upper Saddle River, NJ: Pearson Education, pp. 623–626.

6 **Answer: 1** **Rationale:** Gastric ulcers are usually a result of a disruption of the protective mechanism of the gastric epithelium. Substances that reduce prostaglandin secretion in the gastric mucosa (aspirin, NSAIDs, alcohol) and infection with *H. pylori* are responsible for most peptic ulcer disease. Although certain foods and fluids may possibly aggravate an existing ulcer, they do not cause them. Acetaminophen (Tylenol) is allowed with peptic ulcer disease. **Cognitive Level:** Applying **Client Need:** Physiological Adaptation **Integrated Process:** Nursing Process: Assessment **Content Area:** Adult Health **Strategy:** Review the pathophysiology of gastric ulcers and risk factors. This information will help you identify which answer option increases the risk for developing an ulcer versus increasing the symptoms of an existing ulcer. **Reference:** LeMone, P., Burke, K., & Bauldoff, G. (2011). *Medical-surgical nursing: Critical thinking in patient care* (5th ed.). Upper Saddle River, NJ: Pearson Education, pp. 633–638.

7 **Answer: 1, 3, 4, 5** **Rationale:** Clients receiving enteral feedings should not be placed in the supine position because of the increased risk for regurgitation and aspiration. The nurse should first note that the client is in the semi-Fowler's position. The presence of a gag reflex enables the client to protect the airway. If bowel sounds were absent, the risk for regurgitation and aspiration would be increased so the enteral feedings would need to be discontinued. The rate and type of solution should be checked to reflect the written order. Breath sounds would be a means of detecting whether the client has aspirated and are not a protective measure. **Cognitive Level:** Analyzing **Client Need:** Reduction of Risk Potential **Integrated Process:** Nursing Process: Assessment **Content Area:** Adult Health **Strategy:** The critical word in the question is *protected*. Review the procedure for managing nasoduodenal tube and protecting the airway. Be sure to differentiate prevention from detection. Note also that for any intervention the order should be verified. **Reference:** LeMone, P., Burke, K., & Bauldoff, G. (2011). *Medical-surgical nursing: Critical thinking in patient care* (5th ed.). Upper Saddle River, NJ: Pearson Education, p. 603.

8 **Answer: 1** **Rationale:** Because hemorrhage and bleeding common features of ulcerative colitis, and over time this can lead to significant loss of RBCs, the client should be assessed for possible anemia by checking for low hemoglobin and hematocrit. Steatorrhea is seen in malabsorption syndrome. Thrombocytopenia may occur if the client is treated with immunosuppressants to control the disease. Signs of cholelithiasis are unrelated to ulcerative colitis. **Cognitive Level:** Applying **Client Need:** Reduction of Risk Potential **Integrated Process:** Nursing Process: Assessment **Content Area:** Adult Health **Strategy:** Differentiate the normal findings of ulcerative colitis with the complications of ulcerative colitis. Eliminate any answer options that are inconsistent with these lists or that are unrelated. Select the item that represents the complication. **Reference:** LeMone, P., Burke, K., & Bauldoff, G. (2011). *Medical-surgical nursing: Critical thinking in patient care* (5th ed.). Upper Saddle River, NJ: Pearson Education, pp. 680–681.

9 **Answer: 1** **Rationale:** Diets high in refined foods and low fiber are associated with an increased risk of diverticular disease. Crohn's disease is believed to be genetic or the result of a defect in the immune system. The cause of irritable bowel syndrome is unknown but thought to be related to gastric stimulation. Overuse of laxatives is detrimental to GI health. **Cognitive Level:** Analyzing **Client Need:** Health Promotion and Maintenance **Integrated Process:** Nursing Process: Planning **Content Area:** Adult Health **Strategy:** This item requires knowledge of multiple GI disorders and normal GI function. Compare each statement to what you know to be true about the content area in the answer options. **Reference:** LeMone, P., Burke, K., & Bauldoff, G. (2011). *Medical-surgical nursing: Critical thinking in patient care* (5th ed.). Upper Saddle River, NJ: Pearson Education, pp. 657–662, 681–682, 692–693.

10 **Answer: 1** **Rationale:** Early in a bowel obstruction, the bowel attempts to move the contents past the obstruction and this is heard as high-pitched tinkling bowel sounds. As the obstruction progresses, bowel sounds will diminish and may finally become absent. Bowel sounds in all four quadrants and rumbling bowel sounds are normal. **Cognitive Level:** Analyzing **Client Need:** Physiological Adaptation **Integrated Process:** Nursing Process: Assessment **Content Area:** Adult Health **Strategy:** Eliminate answer options that are normal findings in a GI assessment. The look at the remaining answer options in relation to the timing of their occurrence. Select the answer that represents an early finding. **Reference:** LeMone, P., Burke, K., & Bauldoff, G. (2011). *Medical-surgical nursing: Critical thinking in patient care* (5th ed.). Upper Saddle River, NJ: Pearson Education, pp. 711–713.

Posttest

1 **Answer: 2** **Rationale:** Keeping the client in a high-Fowler's position minimizes the risk of aspiration. Flushing with air will increase abdominal distention and increase discomfort as well as the risk for aspiration. Advancing the tube is only relevant if it is a nasoduodenal tube that has not advanced beyond the pylorus. Plugging the air vent is unnecessary. **Cognitive Level:** Applying **Client Need:** Physiological Adaptation **Integrated Process:** Nursing Process: Implementation **Content Area:** Fundamentals **Strategy:** Focus on the fact that the NG tube bypasses the oropharynx and the gag reflex. This fact then leads you to the conclusion that the airway is compromised. Select the answer option that protects the airway. **Reference:** Berman, A. J., & Snyder, S. (2011). *Kozier and Erb's fundamentals of nursing: Concepts, process, and practice* (9th ed.). Upper Saddle River, NJ: Pearson Education, pp. 1290–1293.

2 **Answer: 2, 4, 5** **Rationale:** Prior to inserting a nasogastric tube the nurse measures from the tip of the nose to the ear and then to the stomach. This approximates the length of the esophagus from nose to stomach. When inserting the tube into the nares the client's head should be slightly hyperextended in order to reduce the curvature of the nasopharyngeal junction. After the tube is inserted the nurse checks placement by aspirating stomach contents through a 60 mL syringe. Smaller syringes used with a small-bore feeding tube may cause the tube to collapse. The nurse checks the pH of the aspirate. Stomach contents should have a pH of 1 to 5. The client should be placed in a Fowler's or higher position to facilitate the gravitational flow of the feeding and to help prevent aspiration of the fluid into the lungs. **Cognitive Level:** Applying **Client Need:** Basic Care and Comfort **Integrated Process:** Nursing Process: Implementation **Content Area:** Fundamentals **Strategy:** Picture the anatomy of the gastrointestinal system and the respiratory system. Consider each option as a true-false question. **Reference:** Berman, A. J., & Snyder, S. (2011). *Kozier and Erb's fundamentals of nursing: Concepts*, process, and practice (9th ed.). Upper Saddle River, NJ: Pearson Education, pp. 1284, 1291.

3 **Answer: 4** **Rationale:** Respiratory distress is an indication that the Blakemore tube has migrated upward into the oropharynx and is obstructing the airway. The other selections will be ineffective as long as the Sengstaken-Blakemore tube is obstructing the airway. **Cognitive Level:** Analyzing **Client Need:** Physiological Adaptation **Integrated Process:** Nursing Process: Implementation **Content Area:** Adult Health **Strategy:** Always provide an open airway. In this case, the Blakemore tube must be removed to open the airway. **Reference:** LeMone, P., Burke, K., & Bauldoff, G. (2011). *Medical-surgical nursing: Critical thinking in patient care* (5th ed.). Upper Saddle River, NJ: Pearson Education, pp. 743–744.

4 **Answer: 2** **Rationale:** A healthy stoma is red to reddish-pink, moist, and shiny. A stoma that appears dark red, bluish, or black indicates ischemia or necrosis. This finding must be reported immediately because the viability of the tissue is at risk. The colostomy is not functional for 2–4 days. No drainage or serous fluid is a normal finding in the immediate postoperative period. **Cognitive Level:** Applying **Client Need:** Physiological Adaptation **Integrated Process:** Nursing Process: Assessment **Content Area:** Adult Health **Strategy:** The stoma is live tissue and should resemble normal bowel. Any stoma deprived of oxygen will take on the characteristics of all tissues with an inadequate oxygen supply. **Reference:** LeMone, P., Burke, K., & Bauldoff, G. (2011). *Medical-surgical nursing: Critical thinking in patient care* (5th ed.). Upper Saddle River, NJ: Pearson Education, pp. 704–705.

5 **Answer: 2, 5** **Rationale:** Left-sided abdominal pain, a palpable mass in the lower left quadrant, abdominal distention and a low-grade fever are consistent with the diagnosis of diverticulitis and do not need to be reported to the health care provider. If perforation occurs, abdominal pain is generalized and the fever will be above 101°F. Other symptoms may include tachycardia, tachypnea, a change in behavior or lethargy, increasing abdominal distention, a decrease or change in quality of bowel sounds, and/or increasing tenderness or guarding. **Cognitive Level:** Analyzing **Client Need:** Physiological Adaptation **Integrated Process:** Nursing Process: Assessment **Content Area:** Adult Health **Strategy:** Distinguish between assessment findings consistent with the admission diagnosis and those that indicate a possible complication. **Reference:** LeMone, P., Burke, K., & Bauldoff, G. (2011). *Medical-surgical nursing: Critical thinking in patient care* (5th ed.). Upper Saddle River, NJ: Pearson Education, pp. 692–695.

6 **Answer: 1** **Rationale:** Undernutrition affects many systems, causing decreases in metabolic function and cell-mediated and humoral immunity, thereby increasing the susceptibility to infection. The client with malabsorption may have

fat-laden diarrhea stools as a presenting symptom. Tumor formation may be a cause of malabsorption syndrome, but does not occur as a result of it. Inflammatory bowel diseases are a cause of malnutrition, not a result of it. **Cognitive Level:** Analyzing **Client Need:** Physiological Adaptation **Integrated Process:** Nursing Process: Diagnosis **Content Area:** Adult Health **Strategy:** Adequate nutrition is needed for all activities of the human body. Eliminate answer options that are symptoms of a problem. Select the answer option that has the broadest view. **Reference:** LeMone, P., Burke, K., & Bauldoff, G. (2011). *Medical-surgical nursing: Critical thinking in patient care* (5th ed.). Upper Saddle River, NJ: Pearson Education, pp. 598–600.

7 **Answer: 4** **Rationale:** Famotidine is a histamine$_2$-receptor antagonist and reduces the secretion of gastric acid. This class of drugs does not have a direct effect on reflux, LES tone, or GI motility. Metoclopramide improves GI motility. Sucralfate coats the ulcer. Antacids neutralize the hydrochloric acid in the stomach. **Cognitive Level:** Applying **Client Need:** Pharmacological and Parenteral Therapies **Integrated Process:** Nursing Process: Planning **Content Area:** Adult Health **Strategy:** List the medications commonly used in GERD and their mechanisms of action. Compare this information to each of the answer options until the action of famotidine is identified. **Reference:** LeMone, P., Burke, K., & Bauldoff, G. (2011). *Medical-surgical nursing: Critical thinking in patient care* (5th ed.). Upper Saddle River, NJ: Pearson Education, pp. 625, 638.

8 **Answer: 2** **Rationale:** Many common substances contribute to decreased LES tone including fatty foods, caffeinated beverages, nicotine, beta-adrenergic blocking agents, calcium channel blockers, nitrates, theophylline, peppermint, alcohol, high levels of estrogen and progesterone, and anticholinergic drugs. Antidepressants, antiestrogen agents, and alpha-adrenergic blockers have no effect on LES tone. **Cognitive Level:** Applying **Client Need:** Pharmacological and Parenteral Therapies **Integrated Process:** Nursing Process: Implementation **Content Area:** Adult Health **Strategy:** Identify how the lower esophageal sphincter contributes to the symptoms of GERD. Select the drug that increases that effect. **Reference:** Osborn, K. S., Wraa, C. E., & Watson, A. (2010). *Medical surgical nursing: Preparation for practice*. Upper Saddle River, NJ: Pearson Education, pp. 1387–1388.

9 **Answer: 3** **Rationale:** There is no known cause of IBS, and diagnosis is made by excluding all the other diseases that cause the symptoms. There is no inflammation of the bowel. Some factors exacerbate the symptoms, including anxiety, fear, stress, depression, some foods and drugs, but these do not cause the disease. **Cognitive Level:** Applying **Client Need:** Physiological Adaptation **Integrated Process:** Nursing Process: Assessment **Content Area:** Adult Health **Strategy:** Differentiate the forms of inflammatory bowel disease and causative factors versus exacerbating factors. **Reference:** LeMone, P., Burke, K., & Bauldoff,

G. (2011). *Medical-surgical nursing: Critical thinking in patient care* (5th ed.). Upper Saddle River, NJ: Pearson Education, pp. 660–661.

10 Answer: 2 Rationale: Sulfasalazine is a GI anti-inflammatory medication that exerts its action by decreasing prostaglandin production in the bowel (which results in decreased inflammation). Peristalsis is decreased by anticholinergic agents. Analgesics affect pain impulses. Endorphin release is not a result of sulfasalazine.

Cognitive Level: Applying **Client Need:** Pharmacological and Parenteral Therapies **Integrated Process:** Nursing Process: Implementation **Content Area:** Adult Health **Strategy:** Review the goals of treatment for inflammatory bowel disease. Select the answer option that works directly to decrease the inflammatory response. **Reference:** LeMone, P., Burke, K., & Bauldoff, G. (2011). *Medical-surgical nursing: Critical thinking in patient care* (5th ed.). Upper Saddle River, NJ: Pearson Education, pp. 684–685.

References

Berman, A., & Snyder, S. (2012). *Kozier & Erb's fundamentals of nursing: Concepts, process, and practice* (9th ed.). Upper Saddle River, NJ: Pearson Education.

D'Amico, D. & Barbarito, C. (2012). *Health & physical assessment in nursing* (2nd ed.). Upper Saddle River, NJ: Pearson Education.

Ignatavicius, D. D., & Workman, M. L. (2013). *Medical-surgical nursing: Critical thinking for collaborative care* (7th ed.) Philadelphia: W. B. Saunders Company.

Kee, J. L. (2010). *Laboratory and diagnostic tests* (8th ed.). Upper Saddle River, NJ: Pearson Education.

Lehne, R. (2010). *Pharmacology for nursing care* (7th ed.). St. Louis, MO: Saunders.

LeMone, P., Burke, K., & Bauldoff, G. (2011). *Medical surgical nursing: Critical thinking in patient care* (5th ed.). Upper Saddle River, NJ: Pearson Education.

Lewis, S., Dirksen, S. Heitkemper, M., Bucher, L. & Camera, I. (2011). *Medical surgical nursing: Assessment and management of clinical problems* (8th ed.). St. Louis, MO: Elsevier.

McCance, K. L., & Huether, S. E. (2010). *Pathophysiology: The biologic basis for disease in adults and children* (6th ed.). St. Louis, MO: Mosby, Inc.

Osborn, K. S., Wraa, C. E., & Watson, A. (2010). *Medical surgical nursing: Preparation for practice.* Upper Saddle River, NJ: Pearson Education.

Smith, S. F., Duell, D. J., & Martin, B. C. (2012). *Clinical nursing skills: Basic to advanced skills* (8th ed.). Upper Saddle River, NJ: Pearson Education.

Musculoskeletal Disorders

Chapter Outline

NCLEX-RN® Test Prep

Use the accompanying online resource, NursingReviewsandRationales, to test yourself with hundreds of NCLEX®-style practice questions.

Objectives

➤ Identify basic structures and functions of the musculoskeletal system.
➤ Describe the pathophysiology and etiology of common musculoskeletal disorders.
➤ Discuss expected assessment data and diagnostic test findings for selected musculoskeletal disorders.
➤ Identify priority nursing problems for selected musculoskeletal disorders.
➤ Discuss therapeutic management of selected musculoskeletal disorders.
➤ Discuss nursing management of a client experiencing a musculoskeletal disorder.
➤ Identify expected outcomes for the client experiencing a musculoskeletal disorder.

Review at a Glance

arthrocentesis a surgical procedure to remove fluid from joint to reduce swelling and pain and/or to obtain fluid for examination using sterile technique

arthrogram injection of contrast media into joint cavity to examine joint structures through a series of x-rays

arthroscopy a surgical procedure used to examine internal structure of a joint using an arthroscope

Bouchard's nodes raised bony growths over proximal interphalangeal joint of hand seen less frequently than Heberden's nodes in osteoarthritis

cancellous bone a spongy bone resulting from structural units fitting loosely together leaving many spaces between thin processes and labyrinth of bone tissue

compact bone a dense structured bone resulting from structural units fitted closely together

compartment syndrome occurs when circulation to a compartment is impeded due to excessive pressure against the nonelastic fascia; compartment pressure exceeds 30 mmHg (normal 10–20 mmHg), resulting in tissue death and nerve injury

countertraction a pulling force exerted in opposite direction to prevent client from sliding to end of bed

crepitation a grating or soft popping sound caused by splinters of a fractured bone or rough joint surfaces rubbing against other structures or by air entering subcutaneous tissue in a compound fracture

degenerative joint disease a slowly progressive disorder of articulating joints, especially weight-bearing joints, primarily affecting middle-aged to older adults

gout a metabolic disorder characterized by elevated uric acid levels in blood resulting in deposition of urate crystals in synovial fluid and joint tissues

Heberden's nodes raised bony growths over distal interphalangeal joints that occur frequently in osteoarthritis and are a common manifestation in women

internal fixation a surgically implanted fracture immobilization device to realign a fracture

laminectomy a surgical incision of lamina primarily done to relieve symptoms related to an intervertebral disc

osteitis deformans also known as Paget's disease, a chronic skeletal bone disease resulting in enlarged and deformed bones

osteomyelitis an acute or chronic infection of bone usually caused by *Staphylococcus aureus* organism

osteoporosis disease characterized by low bone mass and structural deterioration of bone tissue causing bone to become fragile and susceptible to fractures

sprain a stretching and/or tearing of a ligament

strain a stretching or tearing of muscle fibers

traction direct pulling force applied to a fractured extremity that results in realignment of bone

PRETEST

1. The primary care provider determines that a 55-year-old female client is experiencing menopause and is also at risk for osteoporosis. What foods other than milk can the nurse suggest to this client to increase calcium intake?
   1. Seafood, wheat, corn, green vegetables
   2. Chicken, green vegetables, pasta, broccoli
   3. Green vegetables, sardines, salmon with bone, molasses
   4. Fresh fruits, English muffins, black beans, asparagus

2. The nurse is conducting a class on health promotion. Which risk factors identified by the nurse would put a client at risk for developing osteoporosis? Select all that apply.
   1. Menopause
   2. Sedentary lifestyle
   3. Decreased intake of calcium
   4. Use of glucocorticoids
   5. Increased fluid intake

3. Alendronate (Fosamax) is ordered for a client with osteoporosis. Which information should the nurse include in teaching the client about the medication?
   1. Acts as a selective estrogen receptor modulator
   2. Reduces risk of invasive breast cancer
   3. May be obtained as a nasal spray
   4. Inhibits bone resorption

4. The nurse is providing discharge instructions to a client who had a hip replacement. The nurse should teach the client to avoid what activity to prevent dislocation of the hip?
   1. Crossing the legs at the knees
   2. Taking leisurely walks
   3. Sitting in a chair that has arms
   4. Using a raised toilet seat

5. A client with a total hip replacement is concerned about dislocation of the prosthesis. The nurse should include which information in a response?
   1. Activities that involve hip adduction may cause hip dislocation.
   2. Using elevated toilet seats may cause hip dislocation.
   3. Exercises that involve bending are useful in preventing dislocation.
   4. Removing the foam abduction pillow will prevent hip dislocation.

6. A client has undergone a lumbar laminectomy and has just returned to the nursing unit. In performing initial postoperative care, what would be the nurse's highest priority?
   1. Instituting early ambulation
   2. Calculating IV fluid totals
   3. Performing neurovascular checks
   4. Assessing bladder function

7 A client in skeletal traction slides down in the bed so that the feet touch the foot of the bed. What should the nurse do to ensure that the pull of traction remains uninterrupted?

1. Release weights, pull client up in bed, and then reapply weights.
2. Ask provider for a change in the amount of weight ordered.
3. Move client up in bed without releasing pull of traction on the extremity.
4. Elevate client's feet on a pillow.

8 The nurse is preparing a teaching plan for a client who is being discharged following a total hip replacement. The nurse would include which of the following content as part of the teaching plan? Select all that apply.

1. Avoid low, cushioned chairs.
2. Use a device that raises the toilet seat.
3. Avoid bending greater than 90 degrees.
4. Turn at the waist to reach objects.
5. Do not cross the legs.

9 A client with a recently applied plaster leg cast reports unrelieved pain and paresthesia in the affected extremity. The assessment by the nurse reveals diminished pulse, pallor, and increased pain on passive motion. What should the nurse do first?

1. Monitor client for the next hour.
2. Administer an analgesic for pain.
3. Administer an anxiolytic.
4. Notify primary care provider immediately.

10 The nurse is caring for a client who had open reduction and internal fixation (ORIF) of the right femur. The client reports intense pain, swelling, tenderness, and warmth at the site; chills; malaise; and has a temperature of 102.2°F (39°C) and leukocytosis. The nurse concludes that this data is consistent with which complication?

1. Fat embolism
2. Gastrointestinal (GI) bleeding
3. Osteomyelitis
4. Malunion of the bone

➤ *See pages 309–310 for Answers and Rationales.*

I. OVERVIEW OF ANATOMY AND PHYSIOLOGY

A. Skeleton
1. Supports framework of body and protects soft tissue and vital organs and is composed primarily of calcium phosphate and calcium carbonate
2. Bones, joints, and cartilage are primary components of skeleton
3. Serves as storage for calcium, playing a major role in serum calcium balance
4. Serves also as a stable point of attachment for muscles

B. Classification of bones
1. Two major classifications of bones are based on structure—**compact bone** (dense) or **cancellous bone** (spongy)
2. Structural units of compact bone fit closely together resulting in a dense bone composition
3. Structural units of cancellous bone fit loosely together, leaving many open spaces between thin processes and labyrinth of bone tissue
4. A central shaft (diaphysis) and 2 end portions (epiphyseals) characterize long bones (examples: humerus and radius)
5. Short bones are characterized by cancellous bone covered by a thin layer of compact bone (examples: carpals and tarsals)
6. Flat bones are characterized by two layers of compact bone separated by a layer of cancellous bone (examples: skull, ribs, scapula, and sternum)

C. Bone marrow
  1. Soft, spongy, highly cellular blood-forming tissue that fills cavity of bones and is site for hematopoiesis (red blood cell [RBC] production) and storage of RBCs
  2. Responsible for production of RBCs, white blood cells, and platelets
  3. Becomes predominantly fatty with age, particularly in long bones of limb
D. Axial section
  1. Each vertebra is constructed like a ring, set one on top of another with a padding of cartilage between; vertebral rings are studded with bony projections called processes, which function as attachments for muscles and points of articulation with bones
  2. Twelve pairs of ribs attach to thoracic vertebrae; the upper 7 opposing pairs attach at front to sternum; 3 of remaining 5 pairs attach to ribs immediately above by cartilage, and last 2 pairs are unattached
E. Appendicular section: connected to axial skeleton by bones of upper and lower extremities
  1. Shoulder girdle supports arms
  2. Humerus is upper arm bone; ulna and radius are forearm bones
  3. Each innominate bone (hip bone) consists of 3 parts—ileum, ischium, and pubis; innominate bones unite with sacrum and coccyx of vertebral column to form pelvic girdle, which supports legs
F. Joint articulations
  1. Result when 2 bones are joined together; categorized by type of motion
  2. Composed of fibrous connective tissue and cartilage (dense avascular connective tissue) that covers ends of bones making movement smooth
  3. Joint cavity secretes synovial fluid to lubricate joint and reduce friction
  4. Other information about joints
    a. Some joints have no movement after fusion occurs, for example, the skull
    b. Pivot joint permits head to rotate from side to side around a single axis
    c. Hinge joint of elbow, knee, or jaw permits back and forth or up and down movement
    d. Wrist produces a gliding motion in which one bone glides a short distance over another
    e. Shoulder and hip joints are ball and socket joints; ball-shaped end of one bone fits into socket at end of another bone
G. Ligaments and tendons
  1. Ligaments are bands of rigid connective tissue that hold joints together allowing for movement and stability
  2. Ligaments have a relatively poor blood supply, which significantly prolongs healing process after injury
  3. Tendons are bands of fibrous tissue that connect muscles to bones
H. Muscles
  1. Muscle is a tissue that primarily functions as a source of power and pull against bones to make body move
  2. There are 3 primary types of muscle: skeletal muscle (striated, voluntary) moves extremities and external areas of body; cardiac muscle (striated, involuntary) is found in heart; smooth muscle (nonstriated, involuntary) is found in walls of arteries and bowel

II. DIAGNOSTIC TESTS AND ASSESSMENTS

A. Radiologic tests
  1. Diagnostic studies performed using x-rays, with or without injection of contrast media, to detect musculoskeletal problems and monitor effectiveness of treatment
  2. X-ray (radiograph): most common and widely used radiologic test for assessment of musculoskeletal problems and effectiveness of treatment

B. EMG (electromyogram or myogram): records and evaluates electrical activity of muscles during contraction; is used to differentiate between muscle dysfunction and nerve dysfunction
1. Detects abnormal electrical activity in muscle
2. There are 2 different types of EMG: intramuscular (IM) EMG (more commonly used) and surface EMG (SEMG)
3. IM EMG: long, small-gauge needles are inserted through skin into muscle
4. SEMG: electrodes are placed above muscle to detect electrical activity
5. Needles detect electrical activity of muscle and transmit information to electromyogram machine; electrical activity is displayed visually on an oscilloscope or heard audibly through an audiotransmitter (microphone)

C. *Arthroscopy*: a surgical procedure used to examine internal structure of a joint using an arthroscope (a pencil-sized device with optical fibers and lenses), which is inserted into very small skin incisions; device is connected to a video camera to allow for visualization of joint interior
1. Procedure may be used for diagnosis or treatment of musculoskeletal disorders such as osteoarthritis, rheumatoid arthritis, infectious types of arthritis, and internal joint injuries like meniscus tears, ligament strains or tears, and cartilage deterioration
2. Arthroscopic surgery can be done during procedure to repair joint tissue; arthroscopic surgery creates less tissue trauma, less pain, and allows for a rapid recovery
3. Client education: postprocedure
   a. Take analgesics for comfort and limit activity as directed
   b. Observe site for hematoma or bleeding
   c. How to perform neurovascular assessment (temperature, color, capillary refill, movement, and sensation) on affected extremity
   d. Signs and symptoms of infection to report: elevated temperature, warmth at injection site, purulent discharge, and redness

D. *Arthrogram*: contrast media or air is injected into joint cavity to allow for visualization of joint structures; client moves joint through a series of movements while a series of x-rays are taken; assess for allergy to contrast media preprocedure
1. Client education preprocedure: if injected contrast dye is used, inform client that once dye is injected there may be a feeling of warmth, nausea, headache, salty taste in mouth, itching, hives, and rash throughout body (symptoms are usually temporary and will be treated if necessary)
2. Client education postprocedure
   a. Temporary discoloration of skin and urine is normal after injection of dye; increase fluids to eliminate contrast
   b. How to perform neurovascular assessment on affected extremity

E. CT scan (computerized axial tomography): combines x-rays with computer technology to produce a highly detailed, cross-sectional image of internal organs and structures of body
1. Body is visualized from skin to central part of body being examined; recorded image is called a "tomogram"
2. Client education
   a. If ingested contrast medium is used, client should increase fluid intake to assist in elimination of medium
   b. Monitor for evacuation of contrast media and possible constipation
   c. Initial stools may be white in color if barium is used, which is normal until all contrast media is evacuated

F. MRI (magnetic resonance imaging): radiologic technique (without radiation) that uses magnetism, radio waves, and a computer to produce cross-sectional images of body structures
1. Machine is extremely noisy and may cause or exacerbate a claustrophobic sensation
2. Client education

Practice to Pass

The nurse is preparing a client for a CT scan. What information should the nurse include in client teaching about this procedure?

     a. Information about procedure; a mild sedative may be given preprocedure to help decrease any anxiety associated with a claustrophobic feeling

     b. Notify provider of any metallic body parts such as implants, pacemakers, artificial joints, metallic bone plates, prosthetic devices, surgical clips, bullet fragments, metallic clips, or other metal objects within body that can distort MRI image or affect magnetic field

Practice to Pass

It is important that the nurse know that the MRI procedure is contraindicated for which clients?

G. Bone scan: technique used to create images of bones on a computer screen or on a film using a small amount of radioactive material that travels through bloodstream

     1. Radioactive material is especially absorbed in abnormal areas of a bone; degree of radio-contrast absorption is related to amount of blood flow to bone

     2. A camera scans entire body and a recording is made on a special film

     3. Increased radio-contrast absorption is seen with osteomyelitis, osteoporosis, fractures, Paget's disease, and cancer of bone

H. *Arthrocentesis* (joint aspiration) and analysis: fluid is removed from joint to reduce swelling and pain and/or obtain fluid for examination using a sterile needle and syringe

     1. Postprocedure complications are uncommon but may include localized bruising, minor bleeding into joint cavity, and loss of pigment at injection site (septic arthritis is a rare but serious complication)

     2. Client education

        a. If cortisone was injected into joint, monitor for inflammation of injected area, atrophy or loss of pigment at injection site, and increased blood glucose

        b. Follow postprocedure activity restrictions as directed by health care provider

        c. Monitor for postprocedure complications and check dressing for excessive bleeding

III. LABORATORY STUDIES

     A. Antinuclear antibodies (ANA): sensitive screening blood test used to detect autoimmune disease

        1. ANAs destroy nucleus (innermost core of cell that contains DNA) of cells

        2. Test not definitive but suggests presence of auto-antibodies (antibodies directed against body's own tissue)

        3. Present in clients with a number of autoimmune diseases such as rheumatoid arthritis, systemic lupus erythematosus, scleroderma, and others

     B. Calcium (Ca⁺⁺): one of the most abundant electrolytes in body that causes neuromuscular irritability and contractions; adult normal reference value is 9–11 mg/dL but may vary slightly among agencies

        1. Stored in bone and gives bone stability

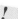

        2. Decreased calcium levels may be found in osteomalacia, inadequate dietary intake of calcium, renal disease, and hypoparathyroidism

        3. Increased calcium levels may be seen in bone neoplasm, multiple fractures, immobilization, renal calculi, and hyperparathyroidism

     C. Phosphorus (2.5–4.5 mg/dL is normal reference range): level is often compared with other electrolytes in body (such as calcium)

        1. Much of total phosphorus in body is combined with calcium in teeth and bones

        2. Decreased levels can be seen with hypercalcemia, starvation, malabsorption syndrome, osteomalacia, and vitamin D deficiency

        3. Increased levels can be seen with healing fractures, metastatic bone tumors, renal failure, and hypocalcemia

     D. Rheumatoid factor (RF) (normal—negative or less than 1:20): screening blood test used to detect antibodies (IgM, IgG, or IgA) found in clients with rheumatoid arthritis; elevated RF level may indicate diseases other than rheumatoid arthritis

E. **Erythrocyte sedimentation rate (ESR)**: normal is less than 20 mm/hr; gender variations exist; nonspecific serologic test that measures rate at which RBCs settle out of unclotted blood in mm/hr; elevated levels indicate inflammatory process in diseases such as rheumatoid arthritis and osteomyelitis

F. **Uric acid** (normal male 4.5–6.5 mg/dL, female 2.5–5.5 mg/dL): generally used to monitor treatment of gout and may be used to diagnose other health problems
   1. Uric acid is end product of purine metabolism; kidneys normally excrete excess uric acid
   2. Hyperuricemia (elevated urine or serum uric acid levels) occurs because of poor renal function, excessive purine metabolism, and/or excessive dietary intake of purine foods
   3. Elevated uric acid level is seen in gout

IV. COMMON NURSING TECHNIQUES AND PROCEDURES

A. **Instructing client on the use of crutches**
   1. Crutch gaits provide a safe method of walking using crutches, alternating body weight on one or both legs and crutches
   2. See Box 9-1 for crutch walking techniques, Box 9-2 for transfer techniques (getting in and out of a chair) using crutches, and Box 9-3 for negotiating stairs while using crutches

---

Box 9-1
Instructions for the Client on the Use of Crutches

4-Point Gait
- Slow gait
- Requires good coordination
- Weight-bearing is on both legs
- Move each foot and crutch forward separately (right crutch, left foot; left crutch, right foot)

2-Point Gait
- Faster than 4-point gait
- Requires more balance
- There is partial weight bearing on each foot
- Arm movements simulate arm movement when walking
- Move left crutch and right foot forward together; move right crutch and left foot forward together

3-Point Gait
- Fast gait
- Two crutches and unaffected leg bear weight alternately
- Weaker leg and both crutches move together followed by stronger leg

Swing-To Gait
- Fast gait
- Used by clients with paralysis of legs and hips
- Prolonged use may lead to atrophy of unused muscles
- Advance crutches forward together, lift body using arms, then swing to meet crutches

Swing-Through Gait
- Fast gait
- Good balance, skill, coordination, and strength required
- Move both crutches forward together
- Lift body using arms, then swing through and beyond crutches

| Box 9-2 | **Getting Into a Chair** |

Transfer Techniques for Clients with Crutches

Getting Into a Chair

1. Use chair with armrests and support back of chair against a wall for stability.
2. Center back part of unaffected leg against chair.
3. Transfer crutches to hand on affected side.
4. Hold crutches by horizontal hand bars.
5. Grasp arm of chair with hand on unaffected side.
6. Lean forward, flex knees and hips, and lower into chair.

Getting Out of a Chair

1. Move forward to edge of chair.
2. Place unaffected leg slightly under or at edge of chair (this position helps client to stand up from chair and achieve balance, since unaffected leg is supported against edge of chair).
3. Grasp crutches by horizontal hand bars using hand on affected side.
4. Grasp arm of chair using hand on unaffected side (body weight is placed on crutches and hand on armrest to support unaffected leg when client rises to stand).
5. Push down on crutches and chair armrest while raising body out of chair.
6. Assume a *tripod position* (crutches out laterally and to front of feet, approximately 6–10 inches, with feet slightly apart creating a wide base of support) for balance before moving.

Box 9-3

Instructions for Clients with Crutches: Negotiating Stairs

Going Up Stairs (stand behind client slightly to affected side for support if needed)

1. Assume tripod position.
2. Transfer weight to crutches and move unaffected leg onto step.
3. Transfer weight to unaffected leg on step and move crutches and affected leg up to step.
4. Repeat steps 2 and 3 until client reaches top of stairs.

Going Down Stairs (stand one step below client on affected side for support if needed)

1. Assume tripod position at top of stairs.
2. Shift weight to unaffected leg.
3. Move crutches and the affected leg down onto next step.
4. Transfer weight to crutches and move unaffected leg to that step.
5. Repeat steps 2 and 3 until client reaches bottom step.

B. *Traction*: direct pulling force applied to a fractured extremity that results in realignment of bone; see Figure 9-1
   1. Reduces fracture, lessens muscle spasms, relieves pain, corrects deformities, promotes rest, and allows for exercise
   2. Skin and skeletal traction are most commonly used; manual traction is only used briefly under health care provider direction
      a. Skin traction (using tape, boots, splints); also called straight traction

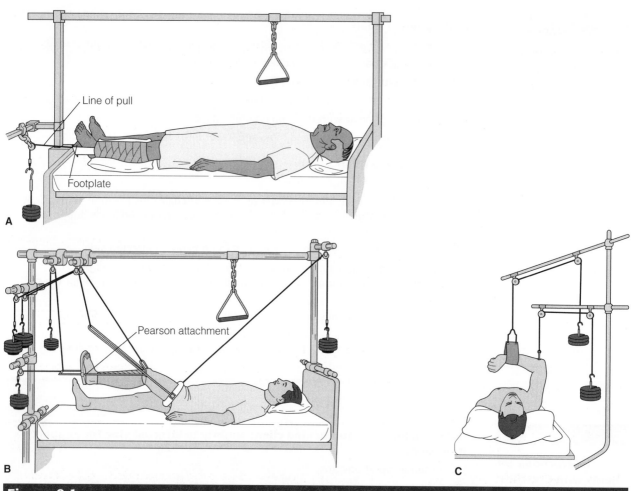

Line of pull

Footplate

A

Pearson attachment

B

C

Figure 9-1

Traction is the application of a pulling force to maintain bone alignment during fracture healing. Different fractures require different types of traction. A. Skin traction (also called straight traction), such as Buck's traction shown here, is often used for hip fractures, B. Balanced suspension traction is commonly used for fractures of the femur, C. Skeletal traction, in which the pulling force is applied directly to the bone, may be used to treat fractures of the humerus.

   1) Assists in reduction of a fracture (does not primarily achieve reduction) and helps decrease muscle spasms

   2) Generally used for short-term treatment (48–72 hours) and is applied directly to skin

   3) Weights range from 5–10 pounds

   4) Most common type is Buck's traction

 b. Skeletal traction (using pins or wires inserted into bones)

   1) Indicated for long-term use

   2) Used to align injured bones and joints or to treat joint contractures and congenital hip dysplasia

   3) Weights range from 5–45 pounds and amounts of weight may be adjusted initially until full fracture reduction is achieved by x-ray results

c. Balanced suspension (traction that is a hanging support to immobilize body part in a desired position)
   1) Used with skeletal traction to improve mobility while maintaining alignment of fracture
   2) Body part is suspended using splints, ropes, and weights
   3) Client able to perform activities such as toileting and personal hygiene; bed linen can be changed without disturbing traction alignment

d. **Countertraction**: pulling force exerted in opposite direction to prevent client from sliding to end of bed; examples of countertraction include client's weight, elevating foot of bed (Trendelenburg), and elevating head of bed with cervical traction

e. See Box 9-4 for nursing care of client in traction

C. **Cast care**: a cast is applied for immobilization to ensure stability of a fracture; see Box 9-5 for associated nursing care

D. **Splinting and immobilization**: like casts, splints are used to immobilize a fractured extremity to ensure stability after closed reduction and external fixation; teach client how to perform neurovascular assessment (color, temperature, capillary refill, and pulses)

Box 9-4	
Nursing Care of the Client in Traction	• Ensure that all ropes, weights, and pulleys are hanging freely, not shredded or torn, in a straight line.
	• Bed linen should be kept off traction ropes.
	• Teach client that weights should not be lifted for any reason (lifting of weights alters the line of pull and could potentially interfere with bone healing).
	• Ensure that prescribed amount of weight is maintained at all times.
	• Avoid jarring bed or equipment.
	• Ensure that knots are not lying on or near the pulley.
	• Perform neurovascular assessment to monitor for superficial nerve damage (radial, median, ulnar, femoral, sciatic, peroneal nerves).
	• Teach client how to perform circulatory assessment on unaffected and affected limb, comparing observations (color, temperature, capillary refill, pulses)
	• Teach client how to perform skin assessment to monitor and prevent skin breakdown on bony prominence and pressure areas.
	• Ensure that body is always kept in proper alignment to prevent complications such as external rotation of the joint, increased pain, and poor healing of the fracture.
	• Teach client how to monitor for infection at pin sites (fever, localized warmth, redness, swelling, abnormal drainage, and odor).
	• Inform client to avoid massaging calves or reddened areas to prevent clot dislodgment caused by venous stasis.
	• Encourage client to increase fluid intake (2,500 mL/day unless contraindicated) and roughage (fresh fruits and vegetables) in diet to prevent constipation, urinary tract infection, and renal calculi.
	• Teach client how to perform deep-breathing and coughing exercises to prevent respiratory complications.
	• Encourage client to use the overhead trapeze (and unaffected leg if possible) to reposition for comfort, shift weight to prevent skin breakdown, perform exercises, and assist with personal care, toileting, and bed linen changes.
	• Encourage client to adhere to exercise regimen to maintain muscle tone, endurance, and prevent bone demineralization.
	• Provide diversional activities and encourage social interaction with family and friends to prevent potential isolation.

Box 9-5	• Teach client that cast made from plaster of Paris should not get wet and that cast padding should not be removed; if cast becomes soiled with feces, clean with a damp cloth or rub baking soda on soiled area to limit odor.
Nursing Care of the Client in a Cast	• Teach client that no foreign objects should be inserted into cast (sticks, food crumbs, etc.) to prevent skin breakdown; teach client how to smooth rough edges.

• Instruct client to avoid covering a new cast with blanket or plastic for extended periods (air cannot circulate, and heat builds up in the cast).

• Turn client from side to side (using palms not fingertips) every 2 hours to facilitate drying for the first 24–72 hours (use of fingertips causes indentation and pressure areas when cast is dry).

• Instruct client to apply ice for the first 24 hours over fracture site to control edema, ensuring that ice is securely contained so cast does not become wet.

• Instruct client to elevate extremity above the level of the heart to promote venous return for the first 24 hours after application.

• Instruct client to perform active range of motion to joints above and below immobilized extremity.

• Teach client about signs and symptoms to report to health care provider: increasing pain in immobilized extremity, excessive swelling and discoloration of exposed limb, burning or tingling under cast, sores, or foul odor under cast.

V. NURSING MANAGEMENT OF CLIENT UNDERGOING MUSCULOSKELETAL SURGERY

A. *Laminectomy*: surgical incision of lamina done primarily to relieve symptoms related to herniated intervertebral disc

1. Assess effectiveness of pain management
2. Perform neurological and neurovascular assessment; monitor bowel and bladder function
3. Assess client for severe headache or leakage of cerebrospinal fluid (CSF), nausea, abdominal discomfort, incontinence, amount and character of drainage on dressing
4. Use *log roll* technique (turning a client as a unit) to turn and reposition client; maintain proper alignment of spine at all times
5. Inform client that bed rest may be maintained for first 24–48 hours after procedure; pillows may be used for comfort under thighs in supine position and between legs in side-lying position
6. Assist client to "rise as a unit" when getting out of bed (especially for first time)
7. Instruct client that paresthesias (numbness and tingling of extremities) may not be relieved immediately after procedure

B. **Internal fixation**: fracture immobilization with a metal device (made of screws, pins, and/or plates) that is surgically inserted to realign and maintain a fracture

1. Inform client that x-rays will be taken at regular intervals to ensure proper alignment of fixation device
2. Instruct client about signs and symptoms to report related to infection: elevated temperature, localized pain and warmth, tenderness, chills, malaise, and changes in neurovascular status of affected extremity

C. **External fixation**: surgical reduction of a fracture using an external fixation device to repair fractures

1. Consists of a frame attached to pins that are inserted into bone at 90-degree angle to long axis of bone; pins are usually inserted above and below fracture site

2. Allows for greater mobility while maintaining immobilization of fracture site

3. Because of presence of pins, care is similar to care of skeletal traction pins, and pin sites need to be assessed for infection; neurovascular status to extremity is also important to assess

D. **Joint replacement, total hip replacement (THR)**

1. THR is frequently performed for client with conditions such as rheumatoid arthritis, malignant bone tumors, arthritis associated with Paget's disease, juvenile rheumatoid arthritis, degenerative joint disease, and hip fractures

2. There are 2 approaches, open or laparoscopic; method is selected based on severity of condition and client status; advantage of laparoscopic approach is shorter anticipated rehabilitation

3. Advantages of THR: substantial relief of pain, improved function and quality of life

4. Teach client about plan for effective pain management and side effects/adverse effects of pain medications

5. Teach client about dislocation precautions

    a. Avoid extremes of internal rotation, adduction, and 90-degree flexion of affected hip for at least 4–6 weeks after procedure

    b. Prevent adduction: use an abduction pillow, avoid crossing legs, avoid twisting to reach for objects behind, avoid driving a car, and avoid taking tub baths for at least 4–6 weeks

    c. Modify equipment to avoid 90-degree hip flexion (raised toilet seats, platform under chair, use of reachers, long-handled shoehorns, and sock pullers)

6. Teach client about signs and symptoms to report to health care provider

    a. Infection: redness, swelling, abnormal drainage, foul odor, and elevated temperature

    b. Deep vein thrombosis (DVT): pain, sudden swelling in affected extremity, enlargement of superficial veins, skin discoloration, and localized warmth

7. Inform client that physical therapy exercises will begin on first postoperative day to restore and maintain range of motion (ROM), muscle strength, and mobility, and to prevent complications such as DVT

8. Instruct client that homecare management program will include:

    a. Ongoing nursing assessment of pain management

    b. Periodic dressing changes and monitoring for infection

    c. Monitoring and adjustment of coagulation status weekly if taking warfarin (Coumadin) and less often if taking enoxaparin (Lovenox), a low-molecular-weight heparin

    d. An exercise program assisted by a physical therapist to assess and restore muscle strength and ROM

9. Instruct client to inform all health care providers (such as dentists) of history of joint replacement surgery so that prophylactic antibiotics can be prescribed as necessary

10. Inform client that periodic x-rays will be required as follow-up throughout lifetime

E. **Amputation**

1. Provide client teaching about effective pain management techniques; signs and symptoms to report: redness, elevated temperature, and/or unusual, foul-smelling drainage; abrasions; and any other signs of skin breakdown

2. Teach client how to care for residual limb: wash daily using warm water and bacteriostatic soap, rinse and gently pat dry thoroughly, expose to air for at least 20 minutes after washing; avoid use of lotions, alcohol, powder, or oils unless prescribed by health care provider; change limb sock daily, wash sock using mild soap and dry flat, and discard sock that is in poor condition

3. Instruct client to perform upper extremity active ROM exercises daily

4. Instruct client to lie prone for 30 minutes 3–4 times/day (if client is able and if part of standard of care) and avoid elevating or sitting with residual limb on pillows to prevent flexion contractures

5. Tell client that pain may persist in amputated extremity (phantom limb pain) and that this is normal and real; the discomfort will be treated with analgesics or other interventions

VI. DISORDERS OF MUSCULOSKELETAL SYSTEM

A. *Osteoporosis* (porous bone)

1. Description
   a. Disease characterized by low bone mass and structural deterioration of bone tissue, causing bone (especially weight-bearing bones such as hip, spine, and wrist) to become fragile and more susceptible to fractures
   b. Affects both women and men; however, women are at greater risk after menopause

2. Etiology and pathophysiology
   a. As people age, bone resorption happens faster than bone formation, which causes bone to lose Ca^{++} and bone density; since most body calcium is stored in bones and teeth, this rapid bone resorption leads to porous bone or osteoporosis
   b. When serum Ca^{++} decreases, body takes stored Ca^{++} from bone

3. Assessment
   a. Risk factors include female gender; increasing age; thin, small body frame; Caucasian or Asian American ethnicity; family history; inadequate dietary intake of calcium and vitamin D; sedentary lifestyle; smoking; excessive alcohol intake; steroid medications; postmenopausal state; chronic liver disease; anorexia; and malabsorption
   b. Females are at a higher risk for osteoporosis than men
      1) Women have smaller body frames, which contribute to less bone density
      2) Bone resorption begins at an earlier age in women and is accelerated in menopause
      3) Breastfeeding and pregnancy deplete skeletal reserves unless calcium intake is increased to match demands
      4) Since currently women often live longer than men, longevity increases likelihood of osteoporosis

4. Priority nursing problems: pain, reduced mobility, potential for injury, insufficient nutrients to meet bodily needs

5. Planning and implementation
   a. Provide client teaching about prevention: take adequate amounts of Ca^{++} throughout lifetime to decrease incidence of osteoporosis; proper nutrition for adequate calcium intake; weight-bearing exercises to force Ca^{++} back into bone; safety measures to prevent falls that can result in fractures; bone mineral density (BMD) tests to measure bone mass in clients at risk for developing osteoporosis
   b. Provide clients with information about recommended daily dietary intake of calcium: Ca^{++} 1,000 mg/day for premenopausal and postmenopausal women taking estrogen replacement therapy (ERT), and 1,500 mg/day for postmenopausal women who are not taking ERT
   c. Provide information about foods high in Ca^{++} and importance of calcium intake with vitamin D: dark, green, leafy vegetables (such as broccoli, bok choy, collard greens, spinach); sardines; salmon with bone; dairy products (such as milk, cottage cheese, cheese, yogurt, and ice cream); Ca^{++} supplements can also be used to supplement dietary intake

  d. Provide information about vitamin D; key source is predominantly sunlight, but may need supplementation if living in moderate temperature or if obese or older adult

 6. Medication therapy

  a. Estrogen replacement therapy (ERT) might be used short-term to prevent osteoporosis after menopause

   1) Usually given in form of a pill or skin patch

   2) Decreases bone demineralization and symptoms of menopause

   3) Can increase risk for breast and endometrial cancer (progesterone may be given with estrogen, called hormone replacement therapy or HRT, to decrease risk)

   4) Client is at risk for developing DVT

  b. Calcitonin (Micalcin, Calcimar): naturally occurring hormone secreted by the thyroid gland; regulates calcium and bone metabolism

   1) Currently available as a nasal spray or injection

   2) Slows bone loss, increases spinal bone density, relieves pain from bone fractures, and reduces risk for spinal and hip fractures

   3) Side effects: flushing of face and hands, urinary frequency, nausea, skin rash (injectable), and nasal discharge/rhinorrhea (nasal spray)

  c. Alendronate (Fosamax): prevents bone resorption; used to treat both men and women with glucocorticoid-induced osteoporosis

  d. Raloxifene (Evista): used to prevent and treat osteoporosis; selective receptor modulator (SERM) that prevents bone loss; side effects are rare but may include hot flashes or DVT

  e. Risedronate sodium (Actonel): bisphosphonate, used to prevent and treat osteoporosis in postmenopausal women and glucocorticoid-induced osteoporosis in both men and women

   1) Slows and stops bone loss, increases mineral density and reduces risk of fractures

   2) Instruct client to take drug with a glass of water at least 30 minutes before first food or beverage of day and avoid eating for at least 30 minutes after taking medication

   3) Remain in an upright position for at least 30 minutes after taking dose

  f. Pamidronate (Aredia) and zoledronic acid (Zometa): parenteral bisphosphonates given at regular intervals to maintain calcium in bone tissue

 7. Client education

  a. Importance of weight-bearing exercises (jogging, walking, swimming, hiking, stair climbing, tennis, dancing, and weight training)

  b. Stop smoking

  c. Avoid excessive intake of alcohol

 8. Expected outcomes: client verbalizes decrease in pain, stops smoking, maintains optimal physical activity, and increases vitamin D and calcium intake

B. _Osteomyelitis_

 1. Description: acute or chronic infection of bone usually caused by _staphylococcus aureus_ organism

 2. Etiology and pathophysiology

  a. Infection can occur from direct or indirect invasion of infectious organisms; see Figure 9-2

  b. Direct invasion generally occurs from invasive procedures such as surgery (joint prosthesis, arthroplasty) and injuries such as fractures

  c. Infection can also be caused by indirect invasion (also referred to as hematogenous dissemination), where infection of bone tissue or joint is caused by spread of infectious organism through bloodstream from a preexisting infectious focus; course and virulence of infection is influenced by blood circulation to affected bone

Practice to Pass

What information should you include when teaching a 38-year-old female client about risk factors associated with osteoporosis and its prevention?

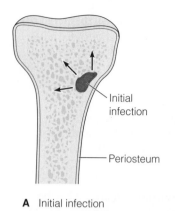
A Initial infection

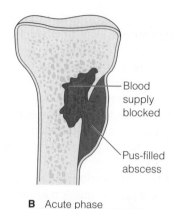
B Acute phase

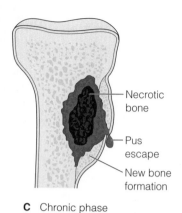
C Chronic phase

Figure 9-2

Osteomyelitis. A. Site of initial infection. Bacteria enter and multiply in the bone and the inflammatory response is initiated, B. Acute phase, in which infection spreads to other parts of the bone. Pus forms, edema occurs, and the vascular supply is compromised. If the infection reaches the outer margin of the bone, the periosteum is lifted, and ischemia and necrosis eventually occur, C. Chronic phase. Necrotic bone separates, a new layer of bone forms around the necrotic bone, and a sinus develops to allow the wound to drain.

  d. Long bones are common sites of infection in children, and spine, hip, and foot are common sites of infection in adults

  e. At-risk populations include children, older adults, and clients with weakened immune systems

  f. Osteomyelitis warrants aggressive immediate treatment with antibiotics or surgery (wound debridement) if infection of bone is extensive

 3. Assessment

  a. Observe for symptoms of local and/or systemic infection: elevated temperature, chills, restlessness, severe bone pain unrelieved by analgesics or rest and aggravated by movement, swelling, redness, and warmth at infection site

  b. Wound culture, bone scan, CT scan, and MRI provide information for diagnosis and assessment of extent of infection

4. Priority nursing problems: pain, fever, reduced mobility, inability to self-manage treatment plan, potential for interrupted skin integrity

5. Planning and implementation

  a. Explain all therapies and interventions to client and family to decrease anxiety and enhance cooperation with plan of care

  b. Use a rating scale to assess pain and evaluate effectiveness of pain management measures

  c. Provide ongoing education and emotional support because seriousness of infection, duration and uncertainty surrounding time for recuperation, potential complications, and associated risk can be a very fearful experience for client and family

  d. Teach client about risk factors for osteomyelitis, which include previous joint replacement surgery and implants

  e. Use sterile technique for all dressing changes and manipulation of affected limb; handle extremity very gently

  f. Avoid activities that increase circulation to affected area or cause edema, pain, and pathologic fractures, such as exercise, application of heat, or keeping extremity in dependent position

  g. Immobilize affected extremity as prescribed by provider and keep body in proper alignment

      h. Monitor temperature at least every 2 hours

      i. Provide cool environment, light clothing, antipyretic medication, antibiotics, and other therapies as prescribed and/or appropriate to keep temperature within client's baseline

      j. Keep client well hydrated to prevent dehydration from insensible water loss

      k. If long-term management is required, provide client with instructions about wound care using sterile technique, medication regimen (including instruction on venous access devices if needed), antibiotic administration, proper diet, rest, follow-up visits, and laboratory tests

      l. Provide information about adverse effects of antibiotic therapy such as ototoxicity and nephrotoxicity (aminoglycosides) and hepatotoxicity (cephalosporins)

      m. Instruct and assist client with interventions to prevent complications associated with immobility (turn and reposition every 2 hours, coughing and deep-breathing exercises, etc.)

  6. Medication therapy: indicated with or without surgical intervention and generally includes antibiotics and analgesics; reinforce information about adverse effects of antibiotic therapy as outlined in previous section

  7. Client education

      a. Importance of taking antibiotic medications as prescribed (for full duration) and to report adverse effects to prescriber

      b. Medication regimen

      c. Importance of rest and proper diet to facilitate healing, and prevent constipation and dehydration

      d. Importance of limb immobilization during treatment

  8. Expected outcomes/evaluation

      a. Client experiences satisfaction with pain management plan

      b. Client's temperature remains within normal range

      c. Physical mobility gradually returns to client's functional baseline

      d. Client states understanding of care plan and confidence in ability to effectively carry out home care program

C. Muscular dystrophy (MD)

  1. Description

      a. Group of genetic childhood disorders characterized by progressive muscle weakness, muscle wasting of symmetrical groups of muscles, and increasing disability and deformity

      b. Types of MD include Duchenne, myotonic, Becker's, limb girdle, and facioscapulohumeral; most common form is Duchenne MD

  2. Etiology and pathophysiology

      a. Inherited sex-linked group of disorders; significant risk factor is family history

      b. Each type differs in regard to age at onset, rate of progression, and pattern of inheritance

      c. Each type of MD affects specific muscle groups

  3. Assessment

      a. Muscle biopsy is primary test to confirm diagnosis (test shows degeneration of muscle fibers)

      b. EMG is used as a diagnostic test that identifies origin of muscle weakness (destruction of muscle or nerve damage; will show a decrease in amplitude)

      c. Creatinine kinase skeletal muscle isoenzyme (CK-MM) is elevated

      d. Ptosis (drooping of eyelid), impaired chewing and swallowing, abnormal gait, fatigue with minimal activity, frequent falls may all be observed and reported by parent or caregiver

      e. Delayed intellectual development is seen with some forms of MD

      f. Muscle contractures and deformities are common

      g. Abnormal curvature of spine (scoliosis or lordosis)

      h. Enlargement of calf muscle (pseudohypertrophy) caused by fatty infiltration causing muscular enlargement

      i. Cardiomyopathy or dysrhythmia may be present with some forms of MD

      j. Progressive muscle weakness, hypotonia (loss of muscle mass), and delayed development of motor skills such as walking may be observed and reported by parent or caregiver

4. Priority nursing problems: potential for aspiration, potential for injury, potential for infection, potential for alteration in respiratory pattern, reduced mobility, potential for interrupted skin integrity, potential for constipation, possible inability to participate in self-care activities, insufficient nutrients to meet bodily needs, possible adverse effects of disuse

5. Planning and implementation

      a. Care is focused on preserving and promoting mobility and preventing complications, there is no cure

      b. Provide support and assist family with decision-making process surrounding:

        1) Development of a home care plan to support as much independence as possible

        2) Modifications in home environment to support client's maximal functional ability

      c. Encourage family to actively involve client in care

      d. Family members may experience a myriad of emotions including fear, guilt, anger and blame; support family to enhance coping with client's progressively worsening disease; refer to local support groups including Muscular Dystrophy Association of America

      e. Assist client and family to cope with progressive, incapacitating, and fatal nature of disease, anticipate client will become wheelchair bound

      f. Encourage family to interact with client based on developmental and not chronological age

      g. Teach family strategies to prevent skin breakdown (frequent skin care and linen changes if incontinent, turn and reposition at least every 2 hours, use of protective skin barrier ointments, and adequate fluid intake)

      h. Perform passive ROM exercises to maintain function in unaffected extremities and prevent/delay contractures in affected extremities

6. Medication therapy: there is no effective pharmacological or other treatment; corticosteroids are often used to increase muscle strength

7. Client education

      a. Health care team members and roles, including those involved in home-care program for client

      b. Offer client soft foods and cut into small pieces to prevent aspiration and choking

      c. Family members should seek genetic counseling (parents, female siblings, maternal aunts, and female offspring)

      d. Assist family in decision making about appropriate clothing and footwear because of contractures and wheelchair-bound status

      e. Provide family with information on community support groups and agencies with respite services to prevent role strain

8. Expected outcomes

      a. Client is free from infection

      b. Client does not experience aspiration

      c. Client maintains as much independence with activities as possible

      d. Client experiences minimal or no complications of immobility (constipation, respiratory infection, contractures, preventable muscle wasting)

    e. Family verbalizes understanding of and confidence with home care program for client

    f. Family experiences minimal or no role strain in caring for client

D. Paget's disease (*osteitis deformans*)

    1. Description: a chronic skeletal bone disease with insidious onset often diagnosed around fourth decade of life; results in enlarged, deformed bones; generally affects skull, long bones, spine, and ribs

    2. Etiology and pathophysiology

        a. Cause of disease unknown; however, viral infection has been hypothesized as a probable etiology

        b. Hereditary factor: may be seen in more than one family member

        c. Early diagnosis and treatment is important to prevent disease progression and deformity

        d. Excessive bone resorption followed by bone formation leads to weakened bone, bone pain, arthritis, deformity, and potential pathologic fractures

        e. Normal bone marrow is replaced by vascular, fibrous, connective tissue that leads to formation of larger, disorganized, and weaker bone tissue

    3. Assessment

        a. X-ray is most definitive diagnostic test

        b. Initial diagnostic tests include serum alkaline phosphatase (elevated level is a positive indicator for disease)

        c. Bone scan may be done after positive serum alkaline phosphatase test (positive result will show characteristic abnormal appearance of bone for Paget's disease such as curved contours and thickened cortex)

        d. Positive bone scan prompts x-ray for definitive diagnosis

        e. Mild form of disease may be undetected because there may be no symptoms

        f. Symptoms include bone pain (most common) and other symptoms, depending on which bones are affected

            1) If skull is affected, headache and hearing loss may be reported as well as increasing head size

            2) Hip pain may be present if pelvis or femur is involved

            3) Bowing of lower extremities producing a waddling gait and curvature of spine may be seen in advanced stages of disease

        g. Arthritis may result because of damage to joint cartilage

        h. Complications are pathologic fractures (may be first indicator of disease) and osteogenic sarcoma (form of bone cancer)

    4. Priority nursing problems: pain, body image alterations, inadequate knowledge, potential for fractures

    5. Planning and implementation

        a. Prognosis is good especially if treatment is started before major deformity occurs

        b. Provide analgesics and muscle relaxants for comfort

        c. Administer medications as directed to control progression of disease (see medication section)

        d. Encourage client to take medication as directed by health care provider since deformity and loss of bone strength will continue without prescribed medications

        e. If skull is affected, assist with diet modification, dentures, and eating utensils since teeth may become weak from the disease

        f. Hearing aid may be recommended if hearing loss results from the disease

        g. Refer client and family to support group

    6. Medication therapy: drugs approved by U.S. Food and Drug Administration (FDA) include the bisphosphonates, etidronate disodium (Didronel), pamidronate disodium (Aredia), alendronate sodium (Fosamax), tiludronate disodium (Skelid), risedronate sodium (Actonel), and calcitonin (Miacalcin)

       7. Client education

          a. Plan for pain management

          b. Take analgesics as prescribed to enhance comfort

          c. Importance of a balanced diet, high in calcium (1,000–1,500 mg/day) and vitamin D (at least 600 units/day); vitamin D can be obtained from exposure to sunlight

          d. Inform health care provider of any history of kidney stones or disease before taking calcium

          e. Participate in an exercise program to maintain skeletal muscle health, ideal body weight, and joint mobility

          f. Sleep on a firm mattress if back discomfort is present; if back brace is needed, instruct client on prevention of skin breakdown under brace (undershirt) and safety measures (no driving with brace)

          g. Modify environment at home to prevent falls that may lead to subsequent fractures

          h. Participate in community support group as needed

       8. Expected outcomes

          a. Client is free of bone pain associated with the disease

          b. Client maintains ideal body weight

          c. Client verbalizes the importance of and adheres to a balanced diet including adequate intake of calcium, vitamin D, and protein

          d. Client verbalizes the importance of adhering to medication regimen to control progression of disease

          e. Client verbalizes an understanding of disease progression and ways to prevent progression

    E. Musculoskeletal trauma

       1. Fractures

          a. Description: a break in continuity of a bone

             1) Fractures may be classified as closed (simple fracture), in which bone breaks but skin remains intact, or open (compound fracture), in which broken ends of bone penetrate skin

             2) Fractures may also be classified by nature of injury (see Table 9-1)

          b. Etiology and pathophysiology

             1) Fractures occur in all age groups, although older adults are more prone to fractures resulting from falls

             2) When a bone breaks, the healing process occurs in 3 phases

                a) An inflammatory response is initiated (inflammatory phase)

                b) Calcium is deposited in area and osteoblasts promote new bone formation (reparative phase)

                c) Ends of fracture reunite (remodeling phase)

Table 9-1   **Classification of Fractures**

Classification	Description of Bone Injury
Avulsion	Fracture results from tearing of supporting tendons and ligaments
Comminuted	Broken bone fragments into more than 2 pieces
Compressed	Bone is crushed from force applied to bone during injury
Impacted	Ends of broken bone are driven into each other
Depressed	Bone structure is broken and pressed inward, such as with skull fracture
Spiral	Break spreads in a spiral fashion along bone shaft; is usually caused by sports injuries
Greenstick	An incomplete break in bone where one side splinters, leaving the other side bent or intact; more common in children

c. Assessment
1) Deformity: deformity may be caused by break in continuity of bone itself and the pull of muscles on fragmented bones
2) Edema and swelling may occur from bleeding into surrounding tissues
3) Pain, which may be severe, is caused by muscle spasms and nerve pressure
4) Crepitus may also be present on palpation; **crepitation** is a soft popping or grating sound created by movement of broken bone fragments
5) Muscle spasms may be noted near fractured bone
6) Ecchymosis or a bluish discoloration of area caused by blood extravasation into surrounding subcutaneous tissues
7) Possibly shock if blood loss is severe
d. Priority nursing problems: potential for reduced tissue perfusion, pain, reduced mobility, potential for infection, inability to endure exercise or activity, potential for interrupted skin integrity
e. Planning and implementation
1) Perform frequent neurovascular assessment, which includes "6 Ps": pain, pallor, polar, paresthesias, pulses, and paralysis
2) Immobilize joints above and below fracture; movement of affected area may cause a closed fracture to become open; immobilize by applying splints
3) Cover open wounds with sterile dressings
4) Manage pain associated with fracture with prescribed analgesics
5) Elevate fractured extremity to reduce swelling and pain
6) Apply ice to affected extremity
7) Assist in fracture reduction; the goal in treating fracture is to reduce and immobilize it
   a) Closed: involves external manipulation to realign bones
   b) Open: involves a surgical procedure to realign the bones
8) Maintain traction as prescribed; see section on nursing care of the client in traction
9) See also section on nursing care of a client in a cast
10) Monitor for major complications
   a) **Compartment syndrome**: impairment of circulation within inelastic fascia caused by external pressure (greater than 30 mmHg) that results in tissue death and nerve injury; external pressure can be created by casts, splints, or dressings; manifestations include unrelieved pain, diminished or absent pulses distal to injury, cyanosis of extremity, tingling or diminished sensation (paresthesia), loss of sensation, pallor, coolness of extremity, and weakness; bivalving may be necessary if cast is too tight
   b) Infection: wound drainage, fever, pain, and odor
   c) Fat embolism: chest pain, dyspnea, tachycardia, decreased O_2 saturation, apprehension, change in level of consciousness (LOC), petechiae on upper trunk and axilla
   d) DVT: calf pain and tenderness, swelling, or edema
f. Medication therapy: includes analgesics and antibiotics
g. Client education
1) Exercise extremities that are not immobilized to prevent muscle atrophy
2) Cast care, splint, and/or traction (see previous discussions)
3) Neurovascular assessments that need to be done
4) Pin care procedure and methods of preventing wound infection
h. Expected outcomes
1) Client verbalizes tolerable or decreased intensity of pain
2) Client is free of complications noted by normal neurovascular findings, no signs of infection, and no skin breakdown under cast
3) Client resumes activities of daily living

Practice to Pass

You are caring for a client in the emergency department who presents with an open fracture of the right tibia. What are your priority interventions for this client?

2. Hip fracture
   a. Description: hip can be fractured at different sites, namely, the head, neck, and trochanteric areas; see Figure 9-3
   b. Etiology and pathophysiology: incidence increases with age; 90% of hip fractures are caused by falls
   c. Assessment
      1) A hip fracture is a medical emergency as most occur at head or neck of trochanter, which compromises blood supply for bone health
      2) Hip fractures are generally sustained from falls; monitor LOC and assess for other injuries
      3) Perform neurovascular assessment on affected extremity
      4) Extremity of affected hip will be shorter than unaffected extremity
      5) Fractured hip will generally externally rotate
   d. Priority nursing problems: pain, reduced mobility, potential for interrupted skin integrity, potential decreased neurovascular status, potential for infection, potential inability to self-manage treatment plan
   e. Planning and implementation
      1) Prepare client for surgical intervention (for example, verify allergies, informed consent)
      2) Explain that an abductor pillow or splint may be needed to prevent disarticulation of femur
      3) Explain that sandbags may be used along external border of affected limb to prevent external rotation
      4) Inform client that sufficient pain medication will be available postoperatively (generally patient controlled analgesia [PCA] is used)
      5) Teach client about pain rating scale to be used postoperatively and encourage client to report any discomfort
      6) Teach client deep-breathing and coughing exercises preoperatively

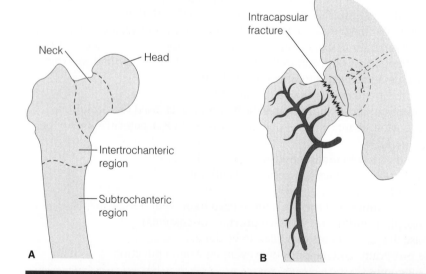
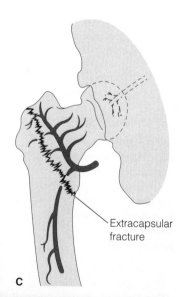

Figure 9-3

A. Hip fractures can occur in the head, neck, or trochanteric regions of the femur, B. An intracapsular fracture affects the femur head or neck, C. An extracapsular fracture occurs across a trochanteric region. All fractures disrupt blood supply to the bone.

7) Use aseptic technique for dressing changes and wound drainage

8) Provide information on therapies and equipment to expect postoperatively (for example, indwelling urinary catheter, PCA, IV therapy, possible traction)

9) Monitor preoperative use of skin traction (Buck's traction) to immobilize the limb and reduce muscle spasms until surgery is ordered

10) Provide diligent postoperative care and employ postoperative precautions to prevent hip dislocation (no hip flexion greater than 90 degrees, internal rotation of affected hip, or adduction of affected hip); these precautions include such items as avoiding low chairs, using raised toilet seat, no excessive bending

f. Medication therapy: analgesics to manage pain

g. Client education

    1) Reinforce deep-breathing and coughing exercises and use of incentive spirometer postoperatively

    2) Reinforce teaching about postoperative course and precautions

h. Expected outcomes: client has effective pain control, cooperates with mobilization precautions, and heals without complications

3. Sprains and strains

a. Description

    1) A **sprain** is a stretch and/or tear of a ligament

    2) A **strain** is a twist, pull, and/or tear that may involve both muscles and tendons

b. Etiology

    1) Direct or indirect trauma (caused by fall, blow to body, muscle exhaustion)

    2) Overuse or prolonged repetitive motion of muscles and tendons

    3) Inadequate rest periods during intensive training

    4) Ankles, knees, and wrist are most vulnerable

    5) Frequently seen in athletes and individuals with poor physical conditioning or who are overweight

c. Assessment

    1) Sprains are classified based on degree of ligament injury

    2) Pain is aggravated by continuous use and influenced by degree of injury

    3) Assess for bruising, edema, joint swelling, muscle spasms, and inflammation at affected site

    4) Assess for changes in neurovascular status (pulse, temperature, capillary refill, and movement) of affected extremity

    5) Decreased mobility in affected extremity

d. Priority nursing problems: pain, reduced physical mobility

e. Planning and implementation

    1) Teach client about RICE approach to recovery

        a) *R*est affected extremity

        b) *I*ce for 15–30 minutes at a time for 2–3 days

        c) *C*ompression (elastic support bandages or adhesive tape)

        d) *E*levation

    2) Perform neurovascular assessment on affected extremity

    3) Encourage client to wrap affected extremity with elastic support bandages before strenuous activities

    4) Inform client that x-rays of injured extremity may be necessary

    5) Administer analgesics as needed

    6) Teach client about importance of stretching and warm-up exercises before athletic activities

    7) Encourage client to adhere to exercise program to regain muscle tone and strength in collaboration with physical therapist

       f. Medication therapy: analgesics, muscle relaxants, and anti-inflammatory agents as necessary

       g. Client education: reinforce information covered above in planning and implementation section

       h. Expected outcomes: client has restored function of affected muscle and tendon, states relief of pain, and states understanding of factors that can precipitate sprains or strains

F. *Gout*

   1. Description: a disorder in which hyperuricemia (elevated serum uric acid) leads to recurring attacks (flares) of acute joint inflammation; primary form is hereditary; secondary form is acquired

   2. Etiology and pathophysiology

       a. Inherited abnormality in body's ability to process uric acid

       b. Hyperuricemia is caused by increased purine synthesis and/or decreased renal excretion of uric acid

       c. Elevated serum uric acid level can also be caused by prolonged fasting and excessive alcohol intake

   3. Assessment

       a. Risk factors: high consumption of meat and seafood, obesity, excessive weight gain, excessive alcohol intake, impaired renal function, hypertension, chemotherapy for leukemia and certain lymphomas, certain thiazide diuretics, aspirin, and tuberculosis medications

       b. Diagnosis includes analysis of synovial fluid, serum uric acid, and 24-hour urine

       c. Joint inflammation is extremely painful and is caused by deposits of uric acid crystals in synovial lining and fluid

       d. Assess for elevated temperature (may not always be present), tenderness and cyanosis of affected extremity, inflammation of small joints (commonly seen in great toe), and multiple joint involvement

       e. Precipitating factors generally include dehydration, fever, injury to joint, and excessive ingestion of alcohol

   4. Priority nursing problems: pain, reduced mobility, potential for inability to maintain health

   5. Planning and implementation

       a. Prevent any bed linen from touching affected extremity because of extreme tenderness (bed cradle and/or footboard can be used)

       b. Instruct client to adhere to activity restriction such as bed rest and immobilization of affected extremity during periods of exacerbation

       c. Monitor uric acid levels to prevent exacerbation and evaluate effectiveness of treatment

       d. Instruct client about precipitating factors for flares

       e. Encourage diet low in purines; avoid foods high in purines such as organ meats, sardines and herring, venison, and goose; other meats (including red meat) also contain purines and should be limited in quantity

   6. Medication therapy: usually includes anti-inflammatory agents (such as NSAIDs or corticosteroids), an antihyperuricemic (such as allopurinol [Zyloprim]) and uricosurics (such as probenecid [Probalan]) colchicine may be used for acute attacks or for prophylaxis

   7. Client education

       a. Reinforce teaching covered in planning and implementation sections above

       b. Action, side/adverse effects of medication

       c. Medications should be taken with meals to avoid gastric irritation

       d. Avoid use of alcoholic beverages when taking medication

e. Drink at least 2.5–3 liters of fluid/day when taking medication

f. Report adverse effect such as gastric irritation, fatigue

g. Discuss complementary therapy use such as vitamin E and acupuncture

8. Expected outcomes

a. Client and family verbalize an understanding of medication regimen and precipitating factors that exacerbate flares

b. Client reports satisfaction with pain management

c. Serum uric levels remain within therapeutic range

G. *Degenerative joint disease* (DJD) or osteoarthritis (OA)

1. Description

a. Slowly progressive disorder of articulating joints, especially weight-bearing joints; most common form of arthritis

b. Commonly affects hand and weight-bearing joints (knees, hips, feet, and back)

c. Breakdown of articular cartilage occurs

d. Injury is usually limited to joint and surrounding tissue

e. Disease ranges from very mild to very severe

2. Etiology and pathophysiology

a. Cartilage degeneration causes bones to rub against each other, causing pain and decreasing function of the joint

b. Risk factors

1) Age (most significant): primarily affects middle-age to older adults

2) Obesity (generally causes arthritis of knees)

3) Repetitive joint injuries caused by sports, accidents, or work-related injuries

4) Genetics (especially seen with OA of hands): client may be born with defective cartilage or slight defect in how joint fits together, and as client ages, joint cartilage continues to progressively degenerate and enzymes (hyaluronidase) are released, which cause further breakdown

3. Assessment

a. Diagnosed by physical exam and a history of symptoms; x-ray confirms disease

b. Joint pain is present with movement and weight-bearing and is relieved by rest

c. There is limited ROM with progressive loss of function

d. There is joint stiffness after rest

e. Crepitation (grating sensation caused by rough joint surfaces rubbing together) occurs

f. **Heberden's nodes** (raised bony growths over distal interphalangeal joints) are present

g. **Bouchard's nodes** (raised bony growths over proximal interphalangeal joints of hand) are noted

4. Priority nursing problems: pain, reduced physical mobility, possible interrupted sleep, reduced ability to engage in self-care, excess nutrients above bodily needs, reduced self-esteem

5. Planning and implementation

a. Encourage client to participate in an exercise program (approved by provider) to maintain joint flexibility and improve muscle strength

b. Encourage client to maintain ideal body weight to prevent excessive stress on joints

c. Instruct client to apply heat/cold therapy to affected joint for temporary pain relief

d. Assist client in planning scheduled rest periods to relieve stress on joints

e. Assist client with activities of daily living (ADL) as needed

f. Provide information about complementary therapies such as visual imagery and relaxation techniques for pain control

Practice to Pass

You are caring for a client diagnosed with gout. The client is being treated with probenecid (Probalan). The client asks, "How will this drug help decrease the pain from my gout?" How would you respond?

6. Medication therapy
   a. Acetaminophen controls mild pain without inflammation
   b. Anti-inflammatory agents such as NSAIDs are also used
   c. If NSAIDs are ineffective in controlling inflammation and pain, corticosteroids may be injected directly into joint
7. Client education
   a. Nature of and treatment of disease
   b. Principles of good body mechanics
   c. Correct use of assistive devices and encourage use as needed
   d. Avoid activities that put excessive stress on joints and cause pain
   e. Plan daily activities to space out tasks to allow for scheduled rest periods
8. Expected outcomes: client experiences satisfaction with pain management, balances rest periods with activity, uses joint protection and energy conservation measures, and maintains joint function

H. Low back pain

1. Description
   a. Pain may result from acute stress on lower back or repeated stress over a period of years
   b. Pain occurs because of degeneration and/or acute injury to tissue of lower back
      1) Caused by sprain or strain of ligaments and muscles
      2) Pain may be felt at site of injury or referred
   c. Overall health of muscles of lower back determines degree of risk for injury as well as speed of recovery
2. Etiology and pathophysiology
   a. Low back pain occurs because of repeated injury and progressive degeneration of spine
   b. Two most common causes of low back pain are mechanical strain (irritation or injury to disc causing degeneration) and herniation of nucleus pulposus (putting pressure on nerve roots)
3. Assessment
   a. Risk factors include but are not limited to degenerative disc disease, poor muscle tone of lower back, sedentary lifestyle, obesity, poor body mechanics, smoking, and stress
   b. Client will report pain caused by a shift of one vertebra on another or pinching and irritation of nerve root
   c. Muscle spasms are a common symptom
   d. Pain does not appear at time of injury but is related to gradual increase of muscle spasms of paravertebral tissue
   e. Straight leg raise test may not be positive with acute injury but pain is present with radiation to buttock and leg along path of sciatic nerve with chronic injury
4. Priority nursing problems: pain, interrupted sleep pattern, possible reduced coping, alterations in body image, inability to self-manage treatment plan
5. Planning and implementation
   a. Goal of treatment is to improve symptoms and slow progression of degenerative process
   b. Bed rest on a firm mattress (and possibly bed boards) may be initially prescribed
   c. Teach and assist client to use a sleeping position consistent with principles of body mechanics (side lying or supine with knees and hips flexed)
   d. Heat and cold therapy may be used as adjuncts for pain relief
   e. Physical therapy consultation will provide a plan for resuming activities and lower-back strengthening exercises
   f. Include client and family in plan of care
   g. Provide emotional support

6. Medication therapy: includes but is not limited to analgesics, NSAIDs, and muscle relaxants; epidural corticosteroid injections may be used if conservative treatment is ineffective

7. Client education
   a. Expected therapeutic effects, side/adverse effects, and contraindications with medication use
   b. Importance of adhering to activity prescription, which may include bedrest if indicated, then gradual increase in activity along with prescribed exercise plan
   c. Importance of maintaining ideal body weight
   d. Physical therapy will be part of the rehabilitation process to help maintain muscle strength and flexibility as well as improve muscle tone
   e. Continued use of heat or cold therapy for comfort
   f. Importance of adhering to the principles of body mechanics to avoid excessive strain on the lower back
   g. Sleep on a firm mattress using position described in section above
   h. Avoid or stop smoking
   i. How to use prescribed brace or corset (if needed) to prevent flexion and extension motions of lower back

8. Expected outcomes
   a. Client experiences satisfaction with pain management
   b. Client adheres to exercise regimen and uses proper body mechanics with all activities
   c. Client experiences progressive muscle strengthening and flexibility and performs at optimal level of function
   d. Client maintains ideal body weight

Case Study

P. J. is a 67-year-old retired nurse who had an open reduction with internal fixation (ORIF) of the right hip yesterday. Vital signs remain stable within the client's baseline. The client is receiving hydromorphone (Dilaudid) via PCA for pain. The client uses the incentive spirometer every hour as instructed. An abduction pillow is positioned between the client's legs.

1. What assessments would you perform on the client at this time?

2. What position constraints must be observed when turning and repositioning this client?

3. What is the purpose of the abduction pillow between the client's legs?

4. What activities would put this client at risk for dislocation of the affected hip?

5. Why is it important to get this client out of bed by postoperative day one?

For suggested responses, see page 623.

POSTTEST

POSTTEST

❶ The nurse is preparing a client for a bone scan. What priority assessment should the nurse perform for this client?

1. History of claustrophobia
2. Presence of intravenous (IV) access
3. Current vital signs
4. Presence of metallic implants such as a pacemaker or aneurysm clips

2 A retired 66-year-old female client is being evaluated for osteoporosis as part of a yearly physical exam. The client states that she is a smoker, watches television for most of the day, and has been hospitalized twice with fractures within the last year. Based on this information, the nurse suspects which condition?

1. Low bone mass leading to increased bone fragility
2. Degeneration of the articular cartilage
3. Recurrent attacks of acute arthritis
4. Personality changes caused by chronic nature of illness

3 The nurse is caring for a client with a herniated lumbar disk. Following laminectomy surgery, how should the nurse turn and reposition the client?

1. Having the client use the side rails of the bed while twisting the upper body
2. Elevating the head of the bed 45 degrees, then turning the legs together toward the floor, bending at the waist.
3. Logrolling the client as a unit, keeping the body in proper alignment.
4. Turning the client's head and shoulders, then hips.

4 The nurse is caring for a client who had a hip spica cast applied 4 hours earlier. While handling the cast to turn the client, the nurse uses the palms of the hands. When asked by family why this method is being used, which reply by the nurse is accurate?

1. To speed-dry the cast
2. To decrease pain from moving
3. To prevent damage to the cast
4. To prevent swelling

5 The nurse is caring for a client with Buck's traction following a hip fracture. Which nursing interventions are appropriate for this client? Select all that apply.

1. Remove weights prior to lifting the client up in bed
2. Maintain countertraction by having weights hang freely
3. Administer analgesics as ordered
4. Monitor neurovascular integrity of the affect leg
5. Increase fluid intake

6 The nurse is preparing to receive a client from the emergency department who has an acute fractured femur as a result of a fall. For which potential complication should the nurse monitor the client?

1. Crush injury
2. Chronic pain
3. Disturbed body image
4. Fat emboli syndrome

7 The nurse observes that an 18-year-old female client has asymmetry of the shoulders and hips, and the hem of her dress is uneven. The nurse suspects that the client may be presenting with which disorder?

1. Congenital hip dislocation
2. Scoliosis
3. Fractured tibia
4. Degenerative disc disease

8 The nurse is caring for a client with skeletal traction. Which priority intervention should the nurse carry out?

1. Evaluate the pin site for unusual redness, swelling, purulent drainage, and foul odor.
2. Measure the distance between the client's hip and the traction.
3. Record the number of times the client exercises the affected limb.
4. Report how the client is coping with immobilization.

9 The nurse is discussing carpal tunnel syndrome with a client who reports experiencing discomfort while at work. Which intervention might the nurse suggest to help relieve the client's discomfort?

1. Take a narcotic analgesic.
2. Apply a splint.
3. Exercise the hand and wrist regularly.
4. Seek alternate employment.

10 A client is admitted following a motor vehicle crash where the left thigh was crushed beneath the vehicle. The nurse should assess the client for which complications? Select all that apply.

1. Acute renal failure
2. Hyperkalemia
3. Hypernatremia
4. Hypertension
5. Fat emboli syndrome

➤ *See pages 310–312 for Answers and Rationales.*

ANSWERS & RATIONALES

Pretest

1 **Answer: 3** **Rationale:** Women of menopausal age are at risk for osteoporosis, and foods high in calcium should be encouraged. A diet with green vegetables, sardines, salmon with the bone, and molasses provides high-quality calcium and is recommended for a client experiencing menopause in order to decrease the risk of osteoporosis. A diet with seafood, wheat, corn, and green vegetables is more concentrated in carbohydrates than proteins containing calcium. A diet with chicken, green vegetables, sardines, and broccoli contains some calcium but is lower than another option. Foods such as fresh fruits, English muffins, black beans, and asparagus are inadequate in calcium. **Cognitive Level:** Analyzing **Client Need:** Health Promotion and Maintenance **Integrated Process:** Nursing Process: Implementation **Content Area:** Adult Health **Strategy:** Recall the relationship between menopause and osteoporosis as well as foods high in calcium to correctly answer this question. **Reference:** LeMone, P., Burke, K., & Bauldoff, G. (2011). *Medical-surgical nursing: Critical thinking in patient care* (5th ed.). Upper Saddle River, NJ: Pearson Education, pp. 213–216.

2 **Answer: 1, 2, 3, 4** **Rationale:** Lack of estrogen in menopause, decreased calcium intake, sedentary lifestyle, and glucocorticoid use are risk factors for the development of osteoporosis. Increased fluid intake is not a risk factor for the development of osteoporosis. **Cognitive Level:** Applying **Client Need:** Health Promotion and Maintenance **Integrated Process:** Nursing Process: Assessment **Content Area:** Adult Health **Strategy:** The wording of the question indicates that more than one option is correct. Evaluate each option as a true or false statement and choose the ones that are true regarding risks for osteoporosis as answers to the question. **Reference:** LeMone, P., Burke, K., & Bauldoff, G. (2011). *Medical-surgical nursing: Critical thinking in patient care* (5th ed.). Upper Saddle River, NJ: Pearson Education, pp. 1339–1342.

3 **Answer: 4** **Rationale:** Alendronate (Fosamax), a bisphosphonate, is a potent inhibitor of bone resorption that preserves bone mass and increases bone density.

Raloxifene (Evista) is an example of a selective estrogen receptor modulator that is used to treat osteoporosis, and which also reduces the risk of invasive breast cancer. Calcitonin (Miacalcin) is dispensed as a nasal spray. **Cognitive Level:** Analyzing **Client Need:** Pharmacological and Parenteral Therapies **Integrated Process:** Nursing Process: Planning **Content Area:** Pharmacology **Strategy:** To answer this question you need to know the mechanism of action for alendronate. Compare the action to each of the answer options to select the correct response. **Reference:** LeMone, P., Burke, K., & Bauldoff, G. (2011). *Medical-surgical nursing: Critical thinking in patient care* (5th ed.). Upper Saddle River, NJ: Pearson Education, pp. 1342–1344.

4 **Answer: 1** **Rationale:** The client with hip surgery should avoid all activities, including crossing the legs at the knees, that will cause hip adduction, internal rotation, and flexion beyond 90 degrees. The focus of the teaching on clients with hip surgery is to avoid dislocation and the risk for further injury. Exercise that does not risk dislocation, such as walking, should be encouraged. Chairs with arms and raised toilet seats assist the client in rising to a standing position. **Cognitive Level:** Applying **Client Need:** Physiological Adaptation **Integrated Process:** Nursing Process: Implementation **Content Area:** Adult Health **Strategy:** Review the care of the client following a hip fracture. Select the answer option that places the least amount of strain on the hip and pelvis. **Reference:** LeMone, P., Burke, K., & Bauldoff, G. (2012). *Medical-surgical nursing: Critical thinking in patient care* (5th ed.). Upper Saddle River, NJ: Pearson Education, pp. 1321–1322.

5 **Answer: 1** **Rationale:** Extremes of internal rotation, adduction, and 90-degree flexion of the hip should be avoided 4 to 6 weeks after surgery to prevent dislocation. The use of elevated seats helps prevent excess flexion of the hip, decreasing the risk of dislocation. Activities involving bending (such as putting on shoes) place the client at risk for dislocation. Abduction pillows are used to prevent external rotation and must be used postoperatively. **Cognitive Level:** Applying

Client Need: Management of Care **Integrated Process:** Nursing Process: Implementation **Content Area:** Adult Health **Strategy:** Review the care of the client following a hip fracture. Select the answer option that places the least amount of strain on the hip and pelvis **Reference:** LeMone, P., Burke, K., & Bauldoff, G. (2011). *Medical-surgical nursing: Critical thinking in patient care* (5th ed.). Upper Saddle River, NJ: Pearson Education, p. 1322.

6 Answer: 3 Rationale: Bleeding and swelling following a laminectomy may cause compression of nerves in the spinal column that can lead to permanent neurological damage and paralysis. Frequent assessment of the client's neurovascular status is essential following laminectomy and includes assessing for pain, pulses, pallor, paresthesia, and paralysis. The health care provider usually orders ambulation and this is not a priority in the immediate postoperative period. Calculation of IV fluid totals is a routine activity at the end of a shift. Although loss of bladder tone may indicate nerve damage, it may also be a residual effect of the anesthesia. Assessing ability to void becomes of prime importance if the client is due to void, usually 6 to 8 hours after last voiding. **Cognitive Level:** Analyzing **Client Need:** Reduction of Risk Potential **Integrated Process:** Nursing Process: Assessment **Content Area:** Adult Health **Strategy:** Edema at the operative site is a common occurrence. When this occurs in the spinal column, innervation is compromised. Select the answer option to best reflect this occurrence. **Reference:** LeMone, P., Burke, K., & Bauldoff, G. (2011). *Medical-surgical nursing: Critical thinking in patient care* (5th ed.). Upper Saddle River, NJ: Pearson Education, pp. 1493–1494.

7 Answer: 3 Rationale: The pull of traction on the affected limb decreases muscle spasm and ensures bone alignment. The client can be moved up in bed as an independent intervention and does not require a provider's order. The weights should never be removed in a client in skeletal traction. Weights are maintained to ensure healing and union of the bone in proper alignment. A change in weight is not indicated. Elevating the client's feet will not correct the situation and may disturb bone alignment. **Cognitive Level:** Applying **Client Need:** Physiological Adaptation **Integrated Process:** Nursing Process: Implementation **Content Area:** Adult Health **Strategy:** Review the principles and purpose for traction. Select the response that is consistent with these principles. **Reference:** LeMone, P., Burke, K., & Bauldoff, G. (2011). *Medical-surgical nursing: Critical thinking in patient care* (5th ed.). Upper Saddle River, NJ: Pearson Education, pp. 1315–1317.

8 Answer: 1, 2, 3, 5 Rationale: Following a total hip replacement, the client must be instructed to avoid activities such as sitting in low, cushioned chairs; crossing legs; and using a standard-height toilet. These activities cause adduction of the legs or greater-than-90-degrees flexion at the hip, leading to possible to dislocation. Turning at the waist violates principles of general body mechanics. **Cognitive Level:** Applying **Client Need:** Health Promotion and Maintenance **Integrated Process:** Nursing Process: Implementation **Content Area:** Adult Health **Strategy:** Select answer options that would maintain the hip in straight alignment and prevent dislocation of the hip prosthesis. **Reference:** LeMone, P., Burke, K., & Bauldoff, G. (2011). *Medical-surgical nursing: Critical thinking in patient care* (5th ed.). Upper Saddle River, NJ: Pearson Education, pp. 1321–1322.

9 Answer: 4 Rationale: Unrelieved pain, diminished pulses, pallor, paresthesias, and pain on passive motion are all symptoms of compartment syndrome. This is a medical emergency because the pressure must be relieved in the affected limb to prevent permanent complications, such as loss of the limb. Monitoring the client allows the ischemia to continue unrelieved, increasing the risk of necrosis. Administering an analgesic or anxiolytic may mask the symptoms and increase the risk of necrosis. **Cognitive Level:** Analyzing **Client Need:** Physiological Adaptation **Integrated Process:** Nursing Process: Diagnosis **Content Area:** Adult Health **Strategy:** The symptoms in the question indicate ischemia of the tissue. If this is prolonged, the limb can be permanently compromised. With this in mind, use critical thinking skills and the process of elimination to reason that it needs to be reported immediately. **Reference:** LeMone, P., Burke, K., & Bauldoff, G. (2011). *Medical-surgical nursing: Critical thinking in patient care* (5th ed.). Upper Saddle River, NJ: Pearson Education, pp. 1310–1311.

10 Answer: 3 Rationale: The elevated temperature, chills, malaise, pain, and leukocytosis are all clinical manifestations of infection; specifically, osteomyelitis. Symptoms of fat embolism include acute respiratory distress and petechial rash. Gastrointestinal (GI) bleeding would be manifested by abdominal tenderness and pain and decreased hemoglobin. Malunion of the bone will not cause an elevated temperature. **Cognitive Level:** Analyzing **Client Need:** Physiological Adaptation **Integrated Process:** Nursing Process: Diagnosis **Content Area:** Adult Health **Strategy:** Describe the prime symptoms associated with each disorder and compare these with the symptoms presented in the question. **Reference:** LeMone, P., Burke, K., & Bauldoff, G. (2011). *Medical-surgical nursing: Critical thinking in patient care* (5th ed.). Upper Saddle River, NJ: Pearson Education, pp. 1310–1316.

Posttest

1 Answer: 2 Rationale: A bone scan involves administering a radioisotope to visualize the bone for diagnostic purposes. It is critical that the nurse ensure that the client has IV access for injection of the radioisotope prior to the procedure. Claustrophobia and metallic implants are relevant for an MRI. While current vital signs are important for any diagnostic test, having IV access is the priority for a bone scan as the tracer substance needs to be injected into the vascular system. **Cognitive Level:** Applying **Client Need:** Reduction of Risk Potential **Integrated Process:** Nursing Process: Implementation **Content Area:** Adult Health **Strategy:** To answer this question correctly, you need to know that the bone scan requires the administration of a radioisotope and how to prepare the client for this procedure. **Reference:** LeMone, P., Burke, K., & Bauldoff, G. (2011). *Medical-surgical nursing: Critical thinking in patient care* (5th ed.). Upper Saddle River, NJ: Pearson Education, p. 1294.

2 **Answer: 1** **Rationale:** Low bone mass, structural deterioration of bone tissue leading to bone fragility, and increased susceptibility to fractures are seen with osteoporosis. The client also has risk factors associated with osteoporosis: smoking, sedentary lifestyle, and being female and postmenopausal. Degenerative changes are associated with frequent exacerbations of arthritis. There is no indication of a personality change in this client. **Cognitive Level:** Applying **Client Need:** Physiological Adaptation **Integrated Process:** Nursing Process: Diagnosis **Content Area:** Adult Health **Strategy:** The stem provides the risk factors and consequences of osteoporosis. Identify the answer option that reflects the pathophysiology of the disease. **Reference:** LeMone, P., Burke, K., & Bauldoff, G. (2011). *Medical-surgical nursing: Critical thinking in patient care* (5th ed.). Upper Saddle River, NJ: Pearson Education, p. 1340.

3 **Answer: 3** **Rationale:** After laminectomy, it is critical that proper body alignment is maintained to prevent postoperative complications such as neurological damage. Logrolling technique ensures that the client turns as a unit. Using the side rail, asking the client to bend at the waist, and turning the client in stages may disrupt the alignment. **Cognitive Level:** Applying **Client Need:** Reduction of Risk Potential **Integrated Process:** Nursing Process: Implementation **Content Area:** Adult Health **Strategy:** This item is testing your knowledge of the principles of care following spinal surgery. Select the answer option that allows the client to maintain strict body alignment. **Reference:** LeMone, P., Burke, K., & Bauldoff, G. (2011). *Medical-surgical nursing: Critical thinking in patient care* (5th ed.). Upper Saddle River, NJ: Pearson Education, pp. 1493–1494.

4 **Answer: 3** **Rationale:** Handling a cast that is not completely dry with the fingertips creates indentations in the cast that can create pressure points within the cast that predispose to breakdown beneath the cast. A wet cast should be exposed to air and allowed to dry slowly. Using the palms of the hands on a cast while turning a client will not affect a client's comfort. Using the palms of the hands while handing a cast will not prevent swelling. **Cognitive Level:** Applying **Client Need:** Reduction of Risk Potential **Integrated Process:** Nursing Process: Implementation **Content Area:** Adult Health **Strategy:** Recall that a fundamental principle of cast care is to prevent impairment to the skin beneath the cast. Select

the answer option that best adheres to this principle. **Reference:** LeMone, P., Burke, K., & Bauldoff, G. (2011). *Medical-surgical nursing: Critical thinking in patient care* (5th ed.). Upper Saddle River, NJ: Pearson Education, pp. 1317–1318.

5 **Answer: 2, 3, 4, 5** **Rationale:** Buck's traction is a skin traction commonly used for hip fractures to stabilize the fracture, reduce muscle spasm, and reduce pain until surgery is performed. It is essential that the weight not be removed to maintain bone alignment. Since neurovascular impairment is commonly associated with a fracture, neurovascular integrity must be evaluated regularly to assure no damage to the vessels or nerves on the affected side. Analgesics should be administered as prescribed for pain management. Fluids should be increased to prevent constipation and renal calculi associated with immobility. **Cognitive Level:** Applying **Client Need:** Physiological Adaptation **Integrated Process:** Nursing Process: Implementation **Content Area:** Adult Health **Strategy:** Focus on the current situation of the client. Select answer options that maintain the traction and prevent complications of this type of therapy and the immobility that accompanies the fracture and treatment. **Reference:** LeMone, P., Burke, K., & Bauldoff, G. (2012). *Medical-surgical nursing: Critical thinking in patient care* (5th ed.). Upper Saddle River, NJ: Pearson Education, p. 1315.

6 **Answer: 4** **Rationale:** Fat emboli syndrome is a potential complication of long bone fractures and occurs when fat globules leave the shaft of the long bone and enter the circulation. There is no evidence that the client experienced soft injury at the time of the fracture. The client has an acute fracture. Once the bone is realigned, pain is significantly relieved. Once the bone is healed, the client should not experience chronic pain. The fracture is temporary and unlikely to change body image. **Cognitive Level:** Analyzing **Client Need:** Physiological Adaptation **Integrated Process:** Nursing Process: Assessment **Content Area:** Adult Health **Strategy:** Identify the potential complications of a long bone fracture. Select the answer option that is specifically related to this type of fracture. **Reference:** LeMone, P., Burke, K., & Bauldoff, G. (2012). *Medical-surgical nursing: Critical thinking in patient care* (5th ed.). Upper Saddle River, NJ: Pearson Education, pp. 1311–1314, 1321.

7 **Answer: 2** **Rationale:** A classic sign of scoliosis is asymmetrical dress or skirt hem caused by unevenness of the affected shoulder and hip, due to a lateral curvature of the spine. The spinal deformity causes the asymmetry. Congenital hip dislocation is diagnosed during infancy. Signs of a fractured tibia would include painful ambulation, not unevenness of the shoulder and hip. Degenerative disc disease is typically experienced by older adults and causes a uniform decline in height. **Cognitive Level:** Applying **Client Need:** Health Promotion and Maintenance **Integrated Process:** Nursing Process: Assessment **Content Area:** Adult Health **Strategy:** Identify the disorders that

ANSWERS & RATIONALES

commonly present in adolescence. The question provides the presentation as one that reflects uneven hips and shoulders. Select the answer option that meets these criteria. **Reference:** LeMone, P., Burke, K. & Bauldoff, G. (2011). *Medical-surgical nursing: Critical thinking in patient care* (5th ed.). Upper Saddle River, NJ: Pearson Education, pp. 1392–1393.

8 **Answer: 1** **Rationale:** The pin in skeletal traction goes directly through the bone, making infection and osteomyelitis a major complication of skeletal traction. The nurse must provide pin site care using aseptic technique to prevent infection. Although maintaining the traction, recording the client's exercise routine, and reporting the client's coping status are important, these actions are not the nurse's priority in relation to the risk of osteomyelitis. **Cognitive Level:** Applying **Client Need:** Reduction of Risk Potential **Integrated Process:** Nursing Process: Planning **Content Area:** Adult Health **Strategy:** Review the principles and risks of skeletal traction. Apply this information to each of the answer options to select the best response. **Reference:** LeMone, P., Burke, K., & Bauldoff, G. (2011). *Medical-surgical nursing: Critical thinking in patient care* (5th ed.). Upper Saddle River, NJ: Pearson Education, pp. 1316–1317.

9 **Answer: 2** **Rationale:** Carpal tunnel syndrome is a repetitive stress injury. The pain associated with carpal tunnel syndrome is caused by pressure on the radial nerve. Splinting the joint relieves the pressure and the related pain. Nonsteroidal medications, not narcotic analgesics,

are used to manage the discomfort. Exercise may worsen the pain. **Cognitive Level:** Applying **Client Need:** Physiological Adaptation **Integrated Process:** Nursing Process: Implementation **Content Area:** Adult Health **Strategy:** Consider the pathophysiology of carpal tunnel syndrome and choose the option that is likely to prevent further aggravation of the symptoms. **Reference:** LeMone, P., Burke, K., & Bauldoff, G. (2011). *Medical-surgical nursing: Critical thinking in patient care* (5th ed.). Upper Saddle River, NJ: Pearson Education, pp. 1308–1309.

10 **Answer: 1, 2** **Rationale:** A client with a crush injury is at risk for muscle breakdown and release of myoglobin into the circulation. This can result in acute tubular necrosis and renal failure. This client is more likely to develop hyperkalemia from cell destruction than hypernatremia, as potassium is released from damaged cells. Hypotension, not hypertension, would be a more likely complication. Since there is no evidence of a fracture, the risk of fat emboli syndrome is low. **Cognitive Level:** Analyzing **Client Need:** Physiological Adaptation **Integrated Process:** Nursing Process: Assessment **Content Area:** Adult Health **Strategy:** Identify the structures that are damaged in a crush injury. Then select the answer option that reflects the extent of this injury. **Reference:** LeMone, P., Burke, K., & Bauldoff, G. (2011). *Medical-surgical nursing: Critical thinking in patient care* (5th ed.). Upper Saddle River, NJ: Pearson Education, pp. 256, 835–839.

References

Berman, A., & Snyder, S. (2012). *Kozier & Erb's fundamentals of nursing: Concepts, process, and practice* (9th ed.). Upper Saddle River, NJ: Pearson Education.

D'Amico, D., & Barbarito, C. (2012). *Health & physical assessment in nursing* (2nd ed.). Upper Saddle River, NJ: Pearson Education, Inc.

Ignatavicius, D. D., & Workman, M. L. (2013). *Medical-surgical nursing: Critical thinking for collaborative care* (7th ed.) Philadelphia: W. B. Saunders Company.

Kee, J. L. (2010). *Laboratory and diagnostic tests* (8th ed.). Upper Saddle River, NJ: Pearson Education.

Lehne, R. (2010). *Pharmacology for nursing care* (7th ed.). St. Louis, MO: Saunders.

LeMone, P., Burke, K., & Bauldoff, G. (2011). *Medical-surgical nursing: Critical thinking in patient care* (5th ed.). Upper Saddle River, NJ: Pearson Education.

Lewis, S., Dirksen, S., Heitkemper, M., Bucher, L., & Camera, I. (2011). *Medical surgical nursing: Assessment and management of clinical problems* (8th ed.). St. Louis, MO: Elsevier.

McCance, K. L., & Huether, S. E. (2010). *Pathophysiology: The biologic basis for disease in adults and children* (6th ed.). St. Louis, MO: Mosby, Inc.

Osborn, K. S., Wraa, C. E., & Watson, A. (2010). *Medical surgical nursing: Preparation for practice*. Upper Saddle River, NJ: Pearson Education.

Smith, S. F., Duell, D. J., & Martin, B. C. (2012). *Clinical nursing skills: Basic to advanced skills* (8th ed.). Upper Saddle River, NJ: Pearson Education.

Integumentary Disorders

Integumentary Disorders

10

Chapter Outline

Anatomy and Physiology of Integumentary System

Assessment of Integumentary System

Lesions of Integumentary System

Common Problems of Integumentary System

Infections of Integumentary System

Inflammatory Disorders of Integumentary System

Malignant Disorders of Integumentary System

Trauma to Integumentary System

Objectives

➤ Identify basic structures and functions of the integumentary system.
➤ Describe the pathophysiology and etiology of common integumentary disorders.
➤ Discuss expected assessment data and diagnostic test findings for selected integumentary disorders.
➤ Identify priority nursing problems for selected integumentary disorders.
➤ Discuss nursing management of a client experiencing an integumentary disorder.
➤ Identify expected outcomes for the client experiencing an integumentary disorder.

NCLEX-RN® Test Prep

Use the accompanying online resource, NursingReviewsandRationales, to test yourself with hundreds of NCLEX®-style practice questions.

Review at a Glance

acne androgenically stimulated inflammatory disorder of sebaceous glands resulting in comedones, papules, pustules, and occasional scarring

actinic keratosis premalignant macules found on skin surface of fair-skinned people often after age 50 but may be present at any age

basal cell carcinoma abnormal cell growth of basal layer of epidermal skin

candidiasis infection caused by *Candida albicans*, a yeastlike fungus that most often causes superficial cutaneous infection

contact dermatitis an eruption of skin related to contact with an irritating substance or allergen

eczema inflammatory response in which skin appears erythemic, scaly, dry, and thickened

macule nonpalpable, flat lesion with color measuring less than 1 cm

nodule elevated firm lesion with a circumscribed border measuring 1 to 2 cm

papule elevated, palpable mass measuring less than 0.5 cm

pediculosis an infestation of skin or hair by species of blood-sucking lice capable of living as external parasites on a human host, such as *Pediculosis capitis* (head) and *Pediculosis pubis* (pubic)

plaque elevated group of papules that have convalesced into one lesion measuring greater than 0.5 cm

pressure ulcers ischemic lesions of skin and underlying tissues caused by external pressure that impairs flow of blood and lymph

psoriasis a genetically determined chronic epidermal proliferative disease

characterized by erythematous, dry scaling patches

pustule elevated, serous (pus)-filled vesicle that can measure any size

scabies a contagious disease caused by infestation of skin by the mite *Sarcoptes scabiei var. hominis*

squamous cell carcinoma a cutaneous malignancy that arises from keratinocytes

Tinea corporis commonly known as ringworm; a fungal infection affecting face, trunk, and extremities with exclusion of palms of hands, soles of feet, and groin

Tinea pedis commonly known as *athlete's foot*; a fungal infection affecting plantar surface of feet

urticaria an itchy rash

vesicle fluid-filled, elevated mass which measures less than 0.5 cm; if greater than 0.5 cm, it is a *bulla*

vitiligo totally white macules where there is absence of melanocytes

wheal elevated erythemic lesion that contains fluid in tissue of skin with an irregular border and variable in size

PRETEST

1 The nurse notes that a client has an elevated lesion that contains clear fluid and measures greater than 1 cm in diameter. This finding is best documented by the nurse as which of the following?

1. Papule
2. Vesicle
3. Bulla
4. Pustule

2 The nurse completes a skin assessment on a client. Which finding is most significant and must be reported immediately to the health care practitioner?

1. Lower leg brown skin color in a client with venous insufficiency
2. An asymmetrical black and brown 7 mm skin lesion on the neck
3. A port-wine stain on the client's forehead
4. Contact dermatitis of the hands appearing after client weeded garden

3 A client with herpes simplex virus 1 makes the remark that she hopes she never gets another lesion on her lip "like this one." What is the nurse's best response?

1. "The chances of getting another lesion on your lip are very low."
2. "Herpes simplex virus 1 can be reactivated by many factors."
3. "The lesions will probably also appear on your genital area."
4. "A red, pinpoint painless rash will continue to develop for the next 2 weeks."

4 The nurse would include which priority intervention in the plan of care for a client diagnosed with herpes zoster?

1. Refrain from sexual activity during an outbreak.
2. Teach to apply benzoyl peroxide at the first sign of an outbreak.
3. Monitor skin integrity for secondary bacterial infections.
4. Maintain a warm environment to decrease intensity of pruritus.

5 The nurse uses the "rule of nines" to calculate the client's percentage of burns according to total body surface area (TBSA). What percentage of TBSA burns should the nurse record for this client?

1. _____ % TBSA

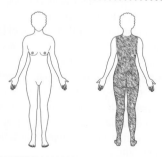

6 The client presents with an increase in the number of white patches across his chest and back. Multiple creams and lotions were not helpful. The nurse concludes that this client's clinical picture is consistent with which condition?

1. Vitiligo
2. Eczema
3. Psoriasis
4. Contact dermatitis

7 When counseling clients regarding fire prevention, the nurse should plan to include which of the following topics?

1. Discussion of the handling of smoking related materials
2. Demonstration of the use of a fire extinguisher
3. Assistance in the planning of an escape route
4. Stress of the need for smoke detectors

8 The nurse is caring for a client with an infected stage IV pressure ulcer with a significant amount of eschar formation. In planning care the nurse considers that which nursing intervention(s) would be appropriate for this client? Select all that apply.

1. Wet–moist saline gauze
2. Reposition every 2 hours
3. Enzymatic debridement
4. Hydrogel dressings
5. Dry gauze dressings

9 The client presents with the pruritic rash shown here. The nurse would ask the client which appropriate question during follow-up assessment?

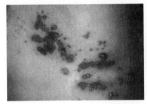
Centers for Disease Control and Prevention

1. "How long has this problem been present?"
2. "Have you recently eaten any new foods?"
3. "Do you spend a great deal of time in the sun?"
4. "Have you recently had a fever blister or cold sore?"

10 In obtaining a health history on a client with a new diagnosis of psoriasis, which finding is significant?

1. Recently tried a new type of food
2. Trauma to the skin from sunburn
3. Contact with an individual with vitiligo
4. Moved houseplants into new pots

➤ *See pages 343–345 for Answers and Rationales.*

I. ANATOMY AND PHYSIOLOGY OF INTEGUMENTARY SYSTEM

A. Epidermis

1. Outer layer of skin structure made up of epithelial cells
2. Epidermis is broken down into 4 layers throughout body, with the exception of palms of hands and soles of feet, which contain 5 layers of cells within epidermal layer

3. Protects body and internal structures from harm by providing a barrier to external environment
4. Contains phagocytes, which protect body from invading bacteria
5. Stores melanin to protect body from harmful ultraviolet rays
6. Converts cholesterol molecules to vitamin D when exposed to sunlight
7. Maintains body's hydration status by preventing water loss and providing a water-repellant layer

B. Dermis

1. Second layer of skin is made up of connective tissue and lymph vessels, blood vessels, and nerve fibers; contains hair follicles, sebaceous glands, and sweat glands
2. Dermis is broken down into 2 layers (papillary and reticular)
   a. Papillary layer: contains capillaries and receptor sites for touch and pain
   b. Reticular layer: contains receptors for deep touch as well as sweat and sebaceous glands
3. Regulates body temperature by dilating and constricting capillaries
4. Serves as a conducting agent to transmit messages from nerve endings to central nervous system (CNS)

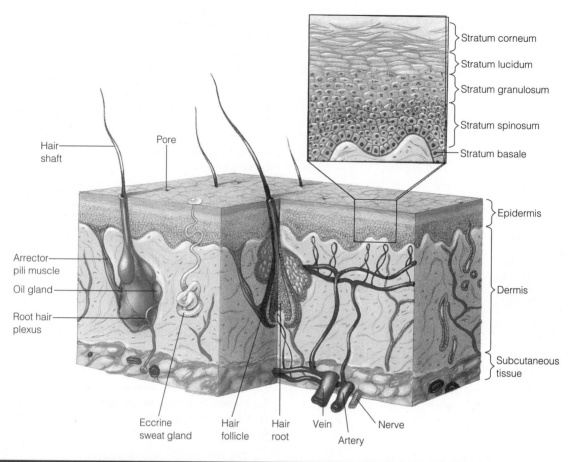

Stratum corneum

Stratum lucidum

Stratum granulosum

Stratum spinosum

Stratum basale

Epidermis

Dermis

Subcutaneous tissue

Hair shaft

Pore

Arrector pili muscle

Oil gland

Root hair plexus

Eccrine sweat gland

Hair follicle

Hair root

Vein

Artery

Nerve

Figure 10-1

Anatomy of the skin

C. Subcutaneous tissue (superficial fascia)
1. Is the layer that lies beneath dermis
2. Is made up of adipose (fat) tissue
3. Assists in connecting skin to structures below subcutaneous tissue

D. Appendages
1. Structures of integumentary system that grow beyond epidermal structure; include hair, nails, and glands
2. Hair: composed of primarily dead cells; hair root begins in bulb of hair follicle and grows from dermis outward; hair root is located under dermis and becomes hair shaft after hair exits dermal layer; protects and pads scalp from external objects as well as serves as a mechanism to maintain body temperature
3. Nails: primarily made up of dead cells that cover nail bed; nail structure begins in epidermis and extends across nail bed; cover dorsum of each digit on hands and feet to protect nail bed of each digit
4. Glands
   a. Apocrine: sweat glands located in axilla, anus, and genital area; function unknown
   b. Eccrine: sweat glands located on forehead, hands, and soles of feet; maintain a stable temperature for body through perspiration when body is overheated
   c. Sebaceous: glands located throughout body that secrete sebum; are highly influenced by increased hormones, especially androgens (see Figure 10-1); lubricate skin and hair and aid in killing bacteria on skin surface

II. ASSESSMENT OF INTEGUMENTARY SYSTEM

A. **Subjective data**

1. Past medical history

   a. Note previous problems with skin, hair, scalp, or nails; discuss duration of symptoms, associated symptoms, treatments used and results

   b. Medical disorders: discuss all body systems (cardiovascular, respiratory, endocrine/metabolic, hepatic, and hematology) that may manifest as a skin disorder; be sure to note any allergies to medications, foods, environment, tape, povidone iodine (Betadine), alcohol, and other substances

   c. Nutrition: note dietary changes, new foods introduced, and fluid intake

   d. External exposure: note new products exposed to skin, such as soaps, lotions, sun, and chemicals; note risks for exposure as part of occupational and social history

   e. Risk factors for skin cancer: male gender, over age 50, family history, too much exposure to UV radiation from sunlight, tanning lamps, or tanning booths; tendency to sunburn, history of sunburn or other skin trauma, light-colored hair or eyes, residence in high altitudes or near equator, exposure to radiation, x-rays, coal, tar, or petroleum products

   f. Sleep–rest: note number of hours of sleep each night and any rest periods

   g. Coping: discuss skin disorders and how skin is affected when stress is experienced; note coping behaviors used and results

2. Current medications: list current medications, onset and dose of medications

3. Recent surgeries or treatments: note any recent surgeries or treatment that may affect skin; for example, phototherapy, radiation therapy

4. Current problem: elicit information regarding current problem; for skin rash, obtain detailed information including date rash began, how it has changed, medications or ointments used, and results of treatment

B. **Objective data**

1. Inspection: ensure good lighting

   a. Note color (pink, yellow, white, purple, bruising, etc.)

   b. For lesions, document color, size, shape, symmetry, and border (see Box 10-1); stretching skin tightly facilitates assessment of lesions

---

Box 10-1	Clients should be informed about how to monitor skin lesions. The "ABCDE" rule is useful in teaching clients how to monitor changes in skin lesions and will assist clients to know when to seek further assessment from the practitioner. The following is the "ABCDE" guideline for monitoring skin lesions:
Characteristics of Skin Lesions	

A = *Asymmetry*: Note any asymmetrical changes of the skin lesion. Lesions are normally symmetrical in shape. Any changes in the symmetry of the lesion need to be evaluated for possible removal.

B = *Border*: The border of the lesion should appear smooth and regular. Note changes in the border that appear rough, irregular and jagged and have the lesion evaluated for possible removal.

C = *Color*: The color of a lesion should stay the same. Lesions that get darker (brown or black), have other variations in color or have more than one color need to be evaluated for possible removal.

D = *Diameter*: The diameter or size of the lesion should be measured and documented. Lesions with diameters greater than 6 mm (size of a pencil eraser) and lesions that change in size/enlarged need to be monitored and evaluated for possible removal.

E = *Elevated or evolving*: The lesion is elevated or evolving (changing).

    c. Inspect hair for color, amount, distribution, lesions, and hygiene

    d. Inspect nails for color, growth pattern, and thickness; inspect nail bed for inflammation or trauma

  2. Palpation

    a. Note texture, temperature, and moisture of skin

      1) Skin is warm and red in inflammation, warm with elevated body temperature

      2) Skin is cool with decreased blood flow as seen with shock (generalized) or arteriosclerosis (localized)

      3) Changes in texture may indicate irritation, trauma, or thyroid dysfunction

      4) Excessively dry skin may indicate hypothyroidism

      5) Oily skin is common in adolescents and young adults

      6) Excess perspiration is seen with shock, fever, increased activity or anxiety

    b. Palpate skin turgor for hydration status

      1) Assess for decreased skin turgor ("tenting") over clavicles by pinching skin together gently and seeing how long it takes to remove to its normal position

      2) Decreased skin turgor is seen with dehydration, but is common in older adults

      3) Increased skin turgor is seen with edema and scleroderma

    c. Palpate lower extremities (tibia and ankle) for edema

      1) Rate as 1+ (slight pitting with no obvious distortion) to 4+ (pit remains with obvious distortion)

      2) Edema is common with cardiovascular disorders, renal failure, trauma, and cirrhosis of liver

    d. For lesions, note location and palpate texture, consistency, and mobility

    e. Palpate hair for texture (coarse, fine); palpate nails for texture and check capillary refill

C. Age-related skin changes

  1. Decreased thickness and miotic activity of epidermis leads to more fragile skin with a greater risk for tears or injury, delayed wound healing, hyperkeratosis, and skin cancers in sun-exposed areas

  2. Increased permeability of epidermis and decreased Langerhans cells leads to increased risk of reactions to irritants and decreased inflammatory response

  3. Decreased number of active melanocytes and hyperplasia of existing melanocytes leads to increased susceptibility to sun exposure, small areas of hyperpigmentation ("liver spots") and hypopigmentation ("age spots")

  4. Decreased vitamin D production leads to increased risk of osteomalacia and osteoporosis

  5. Flattening of dermal–epidermal junction leads to an increased risk of skin tears, purpura, and pressure ulcers

  6. Decreased perfusion leads to drier skin, decreased sensation (pain, touch, temperature, peripheral vibration) and increased risk of injury

  7. Decreased vasomotor response leads to increased risk of hyperthermia and hypothermia

  8. Degeneration of elastic fibers leads to decreased tone and elasticity, with formation of wrinkles

  9. Proliferation of capillaries leads to presence of cherry hemangiomas

  10. Thinning of subcutaneous layer leads to increased risk of hypothermia and pressure ulcers

  11. Redistribution of fatty tissue leads to formation of cellulite, bags over and under eyes, double chin formation, abdominal fat, sagging of breasts, and delayed return to normal when pinched (tenting)

  12. Decreased exocrine and apocrine gland activity decreases perspiration and contributes to dry skin

III. LESIONS OF INTEGUMENTARY SYSTEM

A. Vascular skin lesions
  1. Spider angioma: a flat, bright red spot with radiating blood vessels at edges, commonly found on upper body; varies in size from a tiny dot up to 1.5–2 cm; caused by vascular dilation of blood vessels commonly seen with high estrogen levels, pregnancy, liver disease, and/or vitamin B deficiency
  2. Petechiae: flat red or purple spots, approximately 1–3 mm in diameter that do not change in color when blanched; caused by tiny capillaries that have broken, possibly caused by anticoagulation of blood, liver disease, vitamin K deficiency, or septicemia
  3. Purpura: flat purple/blue-appearing patch, varies in size and shape, caused by a bleeding disorder or broken blood vessels and may appear throughout body
  4. Ecchymosis: flat, irregularly shaped lesion ("bruise") which does not blanch with pressure, caused by release of blood from superficial vessels into surrounding tissue due to trauma, hemophilia, liver disease, or deficiency of vitamin C or K

B. Primary skin lesions (see Figure 10-2)
  1. **Macule**, patch: nonpalpable, flat lesion that has color and measures less than 1 cm; examples: petechiae, freckles, chloasma
  2. **Nodule**, tumor: an elevated solid, hard or soft palpable lesion with a circumscribed border that measures approximately 0.5–2 cm; tumors may have irregular borders and are larger than 2 cm

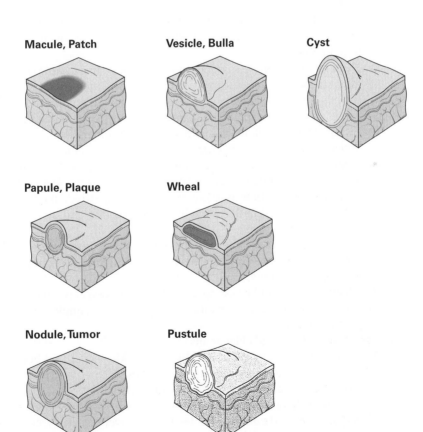

Macule, Patch Vesicle, Bulla Cyst

Papule, Plaque Wheal

Nodule, Tumor Pustule

Figure 10-2

Primary skin lesions

3. **Papule**, **plaque**: elevated, palpable mass, measuring less than 0.5 cm; examples include warts and moles; plaques are groups of papules that form lesions larger than 0.5 cm; examples are actinic keratosis and psoriasis
   a. Management of papules depends on diagnosis, such as cryotherapy for wart removal
   b. Mole removal may be recommended if mole is considered premalignant; different methods of mole removal are available
   c. Excision of mole may be done in an office setting; nursing care before treatment would be to reinforce explanation of procedure to client and obtain history of allergies (povidone iodine [Betadine], alcohol)
4. **Pustule**: elevated, serous (pus)-filled vesicle that can measure any size; examples are **acne** and boils
5. **Vesicle**, bulla: vesicle is a fluid-filled, elevated mass that measures less than 0.5 cm with thin, translucent walls and circumscribed borders; a bulla is greater than 0.5 cm; examples of vesicles are chickenpox, small burns, and herpes virus lesion
6. **Wheal**: variable-sized, elevated erythemic lesion with an irregular border that contains diffuse fluid in tissue of skin; examples are insect bites and hives
7. **Cyst**: elevated, encapsulated, fluid-filled, or semisolid mass originating in subcutaneous tissue or dermis, usually 1 cm or larger; examples are sebaceous cysts

C. **Secondary skin lesions**
   1. Atrophy: dry, thin, taut skin that appears wasted from loss of collagen; an example is aged skin; hydration with fluids and keeping skin well-moisturized with emollients such as Eucerin™ cream are helpful
   2. Crusts: dried pus, serum or blood on skin surface resulting from a vesicle or pustule that has ruptured; examples of crusts are final stages of chickenpox lesions or impetigo lesions
   3. Erosion: moist, superficial indentation of skin; an example of erosion is a scratch mark; therapeutic management includes warm moist compresses to site for comfort, keeping site clean and dry, and cleaning with antibacterial soaps at least 3–4 times a day; may need to apply topical antibiotics if site gets secondary bacterial infection
   4. Fissure: linear break in skin with sharp edges, extending into dermis; examples are athlete's foot or cracks in corner of mouth from chapped lips; therapeutic management for athlete's foot includes antifungal medications and keeping feet cool and dry; encourage use of white, cool socks and avoid allowing feet to sweat; fissures of lips may be treated with topical ointments such as petroleum jelly or Blistex™ ointment
   5. Scales: dry, dead skin that sloughs off skin surface and that may be dry or greasy; examples are dandruff or psoriasis
   6. Scar: a flat irregular area of connective tissue resulting from healing over site of previous injury and may vary in size, color, and shape; examples are healed surgery incisions or acne scars
   7. Ulcers: deep irregularly shaped areas of skin loss; may vary in size and shape and extend into dermis or subcutaneous tissue; examples are chancres and pressure ulcers

D. **Common skin lesions of older adults**
   1. Lentigo: a brown macule resembling a freckle except that border is usually irregular; senile lentigo (liver spots) occurs on exposed skin of older white adults; should be monitored for changes consistent with melanoma
   2. Seborrheic keratosis: benign plaques, beige to brown or even black in color, ranging in size from 3–20 mm in diameter with a velvety or warty surface
   3. Skin tags: soft brown or flesh-colored benign papules
   4. Angiomas (hemangiomas): benign vascular tumors with dilated blood vessels found in middle to upper dermis

5. Telangiectases: single dilated blood vessels, capillaries, or terminal arteries
6. Venous lakes: small, dark blue, slightly raised benign papules
7. Photoaging: skin that has wrinkling, mottling, pigmented areas, loss of elasticity, benign or malignant lesions
8. **Vitiligo**: totally white macules where there are no melanocytes

IV. COMMON PROBLEMS OF INTEGUMENTARY SYSTEM

A. Pruritis

1. Description: a subjective itching sensation producing an urge to scratch
2. Causes: elements in internal or external environment including insects, animals, plants, fabrics, metals, medications, allergies, emotional distress; also occur as secondary manifestations of systemic disorders such as certain types of cancer, diabetes mellitus, liver disease, and renal failure
3. Exacerbating factors: can be triggered by heat and prostaglandins and increases with histamine and morphine
4. Pathophysiology: sensation stimulated in nerve endings of skin; may trigger release of histamine and other chemical mediators that further stimulate itch response; sensation travels to brain where it stimulates a scratching reflex; scratching further irritates skin and causes inflammation, which intensifies itching and may cause secondary effects of skin escoriation and infections
5. Management
   a. Identify and eliminate cause
   b. Antihistamines to reduce itching
   c. Topical or systemic antibiotics if infection present
   d. Topical corticosteroids to reduce itching and inflammation
   e. Therapeutic baths or soaks with agents such as cornstarch, baking soda, coal tar concentrates, colloid substances (oatmeal), or emoillients to reduce itching
   f. Teach measures to reduce dry skin, including to use mild detergent; avoid fabric softeners, perfumes and alcohol containg lotions; cleanse with tepid water and mild soap; apply creams and lotions when skin is slightly damp; increase fluid intake; keep nails trimmed; wear loose clothing; keep environment cool; wear cotton gloves to prevent scratching during sleep

B. *Psoriasis*

1. Description: a chronic, immune skin disorder characterized by raised, reddened, round circumscribed plaques covered by whitish, scaly plaques on scalp, knees, and/or elbows; most affected clients have a family history of disease; exact cause unknown
2. Triggers: sunlight, seasonal changes, hormone fluctuations, steroid withdrawal, drugs (beta blockers, lithium), trauma from surgery, sunburn, or excoriation
3. Therapeutic management
   a. Phototherapy with Ultraviolet-B (UVB) light to reduce growth rate of epidermal cells and hyperkeratosis and/or Ultraviolet-A (UVA) light, which penetrates deeper, 3 times a week
   b. Photochemotherapy using a light-activated (UVA) form of antimetabolite drug methoxsalen (Uvadex) to inhibit DNA synthesis and prevent cell mitosis
   c. Care as discussed in previous section for pruritis and dry skin
   d. Monoclonal antibody therapy may decrease immune response
4. Priority nursing problems: interrupted skin integrity, alteration in comfort, body image alterations

V. INFECTIONS OF INTEGUMENTARY SYSTEM

A. **Bacterial infections**: most commonly caused by *Staphylococcus aureas* and *group-A beta-hemolytic streptococcus*

1. Impetigo: a superficial skin infection that initially appears as an erythemic vesicle and later changes to a honey-colored crusted lesion
   a. Most commonly seen in children but occasionally affects adults
   b. An alteration in skin integrity occurs, and bacteria invade epidermis and cause an infection
   c. Commonly found on face, arms, legs, and buttocks
   d. They may occur as a single lesion or several lesions that have convalesced and appear as a group of lesions

2. Folliculitis: a bacterial infection of hair follicle
   a. Folliculitis can occur at any age and is seen more frequently in males
   b. Found most often on skin on face (beard), legs, and axilla, when found on eyelids is called a stye
   c. Lesion appears as an erythemic, pruritic, mildly tender pustule located at hair follicle; various stages of folliculitis may occur, including a simple pustule, progressing to a furuncle or carbuncle
   d. In severe cases, fever and chills may be present
   e. Contributing factors include poor hygiene, poor nutrition, prolonged skin moisture, tight heavy fabrics on upper legs, and trauma to skin

3. Furuncles and carbuncles: inflammations of hair follicle that often start as folliculitis but spread into dermis
   a. Initially deep, firm, red, painful nodule from 1–5 cm in diameter
   b. Progresses into a large, painful cystic nodule that may drain substantial amounts
   c. Carbuncle is an inflammatory lesion that is formed when several furuncles convalesce to form one larger infected lesion of skin
   d. Common in hot, humid climates

4. Cellulitis: a bacterial infection of dermal and subcutaneous tissues
   a. Occurs because of a break in skin integrity (abrasion, laceration, etc.); this bacterial infection may also occur secondary to a skin lesion
   b. Characterized by an erythemic, swollen, tender-to-touch area of skin at site of entry of bacteria; vesicles may form over area
   c. Associated symptoms include fever, chills, malaise, and anorexia with associated regional lymphadenopathy

5. Methicillin-resistant *Staphylococcus aureus* (MRSA) infection: an infection caused by a form of *S. aureus* that is resistant to broad-spectrum antibiotics
   a. Types include health care–associated (acquired in hospitals and other health care settings) and community associated (acquired in community in otherwise healthy people, believed to be related to overuse or misuse of antibiotics)
   b. Potentially life threatening, begins as a small, raised nodule that rapidly increases in size and may become a deep abscess; cellulitis is often present
   c. Can be present without causing illness, client is colonized and can spread to others

6. Collaborative management of bacterial infections
   a. Encourage good hand hygiene with hot soapy water to prevent spreading bacteria to others; for recurrent lesions, a culture of site is obtained to isolate pathogens
   b. Topical treatment includes cleaning site with warm soapy water 2–3 times a day
   c. Teach importance of taking full course of prescribed antibiotics (see section to follow)
   d. Teach not to share linens and towels; to wash clothes and linens in hot water; not to squeeze or try to open a pimple or boil; and how to properly handle and dispose of dressings

   e. Assess for and teach manifestations of infection, including fever, tachycardia, chills, and malaise

   f. Warm moist heat may be applied to site for comfort; occasionally, incision and drainage of site may be needed in which gram stain, culture, and sensitivity is obtained

7. Medication therapy: topical antibiotics, or for severe cases, systemic antibiotics; MRSA infections may be treated with anti-microbial therapy, including trimethoprim-sulfamethoxazole (Bactrim), minocycline (Minocin), doxycycline (Vibramycin) or clindamycin (Cleocin)

B. Viral infections

1. Herpes simplex virus (HSV): a viral infection that is manifested by vesicles on oral mucosa—mouth or lips, which is HSV Type 1 (also called a cold sore or fever blister) or in genital mucosa (HSV Type 2)

   a. Spread by direct contact of contaminated body fluids (kissing, oral sex, physical contact)

   b. Prodromal symptoms include a burning or tingling sensation, followed by development of erythema, vesicles and pain; initial infection is often severe; malaise and fever are also common symptoms

   c. HSV lives in nerve ganglia and recurrent lesions are seen in response to sunlight, menstruation, injury, or stress

   d. Recurrent infections are more localized and less severe

   e. Oral acyclovir may be used prophylactically and as treatment

2. Herpes zoster (shingles): a viral infection manifested by vesicles with an erythematous base on skin

   a. More than half of cases are seen in adults over age 60; also is more common in immunocompromised clients

   b. Herpes zoster is a reactivation of varicella (chickenpox) virus, which has been dormant for many years in dorsal root ganglia

   c. Vesicles are usually unilateral and follow path of a nerve

   d. Complications include postherpetic neuralgia, loss of vision (when located in ophthalmic division of trigeminal nerve), or disseminated lesions and encephalitis (in immunocompromised clients)

3. Warts: an elevation in epidermal skin layer caused by human papilloma virus (HPV)

   a. Virus may be transmitted from person to person by touch and is commonly seen on hands and feet but can also occur on genitals

   b. Types of warts

      1) Common wart: flesh-colored nodule commonly seen on hands or extremities, but can occur anywhere on body; it commonly appears to have a "black seed" in center of lesion; these warts may come and go, usually lasting approximately 6–12 months without treatment

      2) Flat wart: a tiny flesh-colored node, 1–3 mm in diameter, that may appear in clusters on dorsum of hand or forehead

      3) Plantar wart: a hard nodule found on bottom of foot; it commonly projects into foot from constant pressure applied while walking on nodule; it measures approximately 2–3 cm and is frequently associated with discomfort or pain at site of wart

   c. May resolve without treatment or be treated with medications containing salicylic acid (17%) and lactic acid, cryotherapy, or electrodessication and curettage; immune response may take up to 5 years to develop

4. Nursing diagnoses for viral infections

   a. Acute Pain

   b. Risk for Infection

Practice to Pass

A 25-year-old female comes into the office for evaluation of a lesion on her labia. While interviewing the client, you ask if she has a history of genital herpes. She responds that she was diagnosed with genital herpes when she was 18 years old but states, "I took the medication and got cured." What is your response to her regarding the nature of the virus responsible for herpes infection?

5. Collaborative management of viral infections
   a. Teach measures to relieve pruritus (see earlier section)
   b. Wet dressings or soaks (see earlier section under pruritis)
   c. Teach that virus may be transmitted to others; therefore, care should be taken to avoid persons at risk including immunocompromised and those who have not had chicken pox, especially children or pregnant women
   d. Teach to monitor lesions for secondary bacterial infections
   e. Wear latex condoms to prevent spreading virus from genital infection
6. Medication therapy
   a. Acetaminophen (Tylenol) may be used for comfort as needed; over-the-counter (OTC) products such as or Camphophenique™ may be used for comfort with HSV 1 cold sores
   b. Antiviral medications such as acyclovir (Zovirax), famciclovir (Famvir), or valacyclovir (Valtrex) may be used for herpes zoster infections to check further replication of virus and diminish symptoms if started within 24–48 hours after initial onset of lesions
   c. Zostavax (a weakened form of varicella-zoster virus) may be used for adults aged 60 or older to increase immune system response and prevent outbreaks; contraindicated for people with a weaker immune system

C. **Fungal infections**
1. **Candidiasis**: infection caused by *Candida albicans*, a yeastlike fungus that most often causes superficial cutaneous infections
   a. Risk factors include moist, warm, or interrupted skin integrity, systemic antibiotics, pregnancy, birth control use, poor nutrition, diabetes mellitus or chronic illnesses, and immunosuppression
   b. Types
      1) Oral candidiasis (also called thrush): often seen after antibiotic therapy or in immunocompromised clients; is characterized by white, milky, partially-removable plaques on oral mucosa; associated symptoms may include a burning sensation or decreased taste
      2) Vulvovaginitis: found on vaginal mucosa and can spread to perineum and groin; satellite lesions are usually present; other manifestations include excessive itching and a thick, white, curdlike vaginal discharge
      3) Perineal or diaper and skinfold rash: occurs on perigenital and perianal areas and can extend to inner thighs and buttocks; common in infants and incontinent clients; other areas affected include axilla, umbilical area, and under breasts; erythema, papules, pustules, and a scaling border are characteristic
      4) Balanitis: an inflammation of glans and prepuce of penis that typically presents as flattened pustules with edema, scaling, erosion, burning, and tenderness
      5) Paronychial infection: presents as erythema, edema, and tenderness of nail folds; a creamy, purulent discharge may be expressed with pressure on nail, which usually becomes discolored and has ridging
      6) Candida organisms may also be a causative agent in otitis externa and scalp disorders
   c. Collaborative management of fungal infections
      1) Diagnosis is made by culture of scrapings or by microscopic examination of scaling with potassium hydrochloride (KOH) preparation
      2) Avoid sharing linens or personal items
      3) Use clean towel and washcloth daily
      4) Dry all skinfolds; avoid frequent immersion of hands in water
      5) Wear clean cotton underwear daily

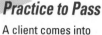

Practice to Pass

A client comes into the office today for removal of a wart. He says he has tried over-the-counter medications for removal; however, about 1–2 months later the wart reappears in the same spot. Now he wants the wart frozen and removed because he is tired of the wart coming back. What is your response?

        6) For vaginal candida, avoid tight clothing and pantyhose, bathe more frequently and dry genital area thoroughly; may need to treat sexual partner at same time to avoid reinfection or have partner use condoms until resolved; avoid douching and change perineal pads frequently

        7) For balanitis, carefully retract foreskin and perform careful cleaning and drying of glans penis

        8) Encourage weight loss for obese clients and maintenance of normal serum glucose levels in diabetic clients to decrease risk of infection

    d. Priority nursing problems: pain, reduced tissue perfusion

    e. Medication therapy

        1) Oral candidiasis: antifungals such as nystatin (generic), clotrimazole (Lotrimin), and in recurrent cases, ketoconazole (Nizoral), fluconazole (Diflucan), or itraconazole (Sporanox); liver function tests must be monitored because of risk of hepatotoxicity

        2) Perineal: topical treatment with nystatin ointments bid

        3) Balantitis: topical treatment with nystatin powder bid

        4) Paronychial: topical undecylenic acid (Fungi-Nail) or 2% gentian violet; for nonresponsive cases, systemic ketoconazole or fluconazole; systemic medications require monitoring of liver function tests because of risk of hepatotoxicity

        5) Hair/scalp: antifungal shampoo

        6) Vulvovaginitis: vaginal creams/suppositories or treat with fluconazole

2. Tinea

    a. Types: for most clinical purposes, classification by anatomic site is preferred

        1) Dermatophytosis (ringworm): a superficial fungal infection of skin

        2) Tinea corporis: a fungal infection of face, trunk, and extremities with exclusion of palms of hands, soles of feet, and groin; also known as ringworm of body

        3) Tinea pedis (athlete's foot): most common of all fungal infections; affects plantar surface of feet with mild to moderate erythema and scaly skin between toes; is often accompanied by pruritus and a foul odor; frequently chronic, absent in winter but reappearing in hot weather

        4) Tinea cruris ("jock itch"): a fungal infection of groin that may extend to inner thighs and buttocks; more common in those who are physically active, obese, or wear tight underclothing

    b. Risk factors

        1) All species of dermatophytes can be causative agents; generally more prevalent in hot and humid climates because moisture is key to development of infection

        2) Use of broad-spectrum antibiotics that kill off normal flora and allow fungi to grow

        3) Diabetes mellitus, immunodeficiencies, nutritional deficiencies, pregnancy, increasing age, and iron deficiency

        4) Tinea pedis risk factors include communal showers and pools; occlusive footwear; excessive sweating; sharing of footwear

    c. It can be spread human-to-human, animal-to-human, and soil-to-human by direct contact; other risk factors include prolonged use of topical steroids or immunosuppression

    d. Clinical manifestations

        1) Classic lesions are annular (ringlike) plaques with an elevated border, sharp margins, and a clearing center

        2) May see interdigital scaling, crusting, and maceration of feet

        3) May occur singly or in groups of 3 to 4

        4) KOH preparation from these lesions is usually positive; woods lamp fluoresces yellow; dermatophyte test media changes medium from yellow to red

   e. Therapeutic management
- **1)** Avoid contact with suspected lesions
- **2)** Topical creams are treatment of choice
- **3)** Clean environment to remove fungal scales
- **4)** Avoid sharing towels or other items that can transmit fungal scales
- **5)** Search out infected animals/pets and treat appropriately
- **6)** Apply creams after bathing and reapply after swimming and exercising
- **7)** Keep skin dry
- **8)** Keep involved areas clean, dry, and exposed to air when possible
- **9)** Wear light cotton socks or underwear and change frequently throughout day
- **10)** Wear sandals or open-toed shoes when possible; avoid plastic footwear and occlusive shoes
- **11)** Dry carefully between toes and in skin folds after showering or bathing
- **12)** Apply drying or dusting powers, topical antiperspirants
- **13)** Put socks on before underwear to avoid spreading to groin
- **14)** Instruct on signs and symptoms of bacterial infection such as pain, increased inflammation, pustules, or purulent exudates

   f. Medication therapy: antifungals in form of powders, creams, shampoos, suspensions, troches, vaginal suppositories, oral tablets, and intravenous solutions
- **1)** Topical drugs to treat superficial fungal infections include ciclopirox (Lopirox, others), clotrimazole (Lotrimin), and econazole (Spectrazole); eradication is slow and treatment may take 2–8 weeks
- **2)** For added benefit, client should wash with an antifungal shampoo such as ketoconazole (Nizoral) prior to using a cream
- **3)** Before an oral antifungal agent such as terbinafine (Lamisil) or nizoral is prescribed, baseline liver function tests and complete blood count (CBC) should be obtained; repeat liver function tests and CBC are recommended at 4–6 weeks and then every 6 months
- **4)** Antifungal powders may be used as an adjunct treatment and aid in keeping areas dry
- **5)** For severe cases: Burow's solution soak for lesions that are oozing, oral griseofulvin (Fulvin), fluconazole (Diflucan), itraconazole (Sporanox), and terbinafine (Lamisil)

D. Parasitic Infections

   1. Pediculosis: an infestation of skin or hair by species of blood-sucking lice capable of living as external parasites on human host
- **a.** Nits/eggs attach to hair shaft by a cement-like/cocoon-like structure and are difficult to remove
- **b.** Lice live up to 30 days and a female can lay up to 100 eggs
- **c.** *Pediculosis capitis* (head louse) is size of a sesame seed, clear in color when hatched but becomes grayish-white to red/brown after maturing
  - **1)** Head lice infestation is very common among school-age children of all socioeconomic backgrounds
  - **2)** Is spread by sharing combs, hats, and scarves
- **d.** *Pediculosis pubis*, also known as "crabs"
  - **1)** Infests genital area
  - **2)** One of the most common sexually transmitted infections; can also be acquired through contact with infested clothing or linens
- **e.** Clinical manifestations
  - **1)** Intensive pruritis is the most common symptom and may result in excoriations
  - **2)** Head lice may resemble dandruff flakes; however, they are not easily brushed off
  - **3)** **Urticaria** (intense itching of skin) with papules may be found at neck or pubic area

    f. Collaborative management

        1) Nits must be mechanically removed; a 50/50 white vinegar/water solution may loosen nits; olive oil may also be used; a nit comb is used to remove nits from hair shafts; lice may also be removed by fingers or tweezers; nits remove more easily by back-combing the hair

        2) To treat eyelashes apply petrolatum to lashes bid for 10 days; lice will either suffocate or slide off

        3) Educate children and parents about mode of transmission (person to person) and preventive measures, such as not sharing combs, brushes, hats, scarves, helmets, headphones, bedding, or sleeping bags

        4) Coats and hats should be hung separately and not touching each other

        5) Sleeping material should be labeled and kept separately in plastic bags, not stacked

        6) All family members need to be examined and treated at same time

        7) Soak personal hair items or any other object in contact with hair in 2% Lysol or pediculocide for 1 hour

        8) Shaving hair is not found to be helpful

        9) Machine wash all washable clothing used in last 48 hours and dry in dryer for at least 20 minutes

        10) Place unwashable items in airtight plastic bags for a period of 1 week to kill lice

        11) Upholstered furniture or pillows may be ironed with a hot iron

        12) Vacuum mattresses, rugs, upholstered furniture, and stuffed animals regularly

    g. Medication therapy

        1) For *pediculosis capitis*: permethrin (Nix), pyrethrin shampoo (Rid), or lindane (Kwell) shampoo left on 5–10 minutes and then washed off; lindane can be repeated in 1 week; due to neurotoxicity of lindane, it should not be used by children, nursing or pregnant women, clients with known seizure disorders, or on open skin

        2) For *pediculosis pubis*: treatment includes lindane, pyrethrin (Rid) or permethrin (Nix) as a shampoo left on for 10 minutes or as a lotion left on for several hours

        3) Co-trimoxazole (Bactrim DS): bid for 3 days has been shown to be effective; a second therapy 10 days later may be necessary to kill emerging nits before they reproduce

2. **Scabies**: a contagious disease caused by infestation of skin by *Sarcoptes scabiei var. hominis* mite

    a. Impregnated mite burrows into skin and remains there for life (approximately 30 days), laying 2–3 eggs per day

    b. Eggs hatch in 3–4 days and reach maturity in 4 days, migrate to skin surface, mate, and repeat cycle

    c. It is more common in people who do not have bathing facilities or access to clothes-washing facilities; incidence is increased in nursing homes and extended care facilities; mites can live in clothing fibers and can be transmitted by contact of infected clothing or bed linens

    d. Pathological findings by skin biopsy of a nodule (although rarely performed) will reveal portions of mite; diagnosis is usually made by clinical presentation of burrows, vesicles, and nodules

    e. Clinical manifestations

        1) Presents as a generalized pruritic rash particularly of hands, wrists, elbows, axillary areas, breasts, abdomen, or genitals

        2) Itching may become intense; increased warmth of skin and nocturnal itching is a classic symptom, since mites tend to have increased movment at night; exposure to hot water or steam also can increase pruritis

        3) Lesions may be erythematous, crusted papules, or purplish nodules, which may be accompanied by flesh-colored, raised burrows (threadlike linear ridges a few millimeters in length with a tiny black dot at one end); clients develop itch approximately 10–14 days after exposure

    f. Collaborative management

        1) Close family members and personal contacts must be treated as well, even if there are no apparent signs or symptoms

        2) All bed clothing, linens, unwashed worn clothing, and stuffed animals should be washed and dried in a hot dryer because heat kills mites

        3) Mites and eggs may be killed by placing items in airtight plastic bags for 7 days since mite cannot live off host more than 3 days; mites can live 24–36 hours in room conditions and longer in humid environments

        4) Relief from itching may not occur for 3–6 weeks after treatment because of hypersensitivity of skin to debris left in burrow

        5) Lotions/creams should be applied from neck down, using a toothbrush to get under fingernails and toenails; lotion is showered off 8–12 hours later

    g. Priority nursing problems: interrupted skin integrity, alteration in comfort

    h. Medication therapy

        1) Permethrin 5% cream (Elimite) is treatment of choice; a second application in 48 hours is sometimes recommended

        2) Crotamiton 10% (Eurax) is less toxic but is also slightly less effective; therefore application for 2 nights is advised

        3) Lindane 1% cream or lotion (Kwell) is the least expensive but has potential for neurotoxicity and should not be used by children, nursing or pregnant women, people with a known seizure disorder, or any widespread excoriations/open skin; treatment may be repeated after 1 week

        4) Systemic antipruritics

        5) May require emollients and midpotency corticosteroids after using scabicide to suppress skin hyperreactivity caused by mites

VI. INFLAMMATORY DISORDERS OF INTEGUMENTARY SYSTEM

  A. Dermatitis

    1. Description: an inflammatory response in which skin appears erythemic; may be acute or chronic; lesions may appear as papules or pustules that can lead to excoriation; pruritus may be present

    2. Types

      a. Atopic dermatitis (**eczema**): scaly, dry, and thickened skin; eczema may appear in various stages, depending on type (e.g., infantile vs. adult); etiology is unknown; eczema is characterized by lymphohistiocytic infiltration of vessels of skin

      b. Seborrheic dermatitis: a common chronic skin condition in areas of active sebaceous glands, such as face, scalp, body folds, sternal area, and axilla; appears as an erythematous scaling lesion that may appear dry or greasy; etiology is unknown but possible causes may be hormonal influence, nutritional deficiency, neurogenic influence, dysfunction of sebaceous glands, and fungal infection

      c. **Contact dermatitis**: an eruption of skin related to contact with an irritating substance or allergen

        1) Irritant dermatitis affects individuals exposed to specific irritants and produces discomfort immediately; common irritants include chemicals, dyes, metals, and detergents

        2) Allergic contact dermatitis affects only those previously sensitized to contact agent; it represents a delayed hypersensitivity reaction; most common are poison ivy, sumac, and oak; latex allergies affect 5–10% of health care providers

    3) Allergic contact dermatitis is an inflammation caused by an external irritant or allergic reaction mediated by IgE; the epidermal reaction is caused by T-lymphocytes; location of rash helps provide clues to offending antigen; there is no specific age or sex affected, but black skin is less susceptible

  d. Exfoliative dermatitis: characterized by excessive peeling or shedding of skin; increased risk with preexisting skin disorders but may also be due to reactions to medications and certain cancers; may also lose hair and nails; high risk for dehydration and infections

3. Priority nursing problems: interrupted skin integrity, alteration in comfort

4. Collaborative management of dermatitis

  a. Bath: advise client not to use harsh soaps; avoid frequent bathing

  b. Apply wet dressings to oozing, pruritic lesions to aid in drying and debridement; cool tap water, Burow's solution 1 to 40 (saline 1 tsp salt per pint of water) and silver nitrate solution can be used

  c. Measures to prevent pruritis (as discussed in earlier section) and frequent use of emollients (Eucerin™, Aquaphor™) is recommended

  d. Remove all triggers, causative agents and/or allergens; avoid skin contact with all wool products and lanolin preparations

5. Medication therapy

  1) Antihistamines such as diphenhydramine (Benadryl)

  2) Severe cases may require short-term topical or oral corticosteroids

  3) Scalp treatment: selenium sulfide 2.5% suspension or coal tar shampoos and topical steroid creams

  4) Topical immunosuppressive modulators are effective for atopic dermatitis but may cause skin cancers and lymphomas

  5) Topical anti-infectives if infection present

B. *Acne*

1. Description: an inflammatory or noninflammatory disorder of hair and sebaceous glands

  a. Noninflammatory lesions present as comedones (pimples, whiteheads, and blackheads)

  b. Inflammatory lesions present as comedomes, erythematous pustules, and cysts

  c. Most common in adolescents and young to middle adults, can also occur in middle and older adults

  d. Principal factors include increased sebum production and inflammation from bacteria and fatty acid constituents of sebum

  e. Rate of sebum production is determined genetically and is increased in presence of androgens; earliest changes in acne may be seen in prepubescent years

2. Clinical manifestations

  a. Lesions may occur on forehead, cheeks, nose, and may extend over central back and chest

  b. Scarring may result from picking at comdedones

  c. See Box 10-2 for staging and grading of acne

3. Collaborative management

  a. Intended to control disease and is not curative

  b. Use a gentle antibacterial soap and wash affected areas with fingertips

  c. Avoid cosmetics containing oil and confine moisturizing lotions to dry patches of skin

  d. Instruct not to pick lesions, which would increase scarring

  e. Usually 6–8 weeks of treatment is needed before obvious improvement occurs

  f. Explain that diet does not cause acne

  g. Promote stress management if acne flares with stress

4. Priority nursing problems: interrupted skin integrity, altered body image

Box 10-2 **Stages and Grades of Acne**	**Stages of Acne** Mild—few to several papules, no nodules, on face/neck only Moderate—several papules to many papules/pustules, few to several nodules on face, back, chest, or upper arms Severe—numerous and/or extensive papules/pustules; many nodules with acne-induced scarring **Grades of Acne** Grade 1—comedonal—closed and open Grade 2—papular—over 25 lesions on face and trunk Grade 3—pustular—over 25 lesions with mild scarring Grade 4—nodulocystic, inflammatory nodules and cysts with extensive scarring

   5. Medication therapy
      a. Topical retinoids are usually prescribed for all types of acne
      b. For mild acne, combination therapy of a topical retinoid plus one or more of the following: benzoyl peroxide, topical antibiotics, or azelaic acid
      c. For moderate acne, topical agents indefinitely and oral antibiotics such as tetracycline for a specified period of time only
      d. Antiandrogens such as birth control pills and spironolactone inhibit sebum production

C. **Insect venom (such as bee, yellow jacket, wasp stings; spider bites)**
   1. Local tissue inflammation and destruction results from poison, allergic reaction from previous sensitization or toxic reaction from large inoculation of poison; stings by yellow jackets, hornets, honeybees, and wasps result in generalized allergic reactions of varying severity in approximately 0.4% of the population
   2. IgE-mediated hypersensitivity to insect venom may be confirmed by skin testing with suitable dilutions of available venom, usually done by an allergist
   3. Clinical manifestations
      a. Local reactions include erythema, pain, heat, swelling, itching, blisters, secondary infection, necrosis, ulceration, and drainage
      b. Toxic reactions include nausea, vomiting, headache, fever, diarrhea, light-headedness, syncope, drowsiness, muscle spasms, edema, and possibly seizures
      c. Systemic reactions include allergic/itching eyes, facial flushing, generalized urticaria, dry cough, chest/throat constriction, wheezing, dyspnea, cyanosis, abdominal cramps, diarrhea, nausea, vomiting, vertigo, chills/fever, stridor, shock, loss of consciousness, involuntary bowel/bladder action, frothy sputum, respiratory failure, cardiovascular collapse, and death
      d. Delayed reactions include serum sickness-like reactions, fever, malaise, headache, urticaria, lymphadenopathy, polyarthritis
      e. Unusual reactions include encephalopathy, neuritis, vasculitis, nephrosis, extreme fear/anxiety
   4. Collaborative management
      a. Done on outpatient or inpatient basis depending on client response
      b. First-aid measures; local treatment; activate emergency services in severe reactions
      c. Over-the-counter antihistamine unless contraindicated
      d. Remove stinger by scraping—do not squeeze with a tweezer—then cleanse the wound
      e. Ice packs to bite or sting—alternate 10 minutes on and 10 minutes off
      f. Elevate and rest affected part

    g. Maintain adequate airway

    h. Persons with known sensitivity should wear medical ID tag

    i. Prevent reexposure in known hypersensitive persons

    j. Educate on risks of increasing severity of responses in the future

    k. Instruct to use insect repellants when outdoors or in infested areas

    l. Instruct on Epi-Pen use if prescribed

  5. Priority nursing problems: pain, potential for injury

  6. Medication therapy

    a. Local analgesics, diphenhydramine (Benadryl), or other antihistamines

    b. Topical or oral steroids

    c. Systemic (depending on severity and reaction type) include epinephrine 1:1000 subcutaneous to combat urticaria, wheezing, angioedema (adult 0.3–0.5 mL/kg); treat shock, if present; diphenhydramine may be prescribed to combat urticaria, wheezing, angioedema; aminophylline for bronchospasm; hydrocortisone if needed for severe urticaria or spider bite; tetanus prophylaxis and antibiotics if needed; diazepam (Valium) 5–10 mg if needed for severe muscle spasms; opioid analgesics for pain if needed

    d. Anti-venom for black widow spider or scorpion

    e. Consider desensitization with immunotherapy in severe cases

    f. Consider prescription to carry Epi-Pen or anaphylactic kit

VII. MALIGNANT DISORDERS OF INTEGUMENTARY SYSTEM

  A. *Actinic keratosis* **(senile or solar keratosis)**

    1. Description: pre-malignant macules found on skin surface of fair-skinned clients 50 years of age or older, but can be seen in high-risk individuals at any age; develop because of chronic exposure of skin to sun; persons with light-skin complexion are at highest risk for actinic keratosis; these lesions are considered pre-malignant lesions; approximately 20% will progress to squamous cell carcinoma

    2. Clinical manifestations: erythematous, rough, and shiny-textured macules that may appear as a single macule or in groups; they are commonly seen on face, ears, scalp, lips, neck, and hands

    3. Collaborative management

      a. Prophylactic treatment is recommended to prevent development of these lesions

      b. Protection from ultraviolet rays in sunlight with clothing and sunscreen use are recommended

      c. Biopsy and removal of lesion is recommended if changes occur to color, border, size, and shape of lesion; see Box 10-1 again

  B. Melanoma (malignant melanoma): a serious skin cancer that arises from melanocytes and causes a large majority of skin cancer deaths

    1. Pathophysiology: melanomas can develop wherever there is pigment, one-third originate in existing nevi (moles); slow growing; benign while confined to epidermis (melanoma *in situ*); when penetration of dermis occurs they mingle with blood and lymph vessels and are capable of metastasis

    2. Precursor lesions: have a greater than normal risk of becoming malignant

      a. Congenital nevi: present at birth

      b. Dysplastic nevi (atypical moles): appear normal during childhood and become dysplastic (abnormal development) after puberty

      c. Lentigo maligna (Hutchinson's freckle): grows slowly; usually seen on one side of face of an older adult who has had a large amount of sun exposure

    3. Types of malignant melanomas include superficial spreading melanoma, lentigo maligna melanoma, nodular melanoma, and acral lentigionous melanoma; types differ primarily by length of time growth of melanoma remains parallel to skin surface and are therefore more curable by surgical excision

4. Diagnosis and staging: suspicious lesions are biopsied; positive results indicate need for further tests to assess level of ivasion of malignant melanoma and presence or absence of metastasis

5. Treatment: research is ongoing and directed toward more specific methods of diagnosis and treatment

   a. Surgery: a wide excision that includes full thickness of skin and subcutaneous tissues with surgical dissection of involved lymph nodes

   b. Immunotherapy: agents such as interferons, interleukins, monoclonal antibodies, bacilli Calmette-Guérin (BCG), levamisole, transfer factors, and tumor vaccines have demonstrated varying response rates; may be used alone, in combination with chemotherapy, or in combination with each other

   c. Radiation therapy: response rates depend on size and thickness of tumor, type of melanoma, and client's general health with results ranging from 0–71%

   d. Biological therapy: used to boost or restore ability of immune system to fight cancer; agents used also have a direct antitumor effect and include monoclonal antibodies, growth factors, and vaccines

6. Priority nursing problems: interrupted skin integrity, anxiety or fear

7. Collaborative management

   a. Teach to keep incision line clean and dry; use principles of asepsis; recognize manifestations of infection

   b. Encourage caloric and protein intake; refer to a dietician if needed

   c. Use active listening, ask open-ended questions, and reflect on client's statements

   d. Encourage active participation in self-care as well as in mutual decision making and goal setting

   e. Provide interventions that decrease anxiety levels, including provision of accurate information, inclusion of family members in teaching, encouragement of discussion of feelings

8. Client education

   a. Schedule regular medical checkups every 3 months for first 2 years

   b. Use of strategies to decrease sun exposure (e.g. minimizing sun exposure, wearing protective clothing, wearing sunscreen with a SPF of 15 or greater, and avoiding tanning booths)

C. **Nonmelanoma skin cancers:** most common malignant neoplasm in fair-skinned Americans; less likely than melanomas to be fatal

1. **Basal cell carcinoma**

   a. Description: an abnormal cell growth of basal layer of epidermal skin; highest risk factor is exposure to ultraviolet rays from sunlight exposure; is a bulky tumor that destroys surrounding tissue; most common (80%) but least aggressive type of skin cancer and rarely metastasizes to other organs; tumors greater than 2 cm in diameter have a high recurrence rate

   b. Clinical manifestations vary based on type

   c. Therapeutic management

      1) Monitor progress of growth of all lesions; lesions that measure greater than 2 cm have a high reoccurrence rate; suspicious lesions are excised and sent for pathological examination

      2) Educate clients regarding importance of monitoring lesions and identifying new lesions early; suggest monthly skin assessment byclient and periodic screening based on symptoms by health care provider

      3) Encourage protection from ultraviolet light exposure by using sunscreen products with SPF greater than 15 and wearing clothing such as hats and clothing to protect skin when outdoors

Practice to Pass

A client tells you that she has a mole that she has noticed for the past year, and she is concerned that it is cancer. What is your immediate response to teach her how to evaluate the mole?

Practice to Pass

A 20-year-old client who comes in to the ambulatory clinic for treatment mentions that her father was just diagnosed with skin cancer. She asks you what she can do to protect herself from developing skin cancer later in life. What strategies would you suggest to reduce her risk of developing skin cancer?

     d. Priority nursing problems: interrupted skin integrity, potential for alteration in body image, fear or anxiety

     e. Medication therapy: topical chemotherapy is applied directly on skin to kill tumor cells; immune response modifiers are applied to skin or injected directly into tumor

2. Squamous cell carcinoma

     a. Description: less common (20%); a malignant tumor of squamous epithelium of skin or mucous membranes; grows quicker, is more aggressive, and is more likely to metastasize than basal cell carcinoma

     b. Clinical manifestations: begins as a small, firm red nodule; as tumor grows, color may change and appear erythemic, sore, and/or even bleed if touched; with continued extension the area around the nodule may become indurated (hardened)

     c. Therapeutic management: immediate removal of tumor by a variety of methods, including cryotherapy, surgical excision, electrodesiccation, or radiotherapy; medications as discussed under basal cell carcinoma; regular examinations for recurrence

3. Kaposi's sarcoma

     a. Description: a rare (less than 1%) skin cancer caused by a virus called Kaposi sarcoma-associated herpesvirus (human herpes virus); most common cancer associated with acquired immunodeficiency syndrome (AIDS)

     b. Clinical manifestations: presents as vascular macules, papules or violet lesions; more brown toned in people with dark skin; initially painless, may become painful as disease progresses into viscera

     c. Therapeutic management: milder forms may improve with initiation of highly active antiretroviral therapy (HAART); rapidly progressing forms are treated with chemotherapy

VIII. TRAUMA TO INTEGUMENTARY SYSTEM

    A. *Pressure ulcers* (bedsores, decubitus ulcers)

     1. Description

       a. Ischemic lesions of skin and underlying tissue caused by external pressure that impairs flow of blood and lymph or from friction and shearing forces that tear and injure vessels

       b. Increasing incidence in all health care settings affecting frail, disabled, acutely ill, or immobile client; results in infection, loss of function, and pain

       c. Considered preventable, the Centers for Medicare and Medicaid will no longer make additional reimbursement payments to hospitals to cover costs to treat pressure ulcers that develop during a hospital stay

      d. Most common sites are over bony prominences, such as elbows, hips, heels, outer ankles, back of head, and base of spine; over 95% of ulcers develop on lower part of body

       e. Causes include an uneven application of pressure over a bony hard site: high pressure applied for 2 hours, shearing forces that develop when a seated person slides toward floor or foot of bed if supine, frictional forces that develop when pulling a client across a bed sheet, and moisture from incontinence or perspiration

       f. Risk factors include immobility, malnutrition, and low body weight, hypoalbuminemia, fecal and/or urinary incontinence, bone fracture, vitamin C deficiency, low diastolic blood pressure, age-related skin changes such as diminished pain perception, thinning of epidermis, loss of dermal vessels, altered barrier properties, reduced immunity and slowed wound healing, anemia, infections, peripheral vascular insufficiency, dementia, malignancies, diabetes, CVA, dry skin, and edema

     2. Clinical manifestations:

       a. Pressure ulcers are staged according to their characteristics; see Box 10-3

Box 10-3	*Stage I*: Non-blanching erythema, warmth, and tenderness are present. Tends to occur over bony prominences and indicates a risk for further breakdown if not reversed.
Pressure Ulcer Stages	*Stage II*: Skin breakdown is limited to partial-thickness dermis and involves more sharply defined erythema and may involve excoriation, blistering, and drainage. Skin temperature is variable and local swelling and edema may be present.
	Stage III: Ulcer formation involves full thickness of dermis and may extend into subcutaneous tissue with crater formation and possible presence of slough, drainage, undermining, and tunneling.
	Stage IV: Ulcer extends beyond deep fascia into muscle, bone, or tendon. Involved area may be larger than visible apparent wound because undermining and tunneling are often present. Severity of wound condition poses risk for osteomyelitis or sepsis.

    b. Diagnostic and laboratory test findings: culture of wound, white blood cell (WBC) count with differential and erythrocyte sedimentation rate (ESR) to determine presence of primary or secondary infection; if no progression of ulcer healing, pre-albumin and albumin levels may be obtained to determine dietary needs

3. Collaboarative management

    a. Remove risk factors if possible

    b. Improve overall nutritional status, including intake of protein, calories, vitamins, and minerals

    c. Clean wound each time dressing is changed to remove dead tissue, excess fluid, and debris; avoid hot water; provide a moist wound environment to promote reepithelialization and healing

    d. Maintain normal body temperature and acidic pH

    e. Never use antiseptics and harsh skin cleansers that may harm tissue

    f. Reposition client at least every 2 hours; avoid placing external force on ulcer

    g. Use pressure-reducing devices such as padding (gel pads), flotation pads, mattress overlays, and specialized (such as air-fluidized, oscillating, or kinetic) beds

    h. Avoid agents that delay wound healing such as topical corticosteroids, hydrogen peroxide, iodine, and hypochlorite

    i. Control fecal and urine incontinence; if incontinence cannot be controlled use underpads or briefs made of materials that absorb moisture and present a quick-drying surface to skin; change frequently; do not place plastic directly against skin; use moisture barrier

    j. Avoid massage over bony prominences

    k. Assess site every 8–12 hours (or whenever dressing change is prescribed); carefully document healing, for example, location; dimensions (length, width, depth) of ulcer; presence of tunneling, undermining, necrotic tissue, or exudate; presence or absence of granulation tissue

    l. Use absorption dressing if wound has large amounts of exudate and change as prescribed

4. Priority nursing problems: interrupted skin integrity, possible alteration in body image, potential for infection, insufficient nutrients to meet bodily needs, potential for fever, possible reduced tissue perfusion, potential for reduced mobility, possible anxiety

5. Medication therapy

     a. Clindamycin (Cleocin) or gentamycin (Garamycin) may be ordered to treat complications such as cellulitis, osteomyelitis, or sepsis

     b. Vitamin C 500 mg bid and zinc sulfate supplements aid healing

     c. Antibiotic prophylaxis will eradicate bacterial component

     d. A 2-week trial of topical antimicrobials should be used only for a clean superficial ulcer that is either not healing or producing a moderate amount of exudates—cultures are necessary to determine whether antifungal or specific antibacterial agents are indicated

     e. Enzymatic debriding agents such as collagenase (Santyl, Granulex), fibinolysin-desoxyribonuclease (Elase), papin (Panafil), or sutilains (Travase) are used with a moisture barrier to protect surrounding tissue

     f. See Table 10-1 to review products that promote healing

6. Client education

     a. Teach caregiver about need for frequent evaluation of client with a history of pressure ulcers, especially if client has limited mobility

     b. Nutritional requirements and meal planning

     c. Early identification of skin redness to prevent breakdown

     d. Skin cleansing routine

     e. Underpads to absorb moisture

     f. Repositioning techniques and frequency

     g. Need to evaluate and ensure continence and access to facilities

     h. Use of mattress overlays, seat cushions or special mattresses

     i. Ways to avoid injuries

7. Evaluation: systematic staging of ulcers on a routine schedule documents healing; a schedule is maintained for mobility, nutritional assessment, and continence, and is altered as necessary; client remains free of possible complications, such as growth of resistant organisms and possible development of gangrene secondary to poor healing

Table 10-1   **Products Used to Treat Pressure Ulcers**

PRODUCT	PURPOSE
Hydrocolloid Dressings (such as DuoDerm)	May be used for stages I, II, III, and IV with minimal exudate. Forms a gel when coming into contact with wound exudate. Forms an occlusive barrier over the ulcer while maintaining a moist environment and preventing infection. Helps prevent friction and shear.
Alginate Dressings (such as SilvaSorb and Sorbsan)	May be used for stages II, III, and IV with moderate to heavy drainage, and in infected and non-infected wounds. Forms a gel when coming into contact with wound exudate. Should not be applied to dry or minimally draining wounds, as dehydration and delay in healing may result.
Hydrofibers (such as Aquacel)	May be used for stage II, III, and IV with moderate to heavy exudate. Can be used with actual or risk for infection. Combines the absorption of the hydrofiber with 1.2% silver as an antimicrobial agent.
Hydrogel Dressings (such as Intrasite gel)	May be used for stages II, III, IV. Rehydrate the wound bed and decrease pain. Promotes autolytic debridement.
Transparent Adhesive Dressings (such as OpSite and Tegrderm)	May be used in shallow I, II, and III ulcers. Provide a moist wound setting, prevent infection, and promote re-epithelialization. Minimize friction and shear.
Wet-to-Dry Dressings	Provide mechanical debridement.
Vacuum-assisted closure (VAC) sponges	Stimulate wound contracture while removing the exudate and wound edema.

Source: LeMone, Priscilla; Burke, Karen M.; Bauldoff, Gerene, *Medical-Surgical Nursing: Critical Thinking in Patient Care,* 5th Edition, © 2011. Printed and Electronically reproduced by permission of Pearson Education, Inc., Upper Saddle River, New Jersey.

B. Burn injury
1. Description
   a. An alteration in skin integrity resulting in tissue loss or injury; caused by heat, chemicals, electricity, or radiation
   b. Risk factors are age (children under 5, adults over 65), careless smoking, alcohol or drug intoxication, physical and mental illness, and occupations involving work with chemicals, gasoline or electricity
2. Types: thermal, chemical, electrical, and radiation
   a. Thermal burns (most common) result from dry heat (flames) or moist heat (steam or hot liquids); cause cellular destruction that results in vascular, bony, muscle, or nerve complications; also lead to inhalation injury if head and neck area is affected
   b. Chemical burns are caused by direct contact with either acidic or alkaline agents; they destroy tissue protein and cause altered tissue perfusion leading to necrosis
   c. Electrical burns vary in severity depending on type and duration of current and amount of voltage—current follows path of least resistance (muscles, bone, blood vessels, and nerves); sources of electrical injury include direct current, alternating current, and lightning; entry and exit wounds tend to be small and mask widespread tissue damage underneath
   d. Radiation burns are usually associated with sunburn or radiation treatment for cancer; are usually superficial and all functions of skin remain intact; extensive exposure to radiation may lead to tissue damage and multisystem injury similar to other types of burns
3. Phases of burn management
   a. Emergent/resuscitative stage lasts from onset of injury through successful fluid resuscitation; during this stage, it is determined whether client is to be transported to a burn center for complex intervention depending on onset of injury, identification of burn source, and complicating factors
   b. Acute stage: begins with start of diuresis and ends with closure of burn wound
   c. Rehabilitative stage: begins with wound closure and ends when client returns to highest level of health restoration
4. Assessment
   a. Classification of burn depth: done according to depth of damaged tissue
      1) Superficial thickness (formerly first-degree): involves epidermis only; is characterized by erythema (pink to bright red), mild local edema, local pain; healing occurs spontaneously in 3–6 days with no scar formation
      2) Superficial partial thickness (formerly second-degree): involves epidermis and dermis, characterized by moist areas that are red in color, blisters form immediately; area will blanch on pressure and is painful because touch and pain receptors are intact; area heals with greater or lesser amounts of scarring within 21–28 days; pigment changes are common
      3) Deep partial thickness (formerly second-degree): involves entire dermis, but extends deeper than a superficial partial thickness burn; hair follicles, sebaceous glands, and epidermal sweat glands are left intact; area has a moist or dry waxy whitish appearance and may be difficult to differentiate initially from full-thickness burns; capillary refill is decreased and sensation to deep pressure is present; less painful than a superficial partial-thickness burn, some areas of both pain and decreased sensation may be present; may heal spontaneously in about 1 month, although skin grafting is often done to close wound, accelerate healing, reduce scarring, and reduce risk of infection; can convert to a full-thickness injury due to necrosis

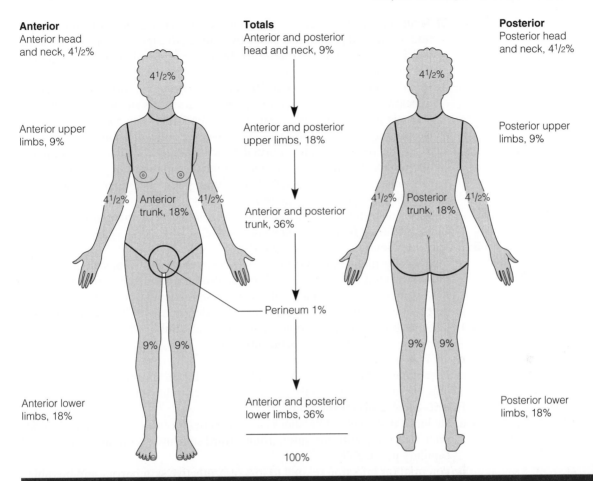

Anterior
Anterior head
and neck, 4¹/₂%

Anterior upper
limbs, 9%

Anterior
trunk, 18%

4¹/₂%   4¹/₂%

Perineum 1%

9%   9%

Anterior lower
limbs, 18%

Totals
Anterior and posterior
head and neck, 9%

Anterior and posterior
upper limbs, 18%

Anterior and posterior
trunk, 36%

Anterior and posterior
lower limbs, 36%

100%

Posterior
Posterior head
and neck, 4¹/₂%

Posterior upper
limbs, 9%

Posterior
trunk, 18%

4¹/₂%   4¹/₂%

9%   9%

Posterior lower
limbs, 18%

Figure 10-3

Rule of nines

4) Full thickness (formerly third-degree): involves destruction of all skin layers with coagulation of subdermal plexus; may extend into subcutaneous fat, connective tissue, muscle and bones; wound may appear pale, waxy, yellow, brown, mottled, charred, or non-blanching red; wound surface is dry, leathery and firm to touch; pain and touch receptors have been destroyed but often also have painful partial-thickness injuries; skin grafting is required to heal

b. Burn size is estimated using "Rule of Nines" (see Figure 10-3) or Lund and Browder method; each method accounts for 100% of total body surface area (TBSA) although Lund and Browder method takes into account client's age when estimating body surface area (BSA)

c. Severity of burn is classified using the American Burn Association criteria as minor burn, moderate uncomplicated burn, and major burn; is based on depth(s) of burn and percent and location of BSA involved

d. Nursing assessment: history of injury (time and cause), first-aid treatment administered, estimated burn extent and depth, age, weight, past medical history and medication history including date of last tetanus prophylaxis; assess for other concurrent injuries

e. Diagnostic and laboratory test findings
1) Complete blood count: elevated hematocrit caused by fluid shifts into interstitium; decreased hemoglobin related to hemolysis; elevated WBCs if infection present

       2) Serum electrolytes: decreased sodium secondary to fluid shifts into interstitium; increased potassium caused by damage to capillary and cell membranes, which later decreases as fluid shifts back to intercellular and intravascular compartments

       3) Renal function tests: elevated BUN caused by dehydration, elevated creatinine indicates renal insufficiency; myoglobin in urinalysis signals acute tubular necrosis, proteinuria and elevated urine specific gravity may be seen

       4) Respiratory function tests: possible elevation or lowering in pH, decreased PCO_2, decreased PO_2, low-normal bicarbonate levels, and oxygen saturations below 95% depending on presence of inhalation injury, hypoxia and acid–base disturbances; chest x-rays refeal atelectasis, pulmonary edema, or acute respiratory distress syndrome (ARDS)

       5) Nutritional status: total protein, albumin, transferrin, and prealbumin; are most useful during rehabilitation phase of care

  5. Medication therapy

    a. Pain management: burn pain is often excrutiating; intravenous medication is given initially around-the-clock and prior to hydrotherapy; may require concurrent use of anxiolytic agents; supplement with non-pharmacological strategies

    b. Antibiotic therapy: systemic infection is leading cause of death in major burn patients; broad-spectrum topical antimicrobials (Sulfamylon, Silvadene, silver nitrate) often used; prophylactic antibiotics

    c. Tetanus prophylaxis

    d. Histamine H_2 blockers (e.g. famotidine [Pepcid]) or proton pum inhibitors (e.g. pantoprazole [Protonix]) to prevent hyperacidity and Curling's ulcer

  6. Priority nursing diagnoses

    a. Reduced tissue perfusion (shock) and potential for intravascular dehydration related to fluid shift into interstitium (third spacing) secondary to increased capillary permeability

    b. Potential for infection related to loss of protective skin barrier and possible exposure to contaminants

    c. Pain related to burns, anxiety, wound care and physical therapy

    d. Insufficient nutrients to meet bodily needs related to increase in caloric requirements (hypermetabolic and catabolic state causes increases of as much as 100% with total caloric needs of 4,000–6,000 kcal per day)

    e. Alterations in respiratory pattern or gas exchange related to inhalation injury, intubation (required for burns of chest, face, or neck), fluid shifts into interstitium of lung tissue or fluid volume overload

    f. Anxiety related to pain, treatments, altered body image and loss of control of health status

    g. Potential for hypothermia related to loss of skin barrier

    h. Reduced physical mobility related to shrinkage of new skin tissue, pain with movement, and contracture formation

    i. Interrupted skin integrity related to burns, decreased movement, pressure garments

  7. Prehospital management

    a. Stop burning process

      1) Thermal burns: douse flames with water or smother them with a blanket, coat, or other similar object; cool a scald burn with use of cool water; remove tar and asphalt with mineral oil or petroleum ointments

      2) Chemical burns: remove clothing and flush copiously with water or other appropriate irrigant after dusting away any dry powder if present; eye irrigation if needed; rescuer should wear protective clothing

3) Electrical burns: remove client from contact with an electrical source only after current has been shut off; begin cardiopulmonary resuscitation if indicated; place in cervical collar and transport on a spinal board

4) Radiation burns: are usually minor, if severe may need trained personnel with protective shielding to rescue

b. Support vital functions

1) CAB: circulation, airway, and breathing

2) Assess for smoke inhalation injury (singed nares, eyebrows, or lashes; burns on face or neck; stridor, increasing dyspnea) and give oxygen (up to 100% as prescribed)

3) Prepare for possible intubation and mechanical ventilation if severe inhalation injury or carbon monoxide inhalation has occurred

4) Assess for signs of shock caused by fluid shifts (increased pulse, falling BP and urine output, pallor, cool clammy skin, deteriorating level of consciousness)

5) Cover to maintain body temperature and prevent further wound contamination and tissue damage

c. Fluid resuscitation is necessary if burns involve 20% or more of total body surface area (TBSA)

1) Modified Brooke formula uses 2 mL × kg × % TBSA burned of lactated Ringers solution over 24 hours

2) Parkland (Baxter) formula uses 4 mL × kg × % TBSA burned of lactated Ringer's solution over 24 hours

3) Both formulas give half of 24 hour total in first 8 hours, and second half over next 16 hours (see Box 10-4 for example of use of Parkland-Baxter formula)

4) Fluids often changed to 5% dextrose in water over second 24 hours

5) Effective if hourly urine output of 0.5 mL/kg/hr for an adult

---

Box 10-4	**Clinical Situation:** *A 34-year-old client who weighs 100 kg has sustained burns to 60% of the total body surface area in a house fire. The client is transported to a major burn center and arrives 2 hours postburn. The client received a total of 2,500 mL of IV fluid during the previous 2 hours.*
Fluid Resuscitation Using Parkland-Baxter Formula	**Calculating Fluid Resuscitation Using Parkland-Baxter Formula:**

1. Multiply 4 mL by weight in kilograms (100) by %TBSA burned (60) to determine total fluid resuscitation volume required in first 24 hours

$$4 \times 100 \times 60 = 24{,}000$$

2. Divide the total volume in half, with first half given during the initial 8 hours, and second half given over the following 16 hours

$$24{,}000 \div 2 = 12{,}000$$

3. Subtract amount already received by client in the first 2 hours from total needed during first 8 hours to determine amount to infuse over next 6 hours

$$12{,}000 - 2{,}500 = 9{,}500$$

4. Divide amount to infuse over next 6 hours by 6 to determine hourly IV rate

$$9{,}500 \div 6 = 1{,}587 \text{ mL/hr}$$

5. After first 8-hour volume is infused, divide the remaining half of the 24-hour volume by 16 to determine the hourly IV rate for the next 16 hours

$$12{,}000 \div 16 = 750 \text{ mL/hr}$$

    d. Other considerations

      1) Remove all rings and jewelry to avoid tourniquet effect caused by swelling/edema of burn site

      2) Provide cardiac monitoring for first 24 hours after electrical burn

8. Emergency and acute care

    a. Fluid resuscitation continues

      1) Be prepared to assist with insertion of pulmonary artery catheter for hemod namic monitoring of central venous pressure (CVP) and pulmonary capillary wedge pressures (PCWP)

      2) Monitor intake and output hourly, weigh daily

      3) Monitor lung sounds to assess tolerance of high-volume fluid resuscitation

    b. Respiratory management

      1) Prevent atelectasis and maintain alveolar oxygen exchange by elevating HOB to at least 30 degrees and turning every 2 hours

      2) Suction frequently, encourage use of incentive spirometer, help cough and deep-breathe at least every 2 hours

      3) Be prepared for immediate intubation and mechanical ventilation

      4) Humidify room air or oxygen to help prevent drying of secretions

      5) Administer bronchodilators and mucolytic agents as prescribed

      6) If carbon monoxide (CO) poisoning has occurred pulse oximetry readings may be false normal or high; monitor carboxyhemoglobin levels and arterial blood gases; hyperbaric oxygen therapy may be needed to replace CO with oxygen

    c. Pain control

      1) Use a consistent pain measurement tool

      2) Medicate before painful procedures

      3) Administer intravenous opioid analgesics as prescribed and combine with non-opioids for pain control (decreased circulation and absorption of medications makes other routes inappropriate)

    d. Wound care management

      1) Surgeries

        a) Escharotomy: eschar (hard crust of dead tissue) can act as a tourniquet and impair circulation; is a sterile surgical incision made longitudinally to release taut skin and allow for expansion

        b) Surgical debridement: excising wound to level of fascia or sequentially to level of viable tissue

        c) Autografting: skin is removed from healthy tissue (donor site) and applied to burn wound; now able to create cultured epithelial autografts from client's own body but problems such as infection and lack of attachment may occur

      2) Biologic and biosynthetic dressings: temporary material that rapidly adheres to wound bed, promotes healing, and may prepare burn wound for permanent autograft coverate

        a) Homograft (allograft) is human skin that has been harvested from cadavers; is in short supply and has high expense; rejected within 14–21 days

        b) Heterograft (xenograft) is skin obtained from an animal (usually a pig); infection rates are high and require frequent dressing changes

        c) Biobrane: synthetic composite material; adheres well to moderately clean wounds

        d) Alloderm: synthetic dermal substance placed in wound under autografts

        e) Skin substitutes: bioengineered and derived from human fibroplast cells

        3) Nonsurgical debridement: removal of all loose tissue, wound debris, and eschar
          a) Mechanical: includes wet to moist dressings, hydrotherapy, irrigation, or scissors and tweezers
          b) Enzymatic: topical agent to dissolve and remove necrotic tissue
        4) Positioning, splints and exercise: prevention of contractures is key
          a) Early physical therapy
          b) Splints to immobilize body parts removed on prescribed schedules
          c) Active and passive range of motion exercises every 2 hours
          d) Exercise program
          e) Move carefully to prevent shearing or dislodgement of skin grafts
          f) Support garments (e.g. Jobst) apply uniform pressure to prevent or reduce hypertrophic scarring

    e. Nutritional therapies
        1) High-calorie, high-protein diet with vitamins and minerals
        2) Enteral feedings or total parenteral nutrition may be required

    f. Infection control
        1) Topical antimicrobial agents as discussed in previous section
        2) Close monitoring for manifestations of topical or systemic infections; an increased body temperature without other manifestations of infection may simply reflect a hypermetabolic response

    g. Psychosocial support
        1) Allow as much control as possible
        2) Encourage expression of feelings
        3) Set short-term, realistic goals
        4) Arrange counseling if necessary
        5) Assist in returning to work, family, and social life
        6) Assess home environment for needs and accessibility

5. Rehabilitative phase of burn management: begins with wound closure and ends when client returns to highest level of health restoration
    a. Considers physiological and psychosocial aspects of recovery, much of which have been covered in previous section; referrals for psychological evaluation and support, physical therapy, occupational therapy, vocational assistance, clergy and home care services may be done as needed
    b. Client education
        1) Environmental safety: use low temperature setting for hot water heater, ensure access to and adequate number of electrical cords/outlets, isolate household chemicals, and avoid smoking in bed
        2) Use of household smoke detectors with emphasis on maintenance, especially annual battery replacement
        3) Proper storage and use of flammable substances
        4) Evacuation plan for family
        5) Signs and symptoms of infection; avoid exposure to people with colds or infections; follow aseptic technique when caring for wounds (graft and donor sites)
        6) Dietary requirements and alternative pain control therapies
        7) Use of sunscreen to protect healing tissue and other protective skin care measures, including splints, pressure support garments, and assistive devices

6. Evaluation: client demonstrates knowledge and understanding of instruction and education about pain management, skin integrity and healing, availability of services for follow-up care

Case Study

A 22-year-old client comes in for evaluation of a skin rash. She thinks she may have psoriasis. For several years, she has experienced a white scaly rash that comes and goes.

1. When performing an initial work-up history, what questions would you ask the client regarding the skin rash?

2. The client asks you to explain what kind of disease psoriasis is and would like you to discuss how the scaly patches develop. What is your response?

3. The client is diagnosed with psoriasis and wants to know how to get rid of the rash

and prevent it from coming back again. What methods do you suggest?

4. She has been prescribed to use topical steroids on her skin. What other over-the-counter products would be useful for her psoriasis?

5. The client would like to go golfing this weekend. What instruction would you give her regarding being outdoors?

For suggested responses, see page 624.

POSTTEST

❶ A client presents with skin lesions that are raised, reddened, round, and covered with silvery white scales. The nurse concludes that the client most likely has which of the following conditions?

1. Eczema
2. Contact dermatitis
3. Psoriasis
4. Poison ivy

❷ A client presents to the primary care clinic reporting frequent scratching and itching of the skin that is worse at night. The nurse should gather additional data that would be consistent with which skin disorder?

1. Scabies
2. Hives
3. Fleas
4. Drug reaction

❸ The nurse teaches guidelines for skin care to a client with acne. Which instruction is appropriate?

1. "Wash the skin with a strong soap and water at least 3 times a day."
2. "Use alcohol-based skin preparations for aftershave lotion."
3. "Eat a regular, well-balanced diet."
4. "Avoid exposing the skin to sunlight."

❹ The nurse is caring for a client with a stage IV pressure ulcer. During the dressing change the nurse notes which characteristics unique to a stage IV ulcer? Select all that apply.

1. Erythema
2. Subcutaneous tissue
3. Bone
4. Muscle
5. Dermis

❺ A client is admitted to the emergency department with partial thickness burns on the scalp, chest, and neck. The client's blood pressure is 96/62 with a heart rate of 86 beats per minute. The nurse notes that the client's voice is slightly hoarse. Which intervention should the nurse implement first?

1. Hang a saline infusion wide open to keep the BP normal.
2. Cleanse the skin with sterile saline to prevent infection.
3. Call the physician and prepare to intubate the client.
4. Observe the client for evidence of distress.

6 The nurse is caring for a client with full-thickness burns on 50% of his body. The spouse asks, "Why does he look so different? He's all puffy." What is the best response by the nurse?

1. "We are giving him a great deal of intravenous solution and that is causing the edema."
2. "It is normal at this stage of a burn injury."
3. "The burn causes his fluids to shift into his tissues and that is causing the puffiness."
4. "When he receives his diuretic, most of the puffiness will go away."

7 The nurse is caring for a client with the skin alteration shown. Which intervention is appropriate? Select all that apply.

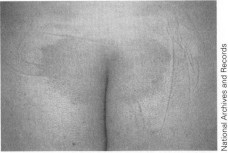

National Archives and Records Administration

1. Apply a hydrogel dressing such as Intrasite gel.
2. Clean the skin gently at regular intervals
3. Massage over bony prominences
4. Offer nutritional supplements and support the patient during mealtimes.
5. Avoid placing the patient in the side-lying position directly on the trochanter.

8 When caring for a client with a burn in the emergent/resuscitative stage of burn injury, which of the following has lowest priority with respect to burn assessment?

1. Extent of burn injury
2. Cause of the burn
3. First-aid treatment given
4. Measures used to debride the burn wound

9 The nurse is gathering intake information from a client in the outpatient clinic who reports discomfort in the vaginal area. Upon questioning, the nurse determines that the client has never been sexually active. The nurse determines that the client is most likely to be infected with which of the following?

1. Herpes virus type 1
2. Herpes virus type 2
3. Candidiasis
4. Herpes zoster

10 A client has a prescription for oral acyclovir as needed to prevent reoccurrences and to treat recurrent outbreaks. The nurse instructs the client to fill the prescription when which disorder is present?

1. Fever blister or cold sore
2. Common wart
3. Tinea pedis
4. Cellulitis

➤ *See pages 345–346 for Answers and Rationales.*

POSTTEST
ANSWERS & RATIONALES

ANSWERS & RATIONALES

Pretest

1 **Answer: 3 Rationale:** A bulla is a raised blister filled with clear fluid and measures greater than 0.5 cm. A papule is solid and firm. A vesicle is also a raised, fluid-filled blister, but measures less than 0.5 cm. A pustule is a vesicle containing purulent exudates. **Cognitive Level:** Applying **Client Need:** Physiological Adaptation **Integrated Process:** Communication and Documentation **Content Area:** Adult Health **Strategy:** Describe each option and then compare the descriptions to the items identified in the question. **Reference:** LeMone, P., Burke, K., & Bauldoff, G.

(2011). *Medical-surgical nursing: Critical thinking in patient care* (5th ed.). Upper Saddle River, NJ: Pearson Education, p. 400.

2 **Answer: 2** **Rationale:** A lesion that has poorly defined edges, asymmetry, color variation but mostly dark black and a diameter greater than 6 mm is characteristic of melanoma and need to be reported immediately. A brownish discoloration to the legs in a client with venous insufficiency is the result of inadequate excretion of metabolites secondary to poor venous return. Birthmarks such as the port-wine stain do not need to be reported to the health care provider. Contact dermatitis may result from an allergic reaction to a plant and can be addressed through client teaching. **Cognitive Level:** Analyzing **Client Need:** Physiological Adaptation **Integrated Process:** Nursing Process: Assessment **Content Area:** Adult Health **Strategy:** When assessing skin lesions apply the ABCDE Rule: Asymmetry, Border, Color, Diameter, Elevation or Evolution. **Reference:** LeMone, P., Burke, K., & Bauldoff, G. (2011). *Medical-surgical nursing: Critical thinking in patient care* (5th ed.). Upper Saddle River, NJ: Pearson Education, p. 430.

3 **Answer: 2** **Rationale:** Herpes simplex virus 1 lies dormant on the nerve ending and may reappear in times of reactivation. Genital herpes lesions are most commonly caused by herpes simplex virus 2. Herpes simplex virus 1 lesions progress from vesicles to pustules, ulcers, and crusting before healing occurs. **Cognitive Level:** Applying **Client Need:** Health Promotion and Maintenance **Integrated Process:** Communication and Documentation **Content Area:** Adult Health **Strategy:** Review the principles of dormancy and the infectious process of the herpes virus. Applying both of these sets of principles will enable you to select the correct answer option. **Reference:** LeMone, P., Burke, K., & Bauldoff, G. (2011). *Medical-surgical nursing: Critical thinking in patient care* (5th ed.). Upper Saddle River, NJ: Pearson Education, p. 416.

4 **Answer: 3** **Rationale:** Herpes zoster is a viral infection of a dermatome section of the skin characterized by eruptions of vesicles over a single dermatome. The client with herpes zoster may experience impaired skin integrity and pruritus in which the client may frequently scratch the lesions, contributing to a secondary bacterial infection. Cool environments should be maintained because heat and scratching will make the pruritus worse. The virus is not transmitted through sexual intercourse. Benzoyl peroxide is used for acne; it is not appropriate for application to herpes zoster lesions. **Cognitive Level:** Applying **Client Need:** Safety and Infection Control **Integrated Process:** Nursing Process: Planning **Content Area:** Adult Health **Strategy:** Recall that herpes zoster causes blisters on the end of the nerve fibers that are painful and itchy. Next, consider that if the blisters rupture, there is an increased risk for a superimposed infection. Review the procedures to prevent a secondary infection if you have the need. **Reference:** LeMone, P.,

Burke, K., & Bauldoff, G. (2011). *Medical-surgical nursing: Critical thinking in patient care* (5th ed.). Upper Saddle River, NJ: Pearson Education, p. 417.

5 **Answer: 36** **Rationale:** When using the rule of nines the body is divided into surface areas that are divisible by 9. Each side of a leg is 9% and each side of the torso is 18%. This client has both posterior sides of the legs (9% + 9%) and 1 side of the torso (18%) for a total of 36% burns. **Cognitive Level:** Applying **Client Need:** Physiological Adaptation **Integrated Process:** Nursing Process: Assessment **Content Area:** Adult Health **Strategy:** Total body percentage must equal 100%. The "rule of nines" cues the reader that the answer will be divisible by 9. **Reference:** LeMone, P., Burke, K., & Bauldoff, G. (2011). *Medical-surgical nursing: Critical thinking in patient care* (5th ed.). Upper Saddle River, NJ: Pearson Education, p. 450.

6 **Answer: 1** **Rationale:** Vitiligo is a slowly progressive depigmentation of the skin caused by disappearance of melanocytes. Eczema is an inflammatory condition in which the skin appears erythemic, dry, scaly, and thickened. Psoriasis is a chronic inflammatory condition in which lesions appear whitish, scaly, and commonly appear on the scalp, knees, and elbows. Contact dermatitis is an eruption of the skin related to contact with an irritating substance or allergen. **Cognitive Level:** Applying **Client Need:** Physiological Adaptation **Integrated Process:** Nursing Process: Assessment **Content Area:** Adult Health **Strategy:** Describe each disorder in the answer options. Compare these descriptions with the one presented in the stem of the question. **Reference:** LeMone, P., Burke, K., & Bauldoff, G. (2011). *Medical-surgical nursing: Critical thinking in patient care* (5th ed.). Upper Saddle River, NJ: Pearson Education, pp. 393–394, 407, 419.

7 **Answer: 1** **Rationale:** Disposal of smoking materials focuses on how to prevent fires. Fire extinguishers, escape routes, and smoke detectors focus on activities after a fire is already present. **Cognitive Level:** Analyzing **Client Need:** Health Promotion and Maintenance **Integrated Process:** Nursing Process: Planning **Content Area:** Adult Health **Strategy:** The critical word in the question is *prevention.* Apply this information to select the best answer option to answer the question. **Reference:** LeMone, P., Burke, K., & Bauldoff, G. (2011). *Medical-surgical nursing: Critical thinking in patient care* (5th ed.). Upper Saddle River, NJ: Pearson Education pp. 446–447.

8 **Answer: 1, 2, 3, 4** **Rationale:** Wet-to-moist dressings provide mechanical debridement of eschar but are not harmful to granulating (healthy) tissue. Turning at least every 2 hours is necessary to prevent the formation of further pressure ulcers. Enzymatic debridement involves the use of a topical agent to dissolve and remove necrotic tissue, as well as lift eschar. Hydrogel dressings may be used for stages II, III, and IV. They rehydrate the wound bed and decrease pain as well as promote autolytic debridement. Dry dressings pull off both newly granulated (healthy) tissue and eschar and should not be used.

Cognitive Level: Analyzing **Client Need:** Physiological Adaptation **Integrated Process:** Nursing Process: Implementation **Content Area:** Adult Health **Strategy:** This infected stage 4 ulcer has areas of necrosis and little granulation tissue. Select the answer options that may be used to treat this type of pressure ulcer and that will not damage new granulation tissue. **Reference:** LeMone, P., Burke, K., & Bauldoff, G. (2011). *Medical-surgical nursing: Critical thinking in patient care* (5th ed.). Upper Saddle River, NJ: Pearson Education, pp. 436–438, 463–464.

9 Answer: 1 Rationale: Questions should be relevant to the probable etiology of the disorder. In this case the client manifests clusters of small vesicles along the route of a nerve characteristic of herpes zoster or shingles. By identifying how long the vesicles have been present the nurse can develop an appropriate plan of care. It is not related to food intake, sun exposure, or herpes simplex cold sores. **Cognitive Level:** Applying **Client Need:** Physiological Adaptation **Integrated Process:** Nursing Process: Assessment **Content Area:** Adult Health **Strategy:** Look for characteristics that distinguish the cause of the rash in order to guide the assessment process. **Reference:** LeMone, P., Burke, K., & Bauldoff, G. (2011). *Medical-surgical nursing: Critical thinking in patient care* (5th ed.). Upper Saddle River, NJ: Pearson Education, pp. 416–417.

10 Answer: 2 Rationale: Psoriasis can often be brought on by sunlight, stress, seasonal changes, hormone fluctuations, steroid withdrawal, certain drugs (beta blockers, lithium, chloroquine), and trauma to the skin from surgery, sunburn or excoriation. About one-third of patients have a family history. Psoriasis is not associated with vitiligo, food allergies, plants or soil. **Cognitive Level:** Applying **Client Need:** Physiological Adaptation **Integrated Process:** Nursing Process: Assessment **Content Area:** Adult Health **Strategy:** Correlate the causes of psoriasis with the information obtained when completing the health assessment. **Reference:** LeMone, P., Burke, K., & Bauldoff, G. (2011). *Medical-surgical nursing: Critical thinking in patient care* (5th ed.). Upper Saddle River, NJ: Pearson Education, pp. 407–408.

Posttest

1 Answer: 3 Rationale: Psoriasis is characterized by the presence of silvery plaques, particularly on the extensor prominences. Eczema is also scaly but can be found throughout the body and has papules and vesicles. Contact dermatitis and poison ivy erupt into vesicles. **Cognitive Level:** Applying **Client Need:** Physiological Adaptation **Integrated Process:** Nursing Process: Assessment **Content Area:** Adult Health **Strategy:** Factual information is needed to answer this question. Based on the appearance of the skin changes, eliminate all options that do not fit that appearance. **Reference:** D'Amico, D., & Barbarito, C. (2012). *Health and physical assessment in nursing* (2nd ed.) Upper Saddle River, NJ: Prentice Hall, p. 223. LeMone, P., Burke, K., & Bauldoff, G.

(2011). *Medical-surgical nursing: Critical thinking in patient care* (5th ed.). Upper Saddle River, NJ: Pearson Education, pp. 407–410, 419.

2 Answer: 1 Rationale: Even though all these problems may cause itching, a classical symptom of scabies is pruritus with worsening at night. The mites tend to have increased movement at night, which accounts for the worsening symptoms at that time. Hives, flea bites, and drug reactions appear at all times, not just at night. **Cognitive Level:** Applying **Client Need:** Physiological Adaptation **Integrated Process:** Nursing Process: Assessment **Content Area:** Adult Health **Strategy:** The symptoms presented in this item occur primarily at night. Delete any answer options that present other times during the day. **Reference:** LeMone, P., Burke, K., & Bauldoff, G. (2011). *Medical-surgical nursing: Critical thinking in patient care* (5th ed.). Upper Saddle River, NJ: Pearson Education, pp. 400, 415.

3 Answer: 3 Rationale: Dietary restrictions were once believed to be necessary to decrease acne, but this has not been clinically relevant or supported in research. Items that irritate or overly dry the skin should not be used. Skin may be exposed to sunlight although sunburn should be avoided. **Cognitive Level:** Applying **Client Need:** Health Promotion and Maintenance **Integrated Process:** Teaching and Learning **Content Area:** Adult Health **Strategy:** Recall that acne is related to clogged pores and stress. Select the answer option that does not reflect these causes. **Reference:** LeMone, P., Burke, K., & Bauldoff, G. (2011). *Medical-surgical nursing: Critical thinking in patient care* (5th ed.). Upper Saddle River, NJ: Pearson Education, pp. 421–422.

4 Answer: 3, 4 Rationale: In stage IV, there is extensive breakdown that exposes the muscle, tendon or bone. There are usually areas of breakdown that extend under the skin and beyond the margins of the wound. Necrosis is often present. In stage I the skin is intact but reddened without blanching. In stage II, skin is lost from the dermis or epidermis. An abrasion, blister, or shallow crater may be present. Subcutaneous tissue is visible with both a stage III and stage IV ulcer. **Cognitive Level:** Applying **Client Need:** Physiological Adaptation **Integrated Process:** Nursing Process: Assessment **Content Area:** Adult Health **Strategy:** Describe the 4 stages of development for a pressure ulcer. Select the options that reflect this description. **Reference:** LeMone, P., Burke, K., & Bauldoff, G. (2011). *Medical-surgical nursing: Critical thinking in patient care* (5th ed.). Upper Saddle River, NJ: Pearson Education, p. 435.

5 Answer: 3 Rationale: Clients with burns around the face are at increased risk of an inhalation injury. The edema that results can be sudden and occlude the airway almost immediately. Most burn centers intubate immediately when the risk of inhalation injury is present. The skin should be cleaned to prevent infection but this clearly is not the priority. The client has a low normal blood pressure and normal heart rate at present. The massive fluid shifts will happen imminently, but maintaining the airway first is the top priority. Observation is not indicated with this type of injury. **Cognitive Level:** Analyzing **Client Need:** Physiological Adaptation **Integrated Process:** Nursing Process: Planning **Content Area:** Adult Health **Strategy:** Apply the ABCs (airway, breathing, and circulation) of emergency management of clients. When the client has a pulse, protect the airway first before attending to other aspects of care. **Reference:** LeMone, P., Burke, K., & Bauldoff, G. (2011). *Medical-surgical nursing: Critical thinking in patient care* (5th ed.). Upper Saddle River, NJ: Pearson Education, pp. 454–455.

6 Answer: 3 Rationale: After a burn, the blood vessels dilate and fluid leaks into the interstitial spaces. This is known as third spacing. The fluid shifts are treated with massive amounts of intravenous fluids to maintain the circulating blood volume, but this is not the initial cause of the edema. It is a normal stage in a burn injury, but the spouse is asking for an explanation. It is a dismissive response. Edema will continue until the fluid is reabsorbed from the interstitium into the intravascular compartment. **Cognitive Level:** Analyzing **Client Need:** Physiological Adaptation **Integrated Process:** Communication and Documentation **Content Area:** Adult Health **Strategy:** Select the option that best reflects the pathophysiology of burns and fluid shifts. The best option directly answers the spouse's question. **Reference:** LeMone, P., Burke, K., & Bauldoff, G. (2011). *Medical-surgical nursing: Critical thinking in patient care* (5th ed.). Upper Saddle River, NJ: Pearson Education, pp. 454–455.

7 Answer: 2, 4, 5 Rationale: Treatment for pressure ulcers includes dressings appropriate for the stage of the ulcer, proper nutrition, proper skin care, prevention of moisture against skin, prevention of prolonged pressure, minimization of friction and shearing forces and proper positioning. **Cognitive Level:** Analyzing **Client Need:** Physiological Adaptation **Integrated Process:** Nursing Process: Implementation **Content Area:** Adult Health **Strategy:** Consider options that prevent injury and options that assist in healing the current damage. **Reference:** LeMone, P., Burke, K., & Bauldoff, G. (2011). *Medical-surgical nursing: Critical thinking in patient care* (5th ed.). Upper Saddle River, NJ: Pearson Education, pp. 435–438.

8 Answer: 4 Rationale: In the emergent/resuscitative stage, the nurse assesses the cause and extent of the burn, initiates fluid resuscitation therapies, and determines first

aid measures that were used. Knowledge of debridement methods is a lower priority because this information does not directly influence the plan of care. **Cognitive Level:** Analyzing **Client Need:** Physiological Adaptation **Integrated Process:** Nursing Process: Assessment **Content Area:** Adult Health **Strategy:** High-priority assessments are those that will directly influence development and implementation of the plan of care. **Reference:** LeMone, P., Burke, K., & Bauldoff, G. (2011). *Medical-surgical nursing: Critical thinking in patient care* (5th ed.). Upper Saddle River, NJ: Pearson Education, pp. 456–457, 463.

9 Answer: 3 Rationale: Candidiasis is a yeast infection that can occur whenever there is a disruption in the balance of normal flora. An example of a causative factor would be antibiotic therapy. Further questioning by the nurse would likely elicit this data. Herpes virus type 1 typically occurs on the lips or oral mucosa. Herpes virus type 2 is a sexually transmitted disease. Herpes zoster usually occurs on the trunk along discrete dermatomes and commonly occurs in immunosuppressed individuals. **Cognitive Level:** Applying **Client Need:** Physiological Adaptation **Integrated Process:** Nursing Process: Diagnosis **Content Area:** Adult Health **Strategy:** Eliminate all answer options that are sexually transmitted or do not cause symptoms in the genital area. **Reference:** LeMone, P., Burke, K., & Bauldoff, G. (2011). *Medical-surgical nursing: Critical thinking in patient care* (5th ed.). Upper Saddle River, NJ: Pearson Education, pp. 413-417.

10 Answer: 1 Rationale: Acyclovir is an antiviral agent appropriate for the prevention and treatment of the herpes simplex virus, also called a *fever blister* or *cold sore*. Common warts are caused by a virus but are treated with acid therapy, cryotherapy or electrodessication. Tinea pedis (athlete's foot) is a fungal infection treated with topical or systemic antifungal medications such as miconazole. Cellulitis is a bacterial infection and is treated with antibiotics specific to the organism. **Cognitive Level:** Analyzing **Client Need:** Pharmacological and Parenteral Therapies **Integrated Process:** Teaching and Learning **Content Area:** Adult Health **Strategy:** Identify the cause of the disorders and select the one that is successfully treated with an antiviral agent. **Reference:** LeMone, P., Burke, K., & Bauldoff, G. (2011). *Medical-surgical nursing: Critical thinking in patient care* (5th ed.). Upper Saddle River, NJ: Pearson Education, pp. 411–416.

References

Berman, A., & Snyder, S. (2012). *Kozier & Erb's fundamentals of nursing: Concepts, process, and practice* (9th ed.). Upper Saddle River, NJ: Pearson Education.

D'Amico, D., & Barbarito, C. (2012). *Health & physical assessment in nursing* (2nd ed.). Upper Saddle River, NJ: Pearson Education, Inc.

Ignatavicius, D. D., & Workman, M. L. (2013). *Medical-surgical nursing: Critical thinking for collaborative care* (7th ed.) Philadelphia: W. B. Saunders Company.

Kee, J. L. (2010). *Laboratory and diagnostic tests* (8th ed.). Upper Saddle River, NJ: Pearson Education.

Lehne, R. (2010). *Pharmacology for nursing care* (7th ed.). St. Louis, MO: Saunders.

LeMone, P., Burke, K., & Bauldoff, G. (2011). *Medical surgical nursing: Critical thinking in patient care* (5th ed.). Upper Saddle River, NJ: Pearson Education.

Lewis, S., Dirksen, S. Heitkemper, M., Bucher, L., & Camera, I. (2011). *Medical surgical nursing: Assessment and management of clinical problems* (8th ed.). St. Louis, MO: Elsevier.

McCance, K. L., & Huether, S. E. (2010). *Pathophysiology: The biologic basis for disease in adults and children* (6th ed.). St. Louis, MO: Mosby, Inc.

National Pressure Ulcer Advisory Panel (2007). Pressure ulcer stages updated by NPUAP. Retrieved from http://www.npuap.org/pr2.htm.

Osborn, K. S., Wraa, C. E., & Watson, A. (2010). *Medical surgical nursing: Preparation for practice* (Vol. Combined). Upper Saddle River, NJ: Prentice Hall.

11 Immunologic Disorders

Chapter Outline

Immunologic System
Altered Immune Responses:
   Hypersensitivity Reactions

Autoimmune Disorders
Immunodeficiency
   Disorders

Tissue Transplants
Infection Precautions

Objectives

➤ Identify basic structures and functions of the immunologic system.
➤ Describe the pathophysiology and etiology of common immunologic disorders.
➤ Discuss expected assessment data and diagnostic test findings for selected immunologic disorders.
➤ Identify priority nursing problems for selected immunologic disorders.
➤ Discuss therapeutic management of selected immunologic disorders.
➤ Discuss nursing management of a client experiencing an immunologic disorder.
➤ Identify expected outcomes for the client experiencing an immunologic disorder.

NCLEX-RN® Test Prep

Use the accompanying online resource, NursingReviewsandRationales, to test yourself with hundreds of NCLEX®-style practice questions.

Review at a Glance

antibody a specific substance produced by B lymphocytes in response to a specific antigen

antigen a protein substance that elicits a specific response that triggers an antibody response

antigen–antibody complexes a binding of antigen–antibody in body to activate immune response by either suppressing, amplifying or causing activation of complement

antihistamine a substance that blocks effects of histamine release in body

atopy incidence of increased allergic reactions as a result of hereditary disposition

cell-mediated immunity recognition of T lymphocytes that are involved in process of autoimmunity to afford protection

colony-stimulating factors a group of proteins that stimulate specific hematologic cell growth to help prevent bone marrow suppression or stimulate a client's response to it

complement fixation an antigen–antibody reaction whereby complement system is activated, causing it to become "fixed"

human leukocyte antigens (HLA) genetic markers found on chromosome 6 that are associated with specific diseases and used for tissue typing

hypersensitivity an exaggerated abnormal response to a specific indicator that leads to an overactive immune response

immunoglobulins a group of 5 structurally distinct humoral antibodies that are secreted in response to specific antigens

major histocompatibility complex (MHC) a group of proteins carrying specific genetic information that plays an active role in autoimmune recognition and tissue rejection

monoclonal antibodies antibodies produced by a specific group of identical cells that are being used to treat hematologic and oncologic disease, both to identify and treat tumors due to their specific targeting effect

myelosuppression inhibition or destruction of blood cells in bone marrow that can lead to immunosuppression

neutropenic precautions institution of specific measures aimed at protecting an individual who is immunosuppressed from potential infection and injury during course of a treatment

opportunistic infection a nonpathogenic infection that becomes pathogenic as a result of an individual's baseline immunosuppressive state

plasmapheresis a process whereby plasma is removed from body and sent through a machine membrane to remove immune complexes that are associated with disease processes

wasting syndrome unexplained weight loss of greater than 10% ideal body weight (IBW) that is associated with a cycle of malnutrition and subsequent wasting that is an AIDS-defining diagnosis

1 Which of the following atypical findings would the nurse look for in an older adult client who presents with an infection?

1. Fever and chills
2. Erythema and edema
3. Behavioral changes and confusion
4. Leukocytosis with elevated neutrophil count

2 A client has an unexplained weight loss of more than 10% of ideal body weight (IBW) and voices nonspecific complaints of fatigue and nausea over the last 6-month period. The nurse should place the highest priority on assessing the client for acquired immunodeficiency syndrome (AIDS) when the client makes which statement?

1. "I have had a low-grade fever for the past week."
2. "I had a blood transfusion several years ago after having surgery."
3. "My stools have changed from a brown color to a pale beige color."
4. "I have this odd purple spot that has developed on the tip of my ear."

3 While obtaining a review of systems the client informs the nurse that he is "highly allergic" to many food items and medications. The nurse concludes that which hypersensitivity reaction would be responsible for this type of clinical presentation?

1. Type 1, IgE mediated hypersensitivity
2. Type 2, cytotoxic hypersensitivity
3. Type 3, immune complex-mediated hypersensitivity
4. Type 4, delayed hypersensitivity

4 A client who receives a positive antinuclear antibody (ANA) test result with a titer level greater than 1:40 does not understand what the test result means and asks the nurse for an explanation. Which response to the client by the nurse would be most appropriate in this situation?

1. "The test result is normal."
2. "The test indicates that you may have an autoimmune disorder, and this result should be discussed in more detail with your physician."
3. "You should have the test repeated to verify its specificity for autoimmune disorders."
4. "Your test result is specific for the detection of systemic lupus, and this should be discussed further with your physician."

5 Which of the following measures would be most appropriate for the nurse to use in helping a client with a past history of anaphylaxis to develop a plan to manage possible allergic reactions?

1. Schedule an appointment for allergy testing using intradermal injections.
2. Ask client to keep a diary of foods consumed and allergic responses for 1 week.
3. Have diphenhydramine (Benadryl) readily available.
4. Have an Epi-Pen (epinephrine) readily available.

6 Hydroxychloroquine (Plaquenil) is prescribed for a client for the treatment of rheumatoid arthritis. The nurse would include which measure as part of client teaching with regard to this medication?

1. Take this medication on an empty stomach to minimize gastric irritation.
2. Have a baseline eye exam performed and follow-up exams every 6 months to monitor for ocular changes.
3. Monitor weight and vital signs as the medication can cause fluid retention and pulse elevations.
4. Be aware that medication can cause drowsiness and do not take it if planning to drive a car.

7 The nurse teaches a client to sneeze into the bend of the elbow. Which link in the chain of infection does this help interrupt? Select the correct area on the image.

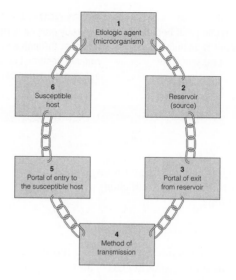

8 A client comes to the office with reports of joint pain. The nurse would assess for which other finding consistent with early clinical manifestations of systemic sclerosis?

1. Raynaud's disease
2. Dysphagia
3. Infections
4. Malabsorption syndrome

9 Which statement indicates to the nurse that the client understands the measures used to treat systemic lupus erythematosus (SLE)?

1. "I will take oral contraceptives to prevent getting pregnant."
2. "I can go visit this weekend with my grandmother who has been ill with a cold."
3. "I can go for a walk on the beach after 3:00 p.m."
4. "I will have a good chance of a cure if I take my immunosuppressive agents as prescribed."

10 The nurse is caring for a client who is admitted with an allergic reaction to a face cream used earlier that day. Which actions should the nurse take with this client? Select all that apply.

1. Wash client's face to remove the allergen.
2. Assess breath sounds for wheezing.
3. Administer interferon with an appropriate order.
4. Administer a bronchodilator with an appropriate order.
5. Administer an antihistamine with an appropriate order.

➤ *See pages 376–378 for Answers and Rationales.*

I. IMMUNOLOGIC SYSTEM

A. Basic structures and functions of immunologic system

1. Lymphoid system
   a. Consists of a communication network of vessels, lymph nodes, lymph node clusters, and circulating and resident lymphocytes that function as a primary component in immune system response
   b. Lymphoid system exists to recover proteins such as albumin for vascular space and to protect bloodstream from invading organisms

    c. Cells of the immune system (neutrophils, macrophages, dendritic cells) carry antigens from interstitial space to lymph nodes for immune surveillance

    d. Lymph nodes

        1) Found throughout body and consist of a small, rounded mass of tissue from which lymph fluid drains

        2) Filter foreign products or antigens from lymph fluid

        3) House and support proliferation of T and B lymphocytes, macrophages, and plasma cells

        4) Presence of antigens in lymph stimulates proliferation of lymphocytes and macrophages

        5) Macrophages destroy antigens by phagocytosis

    e. *Thymus gland*

        1) Assists in T lymphocyte formation, is located in superior mediastinum behind sternum

        2) Gland is large during childhood and atrophies with age because of fat infiltration

        3) Gives rise during childhood to differentiation and maturation of T lymphocytes, which are involved in **cell-mediated immunity**, a part of the process of autoimmunity

        4) Secretes thymosin, a hormone that stimulates lymphopoiesis (formation of lymphocytes or lymphoid tissue); hormone level is stable from birth to age 25 and then gradually decreases

    f. Bone marrow

        1) Sources can be found in iliac crest, sternum, and in bone cavities throughout body

        2) Produces and stores hematopoietic stem cells, from which all cellular components of blood are formed

    g. Tonsils are a group of lymphoid tissue found in palatine area of oropharnyx in mouth; they protect body from inhaled or ingested foreign agents

    h. Mucosa-associated lymph tissue (MALT)

        1) Lymph tissue located at key sites of potential invasion of microorganisms

        2) Specific locators identify source of tissue; for example: bronchial-associated lymph tissue (BALT), gut-associated lymph tissue (GALT), skin-associated lymph tissue (SALT)

    i. Spleen

        1) Located in left upper quadrant of abdomen and is composed of white and red pulp

        2) White pulp is lymphoid tissue composed of B and T lymphocytes

        3) Red pulp is where blood filtration occurs

            a) Phagocytic cells dispose of damaged or aged RBCs and platelets

            b) Filters and removes foreign material (bacteria, viruses, toxins), worn-out cells, and forms of cellular debris

            c) Stores blood and breakdown products of RBCs for future use

2. Leukocytes (white blood cells, WBCs)

    a. All blood cells derive from stem cells (hemocytoblasts) in bone marrow (see Figure 11-1)

    b. WBCs use circulatory system to travel to site of an inflammatory or immune response and attack foreign materials; capable of moving through tissue spaces directly to damaged tissues and infection

    c. Normal WBC count is 4,500–10,000 cells per cubic millimeter (mm^3); level increases when infection is present, decreases when bone marrow activity is suppressed or when increased destruction of WBCs occurs

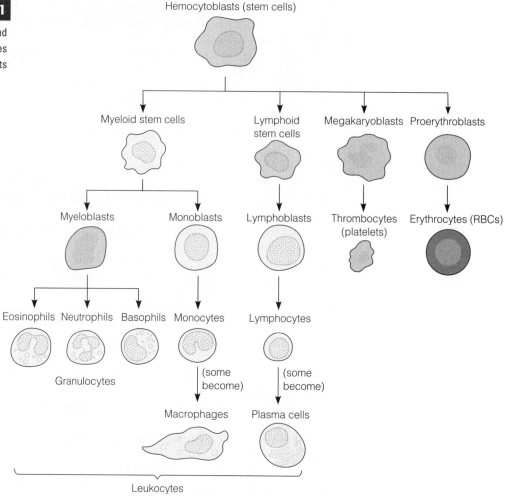

Figure 11-1

The development and differentiation of leukocytes from hemocytoblasts

d. WBCs are divided into 3 major groups:
  1) Granulocytes: comprise greatest total number of WBCs and include 3 types:
    a) Neutrophils (polymorphonuclear leukocytes, PMNs): "first responders," phagocytic cells that engulf and destroy foreign agents; damaged tissues and invading organisms release chemicals that draw them to site of invasion
    b) Eosinophils: less efficient phagocytic cells but able to surround parasites and release toxic enzymes; also involved in **hypersensitivity** responses and inactivate some inflammatory chemicals released during inflammatory process
    c) Basophils: not phagocytic, they contain proteins and chemicals that are released into bloodstream during an acute hypersensitivity reaction or stress response
  2) Monocytes, macrophages, dendritic cells
    a) Drawn to inflamed areas by chemicals that are released from damaged tissue, they initiate immune responses
    b) Are phagocytic; they ingest large foreign matter and cell debris
    c) Monocytes are largest of all WBCs and mature into macrophages after settling into body tissue; macrophages can encapsulate and trap foreign

matter that cannot be phagocytized; monocytes and macrophages also activate immune response against chronic infections

    d) Dendritic cells can capture antigens and carry to lymphoid tissue (antigen presenting cells, APCs) to stimulate production of antigen specific lymphocytes; they also activate T cells against cancer, assist B lymphocytes to produce antibodies, and down-regulate (turn off extra production) the immune system

3) Lymphocytes: are responsible for specific immune response; monitor for and destroy cancer cells; consist of 3 types (see Figure 11-2 Development of T lymphocytes and B lymphocytes from lymphoblasts)

    a) T lymphocytes (T cells): primary agents of cell-mediated (cellular) immune response; destroy intracellular pathogens, including viral-infected cells, cancer cells, and foreign tissue; subdivide into cytotoxic T cells (CD 8 cells), helper T cells (CD 4 cells) and suppressor T cells (CD 8 cells); each type of T cell releases lymphokines (defense mechanisms known as cytokines) that stimulate B cells to become plasma cells and produce antibodies, macrophages to become activated macrophages, and proliferation of killer T cells

    b) B lymphocytes (B cells); after activated by contact with an antigen mature into either plasma cells (secrete antibodies aka immunoglobulins; see Table 11-1 for listing and characteristics of immunoglobulins); primary agents of the antibody-mediated (humoral) immune response, or memory cells (lead to a more rapid response by remembering the original insult)

Figure 11-2

The development and differentiation of lymphocytes from the lymphoid stem cell

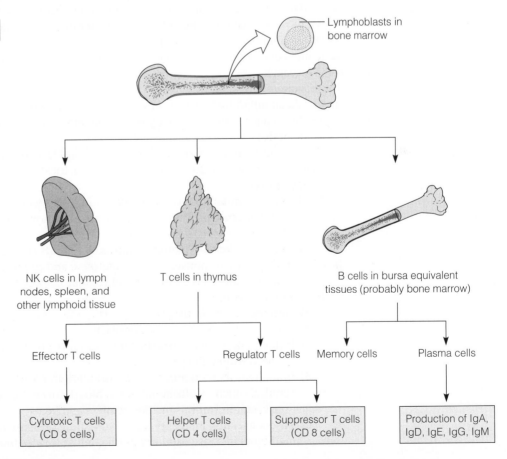

Lymphoblasts in bone marrow

NK cells in lymph nodes, spleen, and other lymphoid tissue

T cells in thymus

B cells in bursa equivalent tissues (probably bone marrow)

Effector T cells

Regulator T cells

Memory cells

Plasma cells

Cytotoxic T cells (CD 8 cells)

Helper T cells (CD 4 cells)

Suppressor T cells (CD 8 cells)

Production of IgA, IgD, IgE, IgG, IgM

Table 11-1	Types of Immunoglobulins	
Class	**Location**	**Characteristics**
IgA	Body secretions Tears, saliva Colostrum and breast milk	Lines mucous membranes Protects body surfaces
IgD	Plasma	Present on lymphocytes
IgE	Plasma Interstitial fluids Exocrine secretions	Allergic/anaphylaxis Bound to mast cells
IgG	Plasma Interstitial fluid	Crosses placenta Complement fixation Secondary immune response
IgM	Plasma	Complement fixation Primary immune response Involved in ABO antigens

  c) Natural killer cells (NK cells, null cells); part of innate immune system and do not require activation to kill cancer cells, virus-infected cells, and cells infected with microbes

 3. Antigens

  a. Substances that are recognized by immune system as foreign ("nonself")

  b. Antigen presenting cell attaches the antigen to itself; specific receptors on a lymphocyte recognize the antigen and generate an immune response (B lymphocytes and/or T lymphocytes)

  c. Lymphocytes (helper T cells, cytotoxic T cells, and/or NK cells) inactivate the antigen

B. Immune response

 1. Innate immune response

  a. Localized inflammatory response; is a generic and nonspecific (activated against any foreign substance that body would encounter; can be from agents outside or inside body)

   1) Acute inflammation: occurs immediately and lasts less than 1–2 weeks; manifestations include erythema (redness); local heat, swelling, pain, and loss of function

   2) Chronic inflammation: is self-perpetuating, lasts weeks to months or years; may result when acute process was ineffective in removing offending agent, for example, *mycobacterium tuberculosis* or from persistent irritation from chemicals, particulate matter or physical irritants (talc, asbestos, silica)

  b. Other nonspecific responses include anatomic and chemical barriers (such as skin and mucous membranes), vascular and cellular responses, and phagocytosis

   1) Vascular response

    a) Damage occurs to tissue cells

    b) Local blood vessels briefly constrict

    c) Inflammatory mediators (histamine, kinins, prostaglandins, leukotrienes) released from damage tissue

    d) Inflammatory mediators cause vasodilation of capillary arterioles and venules, which results in increased blood flow with vasocongestion at site of injury; manifestations include redness and heat

    e) Vasocongestion increases local hydrostatic pressure and inflammatory mediators increase capillary permeability; this results in movement of fluid exudate (containing large amounts of protein) out of capillaries and into interstitial spaces of tissue

f) Protein in fluid exudate draws more water to area (leading to increased edema), brings nutrients needed for tissue healing, dilutes bacterial toxins, and transports cells needed for phagocytosis

g) Increased capillary permeability also enhances release of clotting factors that assist in entrapping bacteria

2) Cellular response

a) Begins within an hour of injury

b) WBCs (neutrophils, monocytes, and macrophages) move from blood vessels into area of inflammation because of chemotactic signals sent by infectious agents, damaged tissues, and activated plasma substances

c) Phagocytosis (engulfment, destruction or digestion of foreign agents or infected cells) begins; during this process particulate matter, bacteria, damaged cells, and inflammatory exudate are removed; constitutes a natural debridement and prepares wound for healing

3) Healing

a) Adequate immune response, nutrition, protein, glucose, and oxygen are critical

b) Clients with diabetes mellitus are at risk for poor healing, most likely due to impaired microcirculation with decreased oxygenation to tissues

c) Clients receiving corticosteroids or chemotherapy have suppressed immune and inflammatory responses, resulting in impaired healing

2. Adaptive immune response

a. Is a specific response in which unique substances (foreign, not-self) lead to activation

b. After an initial exposure to an antigen, a change occurs in host (memory of original exposure) that results in a specific and rapid response to subsequent exposures

c. Immune response is systemic and consists of 2 types of response

1) Antibody-mediated (humoral): recognition of antigens by B lymphocytes

a) B lymphocytes (B cells) are activated by contact with an antigen and by T cells

b) Activated B cell proliferates and differentiates into antibody–producing plasma cells and memory cells

c) Each **antibody** is an immunoglobulin (Ig) molecule that is able to bind to and inactivate a specific antigen through processes of phagocytosis, precipitation, neutralization, lysis, agglutination, or opsonization

d) Subsequent exposures elicit a more rapid and effective response

2) Cell-mediated

a) Infected cells process the antigen and place a marker (**major histocompatibility complex (MHC)**, a group of proteins that play a role in autoimmune recognition and tissue rejection, on outside of cell surface

b) T lymphocytes (T cells) recognize MHC and bind to them

c) T cells synthesize and release cytokines (also called lymphokines and monokines), which are soluble protein mediators of immune response; interleukins, tumor necrosis factor, and interferon are examples of these chemical messengers, which have been used as treatment options in boosting immune response

d) Cytokines enhance inflammatory response, stimulate more B cell response, and stimulate proliferation of killer T cells

e) Protein markers on surface of T-cells help to define specific function receptor sites; these are called CD antigens or clusters of differentiation;

CD markers serve as an important prognostic indicator of immune function and are used to diagnose clients with human immunodeficiency virus (HIV) and acquired immunodeficiency syndrome (AIDS)

    f) Cell-mediated response is responsible for transplant rejection

  3. Acquired immunity

    a. Active acquired immunity: is a long-term response that leads to development of antibodies that offer protection

      1) Can be accomplished by having a disease process or as a response to artificial antigens (such as administration of vaccine or toxoid)

      2) This immunization response can be boosted and maintained via repeated injections

      3) Titer serum levels can be monitored to indicate whether immunity is present

    b. Passive acquired immunity requires that an antibody be introduced, either by maternal transfer (placenta and/or colostrum) or immune serum antibody injection

      1) Promotes a specific response to an antigen

      2) Passive acquired antibodies combine with an antigen or are naturally degraded by body, resulting in a loss of protection

C. Vaccinations

  1. Suspensions of whole or fractionated bacteria or viruses that have been treated to make them nonpathogenic

  2. Recommended for adult clients to maintain optimal health and immune status; do not administer influenza vaccine if client is allergic to eggs; do not administer tetanus antitoxin if client is allergic to horse serum; see Centers for Disease Control Web site for current listing of recommended vaccines for adults and children

  3. A sensitivity test is recommended prior to administration; inject a small amount intradermally; if no reaction occurs after 20 minutes, vaccine can be given

  4. Do not administer if client has an infection because active immunizations will cause a greater inflammatory reaction

  5. Do not administer live virus vaccines (oral polio, MMR) to immunosuppressed clients or individuals who are in close household contact with immunosuppressed persons

  6. Local reactions include redness, swelling, tenderness, and muscle ache

    a. Injecting in dominant arm minimizes this reaction as use and movement of arm facilitates absorption of solution

    b. Applying heat facilitates absorption and decreases tenderness

  7. Clinically important reactions include fever, injection site hypersensitivity, unspecified rash, and injection site edema; these should be reported to the Vaccine Adverse Event Reporting System (VAERS); keep epinephrine 1:1000 available for administration to reduce vasoconstriction or laryngospasms seen with acute anaphylaxis

  8. Monitor client for 20–30 minutes after vaccine administration

II. ALTERED IMMUNE RESPONSES: HYPERSENSITIVITY REACTIONS

  A. The Gell and Coombs Classification of Hypersensitivity Reactions categorizes a reaction according to type, class, and immunity; they include immediate hypersensitivity (type I), cytotoxic reactions (type II), immune complex related (type III), and delayed hypersensitivity (type IV); types I–III provide humoral immunity while type IV is a cell-mediated immunity

  B. The term *hypersensitivity* refers to an abnormal exaggerated immune response to a specific substance that is damaging to body tissues; when the cause is exogenous (from outside body) it is referred to as an allergy

  C. Type I IgE-mediated hypersensitivity

    1. Type I involves an immediate response; however, potential responses can be cumulative; for example, an initial or sensitizing dose may not elicit a strong response, but subsequent contacts, even if not long-term in nature, may cause a stronger response

2. Etiology/pathophysiology: IgE is activated and bound to mast cells, whereby histamine is released; includes allergic asthma, allergic rhinitis (hay fever), allergic conjunctivitis, hives (urticaria) and anaphylactic shock
3. Localized responses are most common
4. Systemic manifestations are more likely with non–oral substances such as insect venom or antibiotics and range from bronchospasm, wheezing, rhinorrhea, and urticaria to angioedema and finally anaphylaxis
5. Alteration of gastrointestinal (GI) mucosa with subsequent absorption of allergen may lead to a systemic reaction; characteristic allergic "gape" and allergic "shiner" can be seen in individuals with **atopy** (allergic reactions stemming from hereditary disposition)
6. Diagnostic and laboratory test findings
   a. Skin and patch testing are performed to determine potential allergens; prick (epicutaneous) testing is done first to avoid a systemic reaction; if this elicits a negative response it is followed by intradermal testing
   b. Radioallergosorbent test (RAST) is a blood test that measures amount of IgE directed toward specific allergies
   c. Food allergy testing involves keeping a diary of foods consumed and allergic responses for 1 week; suspected foods are then eliminated for 1 week to see if symptoms improve
7. Therapeutic management
   a. **Antihistamine** medications such as diphenhydramine (Benadryl) are used to block chemical release of mediators (histamines)
   b. Mast cell degradation inhibitors such as cromolyn sodium (Intal) also are used to block the chemical response
   c. Immunotherapy (hyposensitization, desensitization) incorporates regular injections of gradually increasing doses of an extract of allergen; over time, client develops IgG antibodies to allergen that block allergic response
   d. Decongestants and corticosteroids can help to minimize immune response; however, in potential anaphylactic reactions, use of epinephrine is warranted; an Epi-Pen may be prescribed as appropriate therapy for those at profound risk for hypersensitivity reactions; they are available in both adult and pediatric dosages
   e. In anaphylaxis, administration of warmed intravenous solution may be required to maintain intravascular volume; fluid is warmed to prevent hypothermia from the rapid administration of large amounts of fluid at room temperature
8. Nursing implications
   a. Immediately withdraw offending allergen in presence of documented or suspected reaction
   b. Monitor closely for evidence of Ineffective Airway Clearance or Decreased Cardiac Output as nursing diagnoses
   c. Teach client and family when and how to use an anaphylaxis kit containing epinephrine and antihistamines in injectable, inhaler, and oral forms

D. **Type II: Cytotoxic hypersensitivity**
1. Characteristic type II reaction is a hemolytic transfusion reaction to blood; can also occur from exogenous antigens, such as hemolytic anemia associated with penicillins, cephalosporins and streptomycin; endogenous antigens can also induce autoimmune disorders such as Goodpasture syndrome, Hashimoto's thyroiditis, and autoimmune hemolytic anemia

2. Etiology and pathophysiology
   a. Antigen attaches itself to foreign cell or tissue
   b. Plasma cells produce IgG or IgM antibodies, which bind to antigens
   c. Complement system is activated, resulting in destruction of target cell
3. Clinical manifestations: vary based on affected body system
4. Diagnostic and laboratory test findings: blood type and cross match are ordered prior to any transfusions; further testing with Coombs blood test can identify presence of hemolytic anemia and potential ABO incompatibility
5. Therapeutic management: use of proper identification during blood product administration can help to prevent exposure and sensitization; recognition of certain blood types and awareness that potential drug interactions can cause antigen complex activation can lead to early detection of reactions
6. Nursing implications
   a. Remain in room during first 15 minutes of any blood product administration since clients are more likely to experience a reaction during this time frame
   b. Follow agency policy and procedure for administration of any and all blood products; two RNs must verify blood product before administration

E. **Type III: Immune complex-mediated hypersensitivity**
1. Consists of formation of **antigen–antibody complexes** (a binding together of an antibody and an antigen) in circulation that become deposited in blood vessel walls and extravascular tissues
   a. Leads to activation of serum factors, causing inflammation and activation of complement cascade
   b. Neutrophils release lysosomal enzymes in an attempt to phagocytize the immune complexes; this results in tissue damage
   c. Rheumatoid arthritis and systemic lupus erythematosus are believed to be triggered by type III reactions to antigens (see autoimmune section)
   d. Deposition of antigen–antibody complexes in body tissues can be localized or systemic and therefore can result in more extensive tissue or organ destruction
2. Clinical manifestations
   a. Serum sickness was initially identified after administration of foreign serum (e.g., horse antitetanus toxin); foreign serums are no longer administered but similar responses can be seen to drugs such as penicillin or sulfonamides
   b. May involve a localized inflammatory response with excess IgG causing edema and necrotic lesions and a subsequent systemic response that leads to the deposit and activation of complement throughout body; this can be demonstrated as joint pain, pyrexia, and/or lymphadenopathy
   c. Reactions can be acute or chronic in nature
3. Diagnostic and laboratory test findings
   a. Immune complex assays detect presence of circulating immune complexes; normal result is negative but a negative test does not rule out an immune complex hypersensitivity response
   b. Complement assays reflect decreased levels as complement is "used up" by formation of antigen–antibody complexes
   c. Erythrocyte sedimentation rate (ESR) is elevated due to inflammatory process
   d. Proteinuria may be found on urinalysis if deposits have accumulated in kidneys
4. Nursing implications
   a. Localized inflammatory reactions may develop at site of serum injections after 1 week; this can be followed by a more systemic response involving both regional as well as generalized lymphadenopathies
   b. If symptoms arise, monitor client for potential complications; this is especially important because organ damage can occur and kidneys can be compromised

F. Type IV: Delayed hypersensitivity

1. A form of cell-mediated immunity involving T lymphocytes; it is considered a delayed response (24–48 hours after exposure)

2. Etiology and pathophysiology: exaggerated interaction between antigens and normal cell-mediated mechanisms results in release of inflammatory and immune mediators and recruitment of killer T cells, causing local tissue destruction

3. Clinical manifestations

   a. There is a wide range of presentation from tuberculin response, poison ivy, and contact dermatitis to transplant or graft rejection; edema, ischemia, and eventual tissue destruction may ensue

   b. Latex allergies, seen in 8–13% of health care workers, is initially a type IV hypersensitivity (contact dermatitis) and can progress on subsequent exposure to a type I systemic allergic reaction

4. Diagnostic and laboratory test findings: purified protein derivative (PPD) test result of induration greater than 5 mm identifies type IV hypersensitivity to the tubercle bacillus; abnormal test results indicating declining function of transplanted organ are used to diagnose transplant rejection (see later section)

5. Therapeutic management

   a. Identify potential irritants that can cause contact dermatitis and teach clients to avoid exposure

   b. Screen and educate health care workers periodically about latex sources and symptoms of allergies

   c. Teach health care workers that washing hands after using latex products and using nonlatex gloves whenever possible will limit exposure and decrease the risk of sensitivity developing

6. Nursing implications

   a. Make sure that client avoids offending irritant if a past exposure has been documented

   b. Use topical and oral medications as indicated to alleviate symptom complaints and increase client comfort

Practice to Pass

A client becomes short of breath after eating strawberries. What are your immediate assessments and interventions?

III. AUTOIMMUNE DISORDERS

A. Overview

1. Concept of autoimmunity

   a. Autoimmunity is an abnormal response of immune system whereby it perceives "self" as a threat

   b. May be tissue or organ specific (e.g. Hashimoto's thyroiditis) or systemic (rheumatoid arthritis [RA], systemic lupus erythematosus [SLE])

2. Pathophysiology unclear but may include the following:

   a. Genetic traits: family members of clients with autoimmune disorders are more likely to develop the disorder

   b. Chemical, physical, or biological changes that cause self-antigens to stimulate production of autoantibodies

   c. Release of "hidden" antigens such as DNA or other cell nucleus components into circulation causing an immune response

   d. Antigens such as bacteria or viruses whose antigenic properties closely resemble host tissue, resulting in antibodies that target foreign antigen and host tissue

   e. Defect in normal cellular immune function that allows B cells to produce unlimited numbers of autoantibodies

   f. Initiation of autoimmune response by very slow-growing mycobacteria

   g. More prevalent in females so estrogen may further stimulate immune response

3. Diagnostic testing for autoimmunity
   a. Autoantibody assays, **complement fixation**, and complement assays provide diagnostic information that indicate an autoimmune process rather than a specific disorder
   b. Antinuclear antibody (ANA): detects antibodies produced to DNA and other nuclear material
   c. Lupus erythematosus (LE) cell test: used to detect and monitor SLE; it may be positive with other autoimmune disorders or from medications
   d. Rheumatoid factor (RF): elevated in 80% of clients with RA; may also be elevated in SLE, scleroderma, liver cirrhosis, or Sjogren syndrome
   e. Anti-CCP antibody test: a blood test for an antibody that replaces normal protein in the joints that is specific for RA
4. Treatment for autoimmunity
   a. Immunosuppressive agents, corticosteroids, and anti-inflammatory drugs are given to suppress abnormal immune response
   b. Disease-modifying antirheumatic drugs (DMARDS), such as methotrexate or cyclosporine, help treat clients with RA
   c. Biologicals (biological response modifiers or BMRs), such as infliximab (Remicade), are laboratory-produced proteins that decrease inflammatory process by binding tumor necrosis factor alpha (TNF-α) and interleukin-1 inflammatory elements
   d. Slower-acting anti-inflammatory drugs, such as gold salts, can be toxic and are rarely used
   e. **Plasmapheresis** is used to remove circulating immune complexes; in this treatment, plasma is removed from body, sent through a machine membrane that traps immune complexes, and is returned to client
5. Progression of disease
   a. Autoimmune diseases are characterized by acute exacerbation of a chronic condition
   b. Clients often do not appear ill, making it difficult for others to understand their needs; psychological support is critical

B. Systemic lupus erythematosus (SLE)
1. Description
   a. Chronic inflammatory disease that affects all body systems
   b. Manifestations are variable (mild to fatal) and are believed to result from cell and tissue damage caused by deposits of antigen–antibody complexes in connective tissue
2. Etiology
   a. Genetic component present; certain **human leukocyte antigen (HLA)** genes more likely to be present
   b. Hormonal: primarily affects women of childbearing age (30–50 years of age being most common); estrogen and inhibits suppressor T-cell function leading to an abnormal immune response; reduced levels of androgens that normally inhibit antibody responses; pregnancy and oral contraceptive use can affect estrogen level and therefore may pose an increased risk for disease flare-ups
   c. Environmental: viruses (e.g., Epstein-Barr), bacterial antigens, chemicals, or ultraviolet light may be part of disease activation process
   d. Drug-induced lupus can be found as a response to certain medications such as phenytoin (Dilantin), hydralazine (Apresoline), procainamide (Pronestyl), isoniazid (INH), and penicillamine (Depen); if a client exhibits any signs or symptoms of disease and uses one of these medications, it should be stopped to see whether symptoms disappear

Practice to Pass

A client is diagnosed with an autoimmune disease and wants to know whether this will become a chronic occurrence. What information can you provide to the client that would explain the concept of autoimmune disease?

   e. Ethnic presentations: occur more frequently in those of African American, Hispanic, Asian, and Native American descent
3. Pathophysiology
   a. Disordered T-cell function causes hyperactivity of B cells
   b. Causes large variety of autoantibodies to be produced against normal body components
   c. SLE autoantibodies bind with target tissue to form immune complexes
   d. Immune complexes are deposited in blood vessels, lymphatic vessels, and other tissues
   e. Deposits trigger inflammatory response and cause local tissue damage
   f. Complex deposits often accumulate and cause renal damage
   g. Other commonly affected tissues include musculoskeletal system, brain, heart, spleen, lung, GI tract, skin, and peritoneum
4. Assessment
   a. Clinical manifestations
      1) Joint symptoms and arthritis type manifestations are often early signs and affect more than 90% of clients
      2) Butterfly rash (malar rash) across cheeks and bridge of nose and/or other skin manifestations (photosensitivity, alopecia, or painless mucous membrane ulcerations) occur in majority of clients but at varying times during disease
      3) Hematologic involvement is common and can lead to altered immune responses, which result in increased risk of infection; clients can develop anemia, leukopenia, thrombocytopenia, and even hemolytic anemia
      4) Pleural manifestations include pleuritis, pneumonitis, interstitial fibrosis, and pleural effusions
      5) Renal involvement is a serious consequence of disease progression and occurs in 50% of clients with SLE
      6) Cardiac involvement can include pericarditis, myocarditis, endocarditis, vasculitis, and venous or arterial thrombosis leading to myocardial infarction
      7) Central nervous system involvement can range from subtle behavioral changes to profound psychological disturbances and eventually result in stroke or seizure activity
      8) GI manifestations include anorexia, nausea, abdominal pain, diarrhea, and possible liver enlargement
   b. Diagnostic and laboratory test findings
      1) A positive ANA titer is present in over 95% of clients
      2) Anti-DNA antibody testing is more specific to SLE as it is rarely found in any other disorder
      3) During flare-ups of disease process, complement (C_3 and C_4) may be decreased, while erythrocyte sedimentation rate (ESR) and C-reactive protein (CRP) may be elevated
      4) A positive rheumatoid factor (+RF) may be seen
      5) Complete blood count (CBC) with differential may reveal a normochromic, normocytic anemia with leukopenia and thrombocytopenia
      6) Urinalysis may reveal proteinuria, hematuria, and presence of casts and sediment; creatinine levels may rise as renal involvement progresses
5. Medication therapy
   a. Nonsteroidal anti-inflammatory drugs (NSAIDs) and acetylsalicylic acid (aspirin, ASA) control common joint symptom presentations that most clients experience
   b. Hydroxychloroquine (Plaquenil) treats dermatologic symptoms; it is an anti-malarial that also helps decrease photosensitivity and prevent musculoskeletal

flares; it is critical to monitor client for retinal toxicity; a baseline eye exam should be done along with periodic evaluations (monthly initially and then every 6 months) to monitor ocular status

    c. Glucocorticoids are used to suppress disease activity and clients with severe manifestations may require high doses; dosing can be adjusted in response to flare-ups; oral or IV route is preferred; tapered dose therapy (pulse dose) is initiated as soon as possible to achieve best results at lowest possible dosage and to prevent side effects of steroid therapy

    d. Long-term steroid therapy can result in corticosteroid side effects, including hypertension, infection, osteoporosis, and hypokalemia

    e. Immunosuppressive agents such as cyclophosphamide (Cytoxan) and azathiopine (Imuran) can be given to effectively modulate an immune response; however, there is increased risk for **myelosuppression** (inhibition or destruction of bone marrow) with this treatment regimen, so client must be monitored accordingly

6. Priority nursing problems: potential for infection, interrupted skin integrity, insufficient ability to maintain health

7. Planning and implementation

    a. Teach importance of following prescribed treatment plan and warning signs of a flare of disease: increased fatigue, pain, abdominal discomfort, rash, headache, fever, and dizziness

    b. Teach strategies to limit sun exposure

        1) Avoid going out of doors during hours of greatest sun intensity

        2) Use sunscreen with an SPF of 15 or higher; reapply after swimming, exercising, or bathing

        3) Wear loose clothing with long sleeves and wide-brimmed hats when out of doors

    c. Use aseptic technique and monitor for signs of infection; emphasize importance of avoiding exposure to infections

    d. Collaborate with other health care team members to institute a long-term treatment plan that offers anticipatory guidance and emotional support

    e. Teach importance of preventive health care, including screenings for cholesterol and blood pressure, vaccinations, and eye examinations

    f. Family planning should include alternative birth control methods such as diaphragm and condoms because oral contraceptives can affect estrogen level; pregnancy is not contraindicated but requires close monitoring

    g. Wear a MedicAlert tag identifying condition and therapy such as corticosteroids or immunosuppressants

8. Evaluation: client will be able to identify potential environment risks and prevent exposure to infection, dermatologic eruptions, and stress; monitor underlying disease process and complications that would heighten medical risks; comply with treatment measures aimed at managing symptoms so that activities of daily living (ADLs) can be performed at optimal level

C. Rheumatoid arthritis (RA)

1. Description

    a. A systemic autoimmune disorder that causes inflammation of connective tissue, primarily in joints

    b. Often involves symmetrical inflammation of multiple peripheral joints

    c. Is characterized by periods of remission and exacerbation but is a chronic disease

2. Etiology and pathophysiology

    a. The exact etiology is unknown; genetic factors may combine with environmental factors

    b. Females are 3 times more likely than males to develop the disorder

    c. RA has a bimodal appearance, as there is a juvenile form (JRA), as well as the more commonly seen adult form

    d. Infectious agents may play a role in initiating abnormal immune responses

    e. Pathophysiology

        1) Unidentified antigen causes an aberrant immune response in a genetically susceptible host

        2) Antibodies change to autoantibodies (rheumatoid factors) and attack body tissue (self)

        3) Antibodies bind with target antigens and form immune complexes that prompt an inflammatory response

        4) Inflammatory and immune processes damage synovial membranes resulting in thickening and swelling; this leads to formation of a vascular granulation tissue called pannus

        5) Pannus produces enzymes and proteases that promote further tissue damage; cytokines activate chondrocytes that attack joint cartilage and osteoclasts that demineralize underlying bone

3. Assessment

    a. Clinical manifestations

        1) Initially may see systemic signs of inflammation, including nonspecific aching, fatigue, general malaise, anorexia and weight loss

        2) Progresses to joint swelling with stiffness, warmth, tenderness, and pain; joints feel "boggy" or spongy on palpation because of synovial edema

        3) Characteristic morning stiffness lasting more than 1 hour is also an indication of progression of disease; if present, note onset, duration, and joints involved

        4) May also experience stiffness with prolonged rest during day or after strenuous activity

        5) Persistent inflammation leads to deformities and destruction of joint and supporting structures; weakening of supporting structures results in lack of opposition to muscle pull, causing deformities

        6) Characteristic joint deformities include ulnar deviation of fingers and subluxation of metacarpophalangeal (MCP) joints, swan neck deformity, boutonniere deformity, subcutaneous nodules, and ulnar deviation or drift (see Figure 11-3)

        7) Systemic signs range from fever to splenomegaly and reflect extra-articular findings; rheumatoid nodules often develop in subcutaneous areas subject to pressure and can also develop in heart, lungs, intestinal tract, and dura

        8) RA is associated with a 30% higher risk of cardiovascular mortality, most likely related to systemic inflammation

    b. Diagnostic and laboratory test findings

        1) Rheumatoid factor (RF); elevated in 80% of clients with RA; may also be elevated in SLE, scleroderma, liver cirrhosis or Sjogren syndrome

        2) Anti-CCP antibody test; a blood test for an antibody that replaces normal protein in joints (specific for RA) but may only be present in 50% of individuals with early disease

        3) Elevated ESR, C-reactive protein, and serum complement

        4) CBC with differential may reveal anemia as well as leukocytosis

        5) X-rays of joints are the most specific test for RA and reveal a narrowing of joint spaces and erosive changes at bone margins as disease progresses

        6) Aspiration of synovial fluid reveals characteristic findings such as turbidity, elevated cell counts, and formation of a poor mucin clot

4. Therapeutic management

    a. Goals are to relieve pain, reduce inflammation, slow or stop joint damage, and improve well-being and ability to function

Figure 11-3

Deformities of hands in rheumatoid arthritis

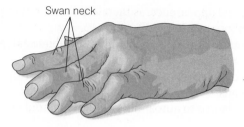

A Swan neck deformity

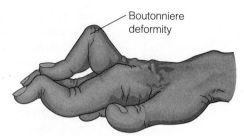

B Boutonniere deformity

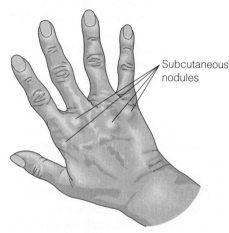

C Subcutaneous nodules

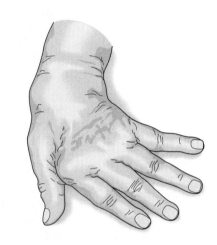

D Ulnar deviation

    b. No cure exists; treatment is done to relieve manifestations

    c. Interdisciplinary approaches with a balance of rest, exercise, physical therapy, and suppression of inflammatory process with pharmacological agents are key measures

5. Medication therapy

    a. ASA and NSAIDs are used to decrease joint inflammation and control symptoms

    b. Low-dose oral corticosteroids reduce pain and inflammation and may slow development and progression of bone erosions; intra-articular corticosteroids may provide temporary relief

    c. Disease-modifying antirheumatic drugs (DMARDs) appear to alter course of disease and reduce destruction of joints; results may not be apparent for several weeks or months; active infection is a contraindication to administration

        1) Nonbiologic DMARDs (see Table 11-2 for DMARD classification) include methotrexate, often the first DMARD used to treat aggressive RA

Table 11-2 **Disease-Modifying Antirheumatic Drug Classification**

Class	Nursing Concerns
Antimalarial	Monitor for adverse effects Instruct client to get eye exam as baseline and every 6 months
Immunosuppressives	Monitor for myelosuppression Maximize effect at lowest dose Monitor for methotrexate interactions with alcohol and other drugs to avoid toxic levels

        2) Biologic DMARDs (e.g., etanercept [Enbrel]) are used for clients who have moderate or high disease activity, have had active RA for a longer period of time, or have failed to respond adequately to nonbiologic DMARDs

    d. Immunosuppressive agents such as azathioprine (Imuran), cyclophosphamide (Cytoxan), and **monoclonal antibodies** are used in clients who are experiencing severe disabling RA or are refractory to other forms of treatment

  6. Priority nursing problems: pain, fatigue, inability to perform usual roles, alteration in body image

  7. Planning and implementation

    a. Support client during diagnosis and as disease progresses; refer to counseling or support groups

    b. Explore use of assistive devices such as a cane, walker, raised toilet seat, grab bars in the bathroom, bath chair, or adapted counter heights for client in a wheelchair

    c. Modify client's schedule as needed to incorporate rest periods and balance with periods of activity

    d. Medicate client as prescribed to achieve pain relief and disease modification; be aware of drug effects and potential interactions as disease process continues

    e. Include nonpharmacologic measures such as use of imagery and biofeedback to provide alternate forms of pain relief

    f. Use heat and cold applications to affected joints to provide relief; these measures should be individualized to afford maximum client comfort

    g. Include foods high in omega-3 fatty acids (current research shows these are beneficial to clients with RA as well as other diseases such as heart disease); suggested food items include fish oils and salmon

    h. Encourage to maintain self-care and usual roles as much as possible

    i. Explain clothing options such as elastic waist pants without zippers, Velcro closures, zippers with large pull-tabs, and slip-on shoes

    j. Teach that immunosuppressive drugs, while given to provide clinical improvement, may also cause myelosuppression and drug toxicity and client needs to monitor for these effects

  8. Evaluation

    a. Client will maintain and preserve function as much as possible during disease progression; assistive devices and alternate environment patterns will assist client in meeting these goals

    b. Client will comply with treatment measures aimed at managing symptoms so that client can perform ADLs at an optimal level

D. Scleroderma: progressive systemic sclerosis (PSS)

  1. Description

    a. Chronic disease characterized by deposition of excess collagen tissue in skin and internal organs

    b. Fibrosis results and leads to inability of involved organs to function normally

    c. CREST syndrome is a specific more limited form of disease called Thibierge–Weissenbach syndrome

        C = Calcium deposits

        R = Raynaud's disease

        E = Esophageal dysmotility

        S = Sclerodactyly (scleroderma digits)

        T = Telangiectasia (spider nevi)

    d. Limited cutaneous systemic sclerosis has less organ involvement and 10-year survival rate is 71%

    e. Diffuse cutaneous systemic sclerosis has more organ involvement and 10-year survival rate is 21%

    2. Etiology and pathophysiology

      a. Results from genetic, immune, and environmental factors; silica and chemical exposure increases risk

      b. Disease usually presents during third to fifth decade of life

      c. Females are affected more often than males

      d. Functional and structural abnormalities of small arteries and arterioles result in progressive vessel obstruction, increased permeability and fibrosis

      e. Autoimmunity and vascular damage also contributes to fibrosis

  3. Assessment

      a. Clinical manifestations

        1) Usual first sign is thickening of skin with diffuse, nonpitting swelling; skin begins to atrophy, becoming taut, shiny, and hyperpigmented; with progressive atrophy, skin becomes tight, leading to loss of skin lines, a pursed-lip appearance and limited mobility of face and hands; telangiectasis (flat, red areas on face, hands and mouth) may appear along with calcium deposits around joints

        2) GI tract changes can lead to dysphagia, esophageal reflux, malabsorption, and bowel obstruction

        3) Cardiovascular changes can present in the form of Raynaud's disease (a vascular disorder with reversible arterial vasospasm), pericarditis and dysrhythmias

        4) Arthralgias (joint pain) are common

        5) Respiratory changes can result from lung restriction caused by fibrosis and pulmonary hypertension

        6) Renal changes lead to development of uremia, malignant hypertension, and eventually renal failure

        7) Scleroderma is often seen in conjunction with Sjogren syndrome, an autoimmune disease affecting lacrimal and salivary glands, causing dry mucous membranes

      b. Diagnostic and laboratory test findings

        1) Biopsy of organs may reveal specific involvement

        2) No single diagnostic test specific for systemic sclerosis

        3) Antinuclear antibody (ANA) titer 1:40 or higher is most sensitive

        4) Skin biopsy may confirm diagnosis

  4. Therapeutic management

      a. Treatment is aimed at supportive and palliative measures

      b. Long-term follow up is indicated to monitor disease progression

      c. Dialysis or transplantation may be indicated if renal function deteriorates

      d. Physical therapy helps to maintain mobility of affected tissues; strengthening and stretching of facial muscles is needed to maintain oral food intake

  5. Medication therapy

      a. Penicillamine to treat scleroderma and pulmonary fibrosis; immunosuppressives and corticosteroids to slow or prevent life-threatening disease

      b. Anti-inflammatory agents are used to treat joint pain

      c. Calcium channel blockers and peripheral alpha$_1$-adrenergic blocking agents are used to treat symptoms of Raynaud's disease

      d. Angiotensin converting enzyme (ACE) inhibitors are used to treat hypertension and prevent development of resultant renal crisis

      e. H$_2$-receptor antagonists and proton pump inhibitors are used to treat esophageal reflux

  6. Priority nursing problems: interrupted skin integrity, insufficient nutrients to meet bodily needs, reduced self-esteem, alteration in body image

7. Planning and implementation
   a. Monitor client for symptoms and medicate as ordered
   b. Develop a support system for client and family members to help them cope with stressors of chronic disease
   c. Teach measures to maintain intact elastic skin, including use of moisturizers, extra protection over joints or bony prominences, and range-of-motion exercises
   d. Provide small, frequent meals with foods that are easy to swallow; keep head of bed elevated after meals and at night to minimize reflux
   e. Discuss need to dress warmly and avoid chilling (local and whole body) that can exacerbate Raynaud's disease
   f. Teach client to avoid temperature changes; encourage use of gloves during activities that involve temperature changes (such as washing dishes)
   g. Explain importance of stopping smoking, as it has vasoconstrictive and respiratory effects that worsen disease
   h. Establish an atmosphere of trust; listen actively, acknowledge concerns and provide referrals as appropriate
8. Evaluation: client will be able to manage symptoms and live more comfortably; will be an active participant in health care team and contribute to decision making on own behalf

IV. IMMUNODEFICIENCY DISORDERS

A. Etiology and pathophysiology

1. Primary immunodeficiency disorders
   a. Caused by a primary defect or deficiency involving B lymphocytes, T lymphocytes, complement or phagocytic cells that results in severe infection that can be recurrent or chronic in nature (refer to Table 11-3 for a listing of selected primary immunodeficiency diseases)
   b. These involve specific genetic alterations in immune response that are seen in infants and young children so genetic counseling is advised
   c. Immunodeficiency is most severe when both antibody-mediated and cell-mediated responses are impaired (combined immunodeficiency)
2. Secondary immunodeficiency disorders
   a. Disease processes cause a secondary immunosuppressive response
   b. Diabetes mellitus, burns, malnutrition, some autoimmune diseases, and acquired immunodeficiency syndrome (AIDS) are examples of precipitating disease processes
   c. Acquired immunodeficiency syndrome (AIDS)
      1) An RNA retrovirus attacks immune system at CD4 antigen, causing cell mutation (reverse transcriptase) that integrates viral DNA into host cell DNA and allows virus to duplicate
      2) Antibodies are produced in response to viral proteins (seroconversion) and are detectable between 6 weeks and 6 months after initial infection

Table 11-3 Selected Primary Immunodeficiency Disorders

Disorder	Immune Cell Problem
Bruton's X-linked disorder	B lymphocytes
DiGeorge syndrome	T lymphocytes
Graft-versus-host disease	B, T lymphocytes
Wiskott–Aldrich syndrome	B, T lymphocytes

        3) Helper T or CD4 cells are primarily infected but also targets macrophages, dendrites, and certain cells of CNS

        4) Primary infection is often followed by a clinical latency period when client may appear asymptomatic but can infect others through contact with blood and/or body fluids

        5) Treatment with highly active antiretroviral therapy (HAART) is used to prevent progression of viral infection to AIDS

        6) Progression is associated with appearance of HIV-associated neoplasms and **opportunistic infections** (infections that occur because of depressed immunologic state)

B. Incidence, prevalence, and prognosis

    1. Primary immunodeficiency diseases are genetically determined and rare; they primarily affect children

    2. Secondary immunosuppression from disease states such as diabetes mellitus or drugs such as chemotherapy are more common but generally less severe in form

    3. Acquired immunodeficiency syndrome (AIDS) resulting from human immunodeficiency virus (HIV) affects adults more than children

        a. Survival rates have improved from 2 years to more than 13 years with use of antiretroviral agents

        b. A majority of people infected with HIV or who have AIDS live in sub-Saharan Africa, and the most common mode of transmission is heterosexual intercourse

        c. Risk factors in the United States

            1) Men who have sex with men (MSM) account for 60% of reported cases

            2) Injection drug use accounts for approximately 25% of cases

            3) Heterosexual intercourse with an infected drug user or exchanging sex for drugs are major risk factors for women

            4) Infection disproportionately affects African Americans

            5) Adults over age 50 account for 29% of persons living with HIV/AIDS in the U.S.; factors include declining immune system function and failure to use protection with sexual activity

            6) Health care workers are most likely to become HIV positive through percutaneous exposure to blood or body fluids through a needle-stick injury or nonintact skin; splashes to eyes or mouth are a much lower risk

C. Prevention of HIV

    1. Identification of infected but undiagnosed individuals

    2. Education on totally safe sex practices

        a. Abstaining from sex

        b. Long term mutually monogamous sexual relations between 2 uninfected people

        c. Mutual masturbation without direct contact

    3. Sex practices that are not totally safe but help to decrease risk

        a. Reduce number of sexual partners

        b. Use latex condoms with every sexual encounter involving vaginal, oral, or anal intercourse

    4. Provide postexposure prophylaxis to health care workers exposed to HIV infection or adults who experience a high-risk exposure to HIV

    5. Teach injection drug users never to share needles, syringes, or other drug paraphernalia

    6. Screen voluntary blood donors and teach HIV-positive clients to abstain from donating blood, organs, or sperm

    7. Treat all clients with standard precautions

    8. Teach HIV-positive clients not to share razors or obtain a tattoo; stress importance of advising all medical personnel providing direct care about the diagnosis

D. Assessment of HIV and AIDS

1. Clinical manifestations

   a. Acute retroviral syndrome (ARS) or primary HIV infection is difficult to diagnose and symptoms include fever, sore throat, arthralgias and myalgias, headache, rash, nausea, vomiting, and abdominal cramping

   b. Asymptomatic infection (latency) lasts from 3 to 15 years

   c. AIDS: CD4 count less than $500/mm^3$ predicts appearance of signs of immunodeficiency, when counts are less than $200/mm^3$ opportunistic infections and cancers are likely

      1) Signs and symptoms of infection and inflammation: fever, chills, cough (nonproductive or productive), respiratory complaints associated with difficulty swallowing or breathing, erythema, edema, or drainage

      2) Diarrhea can be present either because of overwhelming infection caused by offending agents or as a response to antimicrobial therapy

      3) Opportunistic infections are most common manifestation

         a) *Pneumocystis jiroveci* pneumonia (*Pneumocystis carinii*) is most common infection and a major cause of death

         b) Tuberculosis seen in 4% of clients with AIDS

         c) Other infections include herpes virus, CMV, sinusitis, parasitic infections, and candida. *Mycobacterium avium* complex is a major cause of **wasting syndrome** (unexplained weight loss of more than 10% ideal body weight [IBW] that is associated with a cycle of malnutrition and subsequent wasting)

      4) HIV-associated neoplasms: Kaposi's Sarcoma (most common cancer associated with AIDS and often the presenting symptom), lymphomas, and cervical cancer

      5) AIDS dementia complex and neurologic effects from virus and opportunistic infections: fluctuating memory loss, confusion, difficulty concentrating, lethargy, and diminished motor speed

2. Diagnostic and laboratory test findings

   a. CBC with differential detects anemia, leukopenia, and thrombocytopenia

   b. ESR, antibody titers, ANA, ANC (absolute neutrophil count) and culture and sensitivity of pertinent areas may all provide a baseline and allow for identification of potential source(s) of infection

   c. Testing for **immunoglobulins** and complement assay levels provide an overview of immune system function

   d. See Box 11-1 for CDC recommendations for HIV testing

Box 11-1	
CDC Recommendations for HIV Testing of Adults and Adolescents	**1.** All persons aged 13–64, regardless of risk, should receive routine, voluntary screening for HIV in all healthcare settings in which the prevalence of undiagnosed HIV infection is at least 0.1%. **2.** All patients beginning treatment for TB should be screened for HIV. **3.** All patients seeking treatment for sexually transmitted infections should be screened for HIV each time they seek such treatment. **4.** Health care providers should encourage patients and their prospective sex partners to be tested before initiating a new sexual relationship. **5.** Repeat HIV screening should be performed for patients with known risk at least annually. Persons likely to be at high risk include injection-drug users and their sex partners, persons who exchange sex for money or drugs, sex partners of HIV-infected persons, and men who have sex with men (MSM) or heterosexual persons who themselves or whose sex partners have had more than one sex partner since their most recent HIV test.

Source: Centers for Disease Control and Prevention. (2006). *Revised Recommendations for HIV Testing of Adults, Adolescents, and Pregnant Women in Health-care Settings.* Retrieved from www.cdc.gov/ mmwr/preview/mmwrhtml/rr5514al.htm

e. HIV rapid antibody test uses strips embedded with HIV antigen, if there are antibodies to HIV in client's blood the strip turns color; requires confirmation with Western blot antibody test

f. Enzyme-linked immunosorbent assay (ELISA) is the most widely used screening test to detect antibodies to HIV; this test is described as positive or negative

g. Western blot is used to confirm HIV infection because it detects both HIV antibodies and individual viral components that cause reactive bands; this test is described as positive or negative; it is more reliable but more time consuming and more expensive

h. HIV viral load tests measure amount of actively replicating HIV and are used to monitor disease progression and response to antiretroviral medications

i. Absolute CD4 lymphocyte count is the most widely used test to monitor disease progress and guide therapy

j. Other lab and diagnostic tests, such as skin biopsy, serum chemistries, and imaging studies, may be indicated depending on organ/system involvement and disease progression

E. **Therapeutic management**
1. Therapy is most effective when aimed at infection prophylaxis, early treatment of infections, and replacement of immunologic factors
2. Bone marrow transplant (BMT) and/or thymus transplant may be indicated for primary immunodeficiency disorders depending on severity of presentation
3. **Neutropenic precautions** (measures to protect immunosuppressed client) are warranted to prevent further risk for infection and maintain protective isolation as indicated; see discussion later in chapter

F. **Medication therapy**
1. Antimicrobial therapy may be initiated to prevent infection or treat current infection
2. Depending on nature of organism, antifungals may be warranted
3. Gamma globulins may be needed to support and maintain immunoglobulin levels that are currently deficient
4. Use of **colony-stimulating factors** may be warranted to boost immune response
5. HIV specific medication therapy
   a. Combination therapies are most effective and various combinations are now available in one pill; therapy does not eradicate HIV infection and is expensive; taking a brief "holiday" may result in acceleration of viral growth, immune failure, and disease progression
   b. Nucleoside analogue reverse transcriptase inhibitors (NRTIs) are aimed at specific processes to prevent viral replication
   c. Protease inhibitors inhibit specific processes to prevent viral replication; they significantly change metabolism of other medications
   d. Nonnucleoside reverse transcriptase inhibitors (NNRTIs) are used to treat emerging viral mutations and have a risk for liver toxicity and severe rash
   e. Entry inhibitors bind to virus or host cells, thus preventing viral entry into host cell; is administered by injection and very expensive; used for clients who are resistant to HAART regimens
   f. HIV integrase strand transfer inhibitor targets an HIV enzyme; it is approved only for clients with a resistance to HAART regimens

G. **Priority nursing problems**: potential for infection, fatigue, insufficient nutrients to meet bodily needs, inadequate knowledge, interrupted skin integrity, diarrhea, fear, anticipatory grief, alteration in body image, reduced coping ability of client or family, reduced ability of caregiver to perform role

Practice to Pass

A client is concerned about the number of medications that have been prescribed for the treatment of AIDS and states that "there is no way to comply" with this regimen. What information could you provide to the client to support the importance of compliance with the treatment regimen?

H. Planning and implementation
1. For primary immunodeficiency disorders refer clients of childbearing families for genetic counseling
2. Maintain protective isolation as warranted
3. Identify potential infectious sources and establish baseline immune level.
4. Assist client and family members in decisions regarding lifestyle changes to reduce risks of acquiring opportunistic infections
5. Assess social support and usual methods of coping; if possible assign a primary nurse
6. Refer to clergy, social worker, clinical specialist, and/or counselor as appropriate
7. Interact at every opportunity outside of providing specific nursing care treatments; this communicates caring and acceptance without fear of disease
8. Collaborate with health care team members to support the client's ADLs and lifestyle changes during hospitalization and after discharge
9. Administer vaccines, including pneumococcal, influenza, hepatitis B, and *Haemophilus influenza b*
10. Establish an early working relationship with a dietitian to deal with client's altered taste perception and prevent or delay wasting syndrome; monitor nutritional intake and albumin levels
11. Monitor client for potential fluid and electrolyte imbalances that might occur during course of disease process or in response to therapy
12. Keep skin clean and dry using mild, nondrying soaps or oils; apply protective creams to protect from diarrhea

I. Client education
1. Teach client importance of compliance with long-term treatment regimen and adherence to drug regimen; noncompliance could lead to drug resistance over time
2. Stress need for follow-up physical examination and diagnostic tests to monitor disease progression and response to treatment
3. Teach client to identify areas of concern, such as possibility of increased infection caused by disease-related immunodeficiency
4. Discuss confidentiality and release of information concerning health matters in the areas of business and personal relationships
5. Explain use of specific nutrition-related measures:
   a. Small frequent meals and low-fat foods reduce risk of nausea
   b. Fluids between meals instead of with meals
   c. Dry crackers to decrease nausea
   d. Premedicate with antiemetics to decrease nausea
   e. Use of sorbets as palate cleansers
   f. Zinc supplementation to improve taste sensation
   g. Use of plastic utensils instead of metal to reduce unpleasant taste
   h. Soft foods at room temperature will be less painful

J. Evaluation
1. Client maintains health care follow-up visits as recommended
2. Client is actively involved in monitoring for therapeutic response
3. Client is involved in prevention of infection and symptom management in order to limit hospitalizations
4. Client with a primary immunodeficiency is aware that he or she is not infectious to others but is at high risk for infection

Practice to Pass

A male client who is HIV-positive wants to know why oral progesterone (Megace) has been prescribed. What information can you provide related to this medication?

V. TISSUE TRANSPLANTS

A. Overview

1. Include organs (lung, heart, kidney, pancreas, and bone marrow), skin, cornea, bone, heart valves, and islet cells
2. Tissue matching done to obtain an organ with tissue antigens as close as possible to those of recipient
3. Immunosuppression (drugs given to make immune response less effective)
4. Autografts are a transplant of client's own tissue, for example, skin grafts, blood transfusions that client donated prior to need; identical twins are considered isografts
5. Allografts come from members of same species; can be from living donors or cadavers
6. Xenografts come from an animal species, for example, pig skin as a temporary covering for burns

B. Complications

1. Host-versus-graft transplant rejection
   a. Host macrophages present donor antigen to T and B lymphocytes
   b. Killer T cells bind with cells of transplanted organ, resulting in cell lysis
   c. B cells produce antibodies to graft endothelium
   d. May be hyperacute (within 2–3 days) with rapid deterioration of organ function, acute (4 days to 3 months) with inflammation and impaired organ function, or chronic (4 months to years) with a gradual deterioration of organ function
2. Graft-versus-host disease (GVHD)
   a. Immune cells from graft (transplanted tissue) attack host tissue
   b. Most common with bone marrow transplants, liver transplants, or transfusions with nonirradiated blood to immunocompromised clients
   c. Maculopapular pruritic rash begins on palms of hands and soles of feet; if limited to skin and liver prognosis is good; if other organs involved prognosis is poor

C. Medications

1. Antibiotics and antivirals may be given prior to transplantations
2. Post transplantation
   a. Corticosteroids: anti-inflammatory and immunosuppressive activity; significant adverse effects with large doses
   b. Cyclosporine: inhibits T-cell function and normal cell-mediated immune response; blood levels must be monitored closely; is nephrotoxic and hepatotoxic
   c. Azathioprine (Imuran): inhibits cell-mediated and antibody-mediated immunity, especially T-cell activity; bone marrow suppression is common
   d. Monoclonal antibody therapy (muromonab-CD3, OKT3): specifically blocks T-cell generation and function

D. Nursing management of common problems

1. Ineffective Protection: failure of affected organ preoperatively and immunosuppressive drugs postoperatively may decrease immune response and place client at greater risk for infections
   a. Use strict hand hygiene
   b. Initiate reverse or protective isolation procedures as needed
   c. Instruct ill family members and visitors to avoid contact with client
   d. Help ensure adequate nutrient intake
   e. Monitor closely for manifestations of infection and/or adverse effects of medications
2. Anxiety
   a. Provide opportunities to express feelings
   b. Encourage involvement in care
   c. Reduce or eliminate environmental stressors
   d. Provide verbal and written post-transplant care to client and family

VI. INFECTION PRECAUTIONS

A. Tier 1—standard precautions utilized for all clients
1. Hand hygiene
2. Personal protective equipment (gloves, gowns, masks, protective eyewear) when potential contact with blood or body fluid
3. Needles and other sharp objects are not recapped or bent; dispose of in puncture-proof containers
4. Respiratory hygiene/cough etiquette
   a. Cover mouth and nose when sneezing or coughing
   b. Dispose of tissues properly
   c. Separate potentially infected persons from others by at least 3 feet or having them wear a surgical mask

B. Tier 2—transmission-based precautions
1. Used in addition to standard precautions
2. May be used alone or in combination
   a. Airborne precautions: used for serious illnesses transmitted by airborne droplet nuclei smaller than 5 microns
   b. Droplet precautions: used for serious illnesses transmitted by particle droplets larger than 5 microns
   c. Contact precautions: serious illnesses easily transmitted by direct client contact or by contact with items in client's environment

C. Category specific precautions
1. Usage less prevalent
2. Includes strict isolation (total separation of client from all areas of contact), respiratory isolation, and enteric precautions (for intestinal diseases)

D. Disease-specific precautions
1. Private rooms may be needed by clients with specific diseases (such as tuberculosis) to prevent possible spread of infection; clients with the same organism may share a room (called cohorting)
2. Laminar (negative) air flow prevents spread of infection throughout rest of hospital
3. Gowns, face protection, and other self-protection measures are used as appropriate

E. Reverse isolation (protective isolation)
1. Involves measures used to protect clients from risk of exposure due to a compromised immune system; may also be used for clients with burn injury who have lost skin as first line defense against microorganisms
2. Supplies brought into client's room (such as bed linens) are generally sterilized by autoclave or other measures to avoid introducing microorganisms into client's environment
3. Nurse and other staff don gown, mask, gloves, and hair and foot covers before entering room
4. Equipment used in client care is disinfected before being brought into room and remains there throughout time such precautions are in use (avoids risk of introducing microorganisms with moving items in and out of room)

F. Neutropenic precautions
1. Can be employed to prevent risk of infection (as indicated by WBC levels)
2. Client is not allowed to have fresh flowers or plants, raw or undercooked foods, or black pepper, because these items may contain potential gram-negative bacteria
3. Sources of standing water are avoided, such as use of water pitchers; offer client fluids often as liquids should not remain standing in room longer than 15 minutes to avoid accumulation of microbes
4. Invasive procedures and visitors are limited to prevent further exposures

POSTTEST

Practice to Pass

A client has an absolute neutrophil count (ANC) of 500. What are your immediate interventions?

5. Client's temperature is monitored frequently
6. WBC and ANC counts are monitored and client is assessed frequently to detect early signs of infection

G. Other infection control practices

1. Participate in educating others on importance of immunizations and guidelines for use of antibiotics
2. Maintain strict aseptic technique with regard to invasive procedures; maintain aseptic integrity of indwelling systems
3. Teach measures to prevent spread of infection, including:
   a. Avoiding crowds and contact with susceptible persons
   b. Using disposable tissues to contain respiratory secretions
   c. Coughing into the elbow or upper arm when tissues are not available
   d. Using appropriate food-handling precautions
   e. Avoiding contact with or sharing of body fluids
4. Maintain skin integrity by turning and repositioning client; promote respiratory expansion by encouraging coughing and deep breathing, unless coughing is contraindicated for some other reason
5. Dispose of biohazardous equipment according to agency policy

H. Nursing responsibilities

1. Post isolation signs and maintain communication among health care team members, the client, and family/visitors
2. Follow isolation procedures to determine appropriate client placement
3. Transport clients according to isolation procedures
4. Use dedicated equipment for clients on isolation precautions
5. Monitor client's lab values and diagnostic tests
6. Follow up with agency or facility infection control department

Case Study

C. W., a 35-year-old female client, has just been diagnosed with systemic lupus erythematosus and is concerned about the impact of this multisystem disease process. You are the nurse that has been assigned to take care of this client.

1. What background information can you obtain from C. W. that would help you determine how the client is reacting to the diagnosis?
2. When C. W. asks you what "multisystem disease process" means, how would you respond?
3. What diagnostic tests would serve to establish C. W.'s immune baseline?
4. What measures could you include with regard to discharge planning for this client?

For suggested responses, see page 360.

POSTTEST

❶ A client who has tested positive for human immunodeficiency virus (HIV) now presents with a CD4 count of less than 200 cells/mcL and invasive cervical cancer. How would the nurse evaluate these findings in terms of current Centers for Disease Control (CDC) definitions?

1. Client has seroconverted
2. Client continues to remain at HIV-positive status
3. Client is in latent period of the disease process
4. Client has acquired immunodeficiency syndrome (AIDS)

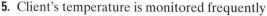

2 A client diagnosed with an autoimmune disorder questions the nurse as to what impact this may have on activities of daily living in the years to come. What is the best response that the nurse can give?

1. "The changes will be subtle at first so it won't be noticeable to others."
2. "It is hard to predict what the disease process has in store for any one individual."
3. "I can hear the concern in your voice. Perhaps we can talk for awhile and discuss some of your concerns."
4. "I would suggest the use of any available remedy that might give you some comfort."

3 The nurse determines that which of the following nursing diagnoses has the highest priority for a client who has rheumatoid arthritis (RA)?

1. Fatigue
2. Chronic Pain
3. Ineffective Role Performance
4. Disturbed Body Image

4 The nurse is caring for a client who has suffered an injury in which the skin is broken. In what order does the nurse anticipate assessing the occurrence of the following pathophysiological responses? Place the options in order.

1. Breach in the barrier of defense
2. Vasodilation of the arterioles and venules
3. Phagocytosis
4. Margination and emigration of leukocytes into the damaged tissue
5. Reconstruction

5 A client who is human immunodeficiency virus (HIV) positive and is taking antiretroviral medications asks why he was told that a change in medication might be needed during the course of treatment. What would be the best explanation for the nurse to give the client?

1. "Antiretroviral medication regimens must be changed to prevent expected toxicity to major organs."
2. "Antiretroviral resistance is a major challenge to long-term management of HIV infection, and drug therapy may change based on research results."
3. "Monotherapy is recommended for the treatment of HIV and must be adjusted."
4. "Your treatment regimen will remain in place and is unlikely to change."

6 A client receives a polio vaccine during a clinic visit. The nurse explains that this will provide what type of immunity to the client?

1. Active natural immunity
2. Active artificial immunity
3. Passive natural immunity
4. Passive artificial immunity

7 The nurse is providing teaching to a client with systemic lupus erythematosus (SLE). Which manifestations are warnings of an acute episode (flare) and should be reported immediately to the health care provider? Select all that apply.

1. Rash
2. Fever
3. Headache
4. Edema
5. Dizziness

8 A client with tuberculosis is being admitted to the medical-surgical unit. Which type of precautions should the nurse institute to protect the client and staff from possible exposure to this infection?

1. Standard precautions
2. Contact precautions
3. Airborne precautions
4. Droplet precautions

9 The nurse has been asked to perform a home assessment on a client who has longstanding rheumatoid arthritis (RA). Which one of the following findings should receive the highest priority for follow-up teaching?

1. Client lives in apartment building that has an elevator
2. Client has installed handrail support in the bathroom
3. Client has area rugs scattered throughout apartment
4. Client keeps medications in a plastic case on kitchen counter

10 After a client is placed on droplet precautions, which of the following actions by the nurse should be given the highest priority for infection control?

1. Using strict aseptic technique
2. Washing of hands before and after giving client care
3. Checking sterile supplies for expiration date
4. Changing intravenous tubing according to hospital policy

➤ *See pages 378–379 for Answers and Rationales.*

ANSWERS & RATIONALES

Pretest

1 **Answer: 3** **Rationale:** Mental status changes ranging from restlessness to confusion comprise one of the most frequent "atypical" signs of infection in older adults. Fever, chills, erythema, and edema are often absent. Leukocytosis with elevated neutrophil count may be present in varying degrees; however, this presentation is considered a typical response. **Cognitive Level:** Applying **Client Need:** Physiological Adaptation **Integrated Process:** Nursing Process: Assessment **Content Area:** Fundamentals **Strategy:** List the common findings associated with an infection. Compare this list with the answer options. Eliminate all answer options that are common in the presence of an infection because of the critical word *atypical* in the question. The correct response is the remaining answer option. **Reference:** LeMone, P., & Burke, K. M. (2011). *Medical-surgical nursing: Critical thinking in patient care* (5th ed., Vol. Single). Upper Saddle River, NJ: Pearson Education, p. 296.

2 **Answer: 4** **Rationale:** Any client who presents with unexplained weight loss and persistent nonspecific complaints of fatigue, nausea, and the presence of a lesion characteristic of Kaposi sarcoma should be evaluated with regard to HIV status. Low-grade fever does not correlate directly with the presence of HIV. Stools which change from brown to a pale beige color are characteristic of a common bile duct obstruction, not of AIDS. A history of blood transfusion may prove to warrant further assessment, but it is not as high of a priority as a symptom of AIDS. **Cognitive Level:** Analyzing **Client Need:** Physiological Adaptation **Integrated Process:** Nursing Process: Diagnosis **Content Area:** Adult Health **Strategy:** The question indicates that whatever is causing the symptoms has been going on for some time. Eliminate answer options that address things of an immediate nature or that address a possible cause for an abnormality. It is most important at this time to get an accurate diagnosis so definitive treatment can be initiated. **Reference:** LeMone, P., & Burke, K. M. (2011). *Medical-surgical nursing: Critical thinking in patient care* (5th ed., Vol. Single). Upper Saddle River, NJ: Prentice Hall, pp. 324–328.

3 **Answer: 1** **Rationale:** Type 1 hypersensitivity involves humorally mediated antigen–antibody reactions. Food allergies and medications can provide a localized as well as systemic response. Clients who have a history of multiple allergies usually have high IgE levels that are a characteristic measure of this type of reaction. Type 2 cytotoxic hypersensitivity involves the formation of IgG or IgM type antibodies against cell-bound antigens such as the ABO or Rh antigen. A hemolytic transfusion reaction to blood of an incompatible type is characteristic of this type of reaction. Type 3 reactions involve the formation of an immune complex of antigen and antibody as seen in vasculitis. Type 4 reactions involve the sensitized T cells and release of lymphokines as in graft rejection. **Cognitive Level:** Applying **Client Need:** Physiological Adaptation **Integrated Process:** Nursing Process: Diagnosis **Content Area:** Adult Health **Strategy:** Review the specific types of immunity and their manifestations. **Reference:** LeMone, P., & Burke, K. M. (2011). *Medical-surgical nursing: Critical thinking in patient care* (5th ed., Vol. Single). Upper Saddle River, NJ: Pearson Education, pp. 308–311.

4 **Answer: 2** **Rationale:** Antinuclear antibodies indicate the presence of an autoimmune disorder. They are not considered specific for systemic lupus, because many other autoimmune disorders have significant numbers of these antibodies. This reported titer is suggestive of the presence of ANA antibodies. The test is abnormal, and more specific diagnostic studies are indicated rather than a repeat of the ANA titer. **Cognitive Level:** Analyzing **Client Need:** Reduction of Risk Potential **Integrated Process:** Nursing Process: Diagnosis **Content Area:** Adult Health **Strategy:** Recall tests that are indicated as a general nonspecific screening mechanism versus testing for specific disorders. **Reference:** LeMone, P., & Burke, K. M. (2011). *Medical-surgical nursing: Critical thinking in patient care* (5th ed., Vol. Single). Upper Saddle River, NJ: Pearson Education, p. 316.

5 **Answer: 4** **Rationale:** Clients with a past medical history of anaphylaxis should have epinephrine readily available for emergencies because it is the drug of choice to alleviate the symptoms of allergic response. Pretreatment with diphenhydramine may be used prior to an exposure if the response is usually mild or exposure is unavoidable. An injectable form may be used in addition to epinephrine for a possible anaphylactic reaction but is not the highest priority. Food allergies are rarely the cause of anaphylactic reactions. An intradermal test is likely to cause a systemic response with another anaphylactic reaction in a client with a previous anaphylactic reaction. The client should have a radioallergosorbent test (RAST) where blood is drawn or a prick test which elicits a local reaction. If a food allergy is suspected as the cause the nurse would not have the client expose themselves to the food and another anaphylactic reaction. **Cognitive Level:** Applying **Client Need:** Physiological Adaptation **Integrated Process:** Nursing Process: Planning **Content Area:** Adult Health **Strategy:** Review the types of allergic response and their manifestations. Compare this information with treatments indicated for each type of reaction. **Reference:** LeMone, P., & Burke, K. M. (2011). *Medical-surgical nursing: Critical thinking in patient care* (5th ed., Vol. Single). Upper Saddle River, NJ: Pearson Education, pp. 308–313.

6 Answer: 2 Rationale: Hydroxychloroquine is an antimalarial agent used in the treatment of rheumatoid arthritis. This medication can cause retinal toxicity with pigmentary retinitis and vision loss, and therefore the client should be closely monitored for this possibility with specified visual exams every 6 months. Gastric irritation, fluid retention, pulse elevations, and drowsiness (drowsiness is not commonly seen with hydroxychloroquine) are not routinely seen with this type of medication. **Cognitive Level:** Applying **Client Need:** Pharmacological and Parenteral Therapies **Integrated Process:** Nursing Process: Implementation **Content Area:** Pharmacology **Strategy:** Specific drug knowledge is needed to answer this question. Review the mechanism of action, common side effects, and preventive measures for hydroxychloroquine if this question was difficult. **Reference:** LeMone, P., & Burke, K. M. (2011). *Medical-surgical nursing: Critical thinking in patient care* (5th ed., Vol. Single). Upper Saddle River, NJ: Pearson Education, pp. 1367–1368.

7 Answer:

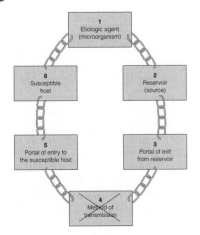

Rationale: Sneezing allows transmission by droplet contact. By sneezing into the bend of the elbow the "method of transmission" link is interrupted. **Cognitive Level:** Applying **Client Need:** Safety and Infection Control **Integrated Process:** Teaching and Learning **Content Area:** Adult Health **Strategy:** Consider the 6 links of the chain of infection and how infection control measures address each link. **Reference:** LeMone, P., & Burke, K. M. (2011). *Medical-surgical nursing: Critical thinking in patient care* (5th ed., Vol. Single). Upper Saddle River, NJ: Pearson Education, pp. 292–293.

8 Answer: 1 Rationale: Arthralgias (joint pain) and Raynaud's disease are common early manifestations of systemic sclerosis. Involvement of visceral organs tends to be slow and insidious and manifestations include dysphagia, pulmonary involvement, dysrhythmias, malabsorption, and renal effects. **Cognitive Level:** Applying **Client Need:** Physiological Adaptation **Integrated Process:** Nursing Process: Assessment **Content Area:** Adult Health **Strategy:** Review common manifestations of each autoimmune disorder. **Reference:** LeMone, P., & Burke, K. M. (2011). *Medical-surgical nursing: Critical thinking in patient care* (5th ed., Vol. Single). Upper Saddle River, NJ: Pearson Education, pp. 1388–1389.

9 Answer: 3 Rationale: The client's understanding is demonstrated by acknowledging the fact that sun exposure should be limited to times other than 10:00 a.m. to 3:00 p.m. because sun exposure can increase the rash. The use of oral contraceptives may cause acute episodes of SLE so alternative methods of birth control should be used. Pregnancy is not contraindicated but close monitoring is needed because acute episodes may occur during pregnancy. Clients should avoid exposure to potential infection. SLE has no cure. It was once considered fatal in most cases but with the use of immunosuppressants the 10-year survival rate is approximately 90%. **Cognitive Level:** Applying **Client Need:** Physiological Adaptation **Integrated Process:** Nursing Process: Evaluation **Content Area:** Adult Health **Strategy:** The core issue of the question is knowledge of appropriate self-care measures that will reduce the risk of a flare-up in the disease. Recall the link between ultraviolet light exposure and the lupus rash and review other causes of exacerbations if this question was difficult. **Reference:** LeMone, P., & Burke, K. M. (2011). *Medical-surgical nursing: Critical thinking in patient care* (5th ed., Vol. Single). Upper Saddle River, NJ: Pearson Education, pp. 1374–1379.

10 Answer: 1, 2, 4, 5 Rationale: The correct approach to working with a client who exhibits an allergy is to remove the offending agent first, and then apply the ABCs. Assess the airway and breathing and administer a bronchodilator as ordered if wheezing is present. Antihistamines may be indicated to block the histamine receptors and their effects, such as itching and angioedema. If severe respiratory distress were present epinephrine would be administered. **Cognitive Level:** Applying

Client Need: Physiological Adaptation Integrated Process: Nursing Process: Implementation Content Area: Adult Health Strategy: Select the answer options that would first prevent further reaction and then reverse the response. Reference: LeMone, P., & Burke, K. M. (2011). *Medical-surgical nursing: Critical thinking in patient care* (5th ed., Vol. Single). Upper Saddle River, NJ: Pearson Education, pp. 313–315, 733.

Posttest

1 **Answer: 4** **Rationale:** AIDS is defined by the presence of opportunistic infections and other diseases indicative of immunodeficiency, HIV-seropositive status and a CD4 count of less than 200/mm^3. Seroconversion can occur up to 1 year after exposure. Once conversion occurs, the client has a positive HIV status until the conditions described previously develop. The latent period is considered to be one in which the individual is asymptomatic. **Cognitive Level:** Applying **Client Need:** Physiological Adaptation **Integrated Process:** Nursing Process: Diagnosis **Content Area:** Adult Health **Strategy:** Select the answer option that incorporates both the CD$_4$ count and the cervical cancer. **Reference:** LeMone, P., Burke, K., & Bauldoff, G. (2011). *Medical-surgical nursing: Critical thinking in patient care* (5th ed.). Upper Saddle River, NJ: Pearson Education, pp. 329–330.

2 **Answer: 3** **Rationale:** A client diagnosed with an autoimmune disease is faced with a lifetime of chronic illness and yet may not appear acutely ill because of the episodic nature of remissions and exacerbations. The nurse promotes a therapeutic relationship by allowing the client to ventilate feelings. It is dismissive to minimize any changes that a client may experience that are unnoticeable to others as they may be quite unsettling to the individual. It is not the role of the nurse to speculate how a disease process will progress. Suggesting that the client use any "available remedy" may lead the client to potential harm or medical quackery. **Cognitive Level:** Applying **Client Need:** Psychosocial Integrity **Integrated Process:** Communication and Documentation **Content Area:** Adult Health **Strategy:** Consider that a goal of the nurse–client interaction is to encourage the client to verbalize concerns related to a diagnosis. Select the answer option that encourages the client to continue providing data to the nurse. **Reference:** Berman, A. J., & Snyder, S. (2011). *Kozier and Erb's fundamentals of nursing: Concepts, process, and practice* (9th ed.). Upper Saddle River, NJ: Prentice Hall, pp. 472–474. LeMone, P., Burke, K., & Bauldoff, G. (2011). *Medical-surgical nursing: Critical thinking in patient care* (5th ed.). Upper Saddle River, NJ: Pearson Education, pp. 315–317.

3 **Answer: 2** **Rationale:** Rheumatoid arthritis causes inflammation, fluid accumulation in the joints, and degenerative changes in the joints. Pain and pain control are the most important elements of care for this client. Fatigue will also be lessened with adequate pain control because it

may allow for better sleep. If the pain is well controlled, the client will be able to function within his or her role. If the pain is well controlled the client has greater independence and self-esteem **Cognitive Level:** Analyzing **Client Need:** Physiological Adaptation **Integrated Process:** Nursing Process: Diagnosis **Content Area:** Adult Health **Strategy:** Select the answer option that is most likely to prevent the client from living independently and being functional. **Reference:** LeMone, P., Burke, K., & Bauldoff, G. (2011). *Medical-surgical nursing: Critical thinking in patient care* (5th ed.). Upper Saddle River, NJ: Pearson Education, pp. 1370–1372.

4 **Answer: 1, 2, 4, 3, 5** **Rationale:** Without a breach in defenses, such as with injury to the skin, the other actions do not occur. Inflammatory mediators are released from damaged tissue and stimulate vasodilation. The cellular phase begins within less than an hour after the injury and is marked by movement of leukocytes into the damaged tissues. The leukocytes need to move to the area before phagocytosis occurs. Particulate matter, bacteria, damaged cells, and inflammatory exudate must be removed by phagocytosis in order for reconstruction to occur. **Cognitive Level:** Applying **Client Need:** Physiological Adaptation **Integrated Process:** Nursing Process: Assessment **Content Area:** Adult Health **Strategy:** Consider the physiology of the innate immune response. **Reference:** LeMone, P., Burke, K., & Bauldoff, G. (2011). *Medical-surgical nursing: Critical thinking in patient care* (5th ed.). Upper Saddle River, NJ: Pearson Education, pp. 274–277.

5 **Answer: 2** **Rationale:** One of the most critical problems with regard to antiretroviral therapy is the emergence of antiretroviral resistance as the HIV virus continues to mutate. Should resistance develop, or research find a more effective drug, therapy will change. Combination therapies have been proven to be more effective in treating disease progression so monotherapy is no longer used. Antiretroviral therapies, in proper dosage, do not cause specific organ toxicity, although they can cause myelosuppression. **Cognitive Level:** Analyzing **Client Need:** Physiological Adaptation **Integrated Process:** Nursing Process: Implementation **Content Area:** Adult Health **Strategy:** This question targets knowledge of viral mutation and how it effects treatment. Select the answer option that best combines both content areas. **Reference:** LeMone, P., Burke, K., & Bauldoff, G. (2011). *Medical-surgical nursing: Critical thinking in patient care* (5th ed.). Upper Saddle River, NJ: Pearson Education, pp. 330–333.

6 **Answer: 2** **Rationale:** Vaccines are administered to client to promote the development of specific antibodies to afford protection. This is an example of active artificial immunity. Active natural immunity implies the development of antibodies in response to a client who had an actual active infection. Passive natural immunity implies the maternal and/or placental transfer of antibodies. Passive artificial immunity implies the specific injection of an immune serum. **Cognitive Level:** Applying **Client Need:** Health Promotion and Maintenance **Integrated Process:** Nursing Process: Diagnosis **Content Area:** Adult Health **Strategy:** Consider the types of possible immunity and select the answer option that reflects the description in the question. **Reference:** LeMone, P., Burke, K., & Bauldoff, G. (2011). *Medical-surgical nursing: Critical thinking in patient care* (5th ed.). Upper Saddle River, NJ: Pearson Education, pp. 281–283.

7 **Answer: 1, 2, 3, 5** **Rationale:** Warning signs of a systemic lupus erythematosus (SLE) flare include increased fatigue, pain, abdominal discomfort, rash, headache, fever, and dizziness. Edema is not a sign of an acute episode of SLE. **Cognitive Level:** Applying **Client Need:** Physiological Adaptation **Integrated Process:** Nursing Process: Assessment **Content Area:** Adult Health **Strategy:** SLE is an autoimmune disorder. Look for manifestations that would indicate problems with immune function. **Reference:** LeMone, P., Burke, K., & Bauldoff, G. (2011). *Medical-surgical nursing: Critical thinking in patient care* (5th ed.). Upper Saddle River, NJ: Pearson Education, pp. 1375–1379.

8 **Answer: 3** **Rationale:** Tuberculosis is transmitted to others via aerosolization. Airborne precautions should be instituted for all clients being admitted with a diagnosis of tuberculosis. Standard precautions should be maintained for all clients in the hospital setting. Contact precautions and droplet precautions do not apply to this disease process. **Cognitive Level:** Applying **Client Need:** Safety and Infection Control **Integrated Process:** Nursing Process: Implementation **Content Area:** Adult Health **Strategy:** First recall how tuberculosis is transmitted. Then select the answer option that best prevents this transmission. **Reference:** LeMone, P., Burke, K., & Bauldoff, G. (2011). *Medical-surgical nursing: Critical thinking in patient care*

(5th ed.). Upper Saddle River, NJ: Pearson Education, pp. 300–301.

9 **Answer: 3** **Rationale:** Individuals with long-standing rheumatoid arthritis (RA) have an increased likelihood of joint deformities and contractures that could increase risk of falls. Scattered area rugs are a potential safety hazard. All of the other assessment findings are considered to be supportive of this client with RA because they enhance mobility, safety, and medication compliance. **Cognitive Level:** Analyzing **Client Need:** Health Promotion and Maintenance **Integrated Process:** Nursing Process: Evaluation **Content Area:** Adult Health **Strategy:** This question is asking you to identify which of the 4 answer options poses a risk to the client. Select the answer option that is most likely to cause injury. **Reference:** LeMone, P., Burke, K., & Bauldoff, G. (2011). *Medical-surgical nursing: Critical thinking in patient care* (5th ed.). Upper Saddle River, NJ: Pearson Education, p. 1373.

10 **Answer: 2** **Rationale:** Regardless of isolation precautions, the basic action by the nurse to prevent infection is hand washing. All of the other options should also be followed but hand washing establishes the first line of defense and is therefore of highest importance. **Cognitive Level:** Applying **Client Need:** Safety and Infection Control **Integrated Process:** Nursing Process: Diagnosis **Content Area:** Fundamentals **Strategy:** This question asks for prioritization of the most important item in reducing the spread of infection. Recall that hand washing is the most important but also the most often neglected or underutilized measure; this will guide you to make the correct selection. **Reference:** LeMone, P., Burke, K., & Bauldoff, G. (2011). *Medical-surgical nursing: Critical thinking in patient care* (5th ed.). Upper Saddle River, NJ: Pearson Education, p. 297.

References

Berman, A., & Snyder, S. (2012). *Kozier & Erb's fundamentals of nursing: Concepts, process, and practice* (9th ed.). Upper Saddle River, NJ: Pearson Education.

D' Amico, D. & Barbarito, C. (2012). *Health & physical assessment in nursing* (2nd ed.). Upper Saddle River, NJ: Pearson Education, Inc.

Ignatavicius, D. D., & Workman, M. L. (2013). *Medical-surgical nursing: Critical thinking for collaborative care* (7th ed.) Philadelphia: W. B. Saunders Company.

Kee, J. L. (2010). *Laboratory and diagnostic tests* (8th ed.). Upper Saddle River, NJ: Pearson Education.

Lehne, R. (2010). *Pharmacology for nursing care* (7th ed.). St. Louis, MO: Saunders.

LeMone, P., Burke, K., & Bauldoff, G. (2011). *Medical surgical nursing: Critical thinking in patient care* (5th ed.). Upper Saddle River, NJ: Pearson Education.

Lewis, S., Dirksen, S. Heitkemper, M., Bucher, L., & Camera, I. (2011). *Medical surgical nursing: Assessment and management of clinical problems* (8th ed.). St. Louis, MO: Elsevier.

McCance, K. L., & Huether, S. E. (2010). *Pathophysiology: The biologic basis for disease in adults and children* (6th ed.). St. Louis, MO: Mosby, Inc.

Public Health Service, U.S. Dept of Health and Human Services, Centers for Disease Control and Prevention, Atlanta, Georgia. Gasner, JS, Hospital Infection Control Practices Advisory Committee

(1996) Guideline for isolation precautions in hospitals. *Infection Control Hospital Epidemiology, 17,* 53–80.

Osborn, K. S., Wraa, C. E., & Watson, A. (2010). *Medical surgical nursing: Preparation for practice* (Vol. Combined). Upper Saddle River, NJ: Pearson Education.

Smith, S. F., Duell, D. J., & Martin, B. C. (2012). *Clinical nursing skills: Basic to advanced skills* (8th ed.). Upper Saddle River, NJ: Pearson Education.

ANSWERS & RATIONALES

12 Cellular Disorders (Oncology)

Chapter Outline

Overview of Anatomy and Physiology

Epidemiology of Cancer

Risk Factors for Development of Cancer

American Cancer Society Recommendations for Early Cancer Detection

Diagnostic Tests and Assessments

Common Effects of Cancer

Common Treatments and Nursing Care

Oncologic Emergencies: Diagnosis and Management

Expected Outcomes for Clients with Cellular Disorders

NCLEX-RN® Test Prep

Use the accompanying online resource, NursingReviewsandRationales, to test yourself with hundreds of NCLEX®-style practice questions.

Objectives

➤ Identify basic structures and functions of cells.

➤ Describe the pathophysiology and etiology of common cellular disorders.

➤ Discuss expected assessment data and diagnostic test findings for selected cellular disorders.

➤ Identify priority nursing problems for selected cellular disorders.

➤ Discuss therapeutic management of selected cellular disorders.

➤ Discuss nursing management of a client experiencing a cellular disorder.

➤ Identify expected outcomes for the client experiencing a cellular disorder.

Review at a Glance

alopecia hair loss that can occur secondary to chemotherapy or radiation

benign neoplasm localized growth, encapsulated, not malignant

bone marrow suppression decrease in number of granulocytes, lymphocytes, and thrombocytes, resulting in anemia and decreased ability to respond to infection or form clots

cancer mutation of normal cells into abnormal cells that proliferate

carcinoma tumor arising from epithelial tissue

cell-kill hypothesis chemotherapy kills a certain percentage of cells during each cell cycle, necessitating several courses of chemotherapy to adequately reduce number of cancer cells

chemotherapy cytotoxic medications used to disrupt cell cycle of cancer cells, resulting in cell death

differentiation normal process by which cells specialize in order to perform certain tasks

extravasation leaking of chemotherapeutic agents into tissues; occurs during intravenous administration and can cause damage to adjacent tissues

malignant neoplasm aggressively growing mass causing tissue death and having ability to metastasize

metastasis spreading of malignant neoplasms through blood or lymph, forming a secondary tumor distant from primary site

sarcoma tumor arising from supportive tissues

stomatitis painful mouth sores

thrombocytopenia decrease in platelet count

tumor also called neoplasm, a mass of new tissue functioning independently, serving no physiologic purpose

tumor markers proteins detected in serum or other body fluids, indicating presence of malignancy

vesicants chemicals causing tissue damage on contact

xerostomia dry mouth

PRETEST

1 A 67-year-old female client refuses to be screened for cancer, stating, "I'm too old to get cancer and if I don't have it by now, I'll never get it." Which of the following should be the basis of the nurse's response to her?

1. Unless symptomatic, screening the client for cancer is not necessary.
2. Screening the elderly for cancer is essential.
3. The incidence of cancer decreases with advancing age.
4. Age is not a significant factor in the development of cancer.

2 A client with cancer is referred to a pain management specialist. In what sequence does the nurse anticipate pharmacological pain management to occur? Put the options in the correct order.

1. Careful assessment of the client's pain
2. Evaluation of the client's functional goals
3. Initiation of opioid pain medications
4. Evaluation of the degree of pain relief
5. Initiation of non-opioid drugs with adjuvants such as antidepressants

3 A client receiving intravenous chemotherapy is experiencing nausea. What would be the best intervention for the nurse to use to reduce the client's discomfort?

1. Administer antiemetics when client begins to report nausea.
2. Offer warm liquids during chemotherapy.
3. Administer antiemetics before chemotherapy.
4. Encourage client to eat a full meal before receiving chemotherapy.

4 When teaching safety precautions to the client with an internal radiation implant, the nurse would include which statement in explanations to the client?

1. No precautions are necessary for internal radiation implants.
2. The client poses a risk of radiation exposure to others.
3. The client must remain in solitary isolation for the entire hospitalization.
4. Visitors should maintain a distance of 3 feet from the client at all times.

5 The nurse is educating a client who will likely experience alopecia as a result of the current chemotherapy treatment. Further instructions are necessary when the client states which of the following?

1. "I will wash my hair every day."
2. "I will pat my hair dry and avoid the use of hairdryers."
3. "My hair will begin to grow back after the chemotherapy is completed."
4. "I will choose a wig or hairpiece before the loss of hair occurs."

6 A client receiving chemotherapy as treatment for leukemia has a white blood cell (WBC) count of 3,900/mm^3. The nurse should teach the client to avoid contact with which family member?

1. 34-year-old nephew with human immunodeficiency (HIV) infection
2. 68-year-old husband with a history of exposure to tuberculosis as a youth
3. 9-year-old grandchild with a recent exposure to chickenpox (varicella)
4. 31-year-old daughter who is 4 months pregnant

7 A 22-year-old female has been seen in the health clinic for a routine physical examination. The nurse determines that she understands health teaching regarding early detection and screening for breast cancer when the client makes which statement?

1. "I should have a breast examination by a health care provider every 3 years."
2. "I should have a breast examination by a health care provider yearly."
3. "I should perform breast self-examination every 3 months."
4. "I should have a mammogram performed yearly."

8 A client is to receive intravenous chemotherapy via a peripherally inserted central catheter (PICC). Which action is the highest priority before the nurse begins the administration?

1. Make client as comfortable as possible.
2. Ensure that catheter is in a vein.
3. Flush catheter with medication to test patency of vein.
4. Administer acetaminophen (Tylenol) prophylactically.

9 A client diagnosed with cancer has been receiving chemotherapy and subsequently develops a platelet count of 95,000/mm^3. The nurse concludes that the client understands instructions to avoid potential complications when the client states to do which of the following?

1. Avoid aspirin and aspirin- (salicylate) containing products.
2. Monitor for fever every 4 hours.
3. Allow for rest periods to avoid fatigue.
4. Brush and floss teeth daily to prevent infection.

10 The nurse is caring for a client receiving chemotherapy prior to a bone marrow transplant. Once the client is placed on thrombocytopenic precautions, which interventions would the nurse utilize for this client? Select all that apply.

1. Place client in a negative pressure room.
2. Avoid intramuscular injections.
3. Have caregivers and visitors wear masks.
4. Avoid rectal temperatures.
5. Avoid using a soft-bristled tooth brush for mouth care.

➤ *See pages 403–404 for Answers and Rationales.*

I. OVERVIEW OF ANATOMY AND PHYSIOLOGY

A. Characteristics of normal cells

1. Normal cell growth (cell cycle) consists of 5 intervals or phases:
   a. G_0: resting phase, not reproducing: some cells are normal while others are undergoing repair or are dying
   b. Interphase: contains 3 subphases that contribute to cell growth and prepare it for reproduction
      1) G_1: cellular production of RNA and protein
      2) S: synthesis of DNA and proteins and new chromosomes appear
      3) G_2: RNA synthesis
   c. Mitosis (M): actual cell division
2. **Differentiation** refers to a process whereby cells develop specific structures and functions in order to specialize in certain tasks
3. Cellular adaptation
   a. *Hypertrophy* refers to an increase in size of normal cells
   b. *Atrophy* refers to shrinkage of cell size
   c. *Hyperplasia* refers to an increase in number of normal cells
   d. *Metaplasia* refers to a conversion from normal pattern of differentiation of one type of cell into another type of cell not normal for that tissue

       e. *Dysplasia* refers to an alteration in shape, size, appearance, and distribution of cells

       f. *Anaplasia* refers to disorganized, irregular cells that have no structure and have loss of differentiation; the result is almost always malignant

B. Evolution of cancer cells

  1. Cancer refers to a disease whereby cells mutate into abnormal cells that proliferate abnormally; *neoplasia* refers to an abnormal cell growth or **tumor**, a mass of new tissue functioning independently and serving no useful purpose

    a. Benign neoplasms are slow-growing, localized, and encapsulated nonmalignant growths with well-defined borders

      1. They are usually easily removed

      2. They generally do not cause tissue damage or other complications unless they interfere with tissue function or circulation

    b. Malignant neoplasms are aggressive growths that invade and destroy surrounding tissues; can lead to death unless treatment is provided

  2. Invasion occurs when cancer cells infiltrate adjacent tissues surrounding neoplasm

  3. Metastasis occurs when malignant cells travel through blood or lymph system and invade other tissues and organs to form a secondary tumor

C. Characteristics of malignant cells

  1. Rapid cell division and growth: regulation of rate of mitosis is lost; cells seem to be "immortal"; they do not stop growing and do not die like normal cells

  2. No contact inhibition: cells do not respect boundaries of other cells and invade their tissue areas

  3. Loss of differentiation: cells lose specialized characteristics of function for that cell type and revert to an earlier, more primitive cell type

  4. Ability to migrate (metastasize): cells move to distant areas of body and establish malignant lesions (tumors) at new site

  5. Alteration in cell structure: differences are evident between normal and malignant cells with respect to cell membrane, cytoplasm, and overall cell shape

  6. Self-survival

    a. May develop ectopic sites to produce hormones needed for own growth

    b. Can develop a connective tissue stroma to support growth

    c. May develop own blood supply by secreting angiotensin growth factor to stimulate local blood vessels to grow into tumor

II. EPIDEMIOLOGY OF CANCER

A. Incidence

  1. Cancer affects every age group, though most cancer and cancer deaths occur in people older than 65 years of age

  2. Cancer is attributable to 25% of all deaths; only cardiovascular diseases cause more deaths than cancer in United States

  3. Highest incidence of all cancer is prostate cancer

  4. Highest cancer incidence in males in order of frequency: prostate cancer, lung cancer, and colorectal cancer, according to American Cancer Society, 2012

  5. Highest cancer incidence in females in order of frequency: breast cancer, lung cancer, and colorectal cancer according to American Cancer Society, 2012

B. Statistics

  1. There are 8 million Americans today who have a history of cancer

  2. Approximately 1 in every 4 deaths in United States is from cancer

  3. Common sites of cancer and their sites of metastasis (see Table 12-1)

Table 12-1	Common Sites of Cancer and Their Sites of Metastasis
Cancer Type	**Sites of Metastasis**
Brain cancer	Other areas of central nervous system
Breast cancer	Regional lymph nodes, liver, lung, vertebrae, and brain
Colon cancer	Lymph nodes, ovaries, liver, lung, brain
Lung cancer	Bone, brain, liver, lymph nodes, spinal cord
Malignant melanoma	Brain, liver, lung, regional lymph nodes, spleen
Prostate cancer	Bladder, bone, liver

III. RISK FACTORS FOR DEVELOPMENT OF CANCER

   A. Age
   1. About 78% of cancer diagnoses occur after age 55 years
   2. Factors attributed to cancer in older adults include hormonal changes, altered immune responses, long-term exposure to promotional agents, a decrease in immune function, stress, and accumulation of free radicals (molecules resulting from body's metabolic and oxidative processes)
   3. Age is identified as the single most important factor related to development of cancer

   B. Gender
   1. Certain cancers are more commonly seen in specific genders
   2. For example, breast and thyroid cancers occur more commonly in females, colon and bladder cancer occurs more commonly in males

   C. Geographic location
   1. Risks for cancer vary according to environment and location
   2. Rates for specific cancer sites, morbidity, and mortality vary from state to state, nation to nation, and in urban versus rural living

   D. Genetics
   1. 15% of cancers may be attributed to a hereditary component and 5% have a strong hereditary component
   2. Cancers demonstrating a familial relationship include breast, colon, lung, ovarian, and prostate
   3. Clients with a genetic predisposition to cancer should be counseled and screened according to American Cancer Society (ACS) guidelines

   E. Immune disturbance
   1. Some viral infections tend to increase risk
   2. Infections associated with cancer include Epstein-Barr, herpes simplex virus types 1 and 2, human herpesvirus-6, human papillomavirus (HPV), hepatitis B, human t-lymphotropic viruses, and cytomegalovirus (CMV)

   F. Chemical agents
   1. Over 1,000 chemicals are known to be carcinogenic
   2. Exposure to chemicals such as asbestos, arsenic, or chemotherapy drugs; some occupations heighten this risk over decades

   G. Race
   1. Cancer can affect any population
   2. Nonetheless, African Americans experience a higher rate of cancer than any other racial or ethnic group and experience highest death rates
   3. Cancer incidence and mortality are lower in Native American men and women than in any other ethnic or racial group

H. Tobacco

1. There is a strong correlation between smoking and lung cancer
2. Other cancers associated with tobacco use include bladder, esophageal, gastric, laryngeal, oropharyngeal, and pancreatic
3. Smokeless tobacco (snuff and chewing tobacco) increases risk of oral and esophageal cancers
4. Long-term exposure to secondhand smoke increases risk for lung and bladder cancers

I. Alcohol

1. Serves as a promoter in liver and esophageal cancers
2. When combined with tobacco, risks for other cancers are even higher

J. Diet

1. Diet has been demonstrated in research to correlate with some cancers
2. Diets high in red meats and saturated fats, low in fiber, and those containing nitrosamines and nitrosindoles found in preserved meats and pickled foods promote certain cancers such as colon, breast, esophageal, and gastric
3. Vegetables, fruits, fiber, folate, and calcium may be protective
4. Excessive frying or broiling of fish and meat may cause the formation of carcinogenic compounds

K. Miscellaneous: stress, poverty, recreational drug use, sun exposure, drugs, hormones, radiation, and obesity also increase risk of cancer

IV. AMERICAN CANCER SOCIETY RECOMMENDATIONS FOR EARLY CANCER DETECTION (AMERICAN CANCER SOCIETY (2011). AMERICAN CANCER SOCIETY GUIDELINES FOR THE EARLY DETECTION OF CANCER. ATLANTA, GA: AMERICAN CANCER SOCIETY.)

A. For detection of breast cancer

1. Beginning at age 20, routinely perform monthly breast self-examinations (BSEs)
2. Women ages 20–39 should have breast examination by a health care provider every 3 years
3. Women age 40 and older should have a yearly mammogram and breast examination by a health care provider
4. Screening MRI is recommended for women with a 20% or greater lifetime risk

B. For detection of colon and rectal cancer

1. All persons aged 50 and older should have one of the following tests that primarily detect cancer
   a. Yearly fecal occult blood test
   b. Yearly fecal immunochemical test (FIT)
   c. Stool DNA test (sDNA), interval dependent upon risk factors
2. All persons aged 50 and older should have one of the following tests that find polyps and cancer (preferred if available)
   a. Flexible sigmoidoscopy every 5 years
   b. CT colonography (virtual colonoscopy) every 5 years
   c. Double-contrast barium enema every 5 years
   d. Colonoscopy every 10 years
3. Moderate or high-risk individuals should have more-frequent testing schedules

C. For detection of cervix or uterine cancer

1. Papanicolaou (Pap) smear
   a. At ages 21–29 years, should be done every 3 years; no human papilloma virus (HPV) testing needed unless Pap smear abnormal
   b. At ages 30–65 years, should be done along with HPV test every 5 years (preferred), but Pap smear may be done alone every 3 years
   c. No testing needed for women over age 65 with negative results for regular Pap smears

2. Post-menopausal women should report unexpected bleeding or spotting to health care provider; those at risk of endometrial cancer might have yearly endometrial biopsy
3. Women who have had a total hysterectomy with removal of cervix may stop screening if surgery was not done as a treatment for cervical cancer

D. For detection of prostate cancer
1. Research has not proven that potential benefits of testing outweigh harms of testing and treatment
2. Screening consists of prostate-specific antigen (PSA) test with or without a digital rectal exam (DRE)
3. African American men and men with a father or brother with prostate cancer before age 65 should consult with health care provider about the pros and cons of testing starting at age 45
4. Other men should talk to health care provider starting at age 50

V. DIAGNOSTIC TESTS AND ASSESSMENTS

A. Classification of cancer
1. **Carcinoma** refers to a tumor that arises from epithelial tissue; name of cancer identifies location; example: basal cell carcinoma
2. **Sarcoma** refers to a tumor arising from supportive tissues; name of cancer identifies specific tissue affected; example: osteosarcoma

B. Staging: TNM tumor system is used for classifying tumors
1. *T* indicates tumor size
    a. *T0* indicates no evidence of tumor
    b. *Tis* indicates tumor in situ
    c. *T1, T2, T3, T4* indicate progressive degrees of tumor size and involvement
2. *N* indicates lymph node involvement
    a. *N0* indicates no abnormal lymph nodes detected
    b. *N1a, N2a* indicate regional nodes involved with increasing degree from N1a to N2a, no metastases detected
    c. *N1b, N2b, N3b* indicate regional lymph node involvement with increasing degree from N1b to N3b, metastasis suspected
    d. *Nx* indicates inability to assess regional nodes
3. *M* indicates distant metastases
    a. *M0* indicates no evidence of distant metastasis
    b. *M1, M2, M3* indicate ascending degrees of distant metastasis and includes distant lymph nodes

C. Tumor markers
1. **Tumor markers** are protein substances found in blood or body fluids
2. Are released either by tumor itself, or by body as a defense in response to tumor (called host response)
3. Generally small amounts are found in normal body tissues or benign tumors but high levels are suspicious and require follow-up; are most useful for monitoring client's response to therapy and for detecting residual disease
4. They are derived from tumor itself, and include the following:
    a. *Oncofetal antigens* are present in fetal tissue but normally suppressed after birth, may indicate an anaplastic process in tumor cells; carcinoembryonic antigen (CEA) and alpha-fetoprotein (AFP) are examples
    b. *Hormones* are present in specified amounts in human body; however, high levels of hormones may indicate a hormone-secreting malignancy; hormones that may be utilized as tumor markers include antidiuretic hormone (ADH), calcitonin, catecholamines, human chorionic gonadotropin (HCG), and parathyroid hormone (PTH)

    c. *Isoenzymes* that are normally present in a particular tissue may be released into bloodstream if tissue is experiencing rapid, excessive growth as a result of a tumor; examples include neuron-specific enolase (NSE) and prostatic acid phosphatase (PAP)

    d. *Tissue-specific proteins* identify type of tissue affected by malignancy; an example is prostate-specific antigen (PSA) used to identify prostate cancer

    e. Proteins, such as serum immunoglobulin and beta-2 microglobulin, that may indicate malignancy or hyperplasia

D. Biopsy/cytology

    1. Histologic and cytologic examination of specimens are performed by pathologist on tissues collected by needle aspiration of solid tumors, exfoliation from epithelial surface, and aspiration of fluid from blood or body cavities

    2. Tissues may be obtained by excisional biopsy, incisional biopsy, and needle biopsy

    3. By examination of these tissues, the name, grade, and stage of a tumor can be identified

E. Laboratory tests: see Table 12-2

F. Other diagnostic studies

    1. Radiologic examinations include routine x-ray imaging, CT, MRI, ultrasonography, nuclear imaging, angiography, and positron emission tomography

    2. Direct visualization procedures such as colonoscopy or bronchoscopy may be done to allow visual identification of organs and permit biopsy of suspicious lesions or masses

G. American Cancer Society's 7 warning signs of cancer (uses acronym CAUTION)

    1. *C*hange in bowel or bladder habits

    2. *A* sore that does not heal

    3. *U*nusual bleeding or discharge

    4. *T*hickening or lump in breast or elsewhere

    5. *I*ndigestion or difficulty in swallowing

    6. *O*bvious change in wart or mole

    7. *N*agging cough or hoarseness

Table 12-2   Laboratory Tests Used for Cancer Diagnosis*

Test	Reference Value	Abnormality Indicated
Acid phosphatase (ACP)	0.0 to 0.8 unit/L	Elevated in prostate, breast, and bone cancer and in multiple myeloma
Adrenocorticotropic hormone (ACTH)	8 to 80 pg/mL	Decreased in adrenal cancer Elevated in pituitary cancer or with tumor that secretes ACTH (bronchiogenic cancer)
Alanine aminotransferase (ALT)	5 to 35 unit/mL (Frankel)	Moderate elevation in liver cancer
Albumin	3.5 to 5.0 g/dL	Decreased in malnutrition, metastatic liver cancer
Alkaline phosphatase (ALP)	20 to 90 unit/L	Elevated in cancer of liver, bone, breast, and prostate; in leukemia; and in multiple myeloma
Alpha-fetoprotein (AFP)	Male and nonpregnant female: < 15 ng/mL	Elevated in germ cell tumors (e.g., seminoma), testicular cancer
Aspartate aminotransferase (AST)	5 to 40 unit/mL (Frankel)	Elevated in liver cancer
Bilirubin	Total: 0.1 to1.2 mg/dL Direct: 0.0 to 0.3 mg/dL	Elevated in liver and gallbladder cancer
Bleeding time	Ivy method: 3 to 7 minutes	Prolonged in leukemia and metastatic liver cancer

(continued)

Table 12-2	Laboratory Tests Used for Cancer Diagnosis (Continued)	
Test	**Reference Value**	**Abnormality Indicated**
Blood urea nitrogen (BUN)	5 to 25 mg/dL	Decreased in malnutrition; increased in renal cancer
Calcitonin	Male: < 40 pg/mL Female: < 20 pg/mL	Elevated to > 500 pg/mL in thyroid medullary cancer, breast cancer, and lung cancer
Calcium (Ca)	4.5 to 5.5 mEq/L 9.0 to 11.0 mg/dL	Elevated in bone cancer and ectopic parathyroid hormone production (paraplastic syndrome)
Carcinoembryonic antigen (CEA)	2.5 ng/mL in nonsmokers 5 ng/mL in smokers > 12 ng/mL neoplasms	Elevated with GI cancers, lung, breast, bladder, kidney, cervical, leukemias Used to evaluate effectiveness of cancer treatment
Chloride (Cl)	95 to 105 mEq/L	Decreased in vomiting, diarrhea, syndrome of inappropriate antidiuretic hormone (SIADH)
C-reactive protein	> 1:2 titer is positive	Elevated in metastatic cancer and Burkitt's lymphoma
Creatinine	0.5 to 1.5 mg/dL	Decreased in malnutrition; elevated in most cancers
Dexamethasone suppression test	> 50% reduction in plasma cortisol	Nonsuppression in adrenal cancer and ACTH-producing tumors, severe stress
Estradiol-serum	Female: 20 to 300 pg/mL Menopausal female: < 20 pg/mL Male: 15 to 50 pg/mL	Elevated in estrogen-producing tumors and testicular tumors
Fibrinogen	200 to 400 mg/dL	Decreased in leukemia and as a side effect of chemotherapy
Gamma glutamyltransferase (GGT)	Male: 10 to 80 international unit/L Female: 5 to 25 international unit/L	Elevated in cancer of liver, pancreas, prostate, breast, kidney, lung, and brain
Fasting blood sugar	70 to 110 mg/dL	Decreased in malnutrition, cancer of stomach, liver, and lung
Haptoglobin	20 to 240 mg/dL	Elevated in Hodgkin's disease and cancer of lung, large intestine, stomach, breast, and liver
Hematocrit (Hct)	Male: 40% to 54% Female: 36% to 46%	Decreased in anemia, leukemia, Hodgkin's disease, lymphosarcoma, multiple myeloma, and malnutrition and as a side effect of chemotherapy
Hemoglobin (Hgb)	Male: 13.5 to 18 g/dL Female: 12 to 16 g/dL 1:3 ratio of Hgb:Hct	Decreased in anemia, many cancers, Hodgkin's disease, leukemia, and malnutrition and as a side effect of chemotherapy
Human chorionic gonadotropin (HCG)	Nonpregnant female <0.01 international unit/L	Elevated in choriocarcinoma
Insulin	5 to 25 microunit/mL	Elevated in insulinoma (islet cell tumor) and insulin-secreting cancers (e.g., lung cancer)
Lactic dehydrogenase (LDH)	100 to 190 international unit/L	Elevated in liver, brain, kidney, muscle cancers, acute leukemia, anemia
Occult blood	Negative	Positive in gastric and colon cancers
Serum osmolality	280 to 300 mOsm/kg H_2O	Decreased in SIADH
Urine osmolality	50 to 1200 mOsm/kg H_2O	Increased in SIADH
Parathyroid hormone (PTH)	400 to 900 pg/mL	Increased in PTH-secreting tumors
Platelet (thrombocyte) count	150,000/mm^3 to 400,000/mm^3	Decreased in bone, gastric, and brain cancer, in leukemia, and as a side effect of chemotherapy
Potassium (K)	3.5 to 5.0 mEq/L	Decreased in vomiting and diarrhea and in malnutrition

Table 12-2	Laboratory Tests Used for Cancer Diagnosis (Continued)	
Test	**Reference Value**	**Abnormality Indicated**
Prostatic-specific antigen (PSA)	0 to 4 ng/mL	Elevated from 10 to 120+ in prostate cancer
Total protein	6.0 to 8.0 g/dL	Decreased in malnutrition, gastrointestinal cancer, Hodgkin's disease; elevated in vomiting, diarrhea, multiple myeloma
Red blood cells (RBCs)	Male: 4.6 to 6.0 million/mm^3 Female: 4.0 to 5.0 million/mm^3	Decreased in anemia, leukemia, infection, multiple myeloma
Sodium (Na)	135 to 145 mEq/L	Decreased in SIADH, vomiting; elevated in dehydration
Uric acid	Male: 3.5 to 8.0 mg/dL Female: 2.8 to 6.8 mg/dL	Increased in leukemia, metastatic cancer, multiple myeloma, Burkitt's lymphoma, after vigorous chemotherapy
White blood cells (WBC)		
Total leukocytes	4500/mm^3 to 10,000/mm^3	Elevated in acute infection, leukemias, tissue necrosis; decreased as a side effect of chemotherapy
Neutrophils	50% to 70%	Elevated in bacterial infection and Hodgkin's disease; decreased in leukemia and malnutrition and as a side effect of chemotherapy
Eosinophils	1% to 3%	Elevated in cancer of bone, ovary, testes, and brain
Basophils	0.4% to 1.0%	Elevated in leukemia and healing stage of infection
Monocytes	4% to 6%	Elevated in infection, monocytic leukemia and cancer; decreased in lymphocytic leukemia and as a side effect of chemotherapy
Lymphocytes	25% to 35%	Elevated in lymphocytic leukemia, Hodgkin's disease, multiple myeloma, viral infections, and chronic infections; decreased in malnutrition, cancer, and other leukemias and as a side effect of chemotherapy

*All values refer to serum values unless otherwise indicated. Values are approximate; check the reference standards specified by your own agency's laboratory.

Source: LeMone, Priscilla; Burke, Karen M.; Bauldoff, Gerene, *Medical-Surgical Nursing: Critical Thinking in Patient Care*, 5th Edition, © 2011. Printed and Electronically reproduced by permission of Pearson Education, Inc., Upper Saddle River, New Jersey.

VI. COMMON EFFECTS OF CANCER

A. **Disruption of function**
1. Caused by obstruction or pressure
2. Can cause anoxia and necrosis of surrounding organs or tissues

B. **Hematologic alterations**
1. Excessive numbers of immature leukocytes may diminish erythrocyte and thrombocyte production in bone marrow
2. Gastrointestinal (GI) tumors may disrupt absorption of vitamin B$_{12}$ and iron
3. Growing tumors accumulate and store purines, depriving bone marrow of needed substances
4. Renal cell carcinomas produce excess erythropoietin, resulting in excess red blood cells and viscous blood that impairs circulation

C. **Infection**
1. Fistulas may develop between organs
2. Tumors may become necrotic and infected
3. Malignant involvement of organs and tissues of immune system can seriously impair immune response

D. Hemorrhage
1. Can be caused by tumor erosion through blood vessels
2. May cause life-threatening hypovolemic shock

E. Anorexia-cachexia syndrome
1. Neoplastic cells divert nutrition to their own use while causing changes that reduce client's appetite
2. Pain, infection, and depression may also contribute to anorexia
3. Widespread catabolism of body's tissue and muscle proteins results in cachexia
4. The normal reduction in metabolic rate seen with starvation does not occur, possibly due to cytokine production

F. Paraneoplastic syndromes
1. Endocrine: cancers set up ectopic sites of hormone production
2. Neurologic: cancers damage nervous system and may cause increased intracranial pressure
3. Can also see hematologic, nephrotic, and cutaneous syndromes

G. Pain
1. More than 60% of clients with cancer experience moderate to severe pain
2. Under-treatment can involve up to 40% of clients
3. Can include acute and chronic pain
4. Causes include direct tumor involvement, chemicals from ischemia or tumor metabolites and toxins, and side effects of treatments
5. It is important to give pain medication on a regular time schedule with additional medication for breakthrough pain
6. When opioid doses are increased gradually, there is no limit to amount that client can receive, as long as adverse reactions can be managed
7. High-dose opioid analgesics should not be stopped abruptly because withdrawal symptoms will appear

H. Physical stress
1. A neoplasm of 1 cm in size can overwhelm most immune systems
2. State of exhaustion often occurs with fatigue, weight loss, dehydration, and altered blood chemistries

I. Psychologic stress
1. May perceive diagnosis as a death sentence, may exhibit denial or intellectualization, or anxiety and stress
2. Possible guilt over past unhealthy behaviors or for delaying seeking treatment
3. Anger, fear, and powerlessness
4. Body image and sexual concerns
5. Use therapeutic communication and help clients become actively involved in managing their life and disease
6. Identify resources such as crisis hotlines and support groups
7. Build on past successful coping behaviors
8. Encourage to continue taking part in activities of life that client enjoys, including maintaining employment as long as possible
9. Answer questions about illness and prognosis honestly but always encourage hope

VII. COMMON CANCER TREATMENTS AND NURSING CARE

A. Surgery
1. Used for diagnosis and staging of 90% of all cancers
2. Is primary treatment for over 60% of cancers; goal is to remove entire tumor and involved surrounding tissue and lymph nodes; may result in loss of function
3. Removal of regional lymph nodes may result in long-term lymphedema (swelling in affected area)

      4. Prophylactic surgery can be done to remove tissues or organs likely to develop cancer

      5. Palliative surgery can be done to increase comfort; decreasing tumor size may also enhance effectiveness of other treatments

      6. Nursing responsibilities focus on preparing client and providing client teaching

B. Radiation therapy

      1. Is used to kill a tumor, reduce tumor size, relieve obstruction, or decrease pain

      2. Causes lethal injury to DNA, so it can destroy rapidly multiplying cancer cells as well as normal cells

      3. Can be classified as internal radiation therapy (brachytherapy) or external radiation therapy (teletherapy)

C. Client undergoing brachytherapy (internal radiation)

      1. Sources of internal radiation

          a. Implanted into affected tissue or body cavity

          b. Ingested as a solution

          c. Injected as a solution into bloodstream or body cavity

          d. Introduced through a catheter into tumor

      2. Side effects of internal radiation

          a. Fatigue

          b. Anorexia

          c. Immunosuppression

          d. Other side effects similar to external radiation (see section that follows)

      3. Priority nursing problems: interrupted tissue integrity, fatigue, anxiety, potential for infection, insufficient nutrients to meet bodily needs, reduced socialization

      4. Client education

          a. Avoid close contact with others until treatment is completed

          b. Maintain daily activities unless contraindicated, allowing for extra rest periods as needed

          c. Maintain balanced diet; may tolerate food better if consumes small, frequent meals

          d. Maintain fluid intake to ensure adequate hydration (2–3 liters/day)

          e. If implant is temporary, maintain bed rest to avoid dislodging implant; may require insertion of indwelling urinary catheter and low-residue diet to prevent straining if internal cervical radiation is being used in female clients

          f. Excreted body fluids may be radioactive; double-flush toilets after use

          g. Radiation therapy may lead to **bone marrow suppression** (refer to precautions for anemia, thrombocytopenia, and immunosuppression later in chapter)

      5. Nursing management of client receiving internal radiation

          a. Exposure to small amounts of radiation is possible during close contact with persons receiving internal radiation; understand the principles of protection from exposure to radiation: time, distance, and shielding

             1) Time: minimize time spent in close proximity to the radiation source; a common standard is to limit contact time to 30 minutes total per 8-hour shift

             2) Distance: maintain maximum distance possible from radiation source; minimum distance of 6 feet used when possible

             3) Shielding: use lead shields and other precautions to reduce exposure to radiation

          b. Place client in private room

          c. Instruct visitors to maintain at least a distance of 6 feet from client and limit visits to 10–30 minutes

          d. Ensure proper handling and disposal of body fluids, assuring containers are marked appropriately

          e. Ensure proper handling of bed linens and clothing

f. In the event of a dislodged implant, use long-handled forceps and place implant into a lead container; *never* directly touch implant

    g. Do not allow pregnant women to come into any contact with radiation sources; screen visitors and staff for pregnancy

    h. If working routinely near radiation sources, wear a monitoring device to measure exposure

    i. Educate client in all safety measures

6. Evaluation: client demonstrates measures to protect others from exposure to radiation, identifies interventions to reduce risk of infection, remains free from infection, achieves adequate fluid and nutritional intake, and participates in activities of daily living (ADLs) at level of ability

D. Client undergoing external radiation therapy (teletherapy)

1. Radiation oncologist marks specific locations for radiation treatment using a semipermanent type of ink or small permanent tattoos

    a. Treatment is usually given 15–30 minutes per day, 5 days per week, for 2–7 weeks

    b. Client does not pose a risk for radiation exposure to other people

2. Side effects of external radiation therapy

    a. Tissue damage to target area (erythema, sloughing, hemorrhage)

    b. Ulcerations of oral mucous membranes

    c. GI effects such as nausea, vomiting, and diarrhea

    d. Radiation pneumonia

    e. Fatigue

    f. **Alopecia** (hair loss)

    g. Immunosuppression

3. Priority nursing problems: potential for infection, interrupted skin integrity, alteration in body image, anxiety, fatigue, reduced socialization

4. Client education for external radiation

    a. Wash marked area of skin with plain water only and pat skin dry; do not use soaps, deodorants, lotions, perfumes, powders, or medications on site for duration of treatment; do not wash off treatment site marks

    b. Avoid rubbing, scratching, or scrubbing treatment site; do not apply extreme temperatures (heat or cold) to treatment site; if shaving, use only an electric razor

    c. Wear soft, loose-fitting clothing over treatment area

    d. Protect skin from sun exposure during and for at least 1 year after completion of treatment; when going outdoors, use sun-blocking agents with sun protection factor (SPF) of at least 15

    e. Maintain proper rest, diet, and fluid intake as essential to promoting health and repair of normal tissues

    f. Hair loss may occur; choose a wig, hat, or scarf to cover and protect head (refer to care of client with alopecia later in chapter)

5. Nursing management of client receiving external radiation

    a. Monitor for adverse side effects of radiation (see preceding section)

    b. Monitor for significant decreases in white blood cell counts and platelet counts

    c. Client teaching (refer to later sections for management of immunosuppression, thrombocytopenia, and anemia)

6. Evaluation: client identifies interventions to reduce risk of infection, remains free from infection, achieves adequate fluid and nutritional intake, participates in activities of daily living (ADLs) at level of ability, and maintains intact skin

E. Client undergoing chemotherapy

1. **Chemotherapy** involves administration of cytotoxic medications and chemicals to promote tumor cell death; intravenous (IV) route is most preferred for administering chemotherapeutic agents, but they may also be administered by oral, intrathecal, topical, intra-arterial, intracavity, and intravesical routes

Practice to Pass

A 38-year-old male client undergoing external radiation for cancer refuses to allow his 5-year-old son to come in close contact with him because he fears exposing the son to radiation. How should you respond to the client?

    a. Chemotherapy disrupts cell cycle in various phases, interfering with cellular metabolism and reproduction

    b. According to **cell-kill hypothesis**, during each cell cycle a fixed percentage of cells are killed by chemotherapy, leaving some tumor cells remaining; this necessitates repeated dosages of chemotherapy in order to reduce numbers of cells, allowing body's immune system to destroy any remaining tumor cells

2. Chemotherapeutic agents are classified according to their mechanism of action (see a pharmacology text for listing of specific chemotherapeutic drugs by category and common side effects); a combination of types is often used

    a. *Alkylating agents* are non-phase-specific and act by interfering with DNA replication; examples include cyclophosphamide (Cytoxan), busulfan (Myleran), and mechlorethamine (Mustargen)

    b. *Antimetabolites* interfere with metabolites or nucleic acids necessary for RNA and DNA synthesis; examples include fluorouracil (5-FU) and methotrexate (generic)

    c. *Cytotoxic (antitumor) antibiotics* disrupt or inhibit DNA or RNA synthesis; examples include bleomycin (Blenoxane) and doxorubicin (Adriamycin)

    d. *Hormones and hormone antagonists* are phase-specific (G1) and act by interfering with RNA synthesis; examples include diethylstilbestrol (DES) and tamoxifen (Nolvadex)

    e. *Plant alkaloids (mitotic inhibitors)*

        1) Vinca alkaloids are phase-specific, inhibiting cell division; examples are vinblastine (Velban) and vincristine (Oncovin)

        2) Etoposide (VePesid) acts during all cell-cycle phases, interfering with DNA and cell division at metaphase

    f. *Miscellaneous agents* may be cell-cycle phase-specific or non-phase-specific and interfere with DNA replication

3. Side effects of chemotherapeutic agents (see Figure 12-1)

    a. Bone marrow suppression (see Figure 12-2)

        1) Decreased WBC count (immunosuppression)

        2) Decreased platelet count (**thrombocytopenia**)

        3) Decreased hemoglobin and hematocrit (anemia)

    b. GI effects: anorexia, nausea, vomiting, and diarrhea

    c. **Stomatitis** (inflammation of the mouth) and mucositis

    d. Alopecia

    e. Fatigue

    f. **Xerostomia** (dry mouth)

    g. Other side effects specific to chemotherapeutic agent

4. Priority nursing problems: potential for infection, fatigue, potential for injury, insufficient nutrients to meet bodily needs, possible dehydration, alteration in body image, reduced socialization

5. Immunosuppression

    a. Client education for immunosuppression

        1) Risk for infection is high when WBC count is low, especially nadir (lowest point during chemotherapy)

        2) Avoid crowds, people with infections, and small children when WBC is low

        3) Use meticulous personal hygiene to avoid infection

        4) Wash hands before and after eating, after toileting, and after contact with other people and pets

        5) Consume a low-bacteria diet high in protein, minerals, and vitamins, especially vitamin C; avoid undercooked meat and raw fruits and vegetables

        6) Be aware of signs and symptoms of infection and report them immediately to health care provider

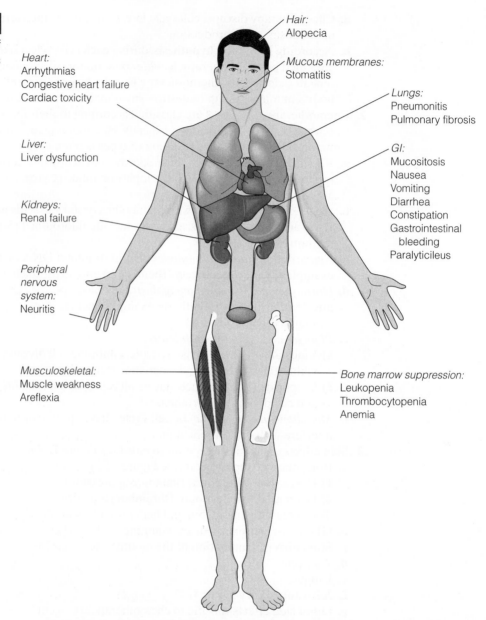

Figure 12-1

Multisystem effects of chemotherapeutic agents

Hair:
Alopecia

Heart:
Arrhythmias
Congestive heart failure
Cardiac toxicity

Mucous membranes:
Stomatitis

Lungs:
Pneumonitis
Pulmonary fibrosis

Liver:
Liver dysfunction

GI:
Mucositosis
Nausea
Vomiting
Diarrhea
Constipation
Gastrointestinal
  bleeding
Paralyticileus

Kidneys:
Renal failure

Peripheral nervous system:
Neuritis

Musculoskeletal:
Muscle weakness
Areflexia

Bone marrow suppression:
Leukopenia
Thrombocytopenia
Anemia

7) Consider dental cleaning prior to initiation of therapy that may cause immunosuppression

8) Protect skin and mucous membranes from injury to maintain first line of defense against infection

b. Nursing management of immunosuppression

1) Monitor laboratory values: CBC with differential, platelets, BUN, liver enzymes

2) Assess for infection; monitor vital signs for early indication of infection: fever, tachycardia, and tachypnea; if bone marrow suppression is present, any usual signs and symptoms of infection may be absent or reduced

3) WBC suppression, malnutrition, impaired skin integrity, tumor necrosis, and presence of disease increase risk for infection

4) Utilize neutropenic precautions (low-bacteria diet, no fresh plants or flowers in room, no pets, no visitors with infections, reverse or protective isolation) when WBC level falls below predetermined level (such as 2,000 mm^3)

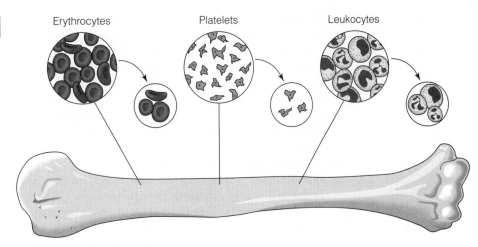

Figure 12-2

Blood cells affected by bone marrow suppression

Erythrocytes   Platelets   Leukocytes

     c. Evaluation of care for immunosuppression: client demonstrates techniques to reduce risk of infection, participates in activities that reduce risk of infection, and remains free from infection

6. Thrombocytopenia

    a. Client education for thrombocytopenia

      1) Monitor stools and urine for bleeding

      2) For shaving, use electric razor only

      3) Avoid contact sports and other activities that may cause trauma

      4) If trauma does occur, apply ice to area and seek medical assistance

      5) Avoid dental work or other invasive procedures

      6) Inform all health care providers of chemotherapy and/or radiation treatments

      7) Avoid aspirin and aspirin-containing products

      8) Safety precautions for oral hygiene: use soft toothbrushes and do not floss

    b. Nursing management of thrombocytopenia

      1) There is a high risk for spontaneous hemorrhage when platelet count is less than 20,000; bleeding precautions are necessary for platelet count less than 50,000

      2) Assess for bleeding, monitor stools and urine for occult blood

      3) Assess skin for ecchymoses, petechiae, and trauma

      4) Educate client about bleeding safety precautions, including instructions to avoid forcefully blowing nose or removing crusts from nose, straining to have a bowel movement, and forceful coughing or sneezing, as these activities increase risk of external and internal bleeding

      5) Avoid intramuscular injections and other invasive procedures; limit venipunctures

      6) Apply pressure to puncture sites for 3–5 minutes; apply pressure to arterial blood gas sites for 15–20 minutes

    c. Evaluation of care for thrombocytopenia: client demonstrates understanding of risks for hemorrhage, participates in activities that reduce risk of hemorrhage, and remains free from complications of bleeding

7. Stomatitis and mucositis

    a. Client education for stomatitis and mucositis

      1) Use a soft toothbrush; mouth swabs may be needed during acute episode; if gums are friable and bleeding, clean teeth with a soft cloth or toothpaste over finger

      2) Avoid mouthwashes containing alcohol; do not use lemon glycerin swabs; if thrombocytopenia is present do not use dental floss

      3) Consider using chlorhexidine mouthwash (Peridex) to decrease risk of hemorrhage and protect gums from trauma

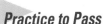

Practice to Pass

You are admitting a client to your hospital unit who is currently receiving chemotherapy for cancer at the outpatient oncology clinic. The client has a decreased platelet count and a decreased leukocyte count. What nursing interventions will you perform for this client?

      4) Assess daily for lesions, infection, bleeding, or irritation

      5) For xerostomia, apply lubricating and moisturizing agents to protect mucous membranes from trauma and infection

      6) May consider using "artificial saliva" and moisturizing agents to help with dryness

      7) Avoid smoking and alcohol, which can further irritate oral mucosa

      8) Teach signs and symptoms of oral infection and to report to health care provider

      9) Drink cool liquids, and avoid hot and irritating foods

      10) Avoid putting sharp instruments in the mouth; use smooth plastic spoons and forks for eating, especially if thrombocytopenia is also present

    b. Nursing management of stomatitis

      1) Assess oral mucous membranes every 4 hours

      2) Teach and implement proper oral care (see client teaching above)

      3) Administer antivirals, antibiotics, antifungals, or numbing agents such as viscous xylocaine as prescribed

    c. Evaluation of care for stomatitis: client participates in techniques to maintain integrity of oral mucosa; oral mucosa remains intact and free from ulcerations and inflammation

  8. Inadequate nutrition and fluid and electrolyte imbalance

    a. Client education for maintaining adequate nutrition, fluid and electrolyte balance

      1) Eat frequent small, low-fat meals

      2) Avoid spicy and fatty foods

      3) Avoid extremely hot foods

      4) Perform oral hygiene before and after meals

      5) Maintain fluid intake as prescribed

      6) Take nutritional supplements as prescribed (vitamins, liquid nutrition)

      7) Maintain a daily journal of food and fluid intake

    b. Nursing management of inadequate nutrition and fluid and electrolyte imbalances

      1) Assess for adequate hydration; for duration of treatment, encourage daily fluid intake of 2–3 liters unless contraindicated

      2) Administer antiemetics *prior* to chemotherapy; around-the-clock prophylaxis may be necessary

      3) Weigh client routinely, monitor for weight loss

      4) Monitor lab values indicative of nutritional status (hemoglobin, hematocrit, albumin, prealbumin)

      5) Monitor for diarrhea or constipation and nausea or vomiting

      6) Encourage adequate nutritional intake with meals that are served attractively, and environment free of noxious stimuli (bedpan, urinal, odors)

      7) Provide nutritional supplements and small frequent meals; increase calories by adding ice cream or frozen yogurt to liquid supplements

      8) Cold and bland semisoft or liquid foods are less irritating to mucosa

      9) Dry, low-fat foods are more readily tolerated when nauseated

    c. Evaluation of nutrition, fluid and electrolyte balance: client participates in activities that maintain nutritional balance, exhibits stable weight, normal lab values, and shows no signs and symptoms of malnutrition

  9. Fatigue

    a. Nursing management of fatigue

      1) Assure client that fatigue is a normal response to chemotherapy and that it does not indicate progression of disease

      2) Encourage client to continue daily activities as much as possible, allowing for rest periods in between

      3) Assist client in self-care needs when indicated

      4) Allow for periods of rest; cluster activities

    b. Evaluation of care for fatigue: client performs self-care, participates in activities at level of ability, and demonstrates techniques to conserve energy

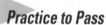

Practice to Pass

A client has lost 7 pounds since beginning chemotherapy. An assessment reveals ulcerations in the mouth, and the client states she experiences severe nausea and occasional diarrhea at home. She eats very little because of the pain, nausea, and diarrhea. What actions will you take?

10. Alopecia (hair loss)
    a. Nursing management of client experiencing alopecia

   1) Chemotherapy and radiation therapy may cause hair loss; alopecia is temporary and hair will grow back, usually beginning about a month after completion of chemotherapy; client should know that texture and color of new hair growth may be different; hair loss during radiation therapy to head may be permanent
   2) Encourage client to choose a wig *before* hair loss occurs in order to match texture and hair color
   3) Care of hair and scalp includes washing hair 2–3 times a week with a mild shampoo; pat hair dry, and do not use a blow dryer or hair dyes
   4) Allow client to express feelings concerning altered body image
   5) Refer to support programs to help diminish feelings of isolation and obtain practical tips for managing problems
   6) Encourage wearing attractive head coverings to both protect head and allow client to feel stylish and well dressed

   b. Evaluation of care for alopecia: client demonstrates understanding and adaptation to body changes and participates in self-care activities

11. Nursing implications for administration of chemotherapy

Practice to Pass

You are administering a chemotherapeutic agent intravenously. The client begins to complain of severe pain at the infusion site. What interventions do you perform?

   a. Access to veins may be obtained by subclavian cathethers, implanted ports, or peripherally inserted catheters; vascular access devices that are peripherally inserted into a large vein or centrally inserted into a major vein, such as subclavian vein, have a lower risk of extravasation or irritation to vein
   b. **Extravasation**, a leaking of chemotherapeutic agents into surrounding tissue, is a major complication of IV chemotherapy; extreme care must be used when administering **vesicant** agents (chemicals causing damage to tissue on contact)
   c. Physicians and nurses should be specially trained to handle and administer chemotherapeutic agents
   d. Vein patency must be assured before administering chemotherapeutic agents
   e. Warning: never test vein patency with chemotherapeutic agents

   f. If extravasation occurs, depending on chemotherapeutic agent, interventions may include injection of an antidote, or application of a cold or warm compress
   g. Assess respiratory and cardiac status; monitor EKG, assess for heart failure, and monitor vital signs
   h. Monitor client closely for anaphylactic reactions or serious side effects; discontinue infusion according to protocol if reactions occur

   i. Monitor IV site closely during administration; observe for pain and other symptoms of infiltration
   j. Provide a calm, quiet environment for client during administration
   k. Chemotherapy agents have potentially carcinogenic effects; wear gloves, a mask, and gown while preparing and administering chemotherapy drugs and disposing of equipment; use care when handling excretory products and teach clients to dispose of their own body fluids safely

F. **Client undergoing a bone marrow transplant (BMT)**
   1. BMT is used primarily in treatment of leukemias, usually in conjunction with radiation or chemotherapy, to stimulate a nonfunctioning marrow or to replace marrow
      a. *Autologous BMT*: client is infused with own bone marrow harvested during remission of disease
      b. *Allogenic BMT*: client is infused with donor bone marrow harvested from a healthy individual
   2. The bone marrow is usually harvested from iliac crests, then frozen and stored until transfusion
   3. Peripheral blood stem cell transplants are an alternative to bone transplants; preparation and risks are similar to those for BMT

4. Before receiving BMT, client must first undergo a phase of immunosuppressive therapy to destroy immune system; infection, bleeding, and death are major complications that can occur during this conditioning phase

5. After immunosuppression, bone marrow or stem cells are transfused by IV route through a central line

6. Side effects of bone marrow transplant
   a. Malnutrition
   b. Infection related to immunosuppression
   c. Bleeding related to thrombocytopenia

7. Priority nursing problems: potential for infection or bleeding, possible insufficient nutrients to meet bodily needs, reduced socialization, anxiety

8. Client education: refer to previous sections on client education for imbalanced nutrition, immunosuppression, and thrombocytopenia

9. Nursing management of client undergoing a bone marrow transplant (BMT)
   a. Monitor for graft-versus-host disease (see immunologic chapter)
   b. Provide private room for client, who will be hospitalized for 6–8 weeks
   c. Encourage contact with significant others by using telephone, computer, and other means of communication to reduce feelings of isolation
   d. Refer to nursing management sections for imbalanced nutrition, immunosuppression, and thrombocytopenia

10. Evaluation: client demonstrates understanding of risks and participates in activities that reduce risk of infection, hemorrhage, and malnutrition; client demonstrates effective coping mechanisms

G. Client undergoing other therapeutic interventions

1. Immunotherapy: biologic response modifiers (BMR)
   a. Enhances person's own immune responses in order to modify biologic processes that result in malignant cells
   b. Used for hematologic malignancies and solid tumors
   c. *Monoclonal antibodies*: antibodies are recovered from an inoculated animal with a specific tumor antigen, and then given to client who has that particular type of cancer; goal is destruction of tumor
   d. *Cytokines*: normal growth-regulating molecules possessing antitumor abilities
      1) Interleukin-2 (IL-2) increases immune response effectiveness and destroys abnormal cells
      2) Interferons are substances produced by cells to protect them from viral infection and replication; interferon-alpha 2b is most commonly used
      3) *Hematopoietic growth factors*, such as granulocyte colony-stimulating factor (G-CSF) and erythropoietin, work to counteract suppression of granulocytes and erythrocytes resulting from chemotherapy
   e. *Natural killer cells* (NK cells): exert a spontaneous cytotoxic effect on specific cancer cells; they also secrete cytokines and provide a resistance to metastasis
   f. Biotherapies have significant side effects and toxicities; monitor for mental slowing, severe flulike symptoms, acute hypertension, and acute alterations in renal, cardiac, liver, or GI function
   g. Combining biotherapy with chemotherapy shows increased tumor destructive activity and treatment responses

2. Photodynamic therapy (PDT)
   a. Used to treat specific superficial tumors such as those of bladder surface, bronchus, chest wall, head, neck, and peritoneal cavity
   b. Photofrin, a photosensitizing compound, is administered IV, where it is retained by malignant tissue
   c. Three days after injection, drug is activated by a laser treatment, which continues for 3 more days

      d. The drug produces a cytotoxic oxygen molecule (singlet oxygen)

      e. During IV administration, monitor for chills, nausea, rash, local skin reactions, and temporary photosensitivity

      f. Drug remains in tissues 4–6 weeks after injection; direct or indirect exposure to sun activates drug, resulting in chemical sunburn; educate client to protect skin from sun exposure

  3. Complementary therapies

      a. Are therapies that clients choose to complement medical treatment

      b. Include botanical agents, nutritional supplements, dietary regimens, mind–body modalities, energy healing, spiritual approaches, and miscellaneous therapies

      c. Provide truthful, nonjudgmental responses to questions or inquiries

      d. Encourage clients to report use to their oncologists to prevent interactions with ongoing medical treatments

VIII. ONCOLOGIC EMERGENCIES: DIAGNOSIS AND MANAGEMENT

A. Type of emergency may vary and only most common types are discussed here; in all cases, immediate notification of health care provider or emergency team is the first step

B. Spinal cord compression

  1. Occurs secondary to pressure from expanding tumors

  2. Early symptoms include back and leg pain, coldness, numbness, tingling, paresthesias; progression leads to bowel and bladder dysfunction, weakness, and paralysis

  3. Early detection is essential: investigate all reports of back pain or neurological changes

  4. Treatment is aimed at reducing tumor size by radiation and/or surgery to relieve compression and prevent irreversible paraplegia; may receive corticosteroids to reduce cord edema

  5. Nursing interventions include early recognition of symptoms, monitoring vital signs, neurological checks, and medication administration

C. Superior vena cava syndrome

  1. Compression or obstruction of superior vena cava (SVC)

  2. Usually associated with cancer of lungs and lymphomas but may also result from thrombus that develops around a central venous catheter

  3. Signs and symptoms are result from blockage of venous circulation of head, neck, and upper trunk

  4. Early signs and symptoms are periorbital edema, facial edema, and jugular vein distention

  5. Symptoms progress to edema of neck, arms, and hands; difficulty swallowing; shortness of breath

  6. Late signs and symptoms are cyanosis, altered mental status, headache, and hypotension

  7. Death may occur if compression is not relieved

  8. Treatment includes high-dose radiation or chemotherapy to shrink tumor and relieve symptoms

  9. Nursing interventions include monitoring vital signs, providing oxygen support, preparing for tracheostomy if necessary, initiating seizure precautions, administering corticosteroids to reduce edema and administering antifibrinolytics if disorder is due to a clot

D. Disseminated intravascular coagulopathy (DIC)

  1. Severe disorder of coagulation, often triggered by sepsis, whereby abnormal clot formation occurs in microvasculature; this process depletes clotting factors and platelets, allowing extensive bleeding to occur; tissue hypoxia occurs from blockage of blood vessels by clots

  2. Signs and symptoms are related to decreased blood flow to major organs (tachycardia, oliguria, dyspnea) and depleted clotting factors (abnormal bleeding and hemorrhage)

  3. Treatment includes anticoagulants to decrease stimulation of coagulation and transfusion of one or more of the following: fresh frozen plasma (FFP), cryoprecipitate, platelets, and packed red blood cells (RBCs)

> **!** ▷

4. Nursing interventions include assessing client, monitoring for bleeding, applying pressure dressings to venipuncture sites, and preventing risk of sepsis

E. Pericardial effusions and cardiac tamponade

1. Pericardial effusion (accumulation of excess fluid in pericardial sac) secondary to metastases or esophageal cancer can lead to compression of heart, restricting heart movement, and resulting in cardiac tamponade
2. Signs and symptoms are related to compression of heart with decreased cardiac output and impaired cardiac function that causes cardiogenic shock or circulatory collapse: anxiety, cyanosis, dyspnea, hypotension, tachycardia, tachypnea, impaired level of consciousness, and increased central venous pressure
3. Pericardiocentesis is performed to remove fluid from pericardial sac
4. Nursing interventions include administering oxygen, maintaining IV line, monitoring vital signs, hemodynamic monitoring, and the administration of vasopressor agents

F. Sepsis and septic shock

1. May result from tumor necrosis, immune deficiency, antineoplastic therapy, malnutrition, and comorbid conditions
2. Gram-negative sepsis progresses to systemic shock and multisystem failure
3. Initial phase is characterized by vasodilation with vascular dehydration, high fever, peripheral edema, hypotension, tachycardia, tachypnea, hot flushed skin with creeping mottling that begins in lower extremities, and anxiety or restlessness
4. Shock progresses to classic signs of hypotension, rapid thread pulse, respiratory distress, cyanosis, subnormal temperature, cold clammy skin, decreased urinary output, and altered mentation
5. Nursing interventions include early recognition and notification of health care provider, oxygen therapy, fluid resuscitation, and administration of vasoactive and inotropic drugs

G. Metabolic emergencies

1. Hypercalcemia results from excessive ectopic production of parathyroid hormone and bone metastasis; symptoms include fatigue, anorexia, and nausea and may progress to include neurological manifestations, cardiac arrhythmias, coma and death
2. Hyperuricemia may result from rapid necrosis of tumor cells after vigorous chemotherapy or from increased uric acid production; uric acid deposits cause renal failure and uremia with nausea, vomiting, lethargy, and oliguria
3. Tumor lysis syndrome is a combination of 2 or more metabolic abnormalities, including hyperuricemia, hyperphosphatemia, hyperkalemia, and/or hypocalcemia
   a. It results from massive and rapid destruction of cancer cells
   b. Manifestations include nausea, vomiting, lethargy, edema, fluid overload, congestive heart failure, cardiac dysrhythmias, seizures, muscle cramps, tetany, syncope, and possible sudden death
   c. Prevention and management includes administration of allopurinol, oral phosphate binders and sodium polystyrene sulfonate (Kayexelate) along with hydration and possible hemodialysis

Practice to Pass

A client with metastatic prostate cancer informs you that he has been experiencing back pain for 3 days and his legs are numb. What assessments should you make and what actions will you take?

IX. EXPECTED OUTCOMES FOR CLIENTS WITH CELLULAR DISORDERS

A. **The 5-year survival rate for all cancers** diagnosed between 2001 and 2007 is 67%, up from 49% in the 1970s; this rate decreases for African Americans and other underserved Americans (American Cancer Society (2012). Cancer facts & figures 2012. Atlanta, Ga: American Cancer Society.)

B. **Over 1.6 million new cancer cases** are expected to be diagnosed in 2012 (American Cancer Society (2012). Cancer facts & figures 2012. Atlanta, Ga: American Cancer Society.)

C. **Approximately 577,190 cancer-related deaths** are expected to occur in 2012; cancer is the second most common cause of death in the US, accounting for nearly 1 of every 4 deaths (American Cancer Society (2012). Cancer facts & figures 2012. Atlanta, Ga: American Cancer Society.)

D. **Lung cancer remains the leading cause of all cancer deaths** in both men and women

Case Study

C. J., a 68-year-old female client on your nursing unit, has recently been diagnosed with cancer of the left breast. This is the first time you have been assigned to the care of this client.

1. You enter C. J.'s room and find her crying. She states, "I can't believe I have cancer." What actions would you take?

2. C. J. asks you what treatments and procedures she will most likely experience. How do you respond to her?

3. Before beginning IV chemotherapy, what information and instructions will you give to C. J.?

4. C. J. reports experiencing severe nausea and vomiting during chemotherapy. What measures can be taken to lessen the severity or control the nausea and vomiting?

5. C. J. expresses concern over the expected alopecia (hair loss) from the chemotherapy. How do you respond to her?

For suggested responses, see pages 624–625.

POSTTEST

1 A client undergoing radiation therapy has a severely depressed white blood cell (WBC) count. The nurse should include which priority nursing intervention in the plan of care?

1. Place client in a private room and maintain strict aseptic technique with all procedures.
2. Encourage client to include fresh fruits and vegetables in the diet.
3. Educate client to avoid shaving with a razor.
4. Encourage frequent visitors to reduce client's feelings of isolation.

2 The nurse is performing an assessment in a local clinic. Based on the history provided by the clients, which client requires an immediate referral for screening and evaluation?

1. Client who reports unintended weight loss of 25 pounds over the past 3 months
2. Client who smokes 2 packages of cigarettes a day
3. Client who reports history of long-term sun exposure
4. Client who consumes diet high in fats and low in fiber

3 The nurse is caring for a client receiving chemotherapy prior to a bone marrow transplant. The client is placed on neutropenic precautions. Which interventions are appropriate for this client? Select all that apply.

1. Restrict young children from visiting.
2. Provide fresh fruit and vegetables with each meal.
3. Transfer client to negative pressure room.
4. Limit visitors to healthy adults.
5. Ensure mask worn by caregivers and visitors.

4 The nurse is making a home visit to a client receiving external radiation therapy on an outpatient basis. Further teaching is necessary when the nurse observes the client doing which of the following?

1. Washing radiation site with plain water and patting skin dry
2. Protecting skin with soft, loose clothing
3. Applying lotion to irritated skin
4. Inspecting skin for damage

5 A hospitalized client with an internal radiation implant calls the nurse to the room to report the implant is dislodged and is lying in the bed. The nurse's actions would include which of the following?

1. Apply gloves and place implant in a biohazard bag.
2. Use long-handled forceps to pick up implant and place it into lead container.
3. Have client pick up the implant and place it into lead container.
4. Notify infection control personnel to dispose of implant.

6 A client with leukemia is undergoing total body irradiation for a bone marrow transplant (BMT). The priority nursing diagnosis for this client is which of the following?

1. Fatigue related to anemia
2. Imbalanced Nutrition: Less than Body Requirements
3. Interrupted Mucous Membranes
4. Risk for Infection

7 The nurse has been asked to do a community presentation on factors that increase the risk for development of cancer. Which factors should be included? Select all that apply.

1. Accumulated stress
2. Human papilloma virus
3. Diets high in whole-grain cereals, raw vegetables and raw fruits
4. Use of estrogen-containing contraceptive pills
5. Autoimmune disorders such as lupus

8 A client who had a mastectomy yesterday refuses to look at the incision. The nurse can best assist the client to cope with a Disturbed Body Image by doing which of the following?

1. Tell client that eventually everyone accepts the loss of a body part.
2. Encourage client to express feelings about loss of body part.
3. Delay wound care until client is prepared to look at wound.
4. Have client assist with the dressing change.

9 In assessing a client receiving chemotherapy, which finding should the nurse recognize as the priority for further evaluation?

1. Dry mucous membranes
2. Large areas of ecchymosis in various sites on body
3. Complaints of fatigue
4. Hair loss on scalp

10 The nurse is evaluating the nutritional status of a client who is receiving chemotherapy as treatment for cancer. On assessment, which finding could potentially affect the client's nutritional intake?

1. Pale and moist mucous membranes
2. Pale skin
3. Ecchymotic areas on forearms
4. Ulcerations of oral mucosa

➤ *See pages 404–406 for Answers and Rationales.*

ANSWERS & RATIONALES

Pretest

1 **Answer: 2** **Rationale:** The incidence of cancer increases with age, making it a significant factor in the development of cancer. Screening is important for early identification because once symptoms develop the disease may have spread. Screening for specific cancers should occur across the life span. **Cognitive Level:** Applying **Client Need:** Health Promotion and Maintenance **Integrated Process:** Nursing Process: Implementation **Content Area:** Adult Health **Strategy:** To answer this question correctly, recall how cancer cells are produced and essential information that is part of theories of aging. Integrating information from these areas enables you to select the correct response. **Reference:** LeMone, P., Burke, K., & Bauldoff, G. (2011). *Medical-surgical nursing: Critical thinking in patient care* (5th ed.). Upper Saddle River, NJ: Pearson Education, pp. 342–343.

2 **Answer: 1, 2, 5, 4, 3** **Rationale:** A successful plan depends upon an accurate assessment of the client's pain as the first step. Noting the client's goals for therapy should be done second to include the client in the plan. Non-opioid analgesics combined with adjuvants relieve many forms of pain, and this would be done third in the treatment of this client. If the client does not get adequate relief other medications should be tried, making evaluation the fourth step. If non-narcotic pain medication does not provide adequate relief the client should be advanced to stronger medications, including narcotics, so this step would occur last. **Cognitive Level:** Applying **Client Need:** Pharmacological and Parenteral Therapies **Integrated Process:** Caring **Content Area:** Pharmacology **Strategy:** Consider the steps of the nursing process, beginning with assessment, and initiate treatment at the lowest level needed to achieve the intended results and progress as needed from there. **Reference:** LeMone, P., Burke, K., & Bauldoff, G. (2011). *Medical-surgical nursing: Critical thinking in patient care* (5th ed.). Upper Saddle River, NJ: Pearson Education, pp. 368–369.

3 **Answer: 3** **Rationale:** Administering antiemetics before chemotherapy helps reduce the severity of nausea. Waiting until the client is experiencing nausea demonstrates lack of planning. Cool foods and liquids are better tolerated and less irritating than warm foods and liquids. Small, frequent meals are more easily tolerated and may reduce the incidence of nausea and vomiting. **Cognitive Level:** Applying **Client Need:** Reduction of Risk Potential **Integrated Process:** Nursing Process: Implementation **Content Area:** Adult Health **Strategy:** The ideal is to prevent a complication rather than wait until it develops. Review the several types of nausea that commonly occur with chemotherapy and their management if this question was difficult. **Reference:** LeMone, P., Burke, K., &

Bauldoff, G. (2011). *Medical-surgical nursing: Critical thinking in patient care* (5th ed.). Upper Saddle River, NJ: Pearson Education, pp. 374–375.

4 **Answer: 2** **Rationale:** Internal radiation is emitted outward to people in close contact as long as the implant is in place. Therefore, the client is a risk to others as long as the radiation implant is present. Therefore, certain precautions to protect others must be taken. The client should have a private room, and visitors should maintain a distance of 6 feet and limit visits to 10 to 30 minutes. The client may not need isolation for the entire period of hospitalization; rather, just for the time the implant is in place. **Cognitive Level:** Applying **Client Need:** Reduction of Risk Potential **Integrated Process:** Nursing Process: Implementation **Content Area:** Adult Health **Strategy:** Differentiate beam radiation from internal radiation. The principle is that anyone exposed to radiation is at risk of being radiated. **Reference:** LeMone, P., Burke, K., & Bauldoff, G. (2011). *Medical-surgical nursing: Critical thinking in patient care* (5th ed.). Upper Saddle River, NJ: Pearson Education, pp. 364–366.

5 **Answer: 1** **Rationale:** Alopecia is hair loss. Washing the hair daily will promote further hair loss, and should be limited to 2 to 3 times per week. Protecting the hair from damage, choosing a wig before loss of hair and identifying that hair will grow back are correct actions taken by the client and do not indicate the need for further instruction. **Cognitive Level:** Applying **Client Need:** Reduction of Risk Potential **Integrated Process:** Nursing Process: Evaluation **Content Area:** Adult Health **Strategy:** Because of the critical words *further instructions*, the question is asking which answer option is a false statement. For this reason, eliminate true statements and then choose the answer option that causes the most mechanical disruption to the follicles. **Reference:** LeMone, P., Burke, K., & Bauldoff, G. (2011). *Medical-surgical nursing: Critical thinking in patient care* (5th ed.). Upper Saddle River, NJ: Pearson Education, pp. 372–373.

6 **Answer: 3** **Rationale:** The client with a low WBC count (normal 5,000–10,000/mm³) is at high risk for infection. The grandchild recently exposed to varicella could be contagious at this point. The nephew with HIV, unless currently infected with another communicable disease, does not pose a risk. There is no indication that the husband has tuberculosis. The pregnant daughter does not pose a risk. **Cognitive Level:** Analyzing **Client Need:** Physiological Adaptation **Integrated Process:** Nursing Process: Implementation **Content Area:** Adult Health **Strategy:** To answer the question, identify the function of WBCs. Then determine the risk and mode of transmission for each answer option. **Reference:** LeMone, P., Burke, K., & Bauldoff, G. (2011). *Medical-surgical* *nursing: Critical thinking in patient care* (5th ed.). Upper Saddle River, NJ: Pearson Education, pp. 373–374.

7 **Answer: 1** **Rationale:** The American Cancer Society recommends a breast examination by a health care provider every 3 years for ages 20 to 39, then yearly from age 40 and older. Breast self-examinations should be performed monthly. Mammograms are recommended yearly beginning at age 40. **Cognitive Level:** Analyzing **Client Need:** Health Promotion and Mainte-nance **Integrated Process:** Nursing Process: Evaluation **Content Area:** Adult Health **Strategy:** Review the screening recommendations for the various cancers to answer this question. **Reference:** LeMone, P., Burke, K., & Bauldoff, G. (2011). *Medical-surgical nursing: Critical thinking in patient care* (5th ed.). Upper Saddle River, NJ: Pearson Education, p. 370.

8 **Answer: 2** **Rationale:** Extravasation of the chemothera-peutic agent, especially if the agent is a vesicant, is a major complication of intravenous administration of chemotherapy. Make sure the catheter is still in the vein and has not infiltrated. Never test the patency of the catheter with the medication, use saline. Making the client comfortable is important, but not a priority. There is no indication to administer acetaminophen. **Cognitive Level:** Applying **Client Need:** Pharmacological and Parenteral Therapies **Integrated Process:** Nursing Process: Planning **Content Area:** Fundamentals **Strategy:** This ques-tion specifically deals with the management of central lines. The critical words in the question are *before beginning the administration*. Recall the specific risks of chemotherapy to the tissues and the need to verify catheter placement to help you to select the most appropriate response. **Reference:** LeMone, P., Burke, K., & Bauldoff, G. (2011). *Medical-surgical nursing: Critical thinking in patient care* (5th ed.). Upper Saddle River, NJ: Pearson Education, pp. 362–364.

9 **Answer: 1** **Rationale:** The client with a low platelet count (thrombocytopenia) is at risk for bleeding. Aspirin further interferes with platelet functioning. Monitoring for fever is necessary for a client with low WBC count, and managing fatigue is necessary for a client with anemia. Flossing is contraindicated in the client with low platelet count. **Cognitive Level:** Analyzing **Client Need:** Reduction of Risk Potential **Integrated Process:** Nursing Process: Evaluation **Content Area:** Adult Health **Strategy:** Knowing the function of platelets is the first step in being able to answer this question. Consider by the client's situation that the platelet count is low and that the client is at risk for bleeding. Eliminate all options that are unrelated to this concept, and choose correctly by recalling the side effects of aspirin. **Reference:** LeMone, P., Burke, K., & Bauldoff, G. (2011). *Medical-surgical nursing: Critical thinking in patient care* (5th ed.). Upper Saddle River, NJ: Pearson Education, pp. 361, 373–375.

10 **Answer: 2, 4** **Rationale:** Thrombocytopenia increases the risk for bleeding because of a low platelet count. These clients should not have rectal temperatures or

intramuscular injections because of the risk for bleeding. Use of a negative pressure room is indicated for an airborne infection. Masks will not protect against bleeding but would be useful as part of neutropenic precautions. Mouth care is important to prevent growth of bacteria in the mouth and a soft toothbrush can be used, although a firm-bristled brush should not. **Cognitive Level:** Applying **Client Need:** Safety and Infection Control **Integrated Process:** Nursing Process: Implementation **Content Area:** Adult Health **Strategy:** The core issue of the question is the ability to recognize the risk of bleeding and appropriately select measures to reduce this risk. Use the process of elimination and nursing knowledge to select answer options that would decrease this risk, being careful not to choose incorrect items because of the negative wording (avoid) in some of the items. **Reference:** LeMone, P., Burke, K., & Bauldoff, G. (2011). *Medical-surgical nursing: Critical thinking in patient care* (5th ed.). Upper Saddle River, NJ: Pearson Education, pp. 375–376.

Posttest

1 **Answer: 1** **Rationale:** The immunosuppressed client is at high risk for infection. A private room, maintaining aseptic technique, and limiting visitors will reduce exposure and risk. Fresh fruits and vegetables may harbor bacteria; serve cooked foods only. The client with a decreased platelet count should be counseled to avoid using razors. **Cognitive Level:** Applying **Client Need:** Safety and Infection Control **Integrated Process:** Nursing Process: Implementation **Content Area:** Adult Health **Strategy:** Select the option that directly reflects the purpose of the WBC and the implications for their loss during radiation. **Reference:** LeMone, P., Burke, K., & Bauldoff, G. (2011). *Medical-surgical nursing: Critical thinking in patient care* (5th ed.). Upper Saddle River, NJ: Pearson Education, pp. 373–374.

2 **Answer: 1** **Rationale:** Cancer cells rapidly divide and grow, thus consuming most of the nutrients ingested. There-fore, an unexplained, rapid weight loss may be the first symptom associated with cancer, and immediate evalua-tion is required. Education regarding health promotion is needed for cigarette smoking, sun exposure, and a high-fat, low-fiber diet. **Cognitive Level:** Analyzing **Client Need:** Health Promotion and Maintenance **Integrated Process:** Nursing Process: Diagnosis **Content Area:** Adult Health **Strategy:** Eliminate answer options that are risk factors. Select the answer option that is an abnormal finding. **Reference:** LeMone, P., Burke, K., & Bauldoff, G. (2011). *Medical-surgical nursing: Critical thinking in patient care* (5th ed.). Upper Saddle River, NJ: Pearson Education, pp. 351–352.

3 **Answer: 1, 4, 5** **Rationale:** Neutropenic precautions are indicated for clients who are immunosuppressed with a low WBC. The goal is to protect them from potential sources of infection until the bone marrow is able to produce sufficient WBC. Visitors should be limited to healthy adults. The client should avoid fresh fruits and vegetables to reduce contact with microbes that could be pathological during an immunosuppressed state. For the same reason, masks should be worn by caregivers and visitors. A negative pressure room is unnecessary. **Cognitive Level:** Applying **Client Need:** Safety and Infection Control **Integrated Process:** Nursing Process: Implementation **Content Area:** Adult Health **Strategy:** Select answer options that would decrease the risk of client contamination when the white blood cell count is severely reduced. **Reference:** Dorman-Wagner, K., Johnson, K., & Hardin-Pierce, M. (2010). *High acuity nursing* (5th ed.). Upper Saddle River, NJ: Prentice Hall, p. 177.

4 Answer: 3 Rationale: Lotion, deodorant, and powders should not be applied to the radiation site during the treatment period to avoid further irritation to the skin. The other options are correct actions and do not indicate a need for further teaching. **Cognitive Level:** Applying **Client Need:** Physiological Adaptation **Integrated Process:** Nursing Process: Assessment **Content Area:** Adult Health **Strategy:** This question is asking for identification of the action that incorrect. Identify the answer option that the client should not do. **Reference:** LeMone, P., Burke, K., & Bauldoff, G. (2011). *Medical-surgical nursing: Critical thinking in patient care* (5th ed.). Upper Saddle River, NJ: Pearson Education, p. 366.

5 Answer: 2 Rationale: Direct handling of the implant causes exposure to radiation and no one should directly touch the implant. Gloves and biohazard bags do not offer protection from radiation. Long-handled forceps should be used to pick up the implant. Lead containers are necessary to prevent exposure to radiation. Infection control personnel have no role in the disposal of the implant, which should be returned to the radiation therapy department after properly being placed in the lead container. **Cognitive Level:** Applying **Client Need:** Safety and Infection Control **Integrated Process:** Nursing Process: Implementation **Content Area:** Adult Health **Strategy:** Radioactive implants pose a hazard to anyone in direct contact. Select the answer option that minimizes exposure to others. **Reference:** LeMone, P., Burke, K., & Bauldoff, G. (2011). *Medical-surgical nursing: Critical thinking in patient care* (5th ed.). Upper Saddle River, NJ: Pearson Education, p. 365.

6 Answer: 4 Rationale: During the conditioning phase additional chemotherapy and total body irradiation is given to eradicate the leukemic cells from the bone marrow. The bone marrow is depressed and without transplantation, the client will die from an infection. Anemia, Impaired Skin Integrity, and Imbalanced Nutrition: Less than Body Requirements may be appropriate diagnoses for clients receiving chemotherapy and radiation, but the risk for infection is the highest priority during this phase. **Cognitive Level:** Analyzing **Client Need:** Physiological Adaptation **Integrated Process:** Nursing Process: Planning **Content Area:** Adult Health **Strategy:** The critical word in the stem is *priority*. This tells you that more than one

option could apply to the client, but that one is more important than the others. Although all cells produced by the bone marrow are suppressed, select the answer option that poses the greatest immediate risk. **Reference:** LeMone, P., Burke, K., & Bauldoff, G. (2011). *Medical-surgical nursing: Critical thinking in patient care* (5th ed.). Upper Saddle River, NJ: Pearson Education, pp. 367, 1089–1093.

7 Answer: 1, 2, 4 Rationale: Accumulated stress weakens the immune response and places an individual at risk for the development of cancer. The human papilloma virus is known to cause malignant melanomas and other cancers. Diets high in fiber are associated with a decreased risk of cancer, not an increased risk. Estrogen-containing contraceptive pills increase the risk of breast cancer but decrease the risk of ovarian cancer. Autoimmune disorders are characterized by overly zealous warding off of foreign invaders and attacks on self, not with the development of cancer. **Cognitive Level:** Applying **Client Need:** Health Promotion and Maintenance **Integrated Process:** Teaching and Learning **Content Area:** Adult Health **Strategy:** Consider each response as a true-false item. **Reference:** LeMone, P., Burke, K., & Bauldoff, G. (2011). *Medical-surgical nursing: Critical thinking in patient care* (5th ed.). Upper Saddle River, NJ: Pearson Education, pp. 347–348.

8 Answer: 2 Rationale: Denial is a protective mechanism, and during this time, the client needs a supportive environment. Allowing the client to express feelings will enable an effective adaptation to this change. Telling the client how they will feel is not a therapeutic communication and places the client's concern on hold. Wound care must be done in order to prevent complications, and the client is obviously not psychologically ready to participate in self-care. **Cognitive Level:** Applying **Client Need:** Psychosocial Integrity **Integrated Process:** Communication and Documentation **Content Area:** Adult Health **Strategy:** The goal of communication is to provide an environment where the client can continue to voice her concerns with safety. Select the answer option that allows the client to maintain her coping mechanism and gradually adjust to the changed body image. **Reference:** LeMone, P., Burke, K., & Bauldoff, G. (2011). *Medical-surgical nursing: Critical thinking in patient care* (5th ed.). Upper Saddle River, NJ: Pearson Education, pp. 372–373.

9 Answer: 2 Rationale: Common side effects of chemotherapy such as dry mucous membranes, fatigue, and hair loss on scalp require follow-up in some way but are not as high of a priority as findings that indicate possible life-threatening problems. Ecchymotic areas may be a sign of decreased platelet count, making the risk of hemorrhage the priority. **Cognitive Level:** Analyzing **Client Need:** Reduction of Risk Potential **Integrated Process:** Nursing Process: Assessment **Content Area:** Adult Health **Strategy:** Eliminate all answer options that are expected in a client receiving chemotherapy. Choose the answer option that infers the greatest risk. **Reference:** LeMone, P., Burke, K., & Bauldoff, G. (2011). *Medical-surgical nursing: Critical thinking in patient care* (5th ed.). Upper Saddle River, NJ: Pearson Education, pp. 371–376.

10 **Answer: 4** **Rationale:** Damage to the mucous membranes, especially oral mucous membranes (stomatitis), leads to painful ulcerations of the mouth, interfering with the client's desire to eat. Pale skin and mucous membranes may be a sign of anemia. Ecchymosis may be indicative

of a low platelet count. **Cognitive Level:** Analyzing **Client Need:** Physiological Adaptation **Integrated Process:** Nursing Process: Assessment **Content Area:** Adult Health **Strategy:** Review common side effects of chemotherapy. Focus on the one that is most likely to interfere with the ability to chew. **Reference:** LeMone, P., Burke, K., & Bauldoff, G. (2011). *Medical-surgical nursing: Critical thinking in patient care* (5th ed.). Upper Saddle River, NJ: Pearson Education, pp. 375–376.

References

American Cancer Society (2011). *American Cancer Society guidelines for the early detection of cancer.* Atlanta, Ga: American Cancer Society.

American Cancer Society (2012). *Cancer facts & figures 2012.* Atlanta, Ga: American Cancer Society.

Berman, A., & Snyder, S. (2012). *Kozier & Erb's fundamentals of nursing: Concepts, process, and practice* (9th ed.). Upper Saddle River, NJ: Pearson Education.

D'Amico, D., & Barbarito, C. (2012). *Health & physical assessment in nursing* (2nd ed.). Upper Saddle River, NJ: Pearson Education, Inc.

Ignatavicius, D. D., & Workman, M. L. (2013). *Medical-surgical nursing: Critical thinking for collaborative care* (7th ed.) Philadelphia: W. B. Saunders Company.

Kee, J. L. (2010). *Laboratory and diagnostic tests* (8th ed.). Upper Saddle River, NJ: Pearson Education.

Lehne, R. (2010). *Pharmacology for nursing care* (7th ed.). St. Louis, MO: Saunders.

LeMone, P., Burke, K., & Bauldoff, G. (2011). *Medical-surgical nursing: Critical thinking in patient care* (5th ed.). Upper Saddle River, NJ: Pearson Education.

Lewis, S., Dirksen, S. Heitkemper, M., Bucher, L., & Camera, I. (2011). *Medical surgical nursing: Assessment and management of clinical problems* (8th ed.). St. Louis, MO: Elsevier.

McCance, K. L., & Huether, S. E. (2010). *Pathophysiology: The biologic basis for disease in adults and children* (6th ed.). St. Louis, MO: Mosby, Inc.

Osborn, K. S., Wraa, C. E., & Watson, A. (2010). *Medical surgical nursing: Preparation for practice* (Vol. Combined). Upper Saddle River, NJ: Prentice Hall.

Smith, S. F., Duell, D. J., & Martin, B. C. (2012). *Clinical nursing skills: Basic to advanced skills* (8th ed.). Upper Saddle River, NJ: Pearson Education.

Endocrine and Metabolic Disorders

13

Chapter Outline

Overview of Anatomy and Physiology

Diagnostic Tests and Assessments

Disorders of Posterior Pituitary Gland

Disorders of Thyroid Gland

Disorders of Parathyroid Gland

Disorders of Adrenal Glands

Disorders of Pancreas

Objectives

➤ Identify basic structures and functions of the endocrine system.

➤ Describe the pathophysiology and etiology of common endocrine disorders.

➤ Discuss expected assessment data and diagnostic test findings for selected endocrine disorders.

➤ Identify priority nursing problems for selected endocrine disorders.

➤ Discuss therapeutic management of selected endocrine disorders.

➤ Discuss nursing management of a client experiencing an endocrine disorder.

➤ Identify expected outcomes for the client experiencing an endocrine disorder.

NCLEX-RN® Test Prep

Use the accompanying online resource, NursingReviewsandRationales, to test yourself with hundreds of NCLEX®-style practice questions.

Review at a Glance

endocrine gland ductless tissue secreting a hormone to regulate body functions

exocrine gland gland whose secretions reach a target via ducts

glycosylated hemoglobin saturation of hemoglobin in the RBC with glucose; serum level greater than 7% indicates inadequate serum glucose regulation in diabetes mellitus; reported as glycosylated hemoglobin, Hb A1C, or glycohemoglobin (GHB)

hormone chemical substance secreted by endocrine tissue that travels in body fluids (usually bloodstream) to effect an action in specific target cells

hyperkalemia excess or elevated level of potassium in blood

hyperglycemia excess or elevated level of glucose in blood

hypersecretion secretion of a chemical above normal level; may be associated with increased (abnormal) function of an endocrine gland

hypocalcemia low level of calcium in blood

hyponatremia low level of sodium in blood

hypophysectomy surgical removal of hypophysis (pituitary gland)

hyposecretion secretion of a chemical below normal level; may be associated with abnormally reduced function of an endocrine gland

ketosis a state in which excessive ketones are produced from incomplete fat metabolism; usually leads to elevated serum and urine ketone levels and causes acidosis

paresthesia abnormal sensation described as tingling, burning, or prickling

photophobia unable to tolerate light

polydipsia excessive thirst

polyphagia eating an abnormally excessive amount of food

polyuria an abnormally large amount of urine output

receptor cell site that is sensitive to a specific stimulus or hormone

sebum lubricating secretion from sebaceous glands of skin

thyroid crisis (thyroid storm) occurrence of life-threatening extreme manifestations of hyperthyroidism: high fever, hypertension, tachycardia, restlessness, and delirium

PRETEST

1 A female client is being given 30 mCi sodium iodide-131 (Iodotope) to treat Graves' disease. What should the nurse do before giving the client her first dose?

1. Assess the client for hypersensitivity by asking if she is allergic to eggs.
2. Instruct the client that she must not get pregnant during treatment.
3. Assess the client's temperature to use as a baseline to evaluate the medication effectiveness.
4. Instruct the client not to drink the medication mixture with a straw in order to ensure she drinks the entire dose.

2 A client is 12 hours status-post (S/P) partial thyroidectomy. For what therapeutic purpose would the nurse ask the client about any numbness or tingling of the face, mouth, or extremities?

1. Early identification of low thyroid hormone
2. Detection of thyroid-induced hypoglycemia
3. Early identification of hypocalcemia
4. Detection of nerve damage related to surgery

3 The client is diagnosed with an allergy to iodine. In addition to client education about foods to avoid, the client should also be taught to report which symptoms associated with endocrine malfunction related to low iodine intake?

1. Diarrhea, weight loss, blurred vision
2. Constipation, weight gain, muscle stiffness
3. Fatigue, dry skin, increased BP
4. Anorexia, dyspnea, weight loss

4 A client with a history of Addison's disease is 20 hours status-post (S/P) colon resection with end-to-end anastomosis for ruptured diverticulum. After noting new onset of lethargy with the current assessment, the nurse should take which important actions next? Select all that apply.

1. Review patient-controlled analgesia (PCA) record for dose history.
2. Assess client for decreased urine output and blood pressure (BP).
3. Check pupils for direct and consensual reaction.
4. Assess results of recent arterial blood gases.
5. Measure the client's recent urinary output.

5 A client with new onset type 1 diabetes mellitus (DM) asks why he needs to check his blood glucose level so frequently. The nurse explains that frequent coverage with insulin to keep the blood glucose level between 70 and 120 mg/dL is important for which reason?

1. Chronic elevated blood glucose levels damage cells and cause multiple organ damage.
2. High glucose levels cause the body to use proteins for energy, causing lactic acidosis.
3. Early identification of hypoglycemia before the onset of symptoms is easier to treat.
4. Carbohydrates are constantly being converted to glucose and transported in the blood by insulin.

6 The nurse has been teaching the client with new onset of syndrome of inappropriate antidiuretic hormone (SIADH) about the disorder. Which statements by the client best indicate the correct understanding of how to manage this disease? Select all that apply.

1. "I should limit my sodium intake to 2 grams daily."
2. "I should report constipation or fatigue to the doctor."
3. "I should drink at least 3,000 mL or 10 glasses of water daily."
4. "I should limit my fluid intake to approximately 800 mL or 4 glasses of water daily."
5. "I should take prescribed diuretics exactly as directed."

7 The client is admitted with decreased level of consciousness (LOC) because of a closed-head injury sustained in a fall while roller skating. Urine output is 500 mL from 6:00 to 11:00 a.m., 1,000 mL from 11:00 to 2:00 p.m., and 350 mL from 2:00 to 3:00 p.m. Which action by the nurse is appropriate at this time?

1. Realize that this is normal urine output and continue to monitor the client.
2. Encourage the client to drink 8 to 10 glasses of fluid daily.
3. Check the urine specific gravity and report any abnormality as well as the urine output.
4. Decrease the IV rate from 100 mL/hr to 25 mL/hr suspecting fluid excess.

8 The client who has acromegaly secondary to excessive growth hormone (GH) states, "I'll be glad to have this surgery; after my pituitary gland is removed I'll be cured; then no more lab tests and pills!" Which statement should the nurse document to reflect the client's current understanding of preoperative teaching?

1. Criteria met: Client correctly verbalized understanding of outcomes
2. Criteria not met: Client needs to know about routine postoperative lab tests done on first postoperative day to evaluate response to surgery
3. Criteria not met: Client needs to know surgery will slow the disease process but client will need regular blood tests and x-rays for approximately 1 year
4. Criteria not met: Client needs to know surgery will stop excess production of growth hormone (GH) and probably other hormones, and thus will need daily replacement medications for life

9 The client is admitted with metabolic acidosis secondary to diabetic ketoacidosis (DKA). Which of the following does the nurse formulate as the priority nursing diagnosis?

1. Impaired Urinary Elimination related to reduced output and muscle function
2. Deficient Fluid Volume related to high urine output
3. Ineffective Breathing Pattern related to hyperventilation
4. Anxiety related to fears of long-term outcomes and discomfort

10 The nurse is caring for a client with type 1 diabetes mellitus (DM) who weighs 138 lbs. The client is prescribed an insulin total daily dose (ITDD) of 0.75 units/kg. Half of the total dose is to be given as a single insulin glargine subcutaneous injection daily. The other half is divided equally into 3 mealtime doses. Assuming no additional mealtime correction insulin is required, how many units of insulin should the nurse administer with supper? Record your answer rounding to the nearest whole number.

1. _____ units

➤ *See pages 438–440 for Answers and Rationales.*

I. OVERVIEW OF ANATOMY AND PHYSIOLOGY

A. Basic structures of endocrine system

1. Both exocrine and endocrine glands originate from glandular epithelial tissue
2. During development of glands intracellular macromolecules are formed (which are chemical substances secreted by gland) and are stored in vesicles called secretory granules
3. **Exocrine glands** secrete substances that reach their target tissue directly or by traveling through a duct; they include sebaceous, salivary, mammary, and sweat glands
4. **Endocrine glands** secrete hormones directly into blood stream; neuronal stimulation, chemical substances, or hormones can control secretion of endocrine glands

5. A **hormone** is a biologically active substance secreted by an endocrine gland that circulates throughout body, affecting function of one or more target organs, tissues, or bodily functions

6. Endocrine gland hormones control a variety of biologic functions

7. Various conditions can cause endocrine gland to hypersecrete or hyposecrete, leading to altered body functions

8. **Hyposecretion** is a condition where an insufficient supply of a substance is secreted

9. **Hypersecretion** is a condition where an excessive amount of a substance is secreted

B. **Basic functions of endocrine system**

1. Exocrine glands provide a vast variety of functions

   a. During lactation, milk is ejected from mammary glands

   b. Salivary glands secrete saliva

      1) Mucus in saliva protects oral mucous membranes, cleanses oral mucosa, and contains lysozyme, an antibacterial-like enzyme

      2) Saliva also contains 2 digestive enzymes, amylase and ptyalin, to initiate starch digestion before it enters stomach

   c. Sweat glands secrete sweat onto skin to regulate body temperature

   d. Sebaceous glands secrete **sebum**, composed of lipids and wax that insulate skin to prevent excess evaporation and conserve body heat

2. Endocrine glands: coordinate and regulate long-term changes in function of all body organs and tissues to maintain homeostasis

3. Hormones: chemical messengers that circulate in bloodstream and alter cellular activities by changing enzymes and proteins in target cells

   a. **Receptor**: specially designed link on a target cell membrane or in cytoplasm for a specific hormone to contact and initiate an action response

   b. Regulation of secretion: effects on target tissue act as a negative feedback controlling mechanism to signal the initiating gland to slow or stop secretion

C. **Major endocrine system glands**

1. Posterior pituitary gland: regulates fluid balance and facilitates childbirth and prostate gland function

   a. Releases antidiuretic hormone (ADH) and oxytocin, which are produced and stored in hypothalamus

   b. ADH, also called vasopressin

      1) Stimulates kidneys to reabsorb water, decreasing urine output, supporting BP and blood volume, and also stimulates peripheral blood vessels to constrict

      2) Release is stimulated by an increased osmolality of blood

      3) Decreased osmolality causes suppression of ADH and increased secretion of renal water

   c. Oxytocin stimulates uterus to contract for childbirth, mammary glands to eject milk, and smooth muscles of prostate gland to contract and eject secretions

2. Anterior pituitary gland: major role of this gland is to produce and release several different hormones (most of which regulate secretion of other hormones)

   a. Thyroid-stimulating hormone (TSH) stimulates synthesis and release of thyroid hormones from thyroid gland

   b. Adrenocorticotropic hormone (ACTH) stimulates release of hormones, especially glucocorticoids, from the adrenal cortex

   c. Follicle-stimulating hormone (FSH) stimulates ovaries and testes

   d. Luteinizing hormone (LH) stimulates ovaries and testes; also called interstitial cell-stimulating hormone (ICSH) in males

   e. Prolactin (PRL) stimulates production of breast milk

   f. Growth hormone (GH), also called somatotropin, stimulates growth of body by signaling cells to increase protein production and by stimulating epiphyseal plates of long bones

3. Thyroid gland: determines rate of cellular metabolism; in children, hormones are responsible for normal development of skeletal, muscular, and nervous systems
    a. Calcitonin targets bone and kidney cells to regulate calcium ion concentrations in body fluids; it also serves as a marker for sepsis and is believed to be a mediator of inflammatory responses
    b. Thyroxine (TX or tetraiodothyronine or T_4), and triiodothyronine (T_3) bind to mitochondria and nucleus of cells to increase rate of ATP production
        1) Secretion is initiated by release of TSH by pituitary gland
        2) Is dependent on an adequate supply of iodine
        3) Negative feedback mechanism; rising levels of these hormones stimulate anterior pituitary gland to stop releasing TSH
4. Parathyroid glands: monitor and maintain circulating concentration of calcium ions
    a. Secrete parathyroid hormone (PTH) to increase serum calcium level and control phosphate metabolism
    b. PTH stimulates osteoclasts, inhibits osteoblasts, promotes absorption of calcium by intestines, increases renal excretion of phosphate and decreases renal excretion of calcium
    c. Is dependent on normal levels of vitamin D
5. Pancreas (islets of Langerhans): regulates blood glucose (BG) concentrations
    a. Alpha cells produce glucagon to signal liver to break down stored glycogen into glucose in response to low glucose level
    b. Beta cells produce insulin that is needed by most cells to transport glucose across cell membranes
    c. Delta cells produce somatostatin that inhibits production of glucagons and insulin
    d. F cells produce pancreatic polypeptide, which is believed to inhibit exocrine (digestive enzyme) activity of pancreas
6. Adrenal medulla: increases cellular energy use and muscular strength endurance, and mobilizes energy reserves
    a. Secretes the catecholamines epinephrine (adrenaline) and norepinephrine (noradrenaline); receptors are on cardiac muscle, skeletal muscle fibers, GI tract, smooth vascular muscle, adipose tissues, and liver
    b. Mobilizes glycogen reserves, metabolizes glucose for ATP, and increases cardiac rate and force of contraction
7. Adrenal cortex: hormones play a vital role for body's survival and affect metabolism of many different tissues
    a. Glucocorticoids: cortisol (hydrocortisone), corticosterone, and cortisone stimulate most cells to increase rate of glucose synthesis, glycogen formation, release of fatty acids, and breakdown of fatty acids; exert an anti-inflammatory effect to suppress immune system
    b. Mineralocorticoids: aldosterone stimulates kidneys to increase reabsorption of sodium and water, and reduces sodium and water loss by sweat glands, salivary glands, and digestive tract; low blood pressure (BP) or low sodium levels activate renin-angiotensin-aldosterone system
8. Female gonads (ovaries): regulate secondary sexual characteristics and reproduction
    a. Estrogens stimulate most cells to develop secondary sex characteristics and behaviors, follicle maturation, and growth of uterine lining
    b. Provides negative feedback to anterior pituitary gland to stop secretion of FSH
    c. Progestins stimulate uterus to prepare for implantation and mammary glands for lactation
9. Male gonads (testes): regulate secondary sexual characteristics and reproduction
    a. Androgens, primarily testosterone, stimulate most cells for protein synthesis, maturation of sperm, secondary sexual characteristics and behaviors
    b. Inhibin is secreted for negative feedback to anterior pituitary gland to stop secretion of FSH

II. DIAGNOSTIC TESTS AND ASSESSMENTS

A. Assessment of endocrine system

1. Dysfunction of any endocrine gland or receptor sites for an endocrine gland hormone causes an alteration of one or more body functions; obtain appropriate health information pertinent to affected gland, such as signs and symptoms of hyper- or hypofunction

2. Physical assessment: use an organized system approach, assessing client's general appearance and proceeding with a head-to-toe assessment

B. Diagnostic studies of endocrine system

1. Refer to Chapter 1 for general information about diagnostic tests

2. Laboratory tests for endocrine disorders (see Table 13-1)

3. Imaging studies (see Table 13-2)

Table 13-1 **Common Laboratory Tests for Endocrine Disorders**

Test	Normal Adult Values	Explanation	Nursing Implications
Pituitary			
Growth hormone (GH)	Less than 5 ng/mL for men Less than 10 ng/mL for women	Used to evaluate growth hormone excess or deficiency. Increased values indicate acromegaly.	The client must be fasting, well rested, and not physically or emotionally stressed.
Water deprivation test	1–5 pg/mL	Increased level indicates SIADH, decreased level means diabetes insipidus.	Tell client to fast for 12 hours and to withhold fluids and smoking at midnight.
Thyroid			
Thyroid-stimulating hormone (TSH)	0.35–5.5 mcg/mL	This is the most sensitive test to evaluate thyroid function by measuring pituitary TSH secretion.	No fluid restriction is required. Avoid shellfish several days before test.
T_3	80–200 ng/dL	Measures triiodothyronine (T_3) and thyroxine (T_4) to evaluate thyroid function. Increased level indicates hyperthyroidism and decreased reflects hypothyroidism.	
T_4	4.5–11.5 mcg/dL		
Parathyroid			
Serum calcium	9–11 mg/dL	This test evaluates parathyroid function and calcium metabolism.	Fasting not required; however, is part of a chemistry panel in which fasting is required.
Serum phosphate	2.5–4.5 mg/dL	It measures serum phosphate. Increased levels in both tests indicate hyperparathyroidism; decreased levels indicate hypoparathyroidism.	
Adrenal			
Cortisol	8 to 10 am 5–23 mcg/dL 4 to 6 pm 3–13 mcg/dL	This test measures total serum cortisol, which evaluates adrenal cortex function. Levels are increased in Cushing's syndrome and decreased in Addison's disease.	Advise client to rest in bed 2 hours before blood is drawn. Explain that two blood samples are drawn—one at 8:00 to 10 a.m., the other at 4 to 6:00 p.m.
Aldosterone	4–30 ng/dL sitting position Less than 16 ng/dL supine position	Levels are drawn to diagnose hyperaldosteronism.	Ask client to be in supine position for 1 hour before test is drawn.

(continued)

Table 13-1	Common Laboratory Tests for Endocrine Disorders (continued)		
Test	**Normal Adult Values**	**Explanation**	**Nursing Implications**
Urinary 17-ketosteroids	5–15 mg/24 hours men 5–25 mg/24 hours women	17-KS are metabolites of testosterone, which are released from adrenal cortex. Levels increase with Cushing's syndrome and decrease in Addison's disease.	Teach client about 24-hour urine collection, which must be iced or refrigerated during collection.
Pancreas			
Fasting blood glucose	70–110 mg/dL	This test measures circulating blood glucose level. Increases are seen in diabetes mellitus, acute pancreatitis; decreased level is seen in Addison's disease.	This test is done fasting.
Glycosylated hemoglobin (Hb A1c)	5.5%–7%	Test used to measure glucose control during the previous 3 months. Levels are increased in newly diagnosed or poorly controlled diabetic. It is not used to diagnose diabetes mellitus.	No fasting is required.
Two-hour oral glucose tolerance test (OGTT)	Less than 125 mg/dL	Determines the level of glucose 2 hours after drinking 75 g of glucose. Glucose level should return to premeal levels, but in diabetics, the level is higher than 200 mg/dL.	Client is NPO for 12 hours before test. Then client must drink entire 100 g of glucose and not eat anything else until blood is drawn.
Urine glucose	Negative	Estimates the amount of glucose in urine, which should be negative.	Collect a fresh urine sample; stagnant urine may alter test results.
Urine ketones	Negative	Measures ketones excreted in urine from incomplete fat metabolism. Positive result means lack of insulin or diabetic ketoacidosis.	Some drugs may interfere with both test results.
Urine test for microalbumin	0.2–1.9 mg/dL	Microalbumin is the earliest indicator for development of diabetic nephropathy. Elevated microalbumin levels increase the risk for end-stage renal disease.	Collect a fresh urine sample and send to laboratory for analysis.

Source: Burke, Karen M.; LeMone, Priscilla; Mohn-Brown, Elaine; EBY, Linda, *Medical Surgical Nursing Care*, 3rd Ed., © 2011, pp. 885, 886. Reprinted and Electronically reproduced by permission of Pearson Education, Inc., Upper Saddle River, New Jersey.

Table 13-2	Imaging Studies	
Test	**Explanation and Purpose**	**Nursing Implications**
Magnetic resonance imaging (MRI)	MRI uses a super magnet and radiofrequency signals to elicit a response from hydrogen nuclei. As a result, tumors of the pituitary gland and hypothalamus can be identified.	Assess for presence of metallic implants, because clients with metal implants cannot have an MRI. Inform client of the need to lie motionless during the test. Be sure all metal objects are removed because the magnetic field can be injurious to anyone within the field.
Computed tomography (CT) scan	Specialized radiographic procedures that produce computer-generated images with significantly more detail than standard x-rays allow. May be done with or without contrast media. Abdominal CT is used to detect tumors of the adrenal gland and pancreas.	If contrast dye used, ask about allergies to iodine and seafood. Client must lie still during the procedure.
Thyroid scan	Iodine-125 is injected IV. A scanner passes over the thyroid making a graph of the radiation emitted. "Cold spots," which do not take up the I-125, indicate malignancy.	Ask about allergies to iodine and seafood. Client may need to withhold thyroid drugs or medications containing iodine for weeks before the study. No fasting is needed.
Radioactive iodine (RAI) uptake test	Iodine-131 or I-125 (capsule or liquid form) is given, then the thyroid is scanned three times. Increased uptake indicates Graves' disease; decreased uptake means hypothyroidism.	Client fasts for 8 hours before the test but can eat 1 hour after radioiodine capsule or liquid has been taken. Thyroid drugs or medications containing iodine are held for weeks before the study.

Source: Burke, Karen M.; LeMone, Priscilla; Mohn-Brown, Elaine; EBY, Linda, *Medical Surgical Nursing Care*, 3rd Ed., © 2011, pp. 885, 886. Reprinted and Electronically reproduced by permission of Pearson Education, Inc., Upper Saddle River, New Jersey.

4. Capillary glucose monitoring
   a. Warm extremity to encourage vasodilation; select digit to be used
   b. Cleanse site with soap and water or 70% alcohol, dry with a gauze sponge
   c. Place at or below heart level to facilitate successful puncture
   d. Avoid squeezing site to enhance blood flow since squeezing causes dilution with tissue fluid
   e. Avoid touching skin with reagent strip; skin oils may affect results
   f. Elevate digit and apply gentle pressure with dry sterile gauze to site until bleeding stops after drop of blood obtained

III. DISORDERS OF POSTERIOR PITUITARY GLAND

A. Syndrome of inappropriate antidiuretic hormone (SIADH)

1. Description: SIADH is an excessive amount of serum ADH, resulting in water intoxication and hyponatremia
2. Etiology and pathophysiology
   a. The usual feedback mechanism does not function to decrease posterior pituitary secretion of ADH with decreased serum osmolality
   b. High levels of ADH leads to renal reabsorption of water and suppression of the renin-angiotensin-aldosterone mechanism, causing renal excretion of sodium
   c. This leads to water intoxication, cellular edema, and dilutional hyponatremia
   d. Water moves from hypotonic plasma and interstitial spaces into cells
   e. Urinary output decreases and urine becomes very concentrated
   f. Causes of SIADH
      1) Malignant tumors (such as oat cell cancer of lung, pancreatic carcinoma, leukemia, and Hodgkin's lymphoma) secrete ADH independent of a normally functioning hypothalamus and feedback mechanisms
      2) Can also be caused by hypersecretion of ADH by hypothalamus resulting from head injury, hydrocephalus, meningitis, encephalitis, pituitary surgery, stroke, brain hemorrhage, or some medications
      3) Positive pressure ventilation and other conditions causing increased intrathoracic pressure may stimulate aortic baroreceptors and cardiopulmonary receptors that trigger the hypothalamus to secrete ADH
      4) Trauma, pain, stress, and acute psychosis may activate the limbic system that, in turn, stimulates hypothalamus to secrete ADH
3. Assessment
   a. General manifestations of fluid volume excess, possibly including increased BP, crackles auscultated in lung fields, distended jugular neck veins, taut skin, weight gain, and intake greater than output
   b. Client may experience thirst despite fluid retention; usually no edema is present, because water is distributed between intracellular and extracellular spaces
   c. Neurologic manifestations are related to swelling of brain cells and include headache, lethargy, progressive altered level of consciousness (LOC), mental status or personality changes, seizures, and coma
   d. Other clinical manifestations include headache, fatigue, anorexia, nausea, muscle aches, abdominal cramps, and small amounts of concentrated amber-colored urine
   e. Diagnostic and laboratory test findings: high urine osmolality (greater than 1,200 mOsm/kg H_2O) and specific gravity greater than 1.032, low serum osmolality (less than 275 mOsm/kg), and decreased hematocrit, BUN and serum sodium (less than 135 mEq/L, also known as **hyponatremia**)
   f. Sodium levels of 116–125 mEq/L lead to changes in LOC, and less than 116 mEq/L may result in seizures, coma, and death

4. Therapeutic management

    a. Limit fluid intake; monitor urine osmolality, serum electrolytes, hematocrit, BUN, sodium and serum osmolality

    b. Supplement sodium intake cautiously orally or by hypertonic (3%) saline IV infusion; correct hyponatremia cautiously to prevent cerebral osmotic demyelination with resultant cerebral edema, brain damage, seizures and possible death

5. Priority nursing problems: fluid overload, alteration in thought processes, pain, potential for injury, insufficient nutrients to meet bodily needs, fatigue, inadequate knowledge

6. Planning and implementation

    a. Restrict oral fluids including ice chips to 800 mL/day to prevent further hemodilution

    b. Flush all enteral and gastric tubes with normal saline (NS) instead of water to replace sodium and prevent further hemodilution

    c. Monitor intake and output (I & O) accurately

    d. Monitor serum sodium, and urine osmolality and specific gravity

    e. Weigh daily; a weight loss of 2 pounds indicates a loss of 1 L of fluid

    f. Assess for changes in LOC, mentation, cognition, nutrition, muscle twitching, and comfort

7. Medication therapy

    a. Demeclocycline (Declomycin): a tetracycline antibiotic with the unique property of creating excessive urine flow

    b. Vasopressin antagonists, especially if client has heart failure

    c. Diuretics such as furosemide (Lasix) to eliminate excessive fluid

8. Client education

    a. Information about SIADH and symptoms to report

    b. Medication may be lifelong depending on cause

    c. Identify hidden sources of water and fluids, such as ice and ice cream, to prevent accidental excessive intake

    d. Plan meal pattern and maintain fluid limitation and sodium prescription

    e. Weigh daily on same scale and report gain of 2 pounds in 1 day

9. Evaluation: client cognition and mentation functions are intact; verbalizes understanding of medications, fluid restriction, sources of water and sodium; demonstrates ability to weigh self and verbalizes to report weight gain; excess fluid is eliminated; lab values normalize; client is free of seizures

B. Diabetes insipidus (DI)

1. Description: results from excessive water loss caused by hyposecretion of ADH or kidneys' inability to respond to ADH; the subsequent **polyuria** (excessive urine output ranging from 4 to 30 L in 24 hours) can lead to severe dehydration if client does not replace lost water

2. Etiology and pathophysiology

    a. Neurogenic DI: renal tubules excrete excessive amounts of water in urine caused by insufficient ADH secretion by posterior pituitary gland

    b. Nephrogenic DI: inability of kidney to respond to ADH

    c. Lithium carbonate and demeclocycline (Declomycin) can cause kidneys to alter response to ADH

    d. Gestational DI: occurs during pregnancy if pituitary is damaged or if placenta destroys ADH too quickly; subsides 4 to 6 weeks after delivery

    e. Dispogenic DI: syndrome caused by disease or damage to part of brain that regulates thirst; clients are not dehydrated but ingest a large volume of water resulting in water intoxication

    f. Primary DI results from an inherited or idiopathic malfunction of posterior pituitary gland

Practice to Pass

The client with SIADH is upset at not being able to drink fluids whenever she wants. How should you respond?

       g. Secondary DI is caused by brain tumors, head trauma, infection, surgery on or near pituitary gland, metastatic tumors from lung or breast, cerebrovascular hemorrhage, granulomatous disease, or cerebral aneurysm

       h. DI can be permanent or transient

  3. Assessment

       a. Assess for a history of head injury, brain surgery, infection, or tumor

       b. Obtain a list of current and past medications

       c. Assess LOC, vital signs (VS) including orthostatic BP, skin turgor, I & O, weight, skin integrity, **polydipsia** (excessive thirst), tenting or sagging skin, bowel sounds, constipation and clear colorless urine; see Figure 13-1 for full listing of multisystem effects of fluid volume deficit

       d. Clinical manifestations: polyuria, excessive thirst, dry tented skin, dry mucous membranes, and severe hypotension leading to cardiovascular collapse (which can occur if the excessive water loss is not replaced)

       e. Diagnostic and laboratory test findings: urine specific gravity less than 1.005, urine osmolality less than 300 mOsm/kg, positive water deprivation test, reduced serum ADH level in primary DI, serum sodium greater than 145 mEq/L, serum osmolality greater than 303 mOsm/kg

  4. Therapeutic management

       a. Water replacement orally is preferred or intravenous (IV) D_5W as needed to normalize lab values

       b. For neurogenic DI, hormone replacement with desmopressin (DDAVP), a synthetic vasopressin; adjunctive medications such as chlorpropamide (Diabinese), or carbamazepine (Tegretol) may act to increase ADH release or effect of ADH on renal collecting duct

       c. For nephrogenic DI, correct underlying disease or stop causative medication; begin a low-salt, low-protein diet to decrease net excretion of solute; administer diuretics to eliminate sodium and decrease glomerular filtration rate (resulting in conservation of urine)

       d. Surgery if a tumor is present

  5. Priority nursing problems: dehydration, reduced cardiac output, potential for interrupted skin integrity, possible constipation, inadequate knowledge

  6. Planning and implementation

       a. Monitor I & O hourly; report urine output greater than 200 mL/hour for 2 consecutive hours or 500 mL over 2 hours; assess for continence and provide easy access to restroom as appropriate

       b. Weigh daily; report weight loss

       c. Monitor urine specific gravity and report if it decreases; monitor serum osmolality and sodium for increases

       d. Encourage fluid intake greater than urine output; provide fluids within reach at all times

       e. Use skin protective barriers with incontinence

  7. Medication therapy: desmopressin (DDAVP) as supplemental ADH, chlorpropamide (Diabinese) or carbamazepine (Tegretol) to potentiate the renal effect of ADH, and replacement IV fluids as needed

  8. Client education

       a. Information about DI, self-administration of medication, and about possible need for lifelong medication

       b. Wear a MedicAlert bracelet listing DI and treatments

       c. Drink fluid equal to amount of urine output, keeping a log of I & O

       d. Weigh self daily, on same scale at same time of day, and report weight loss

       e. Consult health care provider before taking over-the-counter (OTC) medications

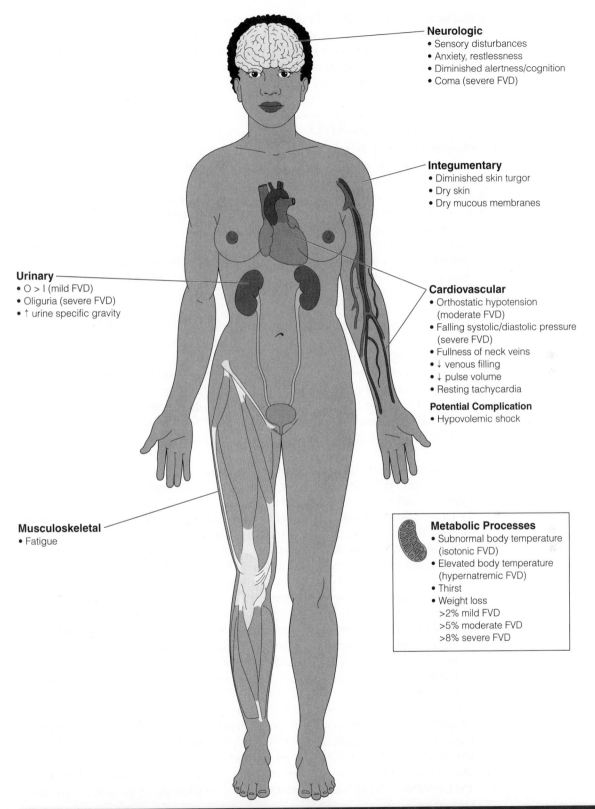

Neurologic
- Sensory disturbances
- Anxiety, restlessness
- Diminished alertness/cognition
- Coma (severe FVD)

Integumentary
- Diminished skin turgor
- Dry skin
- Dry mucous membranes

Urinary
- O > I (mild FVD)
- Oliguria (severe FVD)
- ↑ urine specific gravity

Cardiovascular
- Orthostatic hypotension (moderate FVD)
- Falling systolic/diastolic pressure (severe FVD)
- Fullness of neck veins
- ↓ venous filling
- ↓ pulse volume
- Resting tachycardia

Potential Complication
- Hypovolemic shock

Musculoskeletal
- Fatigue

Metabolic Processes
- Subnormal body temperature (isotonic FVD)
- Elevated body temperature (hypernatremic FVD)
- Thirst
- Weight loss
  >2% mild FVD
  >5% moderate FVD
  >8% severe FVD

Figure 13-1

Multisystem effects of fluid volume deficit

9. Evaluation: intake is within 500 mL of urine output; weight returns to client's baseline; lab values are within normal range, client wears MedicAlert bracelet with appropriate information; skin is intact; bowel function is normal; client verbalizes understanding of medication and self-administers medication correctly; monitors and records intake, output, and weight

IV. DISORDERS OF THYROID GLAND

A. Hyperthyroidism (Graves' disease)

1. Description: excessive secretion of thyroid hormone from thyroid gland, leading to increased basal metabolic rate (BMR), cardiovascular function, gastrointestinal (GI) function, neuromuscular function, weight loss, and heat intolerance; thyroid hormone affects metabolism of fats, carbohydrates (CHOs), and proteins

2. Etiology and pathophysiology
   a. Hyperthyroidism can be caused by excess secretion of TSH from pituitary gland, autoimmune reaction (Graves' disease), thyroiditis (inflammation or viral infection of thyroid gland), tumor, and excessive dose of supplemental thyroid hormone
   b. Graves' disease
      1) Most common form, occurs 5 times more often in women 20–40 years old
      2) Caused by an autoimmune disorder triggering oversecretion of thyroid hormone by thyroid gland
      3) Appears to be a genetic predisposition that can be stimulated by factors such as viral illness or pregnancy
      4) Leads to enlarged thyroid gland (goiter), manifestations of hyperthyroidism, and exophthalmos (forward protrusion of eyeballs related to an accumulation of inflammation by-products in the retro-orbital tissues

3. Assessment
   a. Clinical manifestations: range from very minimal to severe depending on amount and time period of hypersecretion; see Figure 13-2 for multisystem effects of hyperthyroidism
      1) **Thyroid crisis (thyroid storm):** life-threatening emergency occurring in extreme hyperthyroidism; usually occurs with long-term untreated hyperthyroidism or in clients with hyperthyroidism experiencing a stressor such as pregnancy, infection, trauma, or manipulation of thyroid gland during surgery
      2) Common manifestations of thyroid storm are temperature greater than 102°F (39°C), tachycardia, systolic hypertension, dyspnea, abdominal pain, nausea, vomiting, diarrhea, agitation, tremors, confusion, and seizures
      3) Rapid treatment is critical to survival: aspirin for cooling; replacing fluids, glucose, and electrolytes; oxygen; stabilization of cardiovascular function with beta blockers such as propranolol (Inderal); and antithyroid medications to reduce thyroid hormone synthesis and secretion (takes 2 or more weeks for therapeutic effects)
   b. Include in overall assessment: health history, VS, neck (for goiter), eyes (for exophthalmos), respiratory effort, peripheral pulses, energy level, activity tolerance, elimination pattern, oxygenation, weight pattern over weeks, fluid balance, nutritional status, sleep pattern, and comfort
   c. Diagnostic and laboratory test findings: elevated serum T_3, T_4, free T_4; decreased TSH; positive RAI uptake scan and thyroid scan (depending on cause of hyperthyroidism)

4. Therapeutic management: lifelong antithyroid medications (see section to follow), ablative radioactive I-131, or partial or total thyroidectomy)

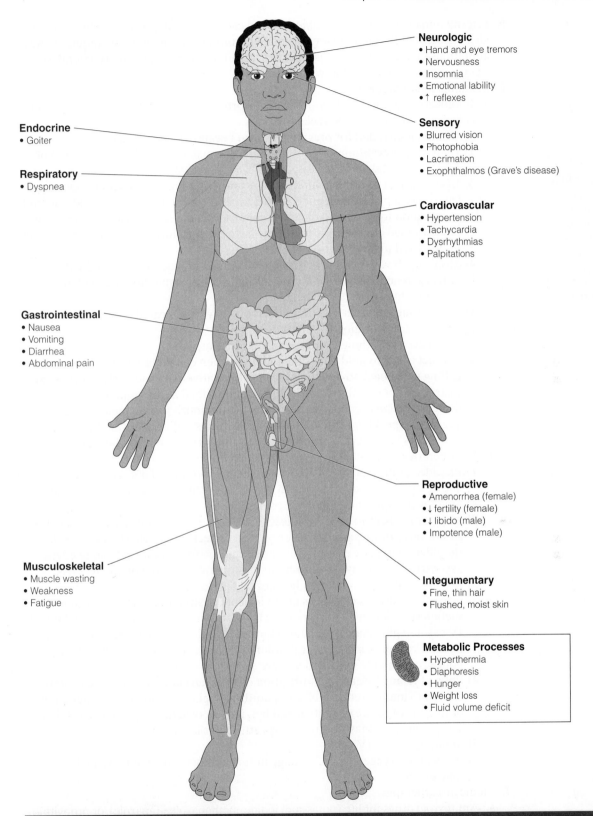

Neurologic
• Hand and eye tremors
• Nervousness
• Insomnia
• Emotional lability
• ↑ reflexes

Sensory
• Blurred vision
• Photophobia
• Lacrimation
• Exophthalmos (Grave's disease)

Cardiovascular
• Hypertension
• Tachycardia
• Dysrhythmias
• Palpitations

Reproductive
• Amenorrhea (female)
• ↓ fertility (female)
• ↓ libido (male)
• Impotence (male)

Integumentary
• Fine, thin hair
• Flushed, moist skin

Metabolic Processes
• Hyperthermia
• Diaphoresis
• Hunger
• Weight loss
• Fluid volume deficit

Endocrine
• Goiter

Respiratory
• Dyspnea

Gastrointestinal
• Nausea
• Vomiting
• Diarrhea
• Abdominal pain

Musculoskeletal
• Muscle wasting
• Weakness
• Fatigue

Figure 13-2

Multisystem effects of hyperthyroidism

5. Priority nursing problems: possible reduced cardiac output, possible disturbances in vision, potential threat to airway, insufficient nutrients to meet bodily requirements, alterations in body image, fever, inability to endure exercise or activity, alteration in sleep pattern, inadequate knowledge

6. Planning and implementation

   a. Radioactive iodine 131: thyroid gland absorbs I-131, which destroys some thyroid cells over a period of 6–8 weeks

      1) Not recommended for pregnant women because it crosses placenta

      2) Radiation precautions are not required for small doses (less than 30 mCi) of I-131; can be taken on an outpatient basis

      3) Instruct client to drink solution with straw to minimize exposure to buccal cavity; use a private toilet and flush 2 times after each use; avoid handling food preparation for others; avoid close contact with other persons for a period of days; arrange alternative care if they have small children; use disposable eating utensils and plates

      4) Monitor lab values, report weight gain, fatigue, decreased pulse and BP

      5) Adverse reactions include thyroiditis and cardiac instability due to liberation of stored thyroid hormone in gland

      6) Total or subtotal (partial) thyroidectomy may be indicated based on situation

   b. Preoperative preparation for thyroidectomy

      1) Teach deep breathing exercises and appropriate cough

      2) Instruct client to hold hands behind neck when coughing, sitting, turning, or getting up or back to bed to reduce postoperative pain and neck muscle strain

      3) Instruct client on self-administration of prescribed antithyroid drugs to decrease vascularity and size of thyroid to minimize risk of hemorrhage

      4) Teach to expect hoarseness due to generalized swelling at suture line; diminishes with healing and is not caused by laryngeal nerve damage

   c. Postoperative care following thyroidectomy

      1) Provide comfort: analgesics, position client in semi-Fowler's position with neck and head supported by pillows to prevent muscle strain, ice collar to wound area for comfort and to prevent edema

      2) Monitor for hemorrhage: tightness of dressing; sanguineous exudate on anterior or posterior neck dressing or on skin of neck, upper chest and upper back, shoulders, and back of neck; auscultate trachea for stridor (indicating edema and narrowed airway); first 24 hours postoperative is time of greatest risk

      3) Promote patent airway: keep head of bed elevated 30 degrees; assess for respiratory distress (stridor is heard in acute obstructions); keep oral and sterile suction supplies and emergency tracheostomy tray (with tracheostomy kit and IV calcium gluconate or calcium chloride) within immediate access; maintain humidification of inspired air if ordered; encourage deep breathing exercises hourly; cough only if needed to clear secretions

      4) Prevent tetany by early identification of **hypocalcemia** (low serum calcium) related to inadvertent damage to parathyroid glands; evidenced by numbness or tingling of toes, extremities, and lips, muscle twitches, positive Chvostek and Trousseau signs; may occur 1–7 days after thyroidectomy

      5) Maintain patent IV site

      6) Assess for laryngeal nerve damage noting ability to speak loudly, quality and tone of voice

7. Medication therapy:

   a. Antithyroid drugs for life (potassium iodide, methimazole [Tapazole], or propylthiouracil [PTU]) to reduce secretion of thyroid hormone or prior to surgery to reduce vascularity and size of thyroid gland and thus reduce thyroid hormone secretion

Practice to Pass

The client with Graves' disease and exophthalmos wants to know why he needs to perform special eye care after having the thyroid gland removed. What is your response?

        b. Analgesics to control pain if surgical treatment is done

        c. Thyroid replacement therapy may be required

8. Client education

    a. For hyperthyroidism

        1) Correct self-administration of medications and that medication use is lifelong

        2) Weigh daily; caloric intake may need to be increased to 4,000 kcal/day if weight loss exceeds 10–17%; eat diet high in CHOs and protein; include between-meal snack

        3) Keep environment cool and free of distractions (stress increases circulating catecholamines, which further increase cardiac workload)

        4) Balance activity with rest periods to decrease cardiac workload

    b. For exophthalmos, instruct client on methods to protect eyes and adapt to altered visual field

        1) Instruct client to have regular eye exams

        2) Instruct client to call practitioner immediately for any change in vision or appearance of eye; closure of eyelids; eye pain; eye exudate, or **photophobia** (sensitivity to light)

        3) Protect eyes with tinted glasses or eye shields since lids do not cover eyes completely and there may be delayed corneal (blink) reflex

        4) Moisten eyes frequently with artificial tears to prevent dry irritation and corneal infection; use caution not to contaminate eyedropper

        5) Soothe dry eye irritation with cool moist compresses

        6) Sleep with head of bed elevated to decrease periorbital fluid accumulation and minimize pressure on optic nerve

        7) Wear eye patches to protect eyes during sleep if lids do not close

    c. Surgical client

        1) Ensure that client understands surgical procedure and expected outcomes

        2) Instruct client to support neck with hands; position neck and head with pillows and maintain semi-Fowler's position; avoid hyperextension and sudden quick movements of head and neck

        3) Instruct on wound care

        4) Instruct client to avoid/minimize talking and coughing until wound is healed to prevent strain on laryngeal nerve and vocal cords

        5) Identify signs of hyperthyroidism and hypothyroidism to report

        6) Identify other conditions to report, including signs of hemorrhage, hypocalcemia, incisional infection, respiratory difficulty and discomfort

    d. Assist client to cope with lifestyle and self-image changes

9. Evaluation: client verbalizes understanding of self-medication administration, eye care, wound care, and symptoms to report; demonstrates support of neck and head; resumes usual social interaction; expresses acceptance of changes and appearance

B. Hypothyroidism

1. Description: occurs when there is an insufficient amount of thyroid hormone (TH) being secreted by thyroid gland, causing decreased BMR, decreased heat production, and various effects on all body systems

2. Etiology and pathophysiology

    a. Primary hypothyroidism accounts for 99% of cases, is 5–7 times more common in women, and 50% of cases are caused by cell-mediated and antibody-mediated (autoimmune) destruction of thyroid gland

    b. Other causes are thyroiditis, subacute postpartum, external irradiation of gland, iatrogenic (30–40%) infections, iodine deficiency, treatment for hyperthyroidism, congenital or idiopathic, medications

      c. The use of iodized salt has reduced rate of iodine deficient hypothyroidism in United States

      d. Secondary hypothyroidism, also called central hypothyroidism, is caused by insufficient secretion of TSH from pituitary gland, TRH deficiency related to disease of hypothalamus, or peripheral resistance to thyroid hormones

  3. Assessment

      a. Hypothyroidism is manifested with varying degrees of symptoms depending on severity of condition; general assessments include health history, LOC, VS, respiratory effort, activity tolerance, and comfort

      b. Clinical manifestations

        1) Depend on length of time and severity of lack of thyroid hormone; slow onset is most common

        2) Thyroid gland gradually enlarges forming a goiter (thickening of gland) in an attempt to secrete more thyroid hormone

        3) Clients with hypothyroidism may have a large number of symptoms, including lethargy, diminished reflexes, periorbital edema, bradycardia, dysrhythmias, hypotension, reproductive problems (menorrhagia and infertility in females and decreased libido in males), coarse dry hair that is easily lost, coarse dry skin, signs of slowed metabolism (hypothermia, fatigue, weight gain, anorexia, constipation), anemia, elevated serum lipids

      c. Assess for myxedema coma, a life-threatening crisis state of hypothyroidism

        1) May be precipitated by trauma, infection, failure to take thyroid replacement drugs, use of CNS depressants, and exposure to cold temperatures

        2) Characterized by non-pitting edema in connective tissues throughout body, puffy face and tongue, severe metabolic disorders (hyponatremia, hypoglycemia, lactic acidosis), hypothermia, cardiovascular collapse, and coma

        3) High mortality if untreated; treatment focuses on addressing precipitating factors; maintaining patent airway; maintaining fluid, electrolyte, and acid–base balance; maintaining cardiovascular status; increasing body temperature; and increasing thyroid hormone levels

      d. Diagnostic and laboratory test findings: decreased T_4 and free T_4, normal T_3, and increased TSH levels (unless secondary hypothyroidism, then TSH levels not elevated)

  4. Therapeutic management: medication to replace T_4

  5. Priority nursing problems: reduced cardiac output, excess nutrients above bodily requirements, constipation, potential for interrupted skin integrity, possible inability to endure exercise or activity, potential for altered sexual function, alteration in body image, reduced temperature, inadequate knowledge

  6. Planning and implementation

      a. Give medication in the morning 1 hour before food intake or 2 hours after food intake to facilitate absorption

      b. Adjust environment with blankets as needed for temperature of comfort; chilling increases metabolic rate, cardiac workload, and oxygen demand

      c. Pace activities with rest periods; instruct client to report shortness of breath, fatigue, dizziness, or any discomfort

      d. Encourage intake of 2,000 mL water daily and a high-fiber diet to promote regular bowel movements

      e. Monitor skin surfaces for redness or lesions; teach client to take baths only as necessary; use warm (not hot) water; use gentle motions when washing and drying skin; use alcohol-free skin oils and lotions

Practice to Pass

Explain why clients with hypothyroidism have increased risk for cardiovascular disease and constipation.

7. Medication therapy
   a. Thyroid hormone replacement, such as dessicated thyroid, levothyroxine (Synthroid), or triiodothyronine (Cytomel)
   b. Raise BMR so increases cardiac output, oxygen consumption and body temperature; monitor for signs of coronary insufficiency
   c. Speeds elimination of vitamin K-dependent clotting factors and thus enhances effects of warfarin (Coumadin)
   d. Effects of insulin may change as thyroid function increases
   e. Potentiates effects of digitalis; monitor for signs of digitalis toxicity
8. Client education
   a. Information about hypothyroidism, the importance of wearing a MedicAlert bracelet, and medication self-administration
   b. Medication is needed for life and should be taken at the same time every morning 1 hour before a meal or 2 hours after a meal; optimal time is 1 hour before breakfast
   c. Withhold medication for heart rate above 100 as if ordered by prescriber, or notify prescriber if this occurs
   d. Take the same brand of medication as brands vary in chemical properties and bioavailability
   e. Report weight gain or loss of 5 pounds, activity intolerance, chest pain, heat or cold intolerance, and sleep pattern disturbance
   f. Report symptoms of hypothyroidism and hyperthyroidism
   g. Maintain a low-fat, calorie-controlled diet
9. Evaluation: client verbalizes appropriate medication self-administration; has stabilized weight; is able to do activities of daily living without fatigue, discomfort, or shortness of breath; has normal sleep and elimination pattern; vital signs are within normal range; skin is intact and elastic; client is wearing appropriate MedicAlert bracelet

V. DISORDERS OF PARATHYROID GLAND

A. Hyperparathyroidism

1. Description: increased parathyroid hormone (PTH) secretion from parathyroid glands located in neck; occurs in older adults; is twice as common in women
   a. Primary hyperparathyroidism: hyperplasia or tumor of one of parathyroid glands, increasing absorption of calcium in GI tract
   b. Secondary hyperparathyroidism: gland enlargement due to chronic hypocalcemia in presence of elevated PTH
   c. Tertiary hyperparathyroidism: parathyroid glands are enlarged and do not respond to changes in serum calcium levels, usually associated with chronic renal failure
2. Etiology and pathophysiology
   a. Increased resorption of calcium and increased excretion of phosphate leads to hypercalcemia and hypophosphatemia
   b. Kidneys increase bicarbonate excretion and decrease acid excretion, leading to metabolic acidosis and hypokalemia
   c. Bones increase rate of calcium and phosphorus release leading to bone decalcification
   d. Hypercalcemia causes calcium deposits in soft tissues, renal calculi, altered neurological function with muscle weakness and atrophy, altered GI function with constipation, abdominal pain, anorexia, and altered cardiovascular system

3. Assessment

   a. General assessments include health history, VS, ECG, elimination pattern, nutritional status, activity–exercise tolerance, cognitive-perceptual and sensory function, and neuromuscular function

   b. Clinical manifestations: may be asymptomatic; polyuria (early sign) and renal calculi, anorexia, constipation, nausea, vomiting, abdominal pain (from peptic ulcer disease), generalized bone pain, pathologic fractures, muscle weakness and atrophy, CNS signs (depressed deep tendon reflexes, paresthesias, depression, psychosis) and cardiovascular changes (dysrhythmias, hypertension, increased sensitivity to digoxin)

   c. Diagnostic and laboratory test findings: elevated serum levels of total calcium; increased PTH; decreased phosphate; possible bone changes on skeletal x-rays and CT scan

4. Therapeutic management

   a. Mild

      1) Increase fluid intake, keep active with weight-bearing exercise to maintain calcium levels and decrease renal calculi formation

      2) Avoid thiazide diuretics, large doses of vitamins A and D, antacids containing calcium, and calcium supplements

   b. Acute

      1) Decrease serum level of calcium with IV normal saline (NS) infusions, diuretics, and phosphate replacement

      2) Surgery to remove involved parathyroid glands

      3) Medications to inhibit bone resorption and reduce hypercalcemia

5. Priority nursing problems: pain, reduced mobility, potential for injury, potential alteration in urinary elimination or constipation, inadequate knowledge

6. Planning and implementation

   a. Promote comfort and safety; client may need to walk with walker to prevent falls

   b. Strain all urine to detect calcium-based urinary stones

   c. Provide 2,000–3,000 mL of fluids daily as tolerated and a high-fiber diet

   d. Encourage progressive activity as tolerated, pacing activity with rest periods

   e. Promote nutrition and fluid and electrolyte balance; weigh daily

   f. Provide pre- and postoperative care as described earlier in section on thyroidectomy

   g. Prevent tetany caused by surgery or aggressive excretion of calcium through early detection of low serum calcium level; watch for numbness and tingling around mouth and fingertips, muscle twitching of extremities, change in voice, and positive Chvostek and Trousseau signs

7. Medication therapy: analgesics to control pain; diuretics and NS by IV infusion to excrete excess calcium; phosphate and calcitonin (Miacalcin) and bisphosphonates such as pamidronate (Aredia) and alendronate (Fosamax) may be used to inhibit bone reabsorption

8. Client education

   a. Instruct client on appropriate self-administration of medications and about hyperparathyroidism

   b. Instruct client about symptoms to report, including those for hypocalcemia, activity intolerance, and infection

9. Evaluation: client verbalizes pain control, understanding of medications, symptoms to report, postoperative care; and demonstrates appropriate wound care

B. **Hypoparathyroidism**

   1. Description: low PTH levels causing hypocalcemia, usually caused by inadvertent damage or surgical removal of all or part of gland during thyroidectomy

2. Etiology and pathophysiology: hypocalcemia raises threshold for excitability in nerve and muscle fibers causing fibers to be easily stimulated; could lead to life-threatening tetany

3. Assessment

   a. General assessments include health history, VS, ECG, elimination pattern, nutritional status, activity–exercise tolerance, cognitive-perceptual and sensory function, neuromuscular function

   b. Clinical manifestations: GI symptoms (abdominal pain, nausea, vomiting, diarrhea, anorexia), signs of hypocalcemia (anxiety, headaches, paresthesias, neuromuscular irritability with tremors, muscle spasms and tetany or seizures), possible difficulty swallowing, possible hoarse voice, sensation of tightness in throat, dry thin hair, patchy hair loss, ridged and brittle finger nails

   c. Diagnostic and laboratory test findings: decreased serum PTH, total calcium, free calcium; increased serum phosphate

4. Therapeutic management: supplemental calcium and vitamin D

5. Priority nursing problems: potential for injury, anxiety, inadequate knowledge

6. Planning and implementation

   a. Promote comfort and safety; client may need to walk with walker to prevent falls

   b. Encourage progressive activity as tolerated, pacing activity with rest periods

   c. Promote nutrition and fluid and electrolyte balance

7. Medication therapy: calcium supplement orally or by IV infusion; vitamin D orally to promote intestinal absorption of calcium

8. Client education

   a. Instruct client about hypoparathyroidism, to wear MedicAlert bracelet listing disease and medications, and about self-administration of medication

   b. Instruct client about symptoms to report (as noted above)

   c. Instruct client about diet high in calcium and vitamin D, identifying minimum daily intake; foods high in calcium include cheese, milk, turnip greens, almonds, collard greens, beans, peanuts, frankfurters, and bologna

9. Evaluation: client verbalizes understanding of disease, medications, diet, and the importance of wearing a medical alert bracelet; demonstrates appropriate meal planning

VI. DISORDERS OF ADRENAL GLANDS

A. Cushing's syndrome (adrenal cortex hypersecretion)

1. Description: hyperfunction of adrenal gland cortex causing elevated serum cortisol or ACTH levels

2. Etiology and pathophysiology

   a. Elevated serum cortisol causes life-threatening changes in physiological, psychological, and metabolic functioning

   b. Incidence is greater in women; usual age of onset is 30–50 years old

   c. Primary Cushing's syndrome (rare) is caused by a tumor of adrenal cortex

   d. Secondary Cushing's syndrome

      1) Disorder of pituitary or hypothalamus gland causing increased ACTH and hyperplasia of adrenal cortex; also called Cushing's disease

      2) An ectopic tissue such as an ACTH-producing cancer of lung, bronchus, or pancreas causes hyperplasia of adrenal cortex

   e. Iatrogenic (most common etiology): long-term use of glucocorticoid medication such as steroids

3. Assessment

   a. General assessments include health history, VS, activity tolerance, skin condition, elimination pattern, nutrition pattern, fluid and electrolyte balance, self-concept, and frequency of BG monitoring

b. Clinical manifestations: generalized weakness with muscle wasting, thin skin that bruises easily, emotional lability (mood swings), skin infections or poor wound healing, striae, hirsutism, hypertension, fluid overload, weight gain, osteoporosis, abnormal fat deposits (truncal obesity, moon facies, fat pad on back of neck), possible amenorrhea, impotence, or decreased libido

c. Diagnostic and laboratory test findings: elevated serum cortisol, sodium, glucose, calcium, and potassium; serum ACTH can be elevated or decreased; elevated urine 17 KS; positive ACTH suppression test; normal BUN

4. Therapeutic management is aimed at etiology and may include the following:
   a. Medications to suppress ACTH by pituitary gland or cortisol secretion by adrenal cortex
   b. Radiation therapy to pituitary gland
   c. Single or bilateral adrenalectomy or **hypophysectomy** (removal of pituitary gland) with cortisol replacement postoperatively
   d. Gradual reduction or withdrawal of corticosteroid drugs and administration of medications on alternate days to help minimize suppression of normal hormone production

5. Priority nursing problems: fluid overload, potential for injury or infection, possible body image alteration, inadequate knowledge

6. Planning and implementation
   a. Assist client to achieve fluid, electrolyte, glucose, and calcium balance
   b. Analyze daily weights and I & O
   c. Promote safety: uncluttered walking area, adequate lighting, assistive walking devices to prevent falls as needed, and use of stable, non-skid shoes/slippers
   d. Assist client to pace activities and rest to prevent fatigue
   e. Prevent infection before and after surgery: use standard precautions, provide aseptic wound care, and promote optimal nutrition with increased intake of protein, vitamin C and vitamin A
   f. Assist client to use effective coping strategies and encourage client to discuss feelings about change in physical appearance
   g. Preoperative care: ensure that client understands the planned surgical procedure, postoperative routines, and expected outcomes
   h. Postoperative care
      1) Promote effective breathing pattern by encouraging hourly client coughing and deep breathing exercises (clients with transsphenoidal surgery should avoid coughing)
      2) Explain that mouth breathing is necessary because of postoperative nasal packing after transsphenoidal surgery
      3) Assist with turning and repositioning every 2 hours, and encourage ankle dorsiflexion exercises hourly
      4) Promote wound healing by minimizing stress on incision line; after adrenalectomy, client should log roll to side to sit up at bedside and should do the reverse to recline; a client with a transsphenoidal incision should avoid blowing nose, sneezing, or coughing unless necessary
      5) Keep HOB elevated 30 degrees, and use aseptic technique for wound care
      6) Examine pituitary surgical wound for cerebrospinal fluid leak (pale yellow fluid that often forms a halo; if tests positive for glucose is most likely cerebrospinal fluid)
   i. Prevent Addisonian crisis related to treatments that stop or sharply decrease cortisol production: give IV normal saline infusion bolus and cortisol per prescriber's order for these symptoms: dry, tenting skin, decreased BP, increased pulse, decreased LOC, anorexia, and weakness

Practice to Pass

Why should the client taking glucocorticosteroids as replacement therapy or to treat an existing disease never miss a dose or suddenly stop taking the medication?

7. Medication therapy: may include metyrapone (Metopirone), which directly inhibits cortisol production and secretion by adrenal cortex; octreotide (Sandostatin), a somatostatin analog that suppresses ACTH secretion; and mitotane (Lysodren), which suppresses adrenal cortex function and decreases metabolism of corticosteroids, thus decreasing serum cortisol

8. Client education
   a. Information about Cushing's syndrome, to wear MedicAlert bracelet listing disease and medications, and self-administration of medication
   b. Symptoms to report to health care provider, such as hyperglycemia and hypoglycemia, and signs of infection
   c. Eat a diet high in protein and vitamins A, B and C to support immune system and support collagen formation needed for repair of body tissues, and take supplemental potassium and calcium
   d. Information about wound care and postoperative cortisol replacement as necessary

9. Evaluation
   a. Client verbalizes understanding of disease, medication, surgical procedure, planned outcomes, and demonstrates appropriate wound care
   b. Client attains and maintains normal cortisol level, glucose level, VS, and is free of infection
   c. Client implements safe behaviors to prevent falls, infection, and other injury

B. **Primary Addison's disease (adrenal cortex insufficiency)**
   1. Description: insufficient level of cortisol because of destruction of adrenal cortex, caused by autoimmune disorder, tuberculosis, septicemia, acquired immunodeficiency syndrome (AIDS), bilateral adrenalectomy, infiltrative diseases, treatment of Cushing's syndrome, and sudden cessation of long-term high dose steroid medication
   2. Etiology and pathophysiology
      a. More common in women age less than 60 years old
      b. Decreased aldosterone and cortisol levels lead to hyponatremia, **hyperkalemia** (high serum potassium), decreased extracellular fluid, decreased intravascular volume, decreased gluconeogenesis, hypoglycemia, and stress intolerance
      c. High ACTH level leads to hyperpigmentation from increased stimulation of melanocytes
   3. Assessment
      a. General assessments include health history, VS, LOC, mentation, skin, energy level, activity tolerance, orthostatic BP, ECG (electrocardiogram), nutrition pattern, and elimination pattern
      b. Clinical manifestations
         1) Include hyperpigmentation of skin (eternal tan), delayed wound healing, cardiovascular changes (tachycardia, dysrhythmias, postural hypotension), dehydration and hypovolemia, weight loss, anorexia, nausea, vomiting, diarrhea, depression, lethargy, emotional lability, confusion, muscle weakness and tremors, and muscle and joint pain
         2) Addisonian crisis: a life-threatening response to sudden withdrawal of steroids or exposure to any form of stress, trauma, or infection is manifested by high fever; weakness; severe, penetrating pain in abdomen, lower back, and legs; severe vomiting; diarrhea; severe hypotension, circulatory collapse, shock, and coma; treated with rapid IV replacement of fluids and glucocorticoids
      c. Diagnostic and laboratory test findings: decreased serum cortisol, glucose, and sodium; increased serum potassium and BUN; changes in ACTH levels (increased for primary adrenal insufficiency but decreased in secondary adrenal insufficiency); decreased urine 17 KS; no increase in cortisol with ACTH stimulation test; CT scan can be positive for intracranial lesions

4. Therapeutic management: replacement of corticosteroids and mineralocorticoids and increased sodium in diet

5. Priority nursing problems: potential for dehydration, potential for electrolyte imbalance (collaborative problem), inadequate knowledge, potential inability to manage treatment regimen

6. Planning and implementation
   a. Maintain fluid and electrolyte balance: analyze lab values, I & O, and daily weight; encourage 3,000 mL of daily oral fluid intake and added sodium in diet
   b. Promote safety: appropriate walking assistive devices, adequate lighting, clear area for walking, and appropriate slippers or shoes

7. Medication therapy: hydrocortisone (Cortef) to replace cortisol; fludrocortisone (Florinef) to replace mineralocorticoids

8. Client education
   a. Information about Addison's disease, symptoms to report (weight gain, easy bruising or bleeding, weakness, dizziness, lethargy, epigastric discomfort, and change in BP or pulse), need for lifelong medication and disease management, need to consult practitioner before taking any OTC medications, self-administration of medication, and plan for medication adjustment targeting stress response
   b. Wear MedicAlert bracelet listing Addison's disease, medications, and contact numbers
   c. Keep intramuscular cortisol available at all times
   d. Eat a diet that promotes immune system function and eat foods to increase sodium intake and decrease potassium intake

9. Evaluation
   a. Client demonstrates normal cognitive and mentation function, fluid and electrolyte balance, elimination function, and usual level of activity tolerance
   b. Client verbalizes understanding of medication, disease, stress management, symptoms to report, and wears MedicAlert bracelet
   c. Client demonstrates understanding of diet plan; has stable VS; is able to perform activities of daily living; has warm, dry, and elastic skin

C. **Adrenal medulla hyperfunction/pheochromocytoma (malignant hypertension)**

1. Description
   a. Increased level of catecholamine secretion in adrenal medulla results in increased sympathetic stimulation
   b. Rapid, acute hypertension occurs
   c. Is life threatening and should be treated within first hour

2. Etiology and pathophysiology
   a. Tumor(s) in adrenal medulla cause chromaffin tissue, located within adrenal medulla, to increase secretion of epinephrine and norepinephrine
   b. Increased levels of these catecholamines result in stimulation of sympathetic nervous system; the most dangerous result is rapid increased vasoconstriction causing acute hypertension
   c. May be precipitated by physical, emotional, or environmental stimuli

3. Assessment
   a. Clinical manifestations: BP will rapidly increase with systolic BP of 200–300 mmHg and diastolic BP of 150–175 mmHg, visual changes, headache, and LOC changes or confusion
   b. Diagnostic and laboratory test findings: urine and blood studies will show increased levels of catecholamines; renal CAT scans or imaging will show presence of tumor on adrenal gland(s)

4. Therapeutic management
   a. Surgical adrenalectomy usually removes one adrenal gland, decreasing catecholamine secretion

b. Medication therapy (see section to follow)
c. Management of stress
5. Priority nursing problems: potential for injury, inadequate knowledge, possible alteration in thought processes
6. Planning and implementation
    a. Preoperative and postoperative care for adrenalectomy
    b. Monitor BP
    c. Monitor for changes in LOC, confusion
7. Medication therapy: alpha- and beta-adrenergic blockers to decrease sympathetic stimulation and BP; drugs to suppress catecholamine synthesis (metyrosine [Demser])
8. Client education: report changes in vision or LOC, facial edema, headaches; take antihypertensive medications on time; avoid physical and emotional stress
9. Evaluation: client verbalizes importance of medication therapy; BP is maintained at normal levels

VII. DISORDERS OF PANCREAS

A. Diabetes mellitus (DM)
1. Description: pancreatic disorder characterized by insufficient or absolute lack of insulin production causing **hyperglycemia** (elevated BG), requiring lifelong lifestyle adjustments, and resulting in multisystem changes in health status (clients with DM are 2-4 times more likely to have heart disease or stroke, and significant incidence of blindness, nontraumatic amputation, and renal failure)
2. Etiology and pathophysiology
    a. The disease affects over 8% of population and is sixth leading cause of death in United States
    b. May be classified as type 1 or type 2
    c. Type 1: results from autoimmune (90%) or idiopathic destruction of beta cells of pancreas; has a genetic predisposition; can occur at any age but usually occurs in children and adolescents; is characterized by a lack of insulin production and resulting hyperglycemia and **ketosis** (ketones in blood resulting from gluconeogenesis of fats)
    d. Type 2: most common form; exact cause remains unknown although several theories are presented, including compromised ability of beta cells to respond to hyperglycemia, abnormal insulin receptors on cells, and peripheral insulin resistance; it has a genetic predisposition, can occur at any age, and is more common in obese clients, older adults, African Americans, Hispanic Americans, and Native Americans; it is characterized by hyperglycemia despite availability of endogenous insulin
3. Assessment
    a. General assessments include health history, cognitive and mentation function, pattern of weight loss or gain, nutrition pattern, elimination pattern, VS, skin/wound healing, eyes/vision, sensory perception, energy level, and activity tolerance
    b. Clinical manifestations
        1) Type 1: polyuria, polydipsia (excess fluid intake), **polyphagia** (increased food intake), weight loss, malaise, and fatigue
        2) Type 2: slower onset of manifestations; polyuria, polydipsia, blurred vision, fatigue, **paresthesias** (numbness, tingling, sensitivity), and skin infections; polyphagia and weight loss are uncommon
    c. See Figure 13-3 for an overview of early and late manifestations of DM
    d. Diagnostic and laboratory test findings: elevated random and/or fasting BG, possible positive serum ketones, elevated **glycosylated hemoglobin**, abnormal oral GTT, urine positive for glucose, and possible positive ketones or acetone

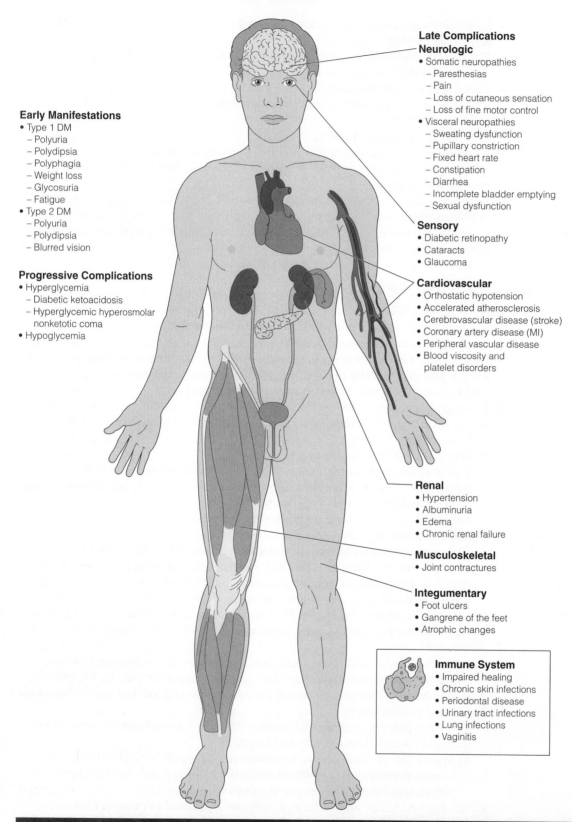

Early Manifestations
- Type 1 DM
  - Polyuria
  - Polydipsia
  - Polyphagia
  - Weight loss
  - Glycosuria
  - Fatigue
- Type 2 DM
  - Polyuria
  - Polydipsia
  - Blurred vision

Progressive Complications
- Hyperglycemia
  - Diabetic ketoacidosis
  - Hyperglycemic hyperosmolar nonketotic coma
- Hypoglycemia

Late Complications

Neurologic
- Somatic neuropathies
  - Paresthesias
  - Pain
  - Loss of cutaneous sensation
  - Loss of fine motor control
- Visceral neuropathies
  - Sweating dysfunction
  - Pupillary constriction
  - Fixed heart rate
  - Constipation
  - Diarrhea
  - Incomplete bladder emptying
  - Sexual dysfunction

Sensory
- Diabetic retinopathy
- Cataracts
- Glaucoma

Cardiovascular
- Orthostatic hypotension
- Accelerated atherosclerosis
- Cerebrovascular disease (stroke)
- Coronary artery disease (MI)
- Peripheral vascular disease
- Blood viscosity and platelet disorders

Renal
- Hypertension
- Albuminuria
- Edema
- Chronic renal failure

Musculoskeletal
- Joint contractures

Integumentary
- Foot ulcers
- Gangrene of the feet
- Atrophic changes

Immune System
- Impaired healing
- Chronic skin infections
- Periodontal disease
- Urinary tract infections
- Lung infections
- Vaginitis

Figure 13-3

Multisystem effects of diabetes mellitus

    4. Therapeutic management: consists of frequent monitoring of blood and capillary glucose, individualized diet plan, oral antidiabetic medication and/or insulin injections, and exercise plan

        a. Diet

            1) Follows the diet that is individualized for each client

            2) Caloric intake is based on individual needs, including possible weight loss needs

            3) Diet should consist of complex CHO in amounts tailored to individual need but ranging from 45–65% of daily diet, avoiding simple sugars; protein at 15–20% of caloric intake; saturated fat less than 10% of calories with cholesterol intake equal to or less than 300 mg/day; sodium intake 2,400–3,000 mg/day (same as for general population); dietary fiber 20–35 gm/day

            4) Diet needs to be tailored to individual and cultural preferences whenever possible to increase adherence

            5) Alcohol intake lowers BG levels and can cause hypoglycemia; it is not encouraged or totally prohibited; recommendation for men is no more than two drinks per day and for women is no more than one drink per day

        b. Oral antidiabetic medications

            1) Are used in type 2 DM only, and are indicated when diet and exercise alone fail to control BG levels

            2) Consist of many different categories; lower BG in different ways, including stimulating or increasing insulin secretion, preventing breakdown of glycogen to glucose by liver, increasing peripheral uptake of glucose by making cells less resistant to insulin, and blocking absorption of CHOs in intestine

            3) Instruct clients taking oral sulfonylureas that concurrent use of alcohol can cause a disulfiram-type reaction (hypoglycemia, flushing, headache, nausea, and abdominal cramps)

            4) Instruct client about risk of metabolic acidosis and to discuss with primary care provider about need to discontinue medicine if severe diarrhea, infection, or dehydration occur

            5) Instruct all clients about manifestations of both hyperglycemia and hypoglycemia, and appropriate corrective actions

        c. Insulin therapy

            1) Is used in type 1 DM or when diet, exercise, and oral agents are insufficient to control type 2 diabetes

            2) Different preparations of insulin are available to maintain near normal BG levels in relation to metabolic demands; insulin is classified according to its source, onset, peak, and duration of action

            3) Insulin is derived from animal (pork pancreas) or biosynthetic human insulin synthesized in the laboratory; standard practice is to prescribe human insulin

            4) Only regular insulin may be given IV; insulin preparations are usually given via subcutaneous (subQ) route; continuous subQ insulin infusion (CSII), also called insulin pump, is available to deliver a basal rate of insulin and allow for additional bolus doses of insulin based on requirements (for example, before a meal); insulin patch, nasal spray, and inhaled aerosolized preparations have been developed but are not yet widely used

            5) Instructions for client receiving insulin

                a) Storage: insulin in use should be stored at room temperature, away from direct sunlight, and should be replaced after 4 weeks; administration of cold insulin causes subcutaneous atrophy (lipoatrophy) or hypertrophy (lipodystrophy), which alters insulin absorption; extra vials of insulin not in use should be stored in refrigerator

  b) Preparation: note date of expiration; discard vial and use a new one if regular insulin appears cloudy; do not shake to avoid inactivation and/or formation of bubbles that lead to dosage errors; roll nonregular insulin gently between hands to evenly disperse suspended particles; draw regular (clear) insulin first when mixing it with other types of insulin; only mix insulins of same concentration (for example, U100 regular and U100 NPH) and from same source

  c) Injection: rotate injection sites to prevent lipoatrophy and lipodystrophy; do not inject insulin in an area that will be involved in exercise, as it will increase rate of absorption, onset and peak action

  d) Monitor for signs of hypoglycemia; have candy or foods with simple CHOs available

  e) If breakfast is delayed, also delay administration of rapid-acting insulin

  f) Monitor and record BG readings 30 minutes before each meal and bedtime as prescribed

  g) Sick day guidelines: BG levels increase with illness, even though food intake decreases; never omit insulin; monitor BG and/or urine ketones at least every 2–4 hours; drink plenty of fluids, try to drink at least one glass of water or other calorie-free, caffeine-free liquid each hour; substitute easily digested liquids or soft foods if solid foods are not tolerated; get as much rest as possible; contact provider for persistent fever, vomiting, shortness of breath, severe pain in abdomen, dehydration, loss of vision, chest pain, persistent diarrhea, BG levels above 250, or ketones in urine

5. Priority nursing problems: reduced coping, reduced ability to maintain health, potential for infection, potential for interrupted skin integrity, potential for injury, body image alteration, inadequate knowledge, altered sexual function

6. Planning and implementation

 a. Promote safety: use appropriate lighting; have client wear protective slippers, socks, and shoes that do not rub or impinge on skin; analyze symptoms, activity tolerance, and coping effectiveness; monitor BG levels; give medication and appropriate food and fluids

 b. Prevent infection: through appropriate skin and foot care, dental health, aseptic injection technique, and fingerstick glucose monitoring technique

 c. Identify appropriate glucose monitoring protocol and medication administration process depending client's vision, finances, finger dexterity, living environment, resources, literacy, lifestyle, personal values, work or school environment, and coping status

 d. Coordinate continuing care as appropriate for client's school, work, and other schedules, such as health club

 e. Promote acceptance and effective coping while living with DM

 f. Promote safety: early identification of hypoglycemia; check BG as scheduled; treat hypoglycemia with 15-gram CHO snack, such as 8 oz skim milk, 5 Lifesaver candies, 3 large marshmallows, 6 oz juice; and need to check BG

 g. Maintain hydration and avoid hyperglycemia; develop sick day protocol and exercise protocol with client

 h. Provide information about the actual and potential physical effects of DM on sexual function, including changes in desire and physical response; men who are impotent may benefit from drugs such as sildenafil (Viagra); women with decreased vaginal lubrication may benefit from use of vaginal lubricants (such as K-Y jelly) or estrogen cream

7. Medication therapy: oral antidiabetic medications and/or insulin by subcutaneous injection as previously discussed

8. Client education
    a. Information about type of DM, symptoms to report, self-administration of medication, BG monitoring, plan for regular exam by practitioner, need to wear MedicAlert bracelet indicating DM and medication prescription, need for lifelong medication management and lifestyle adjustments
    b. Foot care: keep feet clean and dry; inspect feet daily using mirror to see soles; protect feet by wearing shoes (allow ½- to ¾-inch toe room) or slippers at all times; avoid snug-fitting socks or stockings; use cotton or wool socks because they wick perspiration away from skin; cut toenails straight across with a clipper; consider professional care from a podiatrist
    c. Develop with client a plan for sick day management of DM: maintain food and fluid intake, continue to take insulin; increase frequency of BG monitoring, and monitor urine for ketones
    d. Develop with client a diet plan, including considerations for traveling, attendance at parties, sports, and other reasons for altered daily routine
    e. Symptoms of hypoglycemia (restlessness, irritability, weakness, hunger, nausea, pale diaphoretic skin, shakiness or trembling, headache, confusion, inability to concentrate, deteriorating LOC to coma, seizures), actions to take, causes of hypoglycemia, and methods to prevent its occurrence
    f. Prevention and management of acute complications (hyperglycemia, hypoglycemia, diabetic ketoacidosis, and hyperglycemic hyperosmolar nonketotic syndrome [HHNS]) and chronic complications (diabetic retinopathy, nephropathy, cardiovascular complications, peripheral vascular disease, periodontal disease, mood alterations, increased susceptibility to infection, decreased healing and neuropathies)
    g. Develop with client a plan for wellness, including exercise
        1) Daily cardiovascular exercise decreases risk for insulin resistance, reduces risk for complications, and improves BG management
        2) Check BG before exercise; check for urine ketones if fasting BG is 250 mg/dL or higher; call practitioner if ketones are present and avoid exercise
        3) Monitor for signs of hypoglycemia for up to 24 hours after extensive exercise
9. Evaluation
    a. Client verbalizes understanding of DM, medication prescription, need for regular exams, fingerstick glucose monitoring, lifestyle changes, foot care, sick day plan, diet plan, symptoms to report, symptom management, and wellness plan
    b. Client demonstrates effective coping through type of questions, normal glycosylated hemoglobin level, emotional response, and behavior
    c. Client wears appropriate medical alert bracelet, shoes, and clothing
    d. Client demonstrates appropriate meal planning for various situations, foot care, glucose monitoring process, and medication administration
    e. Client carries appropriate protein and CHO supplements to treat hypoglycemia
    f. Client keeps record of BG levels as instructed
    g. Client keeps regular appointments with practitioner

B. Diabetic ketoacidosis (DKA)
    1. Description: life-threatening metabolic acidosis resulting from persistent hyperglycemia and breakdown of fats into glucose, leading to presence of ketones in blood; can be triggered by emotional stress, uncompensated exercise, infection, trauma, or insufficient or delayed insulin administration
    2. Etiology and pathophysiology: hyperglycemia causes uncompensated polyuria, hemoconcentration, dehydration, hyperosmolarity, and electrolyte imbalance; a significant accumulation of serum ketones leads to acidosis; depression of central nervous system from accumulation of ketones and resulting acidosis may cause coma and death if left untreated

Practice to Pass

How does exercise affect glucose and insulin needs of a person with diabetes mellitus (DM)? If the client with DM is planning an intense exercise activity, when should he check his glucose?

3. Assessment
   a. General assessment includes health history, VS, cognitive function and mental status, glucose monitoring log and medication administration, oral intake for past 48 hours, elimination pattern, skin, oxygenation, breath sounds, respiratory effort and pattern, weight, and hourly I & O
   b. Clinical manifestations are primarily related to dehydration and metabolic acidosis: thirst, nausea, vomiting, malaise, lethargy, polyuria, warm dry skin with poor turgor, dry mucous membranes, flushed face, acetone (fruity, alcohol-like) odor to breath, Kussmaul respirations (deep, nonlabored, rapid respirations), abdominal pain, hypotension, rapid and weak pulse
   c. Diagnostic and laboratory test findings: BG greater than 250 mg/dL; plasma pH less than 7.35; plasma bicarbonate less than 15 mEq/L; serum ketones present; urine positive for glucose and ketones; may have abnormal serum sodium and chloride levels and hyperkalemia

4. Therapeutic management: IV fluids, electrolytes, and regular insulin to correct hyperglycemia and acidosis; supportive care as indicated such as NPO status, vasopressors, and possible ventilator to respiratory support
   a. Insulin
      1. A bolus of IV regular insulin is given followed by a continuous IV drip (0.1 unit/kg body weight) until BG drops to 250 mg/dL or pH = 7.30 or higher
      2. Once this is reached, regular insulin is given on a sliding scale according to BG
      3. As an alternative to IV infusion, intramuscular administration of insulin could be given hourly
      4. Bedside BG monitoring is done every 1–2 hours to monitor effectiveness of therapy
   b. Fluid therapy is instituted to treat severe fluid deficit (dehydration) that accompanies DKA
      1) Normal saline solution is usually given at a rate of 500–1,000 mL/hr for first hour, then is decreased to 200–500 mL/hr as tolerated by cardiac and respiratory systems
      2) When BG level reaches 250–300 mg/dL, a 5% glucose solution ($D_5\frac{1}{2}$ NS) is added to prevent hypoglycemia and to prevent cerebral edema
      3) Central venous pressure or hemodynamic monitoring may be necessary to evaluate effectiveness of therapy
   c. Potassium replacement is eventually necessary in DKA
      1) Initial serum potassium (K^+) level is usually elevated
      2) With reversal of acidosis and administration of insulin, K^+ shifts into intracellular compartment and serum level can drop rapidly
      3) Replacement therapy is instituted based on serum K^+ level and urinary output
      4) Electrocardiographic monitoring is initiated to monitor for cardiac changes due to hyper- and hypokalemia and to monitor effects of therapy on serum K^+ level
      5) Other electrolytes such as phosphate will also be replaced based on results of laboratory profiles; bicarbonate is not given routinely in DKA because rapid correction of acidosis can cause severe hypokalemia

5. Priority nursing problems: dehydration, potential for injury, potential for interrupted skin integrity, alteration in respiratory pattern, alteration in sensory perception, inadequate knowledge, anxiety

6. Planning and implementation
   a. Restore fluid, electrolyte, and glucose balance with IV infusions and medications; analyze I & O, BG, urine ketones, VS, oxygenation, and breathing pattern

b. Maintain skin integrity; promote healing of impaired skin; prevent infection by turning and positioning client every 2 hours; provide pressure relief as indicated; manage incontinence and perspiration with skin protective barriers and cleansing; provide appropriate nutrition and oxygen support

c. Promote safety by analyzing VS, client communication, LOC and emotional response, and activity tolerance; implement falls prevention measures

d. Assist client to verbalize concerns and cope effectively with illness and fears

e. Assist client to update MedicAlert bracelet information as appropriate

7. Medication therapy: IV infusion of NS, regular insulin and electrolyte replacement, including potassium replacement as previously described

8. Client education: the nature and causes of DKA (such as excess glucose intake, insufficient medications, or physiological and/or psychological stressors) and any new medications

9. Evaluation

a. Fasting BG is within normal range; serum pH is 7.35 to 7.45; urine is negative for ketones

b. Client's LOC and perceptual function returns to normal; elimination is normal; skin is intact; breathing pattern is normal; and fluid and electrolytes are balanced

c. Client verbalizes understanding of diabetic ketoacidosis, its causes, methods of prevention, and new medications

C. Hyperglycemic hyperosmolar nonketotic syndrome (HHNS)

1. Description: life-threatening metabolic disorder of hyperglycemia usually occurring with type 2 DM and triggered by medications, infection, acute illness, invasive procedure, or a chronic illness

2. Etiology and pathophysiology: increased insulin resistance (caused by one or more triggering situations) along with increased CHO intake lead to hyperglycemia, followed by polyuria, decreased plasma volume, decreased glomerular filtration rate (GFR) leading to glucose retention and sodium and water excretion; hyperosmolarity causes dehydration and reduced intracellular water (cell shrinkage)

3. Assessment

a. General assessments include health history, VS, LOC, cognitive and perceptual function, elimination pattern, skin, breathing pattern, breath sounds, reflexes, sensory and motor function, I & O, weight, electrocardiogram, communication, glucose monitoring log, nutrition pattern, and medications taken within 7 days

b. Clinical manifestations: symptoms gradually occur over 24 hours to 2 weeks and include altered LOC, dry skin and mucous membranes, polydipsia, hyperthermia, impaired sensory and motor function, positive Babinski sign, and seizures; metabolic acidosis is not present because there is sufficient insulin to prevent metabolism of fats

c. Diagnostic and laboratory test findings: elevated serum sodium, serum osmolality greater than 340 mOsm/L, BG greater than 600 mg/dL, abnormal serum potassium and chloride, no serum ketones, and normal serum pH

4. Therapeutic management: determine and treat triggering situation; treat co-existing health deviations; provide fluid and electrolyte replacement; provide regular insulin IV to normalize BG

5. Priority nursing problems: reduced cardiac output, dehydration, fever, alteration in sensory perception, potential for interrupted skin integrity, potential for aspiration, inadequate knowledge

6. Planning and implementation

a. Promote normalized cardiac output, sensory perceptual function, fluid and electrolyte balance, normal body temperature by administering fluids, medications, and analyzing I & O, weight, VS, lab values, sensory function, and cognitive function

b. Maintain intact skin by turning every 2 hours, use of pressure relief aids, nutritional support, use of skin moisturizers and barriers, and management of incontinence

c. Prevent aspiration by using appropriate feeding precautions, elevate head of bed 15–30 degrees during and after feeding for 1 hour; if BP too unstable to elevate head of bed with feeding, then withhold oral feedings

7. Medication therapy: IV infusion of NS to replace fluids and sodium, regular insulin IV to manage the hyperglycemia, and potassium to replace losses and shifts

8. Client education: information about HHNS, symptoms to report, and administration of new medications

9. Evaluation

a. Client returns to normal LOC and perceptual function, elimination function, and breathing pattern; fasting BG is within normal range, and skin is intact

b. Fluid and electrolyte levels are balanced

c. Client verbalizes understanding of HHNS, symptoms to report, and self-administration of new medications

D. Metabolic syndrome

1. Description: a group of metabolic risk factors occurring in a client that together form a strong risk factor for coronary heart disease; closely associated with insulin resistance

2. Risk factors for metabolic syndrome include increased waist circumference, hypertension, elevated serum triglycerides and fasting BG, and low HDL cholesterol

3. Measures to reduce weight, serum triglycerides, BG and to reduce BG should be used

Case Study

You have just finished discharging 2 clients to home when the charge nurse states that you will be receiving a client from surgery following a partial thyroidectomy. You will admit the client from the postanesthesia care unit and will be assigned as the primary nurse. Since you have 2 more work days scheduled, you will be assigned to this client for a total of 3 days.

1. What supplies should you ask the nurse assistant to place in the room?

2. Why should vital signs be assessed every 15 minutes for 2 hours, then hourly for 4 hours then every 2 to 4 hours for 24 hours?

3. What instructions about positioning and transferring the client to the bedside chair should you give to the nurse assistant?

4. What symptoms and signs should you assess?

5. What should the client understand about daily thyroid medication?

For suggested responses, see page 625.

POSTTEST

1 The client is 8 hours status-post (S/P) partial thyroidectomy for Graves' disease. What is the best documentation by the nurse of evaluation of outcome criteria for the nursing diagnosis Risk for Ineffective Airway Clearance?

1. Dressing is clean, dry, and intact; pain minimal and controlled; alert and oriented.
2. Vital signs stable; client supports neck with hand during change of position.
3. No tracheal stridor, speaks clearly, and denies numbness or tingling.
4. Balanced intake and output, vital signs stable, and alert and oriented.

2 Which of the following evaluation data would best lead the nurse to conclude that a client with hyperglycemic hyperosmolar state (HHS) has demonstrated improvement during the first 24 hours?

1. Alert and oriented, balanced intake and output, moist mucous membranes
2. Intake equals output, denies pain and shortness of breath
3. Alert and oriented, blood and urine without ketones, no orthostatic BP
4. Respirations easy and even, eats 50 to 75% of meals, vital signs stable

3 The nurse is caring for a client with type 1 diabetes mellitus. In developing a teaching plan about hypoglycemia as a complication of therapy, which sign or symptom should the nurse include?

1. Shakiness
2. Increased thirst
3. Fever
4. Fruity breath

4 The nurse is caring for a client who is taking 4 units of regular insulin and 30 units of NPH insulin at 8:00 a.m. The nurse keeps which of the following in mind regarding this regimen? Select all that apply.

1. Assess client for hypoglycemia shortly before lunch.
2. Assess client for hypoglycemia at dinnertime.
3. Shake vial of insulin to disperse insulin particles evenly.
4. Administer room temperature insulin only.
5. Neither insulin can be administered intravenously.

5 A postsurgical client is brought back to the nursing unit following a thyroidectomy. Which of the following methods is most reliable for the nurse use to assess for bleeding?

1. Inspect dressing for signs of hemorrhage.
2. Change dressing applied in the operating room.
3. Check latest hemoglobin to determine if there has been a drop in value.
4. Palpate back of neck and shoulders for evidence of bleeding.

6 A diabetic client with the flu asks why he should drink juices, check his fingerstick glucose every 4 hours, and take insulin when he is not eating and is vomiting. What would be the best explanation by the nurse?

1. "You need to prevent dehydration and monitor for hyperglycemia and excessive breakdown of fats for glucose."
2. "You need to check your blood glucose because vomiting could cause hypoglycemia and drinking fluids will prevent dehydration."
3. "Your body uses protein for energy during times of illness, causing increased ketones and hypoglycemia."
4. "If you can substitute water for the juices to prevent dehydration, then you won't need to check your blood glucose levels so often."

7 The client with diabetic ketoacidosis (DKA) is given intravenous (IV) normal saline infusion and regular insulin. In addition to hourly blood glucose monitoring, the nurse would look to what assessment data as early signs of clinical improvement?

1. Respiratory rate of 12 to 15 and normal BP in standing position
2. Temperature and pulse in normal range
3. Improved level of consciousness (LOC) and decreasing urine output
4. Client eats a full meal and respiratory rate is normal

8 The nurse is preparing to discharge a client newly diagnosed with diabetes mellitus. The client states, "I should eat a candy bar or cup of ice cream every time I feel shaky, hungry, or nauseated." What would be the best response by the nurse?

1. "Yes, a candy bar or cup of ice cream is needed to treat the hypoglycemia."
2. "Yes, you should eat the snack, and then have a meal as soon as possible."
3. "No, you should quickly eat a meal; the candy will cause hyperglycemia."
4. "No, these have too much sugar and fat; 5 Lifesavers candy or skim milk would be better choices."

9 The client had a bilateral adrenalectomy for Cushing's disease and is being sent home with a new prescription for hydrocortisone. Which statement by the client best indicates understanding of the drug and associated risks?

1. "I am taking this drug to replace the hormones usually secreted by the adrenal medulla."
2. "I should take this pill every morning before breakfast."
3. "This pill may cause weight gain, so I should exercise more and eat less."
4. "I should call the doctor if I think I am starting a cold, and I should not take aspirin."

10 The nurse is caring for a group of clients. Which client has manifestations characteristic of Cushing's disease?

1. Puffy or edematous facial characteristics
2. Thickening in the neck area
3. Eyes that are bulging
4. A "butterfly" rash on the face

➤ *See pages 440–442 for Answers and Rationales.*

ANSWERS & RATIONALES

Pretest

1 **Answer: 2** **Rationale:** Clients receiving doses of I-131 should not get pregnant during treatment because the radioactive iodine crosses the placenta and can damage the fetus. An egg allergy is irrelevant. Temperature is relevant to assess effectiveness of antibiotics on an active infection. Drinking from a straw is important for liquid iron administration. **Cognitive Level:** Applying **Client Need:** Reduction of Risk Potential **Integrated Process:** Nursing Process: Implementation **Content Area:** Pharmacology **Strategy:** The core issue of the question is specific knowledge of this medication. Consider the mechanism of action and side effects of radioactive iodine to select the correct response. **Reference:** LeMone, P., Burke, K., Bauldoff, G. (2011). *Medical-surgical nursing: Critical thinking in patient care* (5th ed.). Upper Saddle River, NJ: Pearson Education, pp. 496–497.

2 **Answer: 3** **Rationale:** The parathyroid glands, located near the thyroid gland, may have been injured or accidentally removed, resulting in hypocalcemia. Hypocalcemia is life threatening; thus it is important to identify early signs. Numbness and/or tingling of the mouth, face, or extremities are early symptoms of low serum calcium Reduced thyroid hormone levels are expected results of surgery. Hypoglycemia may occur as a result of long-standing untreated hypothyroidism but not as a result of a partial thyroidectomy. Laryngeal nerve damage is a possible complication of a thyroidectomy, but would be detected by hoarseness or weak voice. **Cognitive Level:** Applying **Client Need:** Physiological Adaptation **Integrated Process:** Nursing Process: Assessment **Content Area:** Adult Health **Strategy:** To answer this question, recall anatomy of the neck and adjacent structures and their function. The answer then requires an understanding of the possible complications of a thyroidectomy. **Reference:** LeMone, P., Burke, K., & Bauldoff, G. (2011).

Medical-surgical nursing: Critical thinking in patient care (5th ed.). Upper Saddle River, NJ: Pearson Education, pp. 499–502.

3 **Answer: 2** **Rationale:** Iodine intake is needed for the thyroid gland to produce thyroid hormone. Insufficient iodine intake leads to low thyroid hormone production and symptoms of hypothyroidism, which include constipation, weight gain, and muscle stiffness, among others. The other options are include symptoms characteristic of excess thyroid production. **Cognitive Level:** Applying **Client Need:** Physiological Adaptation **Integrated Process:** Nursing Process: Implementation **Content Area:** Adult Health **Strategy:** Specific knowledge is needed to answer the question. Recall the indications for iodine use and correlate the indications with the symptoms in the answer choices. **Reference:** LeMone, P., Burke, K., & Bauldoff, G. (2011). *Medical-surgical nursing: Critical thinking in patient care* (5th ed.). Upper Saddle River, NJ: Pearson Education, pp. 494–502.

4 **Answer: 2, 5** **Rationale:** Clients with Addison's disease should be assessed for signs of Addisonian crisis or adrenal insufficiency caused by an inadequate supply of corticosteroids. It frequently follows a stressful event such as surgery. Signs of Addisonian crisis include decreased urine output, decreased blood pressure, and altered level of consciousness. While excessive narcotic analgesia could cause lethargy, the Addison's disease must be addressed first because it is potentially life threatening. There is no indication of a central nervous system disorder. Arterial blood gases are done as needed based on client condition, but this assessment is nonspecific for this client. **Cognitive Level:** Analyzing **Client Need:** Physiological Adaptation **Integrated Process:** Nursing Process: Planning **Content Area:** Adult Health **Strategy:** Note that the core issue of the question is an action to take related to Addison's disease and the stress response (in this case a surgical procedure). The postoperative period is relevant in relation to the stress on the body and the body's ability to address that stress. Consider the effects of the sympathetic nervous system as part of the stress response in making your selection. **Reference:** LeMone, P., Burke, K., & Bauldoff, G. (2011). *Medical-surgical nursing: Critical thinking in patient care* (5th ed.). Upper Saddle River, NJ: Pearson Education, pp. 511–512.

5 **Answer: 1** **Rationale:** Research by the National Institute of Health and the American Diabetes Association demonstrates a strong correlation between chronic hyperglycemia and complications of retinopathy, nephropathy, and neuropathy. Thus, there is damage to the eyes, kidneys, and peripheral nerves, respectively. Lactic acidosis occurs with diabetic ketoacidosis and the metabolism of fat. Glucose monitoring is done for detection of hypoglycemia or hyperglycemia. Insulin is needed to carry glucose across the cell membrane into the cell, not to be transported in the blood. **Cognitive Level:** Analyzing **Client Need:** Reduction of Risk Potential

Integrated Process: Nursing Process: Implementation **Content Area:** Adult Health **Strategy:** Consider that knowledge of 2 content areas is needed to answer this question: complications of diabetes and the mechanism of action of insulin. **Reference:** LeMone, P., Burke, K., & Bauldoff, G. (2011). *Medical-surgical nursing: Critical thinking in patient care* (5th ed.). Upper Saddle River, NJ: Pearson Education, pp. 487, 522–523, 526.

6 **Answer: 4, 5** **Rationale:** In syndrome of inappropriate antidiuretic hormone (SIADH) there is excess secretion of ADH, which causes fluid retention, dilutes the plasma, causes suppression of aldosterone, and increases renal excretion of sodium. Water then moves into the cells from the plasma and interstitial spaces causing cellular edema, and dilutional hyponatremia results. The treatment is fluid restriction, possible diuretics, and occasionally hypertonic saline infusion rather than sodium restriction. Constipation and fatigue are unrelated to SIADH. **Cognitive Level:** Applying **Client Need:** Physiological Adaptation **Integrated Process:** Nursing Process: Evaluation **Content Area:** Adult Health **Strategy:** First, consider the role of aldosterone and ADH and the pathophysiology of syndrome of inappropriate antidiuretic hormone (SIADH). Recalling that this disorder is characterized by water retention, choose the option that would serve to counteract water intoxication or fluid overload most directly. **Reference:** LeMone, P., Burke, K., & Bauldoff, G. (2011). *Medical-surgical nursing: Critical thinking in patient care* (5th ed.). Upper Saddle River, NJ: Pearson Education, pp. 516–517.

7 **Answer: 3** **Rationale:** Diabetes insipidus (DI) can develop with head injury, tumors, and other conditions causing increased intracranial pressure. Excessive urine output of 350 mL/hr or more is a classic early symptom of DI. The specific gravity provides valuable information about renal function and response to antidiuretic hormone (ADH). Using critical inquiry to analyze the urine output, specific gravity, and other characteristics of the urine, the nurse assesses for classic signs of DI that can occur following a head injury. The client is excreting large volumes of water and may actually need an increase in fluids to maintain an adequate circulating volume. Giving fluids orally to someone with a decreased LOC increases the risk for aspiration. **Cognitive Level:** Analyzing **Client Need:** Reduction of Risk Potential **Integrated Process:** Nursing Process: Assessment **Content Area:** Adult Health **Strategy:** Assess before treating. First, recall the possible complications of a head injury and their symptoms. Choose the complication directly related to urine output and then determine the response that best addresses the increased urine output. **Reference:** LeMone, P., Burke, K., & Bauldoff, G. (2011). *Medical-surgical nursing: Critical thinking in patient care* (5th ed.). Upper Saddle River, NJ: Pearson Education, pp. 261, 517.

8 **Answer: 4** **Rationale:** Following removal of the pituitary gland, the client requires lifelong hormone replacement of thyroid, glucocorticoids, and gonadotropin. The client has not met the knowledge outcome and the follow-up does not last for only 1 year. Documentation related to the immediate postoperative time does not reflect the client's comments related to long-term outcomes. **Cognitive Level:** Applying **Client Need:** Physiological Adaptation **Integrated Process:** Communication and Documentation **Content Area:** Adult Health **Strategy:** The question has to do with long-term management, so eliminate any answer choices related to the immediate postoperative period. Then differentiate answers that do not reflect ongoing monitoring needed after removal of the pituitary tumor with potential lifelong interruption of pituitary functions. **Reference:** LeMone, P., Burke, K., & Bauldoff, G. (2011). *Medical-surgical nursing: Critical thinking in patient care* (5th ed.). Upper Saddle River, NJ: Pearson Education, pp. 515–516.

9 Answer: 2 Rationale: Diabetic ketoacidosis (DKA) is associated with excessive urine output, dehydration, and hypokalemia, making the nursing diagnosis Deficient Fluid Volume the highest priority. If left untreated, the dehydration can lead to decreased cardiac output and concurrent hypokalemia can lead to cardiac dysrhythmias. The decreased urine output is not caused by Impaired Urinary Elimination. Hyperventilation is a manifestation of the body's attempt to expel excess acid; it does not reflect an Ineffective Breathing Pattern in a client with diabetic ketoacidosis. Anxiety will need to be addressed but this is not the priority diagnosis. **Cognitive Level:** Analyzing **Client Need:** Physiological Adaptation **Integrated Process:** Nursing Process: Diagnosis **Content Area:** Adult Health **Strategy:** The question is directly related to the causes and effects of metabolic acidosis. Recall that diabetic ketoacidosis (DKA) is characterized by significant dehydration and hyperkalemia that could adversely affect cardiac output, while the change in breathing pattern is a compensatory mechanism rather than the primary problem. **Reference:** LeMone, P., Burke, K., & Bauldoff, G. (2011). *Medical-surgical nursing: Critical thinking in patient care* (5th ed.). Upper Saddle River, NJ: Pearson Education, pp. 541–542.

10 Answer: 8 Rationale: Calculate the dosage as shown: 138lbs divided by 2.2 (lbs per kg) = 62.727272 kg × 0.75 units/kg = 47.045454 units/day divided by 2 = 23.522727 divided by 3 = 7.840909. Rounded to the nearest whole number = 8. **Cognitive Level:** Applying **Client Need:** Pharmacological and Parenteral Therapies **Integrated Process:** Nursing Process: Implementation **Content Area:** Adult Health **Strategy:** Convert pounds to kilograms, then complete the calculation. Do not round until the end of the problem. **Reference:** LeMone, P., Burke, K., & Bauldoff, G. (2011). *Medical-surgical nursing: Critical thinking in patient care* (5th ed.). Upper Saddle River, NJ: Pearson Education, p. 531.

Posttest

1 Answer: 3 Rationale: Laryngeal nerve damage can occur as a result of a thyroidectomy manifested by stridor, a weak or a harsh voice. An early sign of edema of the larynx leading to airway obstruction is a tight-fitting dressing. Numbness or tingling or the extremities, lips, or mouth is a sign of hypocalcemia that can lead to respiratory distress due to tetany. The data in the other options are important routine postoperative assessments, but they do not relate specifically to a thyroidectomy and the client's airway. **Cognitive Level:** Applying **Client Need:** Reduction of Risk Potential **Integrated Process:** Nursing Process: Evaluation **Content Area:** Adult Health **Strategy:** This item requires knowledge of the common complications following a thyroidectomy. While all of the answer choices are important in postop care, select the one that is directly related to the surgery performed and to airway clearance. **Reference:** LeMone, P., Burke, K., & Bauldoff, G. (2011). *Medical-surgical nursing: Critical thinking in patient care* (5th ed.). Upper Saddle River, NJ: Pearson Education, pp. 497–499.

2 Answer: 1 Rationale: Hyperglycemic hyperosmolar state (HHS) results from hyperglycemia, causing excessive loss of water and retention of glucose that leads to dehydration, hypernatremia, and hypokalemia. Symptoms are dry, tenting skin, dry mucous membranes, altered level of consciousness, and hyperthermia. Findings that reflect normal fluid volume status and mental status reflect improvement in the client's condition. Ketones are not present in HHS; thus, monitoring for ketones is unnecessary. Pain, shortness of breath, and amount of dietary intake are unrelated to HHS. **Cognitive Level:** Applying **Client Need:** Physiological Adaptation **Integrated Process:** Nursing Process: Evaluation **Content Area:** Adult Health **Strategy:** The pathophysiology of HHS is directly related to dehydration. Select the answer choice that best represents improvement in this condition. **Reference:** LeMone, P., Burke, K., & Bauldoff, G. (2011). *Medical-surgical nursing: Critical thinking in patient care* (5th ed.). Upper Saddle River, NJ: Pearson Education, pp. 542–543.

3 Answer: 1 Rationale: The signs of hypoglycemia include hunger; shakiness; sweating; pale, cool skin; and irritability. These signs may be manifestations of impaired cerebral function from the hypoglycemia. The other options are all signs of hyperglycemia. **Cognitive Level:** Applying **Client Need:** Reduction of Risk Potential **Integrated Process:** Teaching and Learning **Content Area:** Adult Health **Strategy:** Differentiate the presentation for hypoglycemia and hyperglycemia. Select the answer choice that is consistent with the hypoglycemic symptoms. **Reference:** LeMone, P., Burke, K., & Bauldoff, G. (2011). *Medical-surgical nursing: Critical thinking in patient care* (5th ed.). Upper Saddle River, NJ: Pearson Education, pp. 542–543.

4 **Answer: 1, 2, 4** **Rationale:** Regular insulin is rapid acting with an onset of action within 15–30 minutes of administration. Its peak time is about 2–4 hours after administration, which is the most likely time for hypoglycemia to develop. NPH is an intermediate-acting insulin with an onset of action of 1–2 hours, a peak time of 6–8 hours, and a duration of 12–16 hours, so the client could also experience hypoglycemia at dinnertime. Insulin should be administered at room temperature to avoid lipid atrophy caused by cold insulin. Shaking of the insulin vial creates bubbles that lead to dosage error. The vial should be rolled between the hands. Only regular insulin can be administered IV, not NPH insulin. **Cognitive Level:** Applying **Client Need:** Pharmacological and Parenteral Therapies **Integrated Process:** Nursing Process: Implementation **Content Area:** Adult Health **Strategy:** The core issue of the question is knowledge of information related to both NPH and regular insulins. Evaluate each option and select the options that represent true statements. Recall the time for the onset of action and peak action and the correct procedure for administering insulin to help make the correct choices. **Reference:** LeMone, P., Burke, K., & Bauldoff, G. (2011). *Medical-surgical nursing: Critical thinking in patient care* (5th ed.). Upper Saddle River, NJ: Pearson Education, pp. 529–530, 532.

5 **Answer: 4** **Rationale:** The danger of hemorrhage is greatest during the first 24 hours following thyroid surgery. The tendency is for blood to follow gravity and flow down at the sides and posteriorly if hemorrhage occurs in the area of the neck. Inspecting the dressings for signs of hemorrhage may not reveal bleeding. Changing dressings immediately after surgery is not appropriate. A drop in hemoglobin may be a clue to bleeding but is not the best initial assessment action. **Cognitive Level:** Analyzing **Client Need:** Reduction of Risk Potential **Integrated Process:** Nursing Process: Assessment **Content Area:** Adult Health **Strategy:** Eliminate answer choices that are unrelated and take a significant amount of time that could pose a risk to the client. Select the answer choice that is immediate and reflects the placement of the dressing and client positioning. **Reference:** LeMone, P., Burke, K., & Bauldoff, G. (2011). *Medical-surgical nursing: Critical thinking in patient care* (5th ed.). Upper Saddle River, NJ: Pearson Education, p. 499.

6 **Answer: 1** **Rationale:** Starvation-induced ketosis can be prevented by drinking juices that equal the prescribed carbohydrate meal pattern. Fluids are needed to prevent dehydration and hyperosmolality, which could result from large fluid losses from persistent vomiting. The liver breaks down fats, not proteins, to form glucose for energy and ketones, leading to diabetic ketoacidosis (DKA). Vomiting causes loss of fluids and electrolytes, not hypoglycemia. **Cognitive Level:** Applying **Client Need:** Physiological Adaptation **Integrated Process:** Teaching and Learning **Content Area:** Adult Health **Strategy:** Select the answer choice that best reflect the pathophysiology of diabetes.

Both choices in an answer choice must be correct. **Reference:** LeMone, P., Burke, K., & Bauldoff, G. (2011). *Medical-surgical nursing: Critical thinking in patient care* (5th ed.). Upper Saddle River, NJ: Pearson Education, pp. 538–539.

7 **Answer: 3** **Rationale:** Level of consciousness (LOC) responds quickly to early changes in pH and restoration of fluid and electrolyte balance. In addition, urine output decreases as hyperglycemia resolves. The respiratory buffer system takes a few hours to respond to change in pH, and the respiratory rate is likely to come down just into normal range rather than drop to the lower end of normal. Dehydration is usually so severe that several hours of rehydration are needed to reduce pulse and resolve orthostatic BP. Eating a full meal is not an early sign of improvement. **Cognitive Level:** Analyzing **Client Need:** Physiological Adaptation **Integrated Process:** Nursing Process: Evaluation **Content Area:** Adult Health **Strategy:** Recall that the level of consciousness (LOC) is one of the last changes in the development of diabetic ketoacidosis (DKA) and the first to return to normal. Select the answer choice that is consistent with this fact. **Reference:** LeMone, P., Burke, K., & Bauldoff, G. (2011). *Medical-surgical nursing: Critical thinking in patient care* (5th ed.). Upper Saddle River, NJ: Pearson Education, pp. 539–542.

8 **Answer: 4** **Rationale:** The candy bar and ice cream may have too much glucose and fat, potentially leading to hyperglycemia or not being absorbed quickly enough to reverse the hypoglycemia. Immediate absorption of glucose is needed in hypoglycemia, which can be achieved with concentrated simple carbohydrates. A meal would not be absorbed quickly enough to raise the serum glucose. The client should also check the blood glucose within 15 minutes of taking glucose. **Cognitive Level:** Applying **Client Need:** Health Promotion and Maintenance **Integrated Process:** Nursing Process: Implementation **Content Area:** Adult Health **Strategy:** Differentiate the absorption rate for simple versus complex carbohydrates. Select the answer choice with the fastest absorption rate for immediate relief of symptoms. **Reference:** LeMone, P., Burke, K., & Bauldoff, G. (2011). *Medical-surgical nursing: Critical thinking in patient care* (5th ed.). Upper Saddle River, NJ: Pearson Education, pp. 543–544.

9 **Answer: 4** **Rationale:** Hypersecretion of the adrenal cortex (not the medulla) causes Cushing's disease. Normally, the secretion of cortisol is increased in response to stress, infection, or a significant increase in activity. Thus, the replacement dose during illness may need to be adjusted once a client's adrenal glands are removed. Hydrocortisone can irritate gastric mucosa, so clients should not take gastric irritants such as aspirin or nonsteroidal anti-inflammatory drugs (NSAIDs). Hydrocortisone is usually taken twice a day following an adrenalectomy. Weight gain may occur but is primarily related to sodium and water retention and should be reported to the health care provider. **Cognitive Level:** Analyzing **Client Need:** Physiological Adaptation **Integrated Process:** Nursing Process: Evaluation **Content Area:** Adult Health **Strategy:** Identify the hormone secreted by the adrenal medulla and cortex. Eliminate answer choices that refer to the adrenal medulla. Select the answer choice that minimizes the side effects of the hydrocortisone. **Reference:** LeMone, P., Burke, K., & Bauldoff, G. (2011). *Medical-surgical nursing: Critical thinking in patient care* (5th ed.). Upper Saddle River, NJ: Pearson Education, pp. 509, 513.

10 **Answer: 1** **Rationale:** A round "moon" face that appears puffy and edematous is characteristic of Cushing's syndrome. A thickening in the neck area is consistent

with a goiter, which is indicative of a thyroid disorder. Eyes that appear bulging is called exophthalmos and is seen in Grave's disease (hyperthyroidism). A butterfly rash across the bridge of the nose and cheeks is characteristic of systemic lupus erythematosus. **Cognitive Level:** Analyzing **Client Need:** Physiological Adaptation **Integrated Process:** Nursing Process: Assessment **Content Area:** Adult Health **Strategy:** Consider the pathophysiology of Cushing's disease to match the correct characteristic with expected signs and symptoms of the disorder. **Reference:** LeMone, P., Burke, K., & Bauldoff, G. (2011). *Medical-surgical nursing: Critical thinking in patient care* (5th ed.). Upper Saddle River, NJ: Pearson Education, pp. 494, 496, 507, 1375.

References

Adams, M., & Holland, N. (2011). *Pharmacology for nurses: A pathopshysiological approach* (3rd ed.). Upper Saddle River, NJ: Pearson Education.

Berman, A., & Snyder, S. (2012). *Kozier & Erb's fundamentals of nursing: Concepts, process, and practice* (9th ed.). Upper Saddle River, NJ: Pearson Education.

Burke, K. M., Mohn-Brown, E., & Eby, L. (2011). *Medical-surgical nursing care* (3rd ed.). Upper Saddle River, NJ: Pearson Education.

D'Amico, D., & Barbarito, C. (2012). *Health & physical assessment in nursing* (2nd ed.). Upper Saddle River, NJ: Pearson Education, Inc.

Ignatavicius, D. D., & Workman, M. L. (2013). *Medical-surgical nursing: Critical thinking for collaborative care* (7th ed.) Philadelphia: W. B. Saunders Company.

Kee, J. L. (2010). *Laboratory and diagnostic tests* (8th ed.). Upper Saddle River, NJ: Pearson Education.

Lehne, R. (2010). *Pharmacology for nursing care* (7th ed.). St. Louis, MO: Saunders.

LeMone, P., Burke, K., & Bauldoff, G. (2011). *Medical-surgical nursing: Critical thinking in patient care* (5th ed.). Upper Saddle River, NJ: Pearson Education.

Lewis, S., Dirksen, S., Heitkemper, M., Bucher, L., & Camera, I. (2011). *Medical surgical nursing: Assessment and*

management of clinical problems (8th ed.). St. Louis, MO: Elsevier.

McCance, K. L., & Huether, S. E. (2010). *Pathophysiology: The biologic basis for disease in adults and children* (6th ed.). St. Louis, MO: Mosby, Inc.

Osborn, K. S., Wraa, C. E., & Watson, A. (2010). *Medical surgical nursing: Preparation for practice.* Upper Saddle River, NJ: Pearson Education.

Smith, S. F., Duell, D. J., & Martin, B. C. (2012). *Clinical nursing skills: Basic to advanced skills* (8th ed.). Upper Saddle River, NJ: Pearson Education.

Hematologic Disorders

Chapter Outline

Overview of Anatomy and
   Physiology
Diagnostic Tests and
   Assessments

Common Nursing Techniques
   and Procedures
Red Blood Cell Disorders

Platelet and Coagulation
   Disorders
White Blood Cell and Lymphoid
   Tissue Disorders

Objectives

➤ Identify basic structures and functions of the hematologic system.
➤ Describe the pathophysiology and etiology of common hematologic
   disorders.
➤ Discuss expected assessment data and diagnostic test findings for
   selected hematologic disorders.
➤ Identify priority nursing problems for selected hematologic
   disorders.
➤ Discuss therapeutic management of selected hematologic
   disorders.
➤ Discuss nursing management of a client experiencing a
   hematologic disorder.
➤ Identify expected outcomes for the client experiencing a
   hematologic disorder.

NCLEX-RN® Test Prep

Use the accompanying online resource,
NursingReviewsandRationales, to test
yourself with hundreds of NCLEX®-style
practice questions.

Review at a Glance

anergy a decreased reaction to skin
sensitivity tests
bands granulocytes that are less
mature than a fully developed neutrophil
cheilosis one or more cracks in corners of mouth
consumption coagulopathy
another term for disseminated intravascular coagulopathy, a syndrome characterized by abnormal initiation and acceleration
of clotting and simultaneous hemorrhage
culling destruction of red blood cells
erythropoiesis production of red
blood cells
erythromyalgia burning sensation
of fingers and toes
ferritin a measure of iron in plasma,
which is also a direct reflection of total
iron stores

fibrinolysis process whereby a
clot is dissolved after tissue repair is
completed
glossitis smooth, sore, beefy red
tongue
hemarthrosis joint bleeding, swelling, and damage
hemostasis series of reactions that
lead to formation of a platelet plug and
then a clot where there is damage or
injury to an area
hypochromic having less pigmentation; refers to erythrocytes
leukocytosis abnormal elevation of
white blood cell count
leukopenia a decrease in number of
white blood cells
microcytic small in size; refers to
erythrocytes

plethora a ruddy (dark, flushed) color
of face, hands, feet, ears, and mucous
membranes resulting from engorgement
or distention of blood vessels
priapism abnormal, painful, continuous erection of penis
shift to the left an increase in
number of immature neutrophils resulting
from activation of bone marrow to produce
white blood cells in response to infectious processes
thrombocytopenia decrease in
number of platelets

PRETEST

1 A client asks the nurse why vitamin B_{12} is important for red blood cell (RBC) formation. The nurse includes in a response that vitamin B_{12} deficiency causes which change in RBCs?

1. Decreased mean corpuscular volume (MCV)
2. Increased hemoglobin in the RBC
3. Decreased DNA synthesis in the RBC
4. RBC is smaller in shape and deficient in hemoglobin

2 A nurse is discussing the role of hypoxia in red blood cell (RBC) production with a client. Which client statement reflects an accurate understanding of this information?

1. "Hypoxia stimulates the hemoglobin content of the RBC to increase."
2. "Hypoxia stimulates the release of erythropoietin in the kidneys."
3. "Reticulocytes become erythrocytes faster with hypoxia."
4. "RBC destruction is increased with hypoxia, thereby stimulating RBC production."

3 The nurse is caring for a client with leukemia who requires a bone marrow transplant. The nurse teaches the client and family that the following activities take place in what order? Place the options in the correct sequence.

1. Administer high doses of chemotherapy to destroy leukemic cells.
2. Find a donor with closely matched tissue antigens.
3. Administer the donor's bone marrow through a central venous line into the recipient.
4. Monitor for graft-versus-host disease.

4 A client with a hemolytic blood disorder presents to the primary care center with jaundice. The nurse explains to the client that the jaundice is most likely caused by which of the following?

1. Increased bilirubin in plasma
2. Increased haptoglobin in plasma
3. Hepatitis infection
4. Loss of plasma proteins

5 A nurse is evaluating the response of a client with anemia to therapy. Which laboratory test result would the nurse review that best reflects bone marrow production of red blood cells (RBCs)?

1. Hematocrit
2. Hemoglobin
3. Serum ferritin
4. Reticulocyte count

6 The nurse who is assessing a client with vitamin B_{12} deficiency anemia notes that the tongue is inflamed. What other finding should the nurse assess for that is unique to vitamin B_{12} deficiency?

1. Shortness of breath
2. Pallor of the skin
3. Peripheral neuropathies
4. Tachycardia

7 The nurse is teaching a client about measures to increase the absorption of the prescribed oral iron preparation. Which of the following instructions would the nurse give to the client?

1. Take the medicine with milk.
2. Take the pill with a drink that contains Vitamin C.
3. Take the iron with meals.
4. Take the iron shortly after meals.

8 The nurse is caring for a client with a diagnosis of disseminated intravascular coagulopathy (DIC). The client's spouse asks why heparin has been ordered. The nurse's response would incorporate which of the following points? Select all that apply.

1. Maintaining tissue perfusion
2. Preventing occlusion in the microcirculation
3. Preserving the myocardium
4. Dissolving clots that have formed in the large vessels
5. Preventing deep vein thrombosis (DVT) in the legs

9 Which of the following food choices made by a client with anemia best indicates that the nurse's instruction about foods high in iron has been successful?

1. Oranges and grapefruits
2. Spinach and broccoli
3. Eggs, milk, and milk products
4. Liver and muscle meats

10 A nurse is preparing to administer an intramuscular (IM) dose of iron to a client with anemia. Which of the following precautions should the nurse take?

1. Administer drug utilizing a Z track technique.
2. Use a 1-inch, 19-gauge needle.
3. Administer drug deep in the deltoid muscle.
4. Massage area vigorously after administering the iron.

➤ *See Pages 479–480 for Answers and Rationales.*

I. OVERVIEW OF ANATOMY AND PHYSIOLOGY

A. Hematopoietic (blood-producing) system

1. Bone marrow (myeloid)—where blood cells form; all blood cells originate from stem cells in bone marrow (see Figure 14-1)
2. Lymphoid tissues (lymphoid)—where white blood cells mature and circulate

B. Blood components

1. Plasma: straw-colored liquid portion of blood in which cells and platelets are suspended; makes up approximately 50–55% of a blood sample; consists of water (approximately 92%), amino acids, proteins, carbohydrates, lipids, vitamins, hormones, electrolytes, and cellular wastes
2. Serum is essentially same as plasma only without fibrinogen and clotting factors; if whole blood is allowed to clot and clot is removed, remaining fluid is known as serum
3. Blood cells (red and white) along with platelets comprise the remaining blood sample
4. Blood volume is approximately 8% of total body weight
5. Blood functions include transporting oxygen (O_2), nutrients, hormones, and metabolic wastes; protecting against invasion of pathogens; maintaining blood coagulation; and regulating fluids, electrolytes, acids, bases, and body temperature

C. Red blood cells (RBCs)

1. Non-nucleated, biconcave, disc-shaped cells also known as erythrocytes; make up 99% of blood cells; shape serves to increase surface area for diffusion of O_2
2. Production of RBCs, also called **erythropoiesis**, is stimulated by tissue hypoxia; kidneys release erythropoietin in response to tissue hypoxia; this stimulates red bone marrow to produce RBCs (see Figure 14-2)
3. RBCs are released into circulation as reticulocytes, which mature in blood or spleen within 24–48 hours; reticulocyte count serves as an index of erythropoietic activity of bone marrow; normal reticulocyte count is 1% of total RBC count
4. Hemoglobin is contained within RBCs and is the O_2-carrying unit of RBCs; it also carries carbon dioxide to lungs; the rate at which hemoglobin is produced depends upon availability of iron for synthesis
5. Process of destruction of RBCs is called **culling**; an RBC has an approximate life span of 120 days; RBC destruction occurs at same rate as RBC production (1%)
6. Phagocytic cells in liver, spleen, bone marrow, and lymph nodes recognize, ingest, and destroy senescent (aging) RBCs; amino acids (from globulin) and iron from the heme unit are spared; heme unit is converted into bilirubin, which is insoluble in plasma and is called unconjugated or indirect bilirubin; accumulation of indirect bilirubin in plasma causes jaundice; most bilirubin attaches to plasma proteins for transport to liver where it is conjugated with glucorinide; this forms conjugated bilirubin or direct bilirubin, which is water-soluble and is excreted in bile

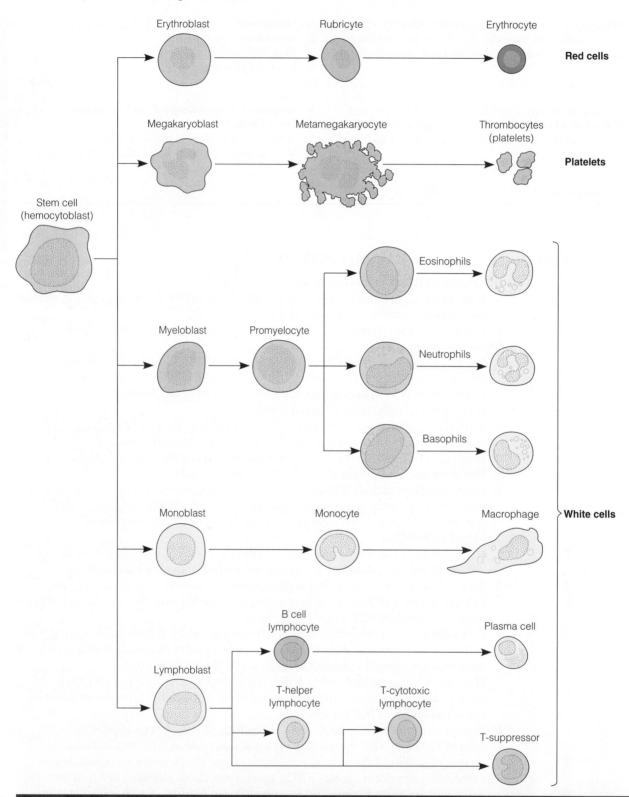

Figure 14-1

Blood cell formation from stem cells. Regulatory factors control the differentiation of stem cells into blasts. Each of the five kinds of blasts is committed to producing one type of mature blood cell. Erythroblasts, for example, can differentiate only into RBCs; megakaryoblasts can differentiate only into platelets.

Bone marrow ———————————————————————————————— **Blood stream** ——→

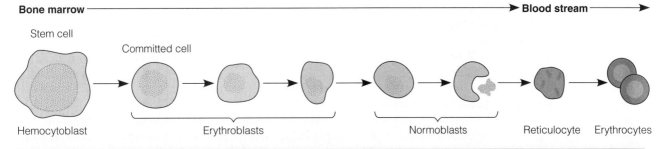

Figure 14-2

Erythropoiesis. RBCs being formed within the bone marrow as erythroblasts. These mature into normoblasts, which eventually eject their nucleus and organelles to form reticulocytes. The reticulocytes mature within the blood or spleen and become erythrocytes.

7. RBCs rely on glucose and the glycolytic pathway for its metabolic needs; depletion of these sources leads to premature RBC death
8. Maturation of RBCs requires certain vitamins and minerals; cyanocobalamin or vitamin B_{12} is referred to as the *maturation factor*; lack of this vitamin causes RBCs to become larger (megaloblasts), oval, and irregular; this morphologic characteristic causes them to have a shorter lifespan; folic acid (pteroyl glutamic acid) is also required for RBC maturation

D. **White blood cells (see also Chapter 11)**
   1. White blood cells (WBCs) are also referred to as leukocytes
   2. There are 2 types of leukocytes: granulocytes and agranulocytes (which includes monocytes and lymphocytes); leukocyte production is stimulated by granulocyte/ macrophage colony stimulating factor (GM-CSF) and granulocyte colony-stimulating factor (G-CSF); granulocytes mature fully before being released into blood stream
   3. Granulocytes contain granules in their cytoplasm and act as phagocytes; 3 types of granulocytes are neutrophils, eosinophils, and basophils, which are referred to as polymorphonuclear leukocytes (PMNs)
      a. Neutrophils: act as phagocytes and are first to arrive at site of injury; an increased number is seen with inflammation; develop from metamyelocytes and become bands; **bands** are granulocytes that are less mature than a fully developed neutrophil; a **shift to the left** describes an increase in immature neutrophils resulting from activation of bone marrow to produce WBCs in response to infectious processes; as bands mature, nuclei become segmented and develop into neutrophils, which is why neutrophils are often referred to as "segs"; a neutrophil's lifespan is 10 hours
      b. Eosinophils are also phagocytes but not as efficient as neutrophils; they are able to engulf antigen–antibody complexes from allergic responses and protect against parasitic infections
      c. Basophils contain histamine, heparin, serotonin, and other inflammatory mediators; these are similar to mast cell activity seen in allergic and inflammatory reactions; basophils have limited phagocytic activity
   4. Monocytes
      a. Large phagocytic cells produced in bone marrow; once they exit circulation, they reside in tissues to become macrophages
      b. Macrophages are responsible for removing dead and senescent cells and are able to engulf microorganisms

    5. Lymphocytes
       a. Originate primarily from lymph nodes and also from bone marrow
       b. There are 2 types of lymphocytes: T lymphocytes and B lymphocytes
       c. T lymphocytes originate from thymus; they are involved in cell-mediated immunity
       d. B lymphocytes are involved in humoral immunity

E. Platelets (thrombocytes)
    1. Most platelets circulate in bloodstream while some are in spleen; approximately 20,000–40,000 new platelets per cubic millimeter (mm^3) of blood are produced each day; life span of platelets is approximately 10 days; production is controlled by thrombopoietin, as number of circulating platelets decrease, release of thrombopoietin increases
    2. Major function of platelets is to maintain hemostasis (control of bleeding) and coagulation; because they are able to plug breaks in blood vessels, they are able to maintain integrity of these vessels
    3. Platelets also release thromboplastin (factor III) necessary for conversion of prothrombin to thrombin (first step of coagulation mechanism)

F. Normal clotting mechanisms
    1. **Hemostasis** and coagulation refer to a series of reactions that lead to aggregation of platelets and clot formation in an area of damage or injury
    2. Clot formation and breakdown involves 5 stages
       a. First 3 stages involve clot formation: vascular spasm, formation of a platelet plug with activation of clotting factors, and formation of fibrin clot (through either the intrinsic or extrinsic pathways; either pathway ends in a common pathway, a process known as coagulation cascade) (see Figure 14-3)
       b. Fourth stage is clot retraction, followed by fifth stage of clot dissolution; **fibrinolysis** is a process whereby a clot is dissolved after tissue repair is completed; plasminogen, which is present in a blood clot, is transformed into plasmin; plasmin dissolves fibrin strands of clot; fibrinolysis continues until blood clot is dissolved

II. DIAGNOSTIC TESTS AND ASSESSMENTS

    A. Red blood cell count (see Table 14-1)
    B. Hemoglobin and hematocrit
       1. Hemoglobin (Hgb) level measures amount of Hgb available in circulation, which is the gas-carrying (O_2/CO_2) capacity of an RBC
       2. Hematocrit is the ratio of RBC volume to volume of whole blood
    C. RBC indexes
       1. MCV (mean corpuscular volume): estimates size of RBC and helps determine causes of anemia; findings include normocytic, microcytic (small), and macrocytic (large)
       2. MCH (mean corpuscular hemoglobin): measures content of Hgb in RBCs from a single cell
       3. MCHC (mean corpuscular hemoglobin concentration): a more accurate measurement of Hgb content of RBC as it measures the entire volume of RBCs
    D. Serum ferritin, transferrin, and total iron-binding capacity (TIBC): these tests are used to evaluate iron levels; ferritin measures iron in plasma, which is also a direct reflection of total iron stores; transferrin is the major iron-transport protein
    E. White blood cell count (WBC)
       1. Abnormal elevation of WBC is referred to as **leukocytosis**
       2. **Leukopenia** is a decrease in number of WBCs; agranulocytosis is severe neutropenia with fewer than 200 cells/mm^3
       3. Differential count refers to breakdown of different types of cells

Figure 14-3

Flow diagram of factor activation leading to clot formation. Clotting may be mediated by chemical factors in either of 2 independent pathways: the longer intrinsic pathway and the "short-cut" extrinsic pathway. Both pathways eventually activate factor X, which begins the series of events leading to clot formation. Once factor X is activated, 4 sequential steps occur: (1) Factor X combines with other factors to form prothrombin activator; (2) prothrombin activator transforms fibrinogen into long fibrin strands; and (3) thrombin also activates factor XIII, which (4) draws the fibrin strands together into a dense meshwork. The complete process of clot formation occurs within 3 to 6 minutes after blood vessel damage.

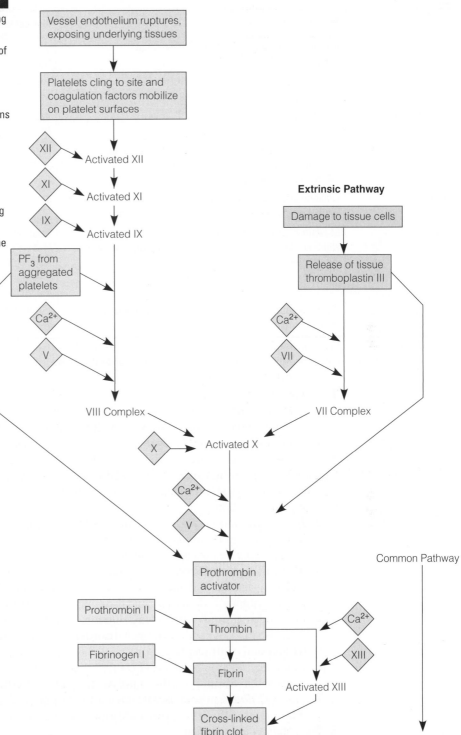

Table 14-1 Complete Blood Count (CBC)

Component	Purpose	Normal Values
Hemoglobin (Hb)	Measures the capacity of the hemoglobin to carry gases	Women: 12–16 g/dL Men: 13.5–18 g/dL
Hematocrit (Hct)	Measures packed cell volume of RBCs, expressed as a percent of the total blood volume	Women: 38%–47% Men: 40%–54%
Total RBC count	Counts number of circulating RBCs	Women: 4–$5 \times 10^6/\mu L$ Men: 4.5–$6 \times 10^6/\mu L$
Red cell indices: MCV 10^6 MCH	Determines relative size of MCV (mean corpuscular volume) Measures average weight of Hb/RBC (MCH = mean corpuscular hemoglobin)	82–98 fl 27–29 pg
MCHC	Evaluates RBC saturation with Hb (MCHC = mean corpuscular hemoglobin concentration)	32%–36%
WBC count	Measures total number of leukocytes (total count) and whether each kind of WBC is present in proper proportion (differential)	Total WBC count: 4000–11,000/μL $(4$–$11 \times 10^9/L)$ WBC differential: Neutrophils: 50%–70% Eosinophils: 2%–4% Basophils: 0%–2% Lymphocytes: 20%–40% Monocytes: 4%–8%
Platelets	Measures number of platelets available to maintain clotting functions	150,000–400,000/μL $(150$–$400 \times 10^9/L)$

Source: LeMone, Priscilla; Burke, Karen M.; Bauldoff, Gerene, *Medical-Surgical Nursing: Critical Thinking in Patient Care*, 5th Ed., © 2011. Reprinted and Electronically reproduced by permission of Pearson Education, Inc., Upper Saddle River, New Jersey.

F. **Coagulation studies**

1. *Bleeding time*: normal range is 1–4 minutes; is used in evaluation of platelet function; extended bleeding times are seen with thrombocytopenia and aspirin therapy
2. *Prothrombin time (PT)*: evaluates speed of blood clotting; normal range is 11–16 seconds; PT evaluates extrinsic coagulation pathway, which includes factors I, II, V, VII, X; International Normalized Ratio (INR) is often used now instead of PT because it is a standardized value (therapeutic range often varies from 2–3 depending on condition)
3. *Partial thromboplastin time (PTT)*: normal range is 60–70 seconds, which evaluates intrinsic coagulation pathway or fibrin clot formation
4. *Activated partial thromboplastin time (APTT)*: normal range is 30–45 seconds; is a modified PTT, preferred because it is quicker to perform; APTT is used in heparin therapy and in evaluation of hemophilia; APTT is increased in anticoagulation therapy, liver disease, vitamin K deficiency, and disseminated intravascular coagulopathy (DIC)
5. *Fibrinogen*: normal range is 150–400 mg/dL; it is a soluble plasma protein that is decreased in DIC and fibrinogen disorders and increased in acute infections, hepatitis, and oral contraceptive use
6. *Fibrin degradation products (FDP)*: normal value is less than 10 mcg/mL; FDP is increased in fibrinolysis, thrombolytic therapy, and DIC
7. *Fibrin D-dimer*: normal is 0-0.5 mcg/mL; D-dimer is the most sensitive indicator to differentiate DIC from primary fibrinolysis; it is elevated in DIC

G. **Bone marrow examination**

1. Evaluates blood-forming tissue to diagnose multiple myeloma, aplastic anemia, Hodgkin's disease, metastatic cancer, and leukemia; is also used to assess effectiveness of therapy for leukemias
2. Specimens obtained during a bone marrow examination may include those obtained by aspiration or biopsy

3. Sites for bone marrow aspiration may include posterosuperior iliac spine, iliac crest, sternum, and tibia

4. Aspiration is the most common procedure for obtaining a marrow sample

5. Client is positioned based on site selected by health care provider; skin and periosteum are anesthetized to decrease pain with anesthetic such as procaine; the marrow aspiration needle is then inserted; after marrow cavity is entered, marrow stylet is removed from needle and a sterile syringe is attached; syringe plunger is drawn back until marrow appears in syringe

6. During withdrawal of aspirate, client will experience sharp pain often described as a burning pain

Practice to Pass

A client undergoes a bone marrow biopsy. What nursing interventions should you implement?

7. After needle is removed, apply a sterile pressure dressing over puncture site for 5–10 minutes, where only minimal bleeding should occur; if client has thrombocytopenia, apply pressure for a longer period; position client supine to enhance pressure to site (prone if posterior iliac crest used)

8. Check agency procedure manual as to disposition of specimens

9. Most clients experience little, if any, pain or discomfort after procedure; some report tenderness and ache at aspiration site for a few days; instruct to monitor for bleeding for 24 hours

10. Procedure for a bone marrow biopsy is essentially same as for aspiration but a small incision is made over bone; the biopsy needle most commonly used is a Jamshidi needle, which allows a second needle, called a stylet, to be inserted within initial biopsy needle and a core of marrow to be collected and withdrawn through sleeve of needle; after the procedure, clients are assessed for bleeding from puncture site

H. Lymphangiography

1. Is visualization of lymph system radiographically after injection of a dye

2. It is used to stage Hodgkin's and non-Hodgkin's lymphoma, assess metastasis to lymph nodes, and identify cause of lymphedema

3. Ask about allergies to iodine or contrast media used in previous x-rays; explain that blue contrast dye may discolor urine and possibly skin for a few days.

4. Have client void prior to procedure

5. Postprocedure monitor for dyspnea, pain, and hypotension; assess incision sites for infection and assess for leg edema

I. Lymph node biopsy

1. Can either be done utilizing a closed needle biopsy done at bedside or an open excisional biopsy performed in operating room

2. Purpose is to obtain lymph tissue for histologic analysis

3. Use sterile technique when changing dressings

III. COMMON NURSING TECHNIQUES AND PROCEDURES

A. Administration of blood and blood products

1. Check agency policy and procedure pertaining to blood transfusion and transfusion of blood products (see Table 14-2)

2. Verify prescription for transfusion, noting blood product ordered, time specified for transfusion (if any), and any medications to be given before transfusion

3. Check for religious or cultural considerations and that client has given consent for receiving blood transfusion; assess for any previous reactions to blood and explain procedure

4. Check that a typing and crossmatch has been performed

Table 14-2	Volume Resuscitation Therapies		
Component	**Indications**	**Advantages**	**Disadvantages**
Ringer's lactate	• Restoration of circulating volume • Replacement of electrolyte deficits	• Good availability • Safe to use • Low cost • Aids in buffering acidosis	• Rapid movement from the intravascular to the extravascular space, leading to three or more times requirement for replacement
Normal saline	• Restoration of circulating volume • Vehicle compatible with administration of blood	• Good availability • Low cost • Safe to use	• Hyperchloremic acidosis associated with prolonged use of sodium solutions
Whole blood	• Replaces blood volume and O_2-carrying capacity in hemorrhage and shock	• Contains RBCs, plasma proteins, clotting factors, and plasma	• Contains few platelets or granulocytes; deficient in clotting factors V and VII • Greatest risks are for incompatibility or circulatory overload • Risk of transmitting blood-borne pathogens
Packed red blood cells (RBCs)	• Restoration of intravascular volume • Replacement of O_2-carrying capacity	• One unit of RBCs should increase the hemoglobin of a 70 kg adult by approximately 1 gm/dl in the absence of volume overload or continuing blood loss.	• Red cells require compatibility testing • Risk of transmitting blood borne pathogens • Should be warmed to prevent hypothermia • Contains little or no clotting factors
Platelets	• Significant thrombocytopenia (platelet count less than 20,000–50,000 per mm^3) • Continued hemorrhage	• Compatibility testing is not required • Typical platelet transfusion should raise the platelets of a 70 kg adult approximately 30,000–50,000/UL	• Post exposure prophylaxis with anti-Rh immune globulin should be considered following Rh+ platelet transfusion to an Rh− woman • Risk of transmitting blood-borne pathogens
Albumin	• Expends blood volume in shock and trauma	• Good availability	• Is not a substitute for whole blood • Risk of hypersensitivity reactions • Risk of transmitting blood-borne pathogens
Fresh frozen plasma (FFP)	• Documented coagulopathy • Restoration of clotting factors • Supplies plasma proteins	• Cross matching and Rh compatibility is not required	• Must be thawed in a 37°C water bath for approximately 30 minutes • Should be ABO compatible • Risk of transmitting blood-borne pathogens
Cryoprecipitate	• Coagulopathy with low fibrinogen • Restoration of fibrinogen	• Rh type not important	• Risk of transmitting blood-borne pathogens • Contains hemagglutinins • If large volume of ABO incompatible cryoprecipitate are administered intravascular hemolysis can occur

Source: LeMone, Priscilla; Burke, Karen M.; Bauldoff, Gerene, *Medical-Surgical Nursing: Critical Thinking in Patient Care*, 5th Ed., © 2011. Reprinted and Electronically reproduced by permission of Pearson Education, Inc., Upper Saddle River, New Jersey.

5. Obtain pretransfusion vital signs, noting especially temperature; report elevation of 100°F or higher prior to obtaining blood from blood bank

6. Ensure intravenous (IV) access with an 18- or 19-gauge catheter; prepare IV equipment with normal saline (dextrose can cause clumping of RBCs and distilled water causes hemolysis); use a Y-tubing with a blood filter

7. Obtain blood from blood bank when an IV access line is available; return blood to blood bank immediately if transfusion is not possible; blood may not be returned to blood bank after 20 minutes; do not keep blood or blood products in nursing unit refrigerator; blood is refrigerated under strict and controlled conditions only in blood bank or in a special blood bank refrigerator on selected specialty nursing units

8. Validate data on blood or blood product with another nurse; client's ID bracelet should match blood bank number on unit of blood

9. Validate with another nurse that client's name, ID number, blood type, and Rh match unit of blood to be transfused

10. Note expiration date indicated on blood product

11. Observe unit of blood for bubbles or discoloration; return blood to blood bank if a break in bag is noted or if signs of contamination are evident

12. Obtain vital signs 15 minutes after transfusion is initiated and immediately after completion of transfusion; any increase of 2°F in client's temperature may indicate a transfusion reaction and should be reported to prescriber

13. Start blood transfusion slowly, administering 25–50 mL (maximum rate of 2 mL/minute) during first 15 minutes (when most untoward reactions occur); stay with client during this period of time; trauma clients in life-threatening situations may require more rapid infusions, rapid infusions may need to be warmed to prevent hypothermia

14. Do not administer any medications through blood transfusion tubing; use tubing specific for blood product being transfused; a blood filter is used to prevent clots and other particles from entering venous system

15. Use only agency-approved blood-warming devices; do not warm blood in hot water or microwave ovens

16. After first 15 minutes increase rate of infusion to 250–500 mL/hour (unless there is a danger of fluid volume overload); blood products should not be infused longer than 4 hours (increasing time at room temperature increases risk of bacterial contamination and deterioration of blood)

17. Discard tubings and bags used for transfusion in a biohazard receptacle

18. Follow agency protocol for any suspected transfusion reactions

B. **Protocol for suspected blood transfusion reaction**
   1. Types of reactions
      a. Febrile reaction: most common reaction; caused by antibodies against donor's WBCs and most commonly occurs in first 15 minutes of transfusion; manifestations include fever and chills; using leukocyte-poor blood helps to avoid this reaction
      b. Hypersensitivity reaction: caused by antibodies against proteins in donor's blood and may occur during or after transfusion; manifested by wheals (urticaria) and itching
      c. Hemolytic reaction: most dangerous transfusion reaction, usually results from ABO (antigen) incompatibility; RBCs clump and block blood flow to vital organs; usually begins after infusion of 100–200 mL of incompatible blood; manifestations include flushing, headache, burning along vein, urticarial, chills, fever, lumbar pain, abdominal pain, chest pain, nausea and vomiting, tachycardia, hypotension, and dyspnea; discontinue transfusion immediately
      d. Other reactions/risks include circulatory overload, electrolyte disturbances, and infectious diseases such as AIDS (rare with current procedures), West Nile virus, hepatitis, or cytomegalovirus

Practice to Pass

Your client is to receive a unit of packed red blood cells. When the unit of blood is delivered to the nursing unit, you are unable to initiate an IV access. What actions should you take?

Practice to Pass

Your client is receiving a unit of packed red blood cells. Twenty minutes after the start of transfusion, the client complains of chills. Describe the actions you would take.

Box 14-1	• *Hemolytic:* Chills, fever, urticaria, tachycardia, chest pain or complaints of chest tightness, shortness of breath, dyspnea, lumbar pain, nausea, vomiting, lung crackles, hematuria, hypotension, wheezing
Signs and Symptoms of Blood Transfusion Reaction	• *Bacterial (pyrogenic):* Hypotension, fever, chills, flushed skin, abdominal pain, pain in extremities, vomiting, diarrhea
	• *Allergic reaction:* Urticaria, pruritus, swelling of the tongue, swelling of the face, difficulty breathing, pulmonary edema, shock
	• *Circulatory overload:* Chest pain, tightness of the chest, cough, lung crackles, pulmonary edema, tachycardia, elevated blood pressure

2. Check specific policy and protocol of agency
3. If blood transfusion reaction is noted or suspected, stop infusion immediately; change IV tubing and keep vein open with normal saline; IV access might be needed for administration of emergency drugs
4. Assess client for other signs and symptoms of transfusion reaction (see Box 14-1)
5. Notify prescriber and blood bank
6. Send unit of blood and tubing used to blood bank; this will help determine cause of reaction
7. Urine and blood samples will be required; follow agency protocol
8. Administer drugs that are prescribed and continue to monitor client
9. Document the reaction and interventions

IV. RED BLOOD CELL DISORDERS

A. Anemia

1. Most common RBC disorder; abnormally low RBC count or reduced Hgb level related to either decreased RBC production or to increased RBC loss or destruction (see Box 14-2)
2. Each type reduces O_2-carrying capacity of blood leading to tissue hypoxia
3. If anemia has gradual onset, fewer symptoms may be seen because compensatory mechanisms have time to occur; symptoms are then noted when there is increased O_2 demand (for example, with exercise or infection)
4. General manifestations characteristic of all types of anemia include fatigue; tachycardia; palpitations; pallor of skin, mucous membranes, conjunctiva and nail beds; increased respiratory rate, and dyspnea on exertion
5. Multiple system effects are common and vary based on the type of anemia (see Figure 14-4, p. 456)
6. Some anemias are referred to as nutritional anemias if commonly caused by dietary deficiency; others are characterized by cell properties such as size (macrocytic, normocytic, or microcytic) or color (normochromic or hypochromic)

B. Blood loss anemia

1. Rapid onset causes a loss of volume as well as O_2-carrying capacity; client may show signs of shock; RBCs are of normal size and shape (normocytic)
2. Chronic loss depletes iron stores so RBCs are microcytic (small) and hypochromic (pale) (see discussion following on iron deficiency anemia)

C. Iron deficiency anemia (IDA)

1. Description: anemia that results when supply of iron is inadequate for optimal formation of RBCs because of excessive iron loss caused by bleeding, decreased dietary intake, or malabsorption; is a type of nutritional anemia in many cases
2. Etiology and pathophysiology

Box 14-2	**Decreased RBC Production**

Pathophysiologic Mechanisms of Anemia

Decreased RBC Production
- Altered hemoglobin synthesis
- Iron deficiency
- Thalassemias
- Chronic inflammation
- Altered DNA synthesis
- Vitamin B_{12} or folic acid malabsorption or deficiency
- Bone marrow failure
- Aplastic anemia (stem cell dysfunction)
- Red cell aplasia
- Myeloproliferative leukemias
- Cancer metastasis, lymphoma
- Chronic infection or inflammation, physical and emotional fatigue

Increased RBC Loss or Destruction
- Acute or chronic blood loss
- Hemorrhage or trauma
- Chronic gastrointestinal bleeding, menorrhagia
- Increased hemolysis
- Hereditary cell membrane disorders
- Defective hemoglobin—sickle cell anemia or trait
- Pyruvate kinase (PK) or G6PD deficiency affecting glycolysis or cell oxidation
- Immune mechanisms and disorders (e.g., blood reaction, hypersensitivity responses, autoimmune disorders)
- Splenomegaly and hypersplenism
- Infection
- Erythrocyte trauma (e.g., due to cardiopulmonary bypass, hemolytic uremic syndrome)

Source: LeMone, Priscilla; Burke, Karen M.; Bauldoff, Gerene, *Medical-Surgical Nursing: Critical Thinking in Patient Care*, 5th Ed., © 2011. Reprinted and Electronically reproduced by permission of Pearson Education, Inc., Upper Saddle River, New Jersey.

    a. Iron deficiency accounts for 60% of anemias in clients over age 65; most common cause of IDA is blood loss from gastrointestinal (GI) or genitourinary (GU) tract

    b. Normal iron excretion is less than 1 mg/day through urine, sweat, bile, feces, and from desquamated skin cells; average woman loses 0.5 mg of iron daily or 15 mg monthly during menstruation (most common cause of iron deficiency in women, while GI bleeding is most common cause in men)

    c. Iron is stored in body as ferritin, an iron-phosphorus-protein complex that contains about 23% iron; it is formed in intestinal mucosa, when ferritin iron joins with apoferritin (a protein); ferritin is stored in tissues, primarily in reticuloendothelial cells of liver, spleen, and bone marrow

    d. Develops slowly through 3 phases: body's iron stores used for erythropoiesis are depleted, insufficient iron is transported to bone marrow and iron deficient erythropoiesis begins, allowing small Hgb-deficient cells to enter peripheral circulation in large numbers; adequate iron in RBC is essential for O_2 molecules to attach

    e. An average diet supplies body with 12–15 mg/day of iron, of which only 5–10% is absorbed

  3. Assessment

    a. Clinical manifestations (usually develop gradually with client not seeking attention until Hgb drops to 7–8 grams/dL)

    b. General manifestations of anemia as previously described, **cheilosis** (cracks in corners of mouth), smooth sore tongue, dizziness, and pica (craving to eat unusual substances such as clay or starch)

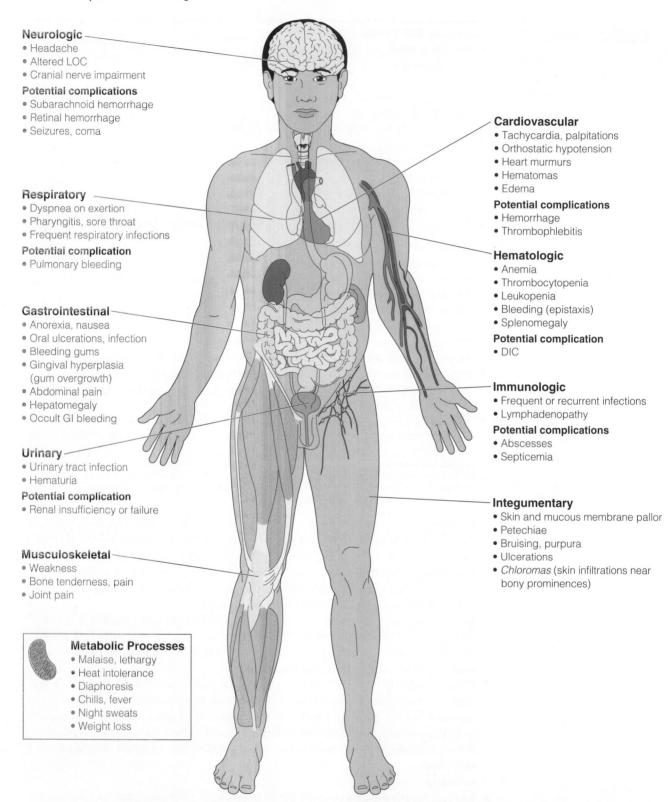

Neurologic
- Headache
- Altered LOC
- Cranial nerve impairment

Potential complications
- Subarachnoid hemorrhage
- Retinal hemorrhage
- Seizures, coma

Respiratory
- Dyspnea on exertion
- Pharyngitis, sore throat
- Frequent respiratory infections

Potential complication
- Pulmonary bleeding

Gastrointestinal
- Anorexia, nausea
- Oral ulcerations, infection
- Bleeding gums
- Gingival hyperplasia
  (gum overgrowth)
- Abdominal pain
- Hepatomegaly
- Occult GI bleeding

Urinary
- Urinary tract infection
- Hematuria

Potential complication
- Renal insufficiency or failure

Musculoskeletal
- Weakness
- Bone tenderness, pain
- Joint pain

Metabolic Processes
- Malaise, lethargy
- Heat intolerance
- Diaphoresis
- Chills, fever
- Night sweats
- Weight loss

Cardiovascular
- Tachycardia, palpitations
- Orthostatic hypotension
- Heart murmurs
- Hematomas
- Edema

Potential complications
- Hemorrhage
- Thrombophlebitis

Hematologic
- Anemia
- Thrombocytopenia
- Leukopenia
- Bleeding (epistaxis)
- Splenomegaly

Potential complication
- DIC

Immunologic
- Frequent or recurrent infections
- Lymphadenopathy

Potential complications
- Abscesses
- Septicemia

Integumentary
- Skin and mucous membrane pallor
- Petechiae
- Bruising, purpura
- Ulcerations
- *Chloromas* (skin infiltrations near
  bony prominences)

Figure 14-4

Multisystem effects of anemia

    c. Diagnostic and laboratory tests

        1) Is considered a **microcytic** and **hypochromic** anemia (small RBC diameter less than 6 with decreased pigmentation) with an increase in red cell size distribution width (RDW)

        2) RBCs are small (microcytic) and pale (hypochromic); mean corpuscular volume (MCV; measures size) is decreased and mean corpuscular Hgb (MCH) and mean corpuscular Hgb concentration (MCHC; calculated value of Hgb present in RBC compared to its size) is decreased; MCV, MCH, and MCHC should be analyzed only when Hgb is low

        3) Low serum iron level and elevated total iron-binding capacity (TIBC) or low serum ferritin levels

4. Therapeutic management

    a. Cause of anemia is usually explored; stools are examined for occult blood; endoscopic exam and other diagnostic procedures may be performed to rule out possible sources of bleeding, which is a common cause of iron deficiency

    b. Increase intake of iron-rich foods (see Box 14-3)

    c. Vitamin supplementation; administration of oral iron preparation in form of ferrous sulfate

    d. Parenteral (IM or IV) administration of iron

    e. Transfusion of packed RBCs and administration of O_2 for signs of hypoxia

5. Priority nursing problems: inability to endure exercise or activity, possible reduced cardiac output, risk for injury, alteration in gas exchange

6. Planning and implementation

    a. Administer oral iron preparation with orange juice or vitamin C to increase absorption; antacids interfere with absorption of iron

    b. High risk of anaphylaxis with IV iron dextran, a lower risk exists with other IV forms and IM forms; administer parenteral iron deep intramuscularly (IM) via Z track method; use separate needles for withdrawing and injecting dose

    c. Identify and implement energy conservation measures, for example, shower chair, sitting to perform tasks, alternate rest and activity periods

    d. Promote quiet environment to facilitate sleep and rest

    e. Monitor for dizziness; suggest position changes be made slowly

    f. Provide and recommend assistance with activities and ambulation as needed, allowing client independence as much as possible

    g. Monitor laboratory studies, for example, Hgb and Hct, RBC count

    h. Administer medications, blood or blood products as indicated; monitor closely for transfusion reactions

    i. Encourage/assist with good oral hygiene before and after meals, using soft bristled toothbrush for gentle brushing of fragile gums

    j. Determine stool color, consistency, frequency, and amount

    k. Encourage fluid intake of 2,500–3,000 mL day

    l. Discuss use of stool softeners, bulk-forming laxatives, mild stimulants, or enemas if indicated; monitor effectiveness

    m. Oral liquid form of iron can stain teeth; clients should use a straw or place spoon at back of mouth to take supplement and rinse mouth thoroughly afterward

Box 14-3		
Sources of Dietary Iron	Organ meats	Beans
	Meat	Molasses
	Green leafy vegetables	Raisins

        n. Caution client that bowel movement may appear greenish black or tarry

        o. Caution regarding possible systemic (allergic) reactions to medication, (for example, flushing, nausea and vomiting, myalgias) and importance of reporting symptoms

        p. Refer to appropriate community resources when indicated, for example, social services for food stamps, Meals on Wheels

  7. Medication therapy

        a. Usual therapy is oral ferrous sulfate ($FeSO_4$) for 6 months and is given 1 hour before meals; other oral forms may include ferrous gluconate (Fergon) and ferrous fumarate (Ircon, Femiron)

        b. If client is unable to tolerate oral therapy, iron dextran (INFeD) may be given by deep IM (Z track) route or as IV therapy; there is risk of anaphylaxis with parenteral administration; therefore, before a full dose is given a small test dose is administered

        c. Transfusion of packed RBCs may be necessary if anemia is severe

  8. Client education

        a. Maintain good nutrition; older adults and those with limited economic means may have dietary deficiencies requiring referrals to appropriate agencies (for example, Meals on Wheels)

        b. Take iron on an empty stomach; absorption of iron is decreased with food but if taken on an empty stomach it causes GI upset; absorption may be enhanced when taken with an acidic beverage (such as one with vitamin C), but avoid grapefruit juice

        c. Stools will appear black with oral intake of iron

        d. Report to health care provider persistent GI symptoms secondary to iron intake for possible administration of enteric coated version

        e. Iron preparations cause constipation; addition of a stool softener may be helpful; other measures such as increasing oral intake of fluids and fiber and increased ambulation or activity will prevent constipation

        f. Review required diet alterations to meet specific dietary needs; foods high in iron include organ meats (beef or calf's liver, chicken liver), other meats, beans (black, pinto, and garbanzo), leafy green vegetables, raisins, and molasses

  9. Evaluation: client verbalizes dietary sources of iron, demonstrates increasing activity tolerance and reports decrease in or resolution of symptoms

D. Vitamin B$_{12}$ deficiency (pernicious) anemia

  1. Description: a megaloblastic anemia that results from impaired DNA synthesis related to a lack of vitamin B_{12} and characterized by macrocytic RBCs; can be related to inadequate intake or poor absorption from a lack of intrinsic factor (pernicious anemia)

  2. Etiology and pathophysiology

        a. Pernicious anemia results from body's inability to absorb vitamin B_{12} because of a lack of intrinsic factor, a substance secreted by the parietal cells of the gastric mucosa

        b. Inevitably develops after total gastrectomy because intrinsic factor is secreted by gastric mucosa; 15% of clients develop after partial gastrectomy or gastrojejunostomy; other risk factors include ulcerative diseases, alcoholism, and vegetarian diets

        c. Inadequate vitamin B_{12} alters structure and disrupts function of peripheral nerves, spinal cord, and brain

        d. Inadequate vitamin B_{12} impairs cellular division and maturation, especially in rapidly proliferating RBCs

  3. Assessment

        a. Clinical manifestations may include slight jaundice; smooth, sore, beefy red tongue (**glossitis**); diarrhea; paresthesias (altered sensations such as numbness or tingling in extremities); and impaired proprioception (difficulty identifying one's position in space, which may progress to difficulty with balance)

     b. Diagnostic and laboratory tests

       1) Macrocytic anemia (RBC diameter greater than 8) with increase in MCV and MCHC

       2) Gastric secretion analysis reveals achlorhydria: absence of free hydrochloric acid in a pH maintained at 3.5

       3) A 24-hour urine for Schilling test (a vitamin B_{12} absorption test that indicates if a client lacks intrinsic factor by measuring excretion of orally administered radionuclide labeled B_{12}) confirms diagnosis of pernicious anemia

  4. Therapeutic management

     1) Review required diet alterations to meet specific dietary needs; if deficiency is caused by a vegetarian diet, fortified soy milk may be added to diet, or oral supplements of vitamin B_{12} may be added

     2) If deficiency is caused by gastric malabsorption such as deficiency of intrinsic factor, lifelong replacement therapy is required; a parenteral injection of vitamin B_{12} is required and in some situations megadoses or oral vitamins may be given

  5. Priority nursing problems: fatigue, potential for injury, inability to endure exercise or activity, oral mucous membrane breakdown

  6. Planning and implementation: the major nursing consideration for client with this type of anemia is client education regarding nutrition and medications (see section h. below); assess client carefully for neurologic deficits and incorporate into plan of care interventions to prevent injury

  7. Medication therapy: parenteral vitamin B_{12}, 100–1000 mcg subcutaneously (subQ) daily for 7 days, then once a week for 1 month, then monthly for life is usually prescribed

  8. Client education

     a. A burning sensation that is felt after a parenteral dose of vitamin B_{12} is temporary

     b. Include in diet sources of vitamin B_{12} such as dairy products, animal proteins, and eggs

     c. It is important to have continued treatment with regularly scheduled dose of parenterally administered vitamin B_{12}

  9. Evaluation: client reports resolution of paresthesias and increased tolerance of activity; no injuries are sustained secondary to loss of balance

E. Folic acid deficiency anemia

  1. Description: anemia caused by a deficiency of folic acid resulting in interruption of DNA synthesis and normal maturation of RBCs

  2. Etiology and pathophysiology

     a. Causative etiology: poor nutrition, malabsorption syndrome, medications that impede folic acid absorption (oral contraceptives, antiepileptics, methotrexate [MTX]), alcohol abuse, and anorexia

     b. Pregnant women, infants, and adolescents are also at risk during periods of rapid growth

     c. Clients on hemodialysis and those receiving total parenteral nutrition are also at risk for folic acid deficiency

  3. Assessment

     a. General manifestations of anemia as previously described

     b. GI symptoms are similar to B_{12} deficiency, but usually more severe (glossitis, cheilosis, and diarrhea)

     c. Neurological symptoms seen in B_{12} deficiency are not seen in folic acid deficiency and therefore assist in differentiating these 2 types of anemia

     d. Diagnostic and laboratory tests

       1) Fragile, macrocytic (megaloblastic) RBCs (diameter greater than 8)

       2) MCV high with low Hgb

       3) Low serum folate level

4. Therapeutic management: includes dietary counseling and administration of folic acid
5. Priority nursing problems: constipation, diarrhea, potential for infection, alteration in gas exchange or ability to tolerate activity
6. Planning and implementation
   a. Identify and implement energy-saving techniques, for example, shower chair, sitting to perform tasks; alternate activity and rest periods
   b. Monitor for dizziness, suggest position changes be made slowly
   c. Provide or recommend assistance with activities and ambulation as needed, allowing client independence as much as possible
   d. Monitor laboratory studies, for example, Hgb/Hct, RBC count
   e. Encourage and assist with oral hygiene before and after meals, using soft-bristled toothbrush for gentle brushing of fragile gums
   f. Refer to appropriate community resources when indicated, e.g., social services for food stamps, Meals on Wheels, Alcoholics Anonymous
7. Medication therapy: oral folate, 1–5 mg/day for 3–4 months; give folate along with vitamin B_{12} when both are deficient; folic acid supplements are recommended for women who are pregnant or may become pregnant to prevent neural tube defects
8. Client education
   a. Discuss dietary sources of folic acid such as green leafy vegetables, asparagus, fish, citrus fruits, yeast, dried beans, grains, nuts, and liver
   b. Discuss strategies to decrease pain associated with glossitis such as eating bland and soft foods
9. Evaluation: client verbalizes decrease in or resolution of symptoms and selects foods that are high in folic acid

F. **Bone marrow suppression anemia: aplastic anemia**
1. Description: aplastic anemia results from a decreased production of bone marrow elements, namely RBCs, WBCs, and platelets
2. Etiology and pathophysiology
   a. Affects all age groups and both genders
   b. Two classifications of aplastic anemia include congenital or acquired; congenital aplastic anemia is caused by a chromosomal alteration; acquired form may be caused by radiation, chemical agents and toxins, drugs, viral and bacterial infections, pregnancy, and idiopathic (in about 50% of cases, the cause is unknown)
   c. There is a decrease or cessation of production of RBCs (anemia), WBCs (leukopenia), and platelets (**thrombocytopenia**); may result from damage to bone marrow stem cells, bone marrow itself, and replacement of bone marrow with fat; depending on causative factor, anemia may be acute or chronic
3. Assessment
   a. Clinical manifestations: general manifestations of anemia, infections of skin and mucous membranes because of WBC deficiency, bleeding from gums, nose, vagina, or rectum from platelet deficiency, purpura (bruising), and possible retinal hemorrhage
   b. Diagnostic and laboratory tests
      1) Blood counts reveal pancytopenia (decreased RBC, WBC, and platelets); RBCs may be normochromic and normocytic or large with increased mean corpuscular volume
      2) Decreased reticulocyte count
      3) Bone marrow examination reveals decrease in activity of bone marrow or no cell activity
4. Therapeutic management: includes identification of cause of bone marrow suppression, bone marrow transplantation, immunosuppression, transfusion of leukocyte-poor RBCs, and splenectomy

Practice to Pass

A client with folic acid deficiency anemia asks you why he developed this type of anemia. What would your response be?

5. Priority nursing problems: potential for infection or bleeding, fatigue
6. Planning and implementation
   a. Institute reverse isolation
   b. Limit visitors and potential sources of infection
   c. Monitor for evidence of bleeding
   d. Avoid invasive procedures including rectal temperatures
   e. Provide frequent rest periods and monitor tolerance to activities
7. Medication therapy
   a. Agents that suppress lymphocyte activity such as antilymphocyte globulin (ALG), antithymocyte globulin (ATG), and cyclosporine (Sandimmune)
   b. Immunosuppressants such as prednisone and cyclophosphamide (Cytoxan)
   c. Prophylactic antibiotic therapy
8. Client education
   a. Prevent infection by avoiding crowds, maintaining good hygiene, handwashing, and eliminating uncooked foods from diet
   b. Prevent bleeding or hemorrhage by using a soft toothbrush, avoiding contact sports, and use of an electric razor
   c. Avoid drugs that increase bleeding tendency such as aspirin
   d. Balance activity with adequate rest periods to avoid fatigue
   e. Symptoms to report to the health care provider include signs of infection, bleeding, and increasing intolerance to activity
9. Evaluation: client verbalizes ways to prevent infection, bleeding, and fatigue and does not develop infection or hemorrhage

G. **Hemolytic anemias**
   1. Description: characterized by premature destruction (lysis) of RBCs, iron and by-products remain in blood; normocytic and normochromic RBCs with increases in reticulocytes (immature RBCs)
   2. Etiology and pathophysiology: can be related to external factors (drugs, bacteria, toxins, trauma or burns, mechanical damage from prosthetic heart valves) or internal factors (hereditary defects)
   3. Assessment: general symptoms of anemia as previously presented
   4. Therapeutic and nursing management: similar to other forms of anemia; remove external cause if possible; blood transfusions to increase red cell count

H. **Sickle cell disease**
   1. Definition: a hereditary, chronic form of hemolytic anemia
   2. Etiology and pathophysiology
      a. Approximately 7–13% of African Americans are heterozygous (carriers) for sickle cell anemia, thereby inheriting one affected gene (sickle cell trait)
      b. Approximately 1% or less of African Americans are homozygous (identical genes) for disorder, thereby inheriting a defective gene from both parents; will develop sickle cell disease and are likely to experience sickle cell crisis
      c. Sickle cell trait (heterozygous state) is a generally mild condition that produces few, if any, manifestations unless stressed by severe hypoxia
      d. Sickle cell anemia is caused by an autosomal genetic defect (one gene affected) that results in synthesis of Hgb S
      e. Produced by a mutation in beta chain of Hgb molecule through a substitution of amino acid valine for glutamine in both beta chains
      f. During times of decreased O_2 tension in plasma, Hgb S causes RBCs to elongate, become rigid, and assume a crescent, sickled shape causing cells to clump together and obstruct capillary blood flow; this causes ischemia and possible tissue infarction

      g. Conditions likely to trigger a sickle cell crisis include hypoxia, low environmental and/or body temperature, excessive exercise, high altitudes, or inadequate O_2 during anesthesia

      h. Other causes of sickle cell crisis include elevated blood viscosity or decreased plasma volume, infection, dehydration, increased hydrogen ion concentration (acidosis), and/or any condition that causes hypoxia

      i. With normal oxygenation, sickled RBCs resume their normal shape; repeated episodes of sickling and unsickling weaken RBC membranes, causing cells to hemolyze and be removed

      j. Crisis is extremely painful and can last from 4–6 days

3. Assessment

    a. Clinical manifestations

      1) Pallor, fatigue, and irritability

      2) Jaundice r/t excess heme units that exceed liver's ability to conjugate and excrete bile

      3) Hands, feet, large joints, and surrounding tissue may become swollen during crisis

      4) Priapism (abnormal, painful, continuous erection of penis) may occur if penile veins are obstructed

      5) Severe pain

      6) Complications include abdominal pain related infarct of abdominal organs and structures; aseptic necrosis of bones related to inactivity that affects bone marrow; stroke related to cerebral vessel occlusion; skin ulcers; acute chest syndrome; liver or renal insufficiency; sequestration crises (pooling of large amounts of blood in liver and spleen, which is believed to be cause of death in early childhood)

    b. Diagnostic and laboratory tests

      1) Anemia with sickled cells noted on a peripheral smear

      2) Hemoglobin electrophoresis: a blood test that causes Hgb molecule to migrate in solution in response to electric currents to determine presence and percentage of Hgb S; used for a definitive diagnosis

      3) Elevated serum bilirubin levels

      4) Elevated reticulocyte count

4. Therapeutic management

    a. Bone marrow transplantation

    b. Blood transfusions

    c. Management of pain

    d. Use of chemotherapy drug hydroxyurea (Droxia) to increase Hgb F and decrease sickling

    e. Adequate hydration and oxygenation

5. Priority nursing problems: pain, reduced tissue perfusion, alteration in gas exchange, potential for infection, inadequate knowledge

6. Planning and implementation

    a. Clients who are in crisis should have the following included in their care

      1) Management of pain

      2) Administration of O_2

      3) Promotion of hydration to decrease blood viscosity; a client in crisis should have an oral intake of 4–6 liters/day or IV fluids of 3 liters/day (plus oral intake)

      4) Monitoring for complications such as vaso-occlusive disease (thrombosis), hypoxia, CVA, renal dysfunction, priapism leading to impotence, acute chest syndrome (fever, chest pain, cough, pulmonary infiltrates, and dyspnea), and substance abuse

      5) Management of infection

    b. Refer to appropriate agency for genetic counseling and family planning

    c. Administer care with attention to culture, avoiding racial bias or cultural insensitivity

7. Medication therapy

    a. Nifedipine (Procardia) may be used for priapism

    b. Hydroxyurea (Droxia) to increase Hgb F and decrease sickling

    c. Opioid analgesics during acute phase of sickle cell crisis, often in large doses

    d. Broad-spectrum antibiotics to manage acute chest syndrome

    e. Folic acid supplements

8. Client education

    a. Utilize strategies to prevent sickle cell crisis

        1) Maintain an oral intake of at least 4–6 liters/day and avoid conditions that might predispose to dehydration

        2) Avoid high altitudes

        3) Prevent and promptly treat infections

        4) Use stress-reduction strategies

        5) Avoid exposure to cold

        6) Avoid overexertion

    b. Adhere to vaccination schedules for pneumococcal pneumonia, *haemophilus influenza* type B, and hepatitis B

    c. Recognize importance of regular medical follow-up

9. Evaluation: client verbalizes pain relief, does not develop infection, adheres to vaccination schedule, and identifies precipitating factor(s) leading to crisis state

I. Polycythemia

1. Description: an increase in number of circulating RBCs and concentration of Hgb in blood; also known as polycythemia vera, PV, or myeloproliferative red cell disorder; polycythemia can be primary or secondary

2. Etiology and pathophysiology

    a. Primary

        1) Common in men of European Jewish descent

        2) Neoplastic stem cell disorder characterized by increased production of RBCs, granulocytes, and platelets

        3) With overproduction of RBCs, increased blood viscosity results in congestion of blood in tissues, liver, and spleen

        4) Thrombi form, acidosis develops, and tissue infarction occurs as a result of diminished circulatory flow of blood caused by increased viscosity

    b. Secondary

        1) Most common form of polycythemia vera

        2) Disturbance is not in RBC development but in abnormal increase of erythropoietin, causing excessive erythropoiesis

        3) Increased RBC production is often a physiologic response to hypoxia, which stimulates release of erythropoietin in kidney; may also be due to kidney disease or erythropoietin-secreting tumors

        4) Chronic hypoxic states may be produced by prolonged exposure to high altitudes, pulmonary diseases, hypoventilation, and smoking

        5) Results of increased RBC production include increased viscosity of blood, which alters circulatory flow

    c. Relative

        1. Increased RBC count due to fluid deficit

        2. Hematocrit is elevated because of increased cell concentration

        3. Condition is corrected by rehydration

3. Assessment

    a. Clinical manifestations

Practice to Pass

A client with sickle cell trait asks you the implications if she marries someone with sickle trait. How should you respond?

1) **Plethora**: a ruddy (dark, flushed) color of face, hands, feet, ears, and mucous membranes resulting from engorgement of blood vessels
2) Hypertension, headaches, vertigo, blurred vision, and tinnitus
3) Distended superficial veins
4) Itching unrelieved by antihistamines
5) Symptoms associated with impaired tissue oxygenation including angina, claudication, or dyspnea
6) **Erythromyalgia**, or burning sensation of fingers and toes
7) Splenomegaly in majority of those with primary polycythemia vera, does not develop with secondary polycythemia
8) Epistaxis, GI bleeding
9) Complications such as thrombosis and hemorrhage are possible with resulting transient ischemic attacks, angina, peripheral vascular disease, GI bleeding, and portal hypertension

b. Diagnostic and laboratory tests
1) Laboratory studies reveal decreased MCHC and elevations in Hgb, RBC count, WBCs and basophils, platelets, leukocyte alkaline phosphatase, uric acid, cobalamin level, and histamine level
2) Bone marrow examination shows hyperplasia of all hematopoietic elements with primary polycythemia but only red stem cell hyperplasia with secondary polycythemia

4. Therapeutic management
a. Management of underlying condition (such as COPD) causing chronic hypoxia
b. Repeated phlebotomy to decrease blood volume; goal is to keep hematocrit less than 45–48%
c. Hydration to decrease blood viscosity

5. Priority nursing problems: reduced tissue perfusion, pain, potential for infection

6. Planning and implementation
a. Assist in phlebotomy
b. Measures to relieve pruritus including cool and tepid baths
c. Maintain accurate monitoring of fluid intake and output
d. Nursing measures to prevent thrombotic events including early ambulation, passive leg exercises when on bed rest, avoid crossing legs, antiembolism stockings or pneumatic boots, foot pump exercises, and maintaining adequate hydration
e. Administer scheduled medications, including anticoagulants, to prevent complications

7. Medication therapy
a. For primary polycythemia: myelosuppressive agents to inhibit bone marrow activity including hydroxyurea (Hydrea), melphalan (Alkeran), and radioactive phosphorus
b. Allopurinol (Zyloprim) to manage gout
c. Antiplatelet agents to prevent thrombotic complications
d. Anticoagulants to prevent thrombus formation (heparin [Liquaemin], sodium warfarin [Coumadin]) or a daily aspirin tablet
e. Antihistamines to relieve itching

8. Client education
a. Importance of maintaining good hydration; drink 3 liters of fluid or more per day
b. Information about disease and ways in which it can be controlled, such as smoking cessation
c. Signs and symptoms of complications, including signs of vaso-occlusive states (MI, CVA) and bleeding that require immediate medical attention
d. Prevent bleeding by using an electric razor, soft-bristled toothbrush, not flossing, and avoiding use of aspirin and aspirin-containing products
e. Regular medical check-ups are important

      f. Avoid products that contain iron

      g. Discuss ways of preventing thrombosis

   9. Evaluation: hematocrit is within normal range; client is free of complications associated with thrombus formation; client maintains adequate hydration

V. PLATELET AND COAGULATION DISORDERS

A. Thrombocytopenia

   1. Definition: a decrease in number of circulating platelets or a platelet count of less than 100,000/mm^3 resulting in inadequate hemostasis

   2. Etiology and pathophysiology

      a. A decrease in number of circulating platelets may result from 3 mechanisms: decreased production, increased destruction or sequestration in spleen

      b. Cause of decreased production of platelets may be inherited or acquired

      c. Increased platelet destruction may be caused by an immune system defect (immune thrombocytopenic purpura or ITP); platelets become coated with an antibody and are recognized as foreign and are destroyed when they reach spleen; platelets normally have a circulating life of 8–10 days that is shortened by this immune response; acute form of ITP is more common in children, whereas chronic form is more common in women ages 20–50 years

      d. Other causes of increased platelet destruction include non–immune related factors such as infection, aplastic anemia, bone marrow malignancy, radiation therapy, or drug-induced effects (most commonly heparin)

      e. A decrease in number of functional platelets leads to bleeding disorders; spontaneous bleeding and hemorrhage from minor trauma can occur with levels less than 20,000/mL; potentially fatal cerebral and pulmonary hemorrhage can occur when platelet count drops below 10,000/mm^3

   3. Assessment

      a. Clinical manifestations

         1) Petechiae and purpura most commonly found in anterior thorax, arms, neck, and ankles

         2) Epistaxis, gingival bleeding, menorrhagia, hematuria, and GI bleeding

         3) Signs of internal hemorrhage

         4) With heparin-induced thrombocytopenia (HIT) may see manifestations of arterial occlusion or of venous thrombosis

      b. Diagnostic and laboratory tests

         1) Decreased Hgb and hematocrit if bleeding is present

         2) Decreased platelet count

         3) Prolonged bleeding time

         4) Bone marrow examination to determine etiology; may reveal decreased platelet activity or increased megakaryocytes

   4. Therapeutic management

      a. Treatment of underlying cause or removal of causative agent

      b. Use of immunosuppressive and chemotherapeutic agents in cases of ITP

      c. Platelet transfusions if there is active bleeding; little benefit in ITP

      d. Splenectomy in ITP

      e. Plasmapheresis to remove autoimmune complexes in autoimmune ITP or acute thrombotic TP

      f. Immunoglobulins for immunosuppression

      g. Non-heparin anticoagulant such as lepirudin (Refludan) or argatroban to prevent thrombus in HIT

   5. Priority nursing problems: potential for bleeding, fatigue, potential for oral mucous membrane breakdown

    6. Planning and implementation

      a. Institute bleeding (thrombocytopenic) precautions

        1) Avoid intramuscular or subcutaneous injections

        2) Avoid indwelling urinary catheters

        3) If absolutely necessary use smallest gauge needles for injections or venipunctures; apply pressure on injection sites for 5 minutes or until bleeding stops; apply pressure to arterial blood gas sites for 15–20 minutes

        4) Discourage straining at stool, vigorous coughing, and nose blowing

        5) Avoid rectal manipulation such as rectal temperatures, suppositories, or enemas

        6) Discourage use of razors; use only electric shavers

        7) Use soft-bristled toothbrush or toothettes and avoid flossing

        8) Pad side rails if necessary and avoid tissue trauma

        9) Avoid use of aspirin and drugs that interfere with blood coagulation

      b. Monitor for signs of bleeding; test stools for occult blood

      c. Monitor CBC and platelet counts

      d. Administer platelets as ordered

      e. Monitor response to therapy

    7. Medication therapy

      a. Steroids and immunoglobulins may be used to suppress immune response in ITP (prednisone [Deltasone], methylprednisolone [Solu-medrol], and IV immunoglobulin [IVIG])

      b. Immunosuppressive agents such as vincristine (Oncovin) and cyclophosphamide (Cytoxan)

      c. Platelet growth factor such as oprelvekin (Neumega)

    8. Client education

      a. Monitor for signs of bleeding and contact primary care provider if bleeding occurs

      b. Use bleeding precautions such as use of soft-bristled toothbrush, avoidance of flossing, prevention of tissue trauma and injury including vigorous sexual activity, and using an electric razor for shaving

      c. Avoid drugs that contain aspirin and others that interfere with coagulation

      d. Follow medication dosing schedule and report adverse effects

      e. Importance of regular medical follow-up and platelet monitoring

    9. Evaluation: there is no evidence of bleeding; client has increased platelet count, verbalizes knowledge of medication actions and precautions and how monitor for signs of occult bleeding

B. Hemophilia

    1. Description: a group of hereditary clotting factor disorders characterized by prolonged coagulation time that result in prolonged and sometimes excessive bleeding

    2. Etiology and pathophysiology

      a. Hemophilia A and B are X-linked recessive disorders transmitted by female carriers, displayed almost exclusively in males

      b. *Hemophilia A* (classic hemophilia) is a deficiency in factor VIII (an alpha globulin that stabilizes fibrin clots) and is most common form of hemophilia

      c. *Hemophilia B* (Christmas disease) is a deficiency in factor IX (a vitamin-dependent beta globulin essential in stage 1 of intrinsic coagulation system as an influence on amount of thromboplastin available)

      d. Despite difference in factor deficiency, hemophilia A and B are clinically identical

      e. In clients with hemophilia A and B, platelet plugs form at site of bleeding, but deficiency in clotting factor impairs coagulation response and capacity to form a stable clot

    f. *Von Willebrand's disease* is a related disorder caused by a deficiency of von Willebrand factor (vWF), which is necessary for factor VIII activity and platelet adhesion; this disorder affects men and women equally; it is often diagnosed following surgery or a dental extraction and bleeding is prolonged but rarely severe

    g. Factor XI deficiency (hemophilia C) is usually a mild disorder identified when postoperative bleeding is prolonged

3. Assessment

    a. Clinical manifestations

       1) Persistent and prolonged bleeding from small cuts and injuries

       2) Epistaxis (nosebleeds)

       3) Subcutaneous ecchymosis and subcutaneous hematomas with minor trauma such as an injection

       4) Gingival bleeding

       5) GI bleeding, which may be manifested by hematemesis (vomiting blood), occult blood in stools, gastric pain, or abdominal pain

       6) Urinary tract bleeding (hematuria)

       7) Pain, paresthesias, or paralysis resulting from nerve compression of hematomas

       8) Hemarthrosis (joint bleeding, swelling, and damage)

    b. Diagnostic and laboratory tests

       1) Specific factor assays are used to determine type of hemophilia present (decreased factor VIII in hemophilia A, vWF in von Willebrand disease, factor IX in hemophilia B, and factor XI in hemophilia C)

       2) APTT is increased in all types of hemophilia

       3) Bleeding time is prolonged in von Willebrand's disease

4. Therapeutic management

    a. Treatment consists of replacing deficient coagulation factor(s); fresh frozen plasma (FFP) replaces all clotting factors (including factors VIII and IX) and may be administered until a definitive diagnosis is made

    b. Hemophilia A: cryoprecipitate containing 8–100 units of factor VIII per bag at 12-hour intervals until bleeding ceases; freeze-dried concentrate of factor VIII may also be given; heat treatment is used to reduce risk of transmitting disease; use of recombinant DNA technology eliminates risk of viral disease transmission but is limited by cost

    c. Hemophilia B: plasma or factor IX concentrate given q 24 h or until bleeding ceases; contains other proteins so has a risk of thrombosis with recurrent use; monoclonal purification or production by recombinant technology lowers risk of stimulating thrombus formation

    d. Von Willebrand's disease: cryoprecipitate containing 8–100 units of factor VIII per bag at 12-hour intervals until bleeding ceases; desmopressin (DDAVP) IV may also be used to stimulate release of factor VIII for several hours

    e. Factor XI deficiency: FFP

    f. Supportive treatment for hemarthrosis (bleeding into joints) including arthrocentesis and physiotherapy

    g. Control of topical bleeding with hemostatic agents, pressure, and application of ice

    h. Management of complications associated with hemorrhage

5. Priority nursing problems: potential for bleeding, reduced cardiac output, dehydration, potential inability to maintain treatment regimen

    a. Teach client and family about disease and therapeutic regimen

    b. Refer for genetic counseling and family planning

    c. Refer to National Hemophilia Foundation for support and counseling

    d. Monitor for signs of complications including hemarthrosis and intracranial bleeding

      e. Assist in management of pain associated with hemarthrosis; measures include joint immobilization, application of ice, and administration of analgesics; aspirin and drugs affecting coagulation are avoided

      f. Control bleeding and maintain hemostasis through direct pressure, and application of ice or topical hemostatic agents (absorbable gelatin sponge, microfibrillar collagen hemostat, or topical thrombin)

      g. Administer medications as prescribed

  7. Medication therapy: see therapeutic management

  8. Client education

      a. Signs and symptoms requiring immediate medical attention, which includes severe joint pain, trauma or injury, and signs of uncontrolled internal bleeding

      b. Bleeding precautions as described in previous section

      c. Stress importance of wearing a MedicAlert bracelet indicating hemophilia

      d. Maintain good dental hygiene to decrease necessity of invasive dental procedures

      e. Adhere to scheduled visits and follow-up care with primary health provider

  9. Evaluation

      a. Client identifies strategies to prevent injury and bleeding precautions

      b. There is no evidence of internal bleeding including hemarthrosis

      c. Client and family seek support from local chapter of National Hemophilia Society

C. Disseminated intravascular coagulopathy

  1. Description: disseminated intravascular coagulopathy (DIC) or **consumption coagulopathy** is a syndrome characterized by abnormal initiation and acceleration of clotting and simultaneous hemorrhage; paradoxical bleeding then occurs from consumption of clotting factors and platelets; syndrome is usually precipitated by an underlying pathologic condition (most commonly sepsis)

  2. Etiology and pathophysiology

      a. Mortality rate associated with DIC is as high as 80% with most frequent sequela being hemorrhage

      b. Syndrome is precipitated by conditions such as widespread tissue damage, hemolysis, hypotension, hypoxia, and metabolic acidosis (see Box 14-4)

      c. Underlying condition causes initiation and widespread formation of clots in vascular system either through activation of factor XII, factors II and X, or release of tissue thromboplastin; substances necessary for clotting are used at a more rapid rate than they can be replaced

      d. As clotting continues, the fibrinolytic pathway is activated to dissolve clots formed; clotting factors become depleted while fibrinolysis continues; platelets decrease, clotting factors II, V, VIII, and fibrinogen are depleted

      e. Fibrin degradation products (FDP) are released as a result of fibrinolysis; these are potent anticoagulants used to lyse clots further, worsening bleeding

Box 14-4		
Risk Factors for DIC	Venomous snakebite	Tissue necrosis
	Sepsis	Drug reactions
	Trauma	Liver disease
	Obstetric complications	Acute hemolysis
	Neoplasms	Extensive burns
	Vascular disorders	Prosthetic devices
	Hypoxia	

f. With depletion of clotting factors and increase in fibrin degradation products, stable blood clots no longer form and hemorrhage occurs

g. There is a chronic form that may be asymptomatic or present with peripheral cyanosis, thrombosis, and pregangrenous changes in fingers and toes, nose, and genitalia

3. Assessment

a. Clinical manifestations (see Box 14-5)

b. Diagnostic and laboratory tests

1) PT, PTT, and thrombin time are prolonged

2) Fibrinogen and platelets are decreased (as they decline, risk of bleeding increases)

3) Fibrin split (degradation) products are elevated

4) Factor assays (factors V, VII, VIII, X, XIII) are reduced

5) D-dimer is elevated

4. Therapeutic management

a. Priority is to treat underlying medical condition that precipitated DIC

b. Supportive treatment for manifestations of DIC such as control of bleeding; life-threatening hemorrhage may be treated with specific blood components based on identified deficiency: platelets for thrombocytopenia, cryoprecipitate to replace fibrinogen and factors V and VII, and FFP to replace all clotting factors except platelets

c. Use of heparin or antithrombin III (AT-III) to control intravascular clotting; their use is controversial and contraindicated with severe bleeding; long-term heparin therapy may be necessary for clients with chronic DIC

5. Priority nursing problems: alteration in gas exchange, reduced tissue perfusion, risk for dehydration, pain, reduced cardiac output

6. Planning and implementation

a. Assess client carefully for evidence of bleeding and reduced tissue oxygenation

b. Institute thrombocytopenic precautions (refer to previous discussion on thrombocytopenia)

Box 14-5

Clinical Manifestations of DIC

Integumentary	**Nervous System**	**Respiratory**
Decreased skin temperature	Vision changes	Dyspnea
Pallor	Dizziness	Tachypnea
Purpura	Headache	Orthopnea
Ecchymoses	Irritability	Decreased breath sounds
Hematomas	Anxiety	Chest pain
Acral cyanosis	Confusion	**Genitourinary**
Altered sensation	Seizures	Hematuria
Superficial gangere	**Gastrointestinal**	Oliguria
Gingival bleeding	Abdominal distention	**Cardiovascular**
Bleeding from puncture sites	Occult blood in stool or vomitus	Decreased pulses
Musculoskeletal	Hemoptysis	Decreased capillary filling time
Joint pain	Melena	Tachycardia
Bone pain	Abdominal pain	Venous distention
Weakness		

       c. Monitor intake and output hourly

       d. Administer blood products as indicated by health care provider

       e. Monitor for signs of complications such as renal failure, pulmonary embolism, stroke, and acute respiratory distress syndrome

       f. Monitor effectiveness of therapy and pharmacologic interventions

       g. Provide emotional support to client and family

7. Medication therapy

       a. Heparin and antithrombin III, although their use is controversial; these drugs are usually indicated to manage thrombosis

       b. Epsilon aminocaproic acid (Amicar) to inhibit fibrinolysis

       c. Blood products (FFP, platelets, and cryoprecipitate)

       d. Vasopressors to support blood pressure

8. Client education

       a. Information about the syndrome, treatments, and interventions

       b. Report symptoms of complications including abdominal pain, headache, visual disturbances, and pain

       c. Use thrombocytopenic precautions (see client education in the discussion of thrombocytopenia)

9. Evaluation: client's hemodynamic status is maintained; peripheral pulses remain intact; skin remains intact

VI. WHITE BLOOD CELL AND LYMPHOID TISSUE DISORDERS

A. Neutropenia

1. Description: refers to a decrease (less than $2,000/mm^3$) in neutrophil count (part of overall WBC count) from either decreased production or increased destruction; neutrophils play a major role in phagocytosis of disease-producing microorganisms; consequently, a decrease in their numbers increases risk for infection

2. Etiology and pathophysiology

       a. Neutropenia is not a disease but a syndrome

       b. Neutropenia may occur as a primary hematologic disorder but may also be caused by drugs, autoimmune disorders, infections, and other medical conditions such as severe sepsis and nutritional deficiencies

       c. If the WBC count is decreased, or if immature WBCs predominate in circulation, normal phagocytic function of WBCs is impaired; when phagocytic activity is decreased, neutropenic client is susceptible to both exogenous and endogenous sources of infection; minor infections may progress to more serious sepsis

       d. Neutrophils constitute about 70% of total circulating WBCs; normally, neutrophil count is above $2,000/mm^3$; the absolute neutrophil count (ANC) is determined by the following formula:

$$\frac{\% \text{ neutrophils} + \% \text{ bands}}{100} \times \text{total WBC count} = \text{ANC}$$

3. Assessment

       a. Clinical manifestations: there are no real symptoms associated with neutropenia

       b. Diagnostic and laboratory tests

          1) Neutrophil count less than $2,000$ cells$/mm^3$

          2) Bone marrow exam to determine cell morphology helps distinguish etiologic factor causing the neutropenia

4. Therapeutic management

       a. If etiology is drug induced, discontinuation of medication is indicated

       b. Corticosteroids are used if etiology is immunologic

        c. If the etiology is decreased production, growth factors (granulocyte/ macrophage colony stimulating factor (GM-CSF) may be used

        d. If client develops a fever, identification and treatment of infection is instituted

    5. Priority nursing problems: potential for infection, inadequate knowledge, anxiety

    6. Planning and implementation

        a. Monitor for signs of infection; monitor temperature elevations

        b. Obtain cultures from suspected sites of infection

        c. Administer antibiotics as prescribed and evaluate their effectiveness

        d. Administer medications that stimulate production of neutrophils

        e. Enforce strict hand hygiene by all individuals in contact with client

        f. Institute reverse isolation; use private room with HEPA filtration if possible

        g. Avoid invasive procedures

        h. Fresh flowers, fruits, and standing water are not permitted in client's room

    7. Medication therapy: growth factors such as G-SF (Neupogen) or GM-CSF (Leukine) are given to increase neutrophil count

    8. Client education

        a. Information about condition and rationale for therapeutic interventions

        b. Report elevated temperature and associated signs of fever

        c. Instruct client and those who come in contact with client to use strict hand hygiene and reverse isolation procedure

        d. Maintain good personal hygiene to reduce risk of infection

        e. Use dietary measures to reduce or eliminate microbes in food, such as no fresh fruit, raw vegetables, or raw or undercooked meat

    9. Evaluation: absolute neutrophil count normalizes; client is free of infection; client and family verbalize methods of limiting exposure to pathogens

B. Leukemia

    1. Definition: a group of malignant disorders of blood-forming tissues in bone marrow, spleen, and lymph system characterized by unregulated proliferation of WBCs and their precursors

    2. Etiology and pathophysiology

        a. Types of leukemia are classified by type of WBC affected (granulocyte, lymphocyte, monocyte) and duration of disease (acute or chronic)

           1) Acute: majority of leukemic cells are primitive (immature)

           2) Chronic: leukemic cells are mostly mature (well differentiated) (see Table 14-3)

           3) Lymphocytic leukemias involve immature lymphocytes and their precursor cells in bone marrow with infiltration of spleen, lymph nodes, CNS, and other tissues

           4) Myeloid leukemias involve myeloid stem cells in bone marrow and interfere with maturation of all types of blood cells

        b. Classifications

           1) Acute lymphocytic or lymphoblastic leukemia (ALL)

              a) Peak incidence at 2–4 years of age

              b) Malignant cells resemble immature lymphocytes but do not mature or function effectively to maintain immunity

              c) Normal hematopoiesis is suppressed, leading to thrombocytopenia, leukopenia, and anemia

           2) Chronic lymphocytic leukemia (CLL)

              a) Least common type

              b) More common between ages 50–70 years

              c) Abnormal and incompetent lymphocytes proliferate and accumulate in lymph nodes and spread to other lymphatic tissues and spleen; most circulating cells are mature lymphocytes but do not produce adequate antibodies to maintain normal immune function

Table 14-3	Major Types of Leukemia		
Classification	**Characteristics**	**Manifestations**	**Treatment**
Acute lymphoblastic leukemia (ALL)	Primarily affects children and young adults; leukemic cells may infiltrate CNS	Recurrent infections; bleeding; pallor, bone pain, weight loss, sore throat, fatigue, night sweats, weakness	Chemotherapy; bone marrow transplant (BMT), or stem cell transplant (SCT)
Chronic lymphocytic leukemia (CLL)	Primarily affects older adults; insidious onset and slow, chronic course	Fatigue; exercise intolerance; lymphadenopathy and splenomegaly; recurrent infections, pallor, edema, thrombophlebitis	Often requires no treatment; chemotherapy; BMT
Acute myeloid leukemia (AML)	Common in older adults, may affect children and young adults. Strongly associated with toxins, genetic disorders, and treatment of other cancers	Fatigue, weakness, fever; anemia; headache, bone and joint pain; abnormal bleeding and bruising; recurrent infection; lymphadenopathy, splenomegaly, and hepatomegaly	Chemotherapy; SCT
Chronic myeloid leukemia (CML)	Primarily affects adults; early course slow and stable, progressing to aggressive phase in 3 to 4 years	Early: weakness, fatigue, dyspnea on exertion; possible splenomegaly Later: fever, weight loss, night sweats	Interferon-α; chemotherapy with imatinib mesylate (Gleevac), SCT

Source: LeMone, Priscilla; Burke, Karen M.; Bauldoff, Gerene, *Medical-Surgical Nursing: Critical Thinking in Patient Care*, 5th Ed., © 2011. Reprinted and Electronically reproduced by permission of Pearson Education, Inc., Upper Saddle River, New Jersey.

      d) Slow onset, often diagnosed during a routine physical exam

   3) Acute myeloid leukemia (AML)

      a) All age groups are affected with a peak incidence at age 60; accounts for 80% of acute leukemia cases in adults

      b) There is uncontrolled proliferation of myeloblasts (precursors of granulocytes); they accumulate in bone marrow

      c) Manifestations from neutropenia and thrombocytopenia; anemia is a late manifestation

   4) Chronic myeloid leukemia (CML)

      a) Uncommon in people under 20 years of age; incidence rises with age

      b) Uncontrolled proliferation of granulocytes results in increased circulating blast (immature) cells; marrow expands into long bones because of this proliferation and also extends into liver and spleen

      c) In most cases a characteristic chromosomal abnormality (Philadelphia chromosome) is present

      d) Has slow onset, often diagnosed with a routine blood test; progression over 3–4 years to a more aggressive phase that evolves into acute leukemia called terminal blast crisis phase

  c. Abnormal or immature WBCs do not function properly because of massive proliferation of these abnormal immature cells; they can continue to multiply, infiltrate, and damage bone marrow, spleen, lymph nodes, liver, kidneys, lungs, gonads, skin, and central nervous system (CNS)

  d. Normal bone marrow becomes diffusely replaced with abnormal or immature WBCs, interfering with bone marrow's ability to produce other types of cells such as RBCs and platelets; bone marrow becomes functionally incompetent with resulting bone marrow suppression

      e. Acute leukemia has a rapid onset, progresses rapidly, with a short clinical course; left untreated, death will result in days or months; the symptoms of acute leukemia relate to depressed bone marrow, infiltration of leukemic cells into other organ systems, and hypermetabolism of leukemia cells

      f. Chronic leukemia has a more insidious onset with a more prolonged clinical course; clients are usually asymptomatic early in disease; life expectancy may be more than 5 years; symptoms of chronic leukemia relate to hypermetabolism of leukemia cells infiltrating other organ systems; cells in this type of leukemia are more mature and function more effectively

3. Assessment

    a. Clinical manifestations

      1) Fever and night sweats

      2) Bleeding, ecchymosis, gingival bleeding or epistaxis (nose bleed)

      3) Lymphadenopathy

      4) Pallor, weakness, and fatigue

      5) Pruritic vesicular lesions

      6) Anorexia and possible weight loss

      7) Shortness of breath and decreased activity tolerance

      8) Bone or joint pain

      9) Visual disturbances

     10) Splenomegaly or hepatomegaly

    b. Diagnostic and laboratory tests

      1) Increased WBC (in CLL and CML)

      2) A normal, decreased, or increased WBC with decreased neutrophils (in ALL and AML)

      3) Decreased RBCs, Hgb, Hct, and platelets (all types)

      4) Decreased reaction to skin sensitivity tests (**anergy**)

      5) Bone marrow tests reveal excessive blast cells in AML

      6) Philadelphia chromosome found in 90–95% of clients with CML; BCR/ABL gene is present in virtually all clients with CML

      7) Bone marrow biopsy and aspirate is the definitive diagnostic test

4. Therapeutic management

    a. Induction of remission with chemotherapy and radiation therapy with use of colony-stimulating factors to "rescue" bone marrow and support neutrophil maturation

    b. Bone marrow and stem cell transplantation (see Chapter 12)

5. Priority nursing problems: potential for infection or bleeding, insufficient nutrients to meet bodily needs, fatigue, inability to endure exercise or activity, pain, anticipatory grief

6. Planning and implementation

    a. Review and institute care for a client receiving chemotherapy (see Chapter 12)

    b. Review and implement nursing care of a client undergoing radiation therapy (see Chapter 12)

    c. Assist in bone marrow biopsy; apply pressure to site for 5–10 minutes or until bleeding stops; frequently assess site for signs of bleeding up to 4 hours after procedure

    d. Institute neutropenic and bleeding precautions (see previous discussion)

    e. Plan activities to prevent fatigue; provide measures for uninterrupted rest and sleep

    f. Provide for diversionary activities

    g. Maintain good nutrition; enlist assistance of a dietitian in meeting client's nutritional needs

    h. Assist client in maintaining good personal hygiene; institute measures to promote oral hygiene

    i. Refer client and family to appropriate agencies such as Meals on Wheels, American Cancer Society, and Leukemia Society

    j. Provide emotional support to client and family; refer to appropriate agency, organization, or professional for counseling and support

    k. Administer drugs that are prescribed and monitor for side effects

    l. Monitor laboratory results to evaluate effectiveness of interventions and therapy

    m. Prepare client for bone marrow transplantation if this is included in treatment plan

7. Medication therapy

    a. Chemotherapeutic drugs include alkylating agents (Busulfan [Myleran]), anthracyclines (doxorubicin [Adriamycin]), antimetabolites (fludarabine [Fludara]), corticosteroid (prednisone [Deltasone]), plant alkaloids (vincristine [Oncovin]) and others

    b. Broad spectrum antibiotics, antifungals

8. Client education

    a. Precautions to prevent bleeding (see previous discussion)

    b. Neutropenic precautions (also previously discussed)

    c. Maintain good oral hygiene including measures to keep oral cavity moist; rinse mouth with saline, lubricate lips and oral mucosa with water-soluble lubricants every 2 hours; avoid alcohol-based mouthwash solutions; use sponge-tipped applicators for oral hygiene if neutrophil and platelet counts are low

    d. Use measures to prevent peri-rectal complications; wash and clean peri-rectal area thoroughly after each bowel movement

    e. Information about therapeutic plans and interventions

9. Evaluation: client has no infection or bleeding episodes, reports adequate pain control, and tolerates activities of daily living

C. Malignant lymphomas

1. Definition: lymphoma is a group of malignant neoplasms that affects lymphatic system resulting in proliferation of lymphocytes; closely related to lymphocytic leukemias; most common types are Hodgkin's disease and non-Hodgkin's lymphoma

2. Etiology and pathophysiology

    a. Hodgkin's disease

        1) More common in men and has 2 peaks; first is at 15–35 years of age and second at age 55–75 years; incidence is higher in whites than in African Americans

        2) Cause is unknown, although several factors have been identified to contribute to development of disease; these factors include infection with Epstein-Barr virus (EBV), genetic factors, and exposure to toxins

        3) Hodgkin's disease is characterized by presence of Reed-Sternberg cell, a multinucleated and gigantic tumor cell thought to be of lymphoid origin

        4) Tumor originates in a lymph node (in majority of cases from cervical nodes) and infiltrates spleen, lungs, and liver

        5) Is a more curable cancer with 60–90% of people with localized disease achieving cure with a normal life span

    b. Non-Hodgkin's lymphoma

        1) Most common form of lymphoma; affects usually adults from age 50–70 years; is more common in men than women and in whites

        2) There is no known cause, but incidence of non-Hodgkin's lymphoma is linked to viral infections, immune disorders, genetic abnormalities, exposure to chemicals, and infection with *Helicobacter pylori*

        3) Non-Hodgkin's lymphoma has a similar pathophysiology to Hodgkin's disease, although Reed-Sternberg cells are absent and method of lymph node infiltration is different

        4) In most cases, disease involves malignant B cells; lymphoma usually originates outside lymph nodes; lymphoid tissues that are involved become infiltrated with malignant cells, which crowd out normal cells

3. Assessment

  a. Clinical manifestations

    1) Hodgkin's disease

      a) Usually begins with a firm and painless enlargement of one or more lymph nodes on one side of neck (cervical or subclavicular regions)

      b) Systemic manifestations are associated with a poorer prognosis; these include fatigue and weakness, fever, night sweats, and unintentional 10% or greater weight loss

      c) Late symptoms that may indicate spread of disease include pruritus, anemia, malaise, splenomegaly and possible involvement of lungs and GI tract

    2) Non-Hodgkin's lymphoma

      a) Painless lymph node enlargement

      b) Systemic manifestations discussed with Hodgkin's lymphoma may be present but are less common

      c) Organ system involvement may cause abdominal pain, nausea, and vomiting

      d) Nervous system involvement, especially CNS, may cause peripheral neuropathy, cranial nerve palsies, headaches, visual disturbances, changes in mental status, and seizures

  b. Diagnostic and laboratory tests

    1) Hodgkin's disease

      a) Normocytic, normochromic anemia

      b) Neutrophilia, monocytophilia, and lymphopenia

      c) Presence of Reed-Sternberg cells in excisional bone biopsy confirms Hodgkin's disease

      d) Mediastinal lymphadenopathy revealed by chest x-ray, CT scan, and radioisotope studies

      e) Mediastinal mass and pulmonary infiltrates may be seen on chest x-ray

      f) Absent or decreased response to skin sensitivity testing known as anergy

    2) Non-Hodgkin's lymphoma

      a) Lymphocytopenia

      b) X-ray may reveal pulmonary infiltrates

      c) Lymph node biopsy helps to identify cell type and pattern

      d) Pancytopenia late in disease

4. Therapeutic management

  a. Hodgkin's disease

    1) Lymphangiography is used to evaluate abdominal nodes

    2) Staging laparotomy is performed to obtain specimen of retroperitoneal lymph nodes and to remove spleen

    3) Staging of disease determines extent of disease and appropriate therapy is instituted; stage I indicates involvement of a single lymph node region; stage IV (for Hodgkin's disease only) indicates diffuse or disseminated involvement of 1+ extralymphatic organs, with or without lymph node involvement (liver, lung, marrow, skin); absence of systemic symptoms is indicated by an A; presence of systemic symptoms indicated by a B

    4) Radiation therapy for stages IA, IB, IIA, and IIB

    5) Combination chemotherapy for stages III, IV, and all B stages

    6) Combination radiation and chemotherapy for stages IA and IB

  b. Non-Hodgkin's lymphoma

    1) Staging of disease is based on data obtained from CT scans and bone marrow biopsies

        2) Combination chemotherapy is used

        3) Radiation alone or in combination with chemotherapy for stage I and II

        4) Biologic therapy with alpha interferon, interleukin-2, and tumor necrosis factor

    c. Other therapies

        1) Immunotherapy: administration of rituximab (Rituxan), a monoclonal antibody against the CD20 antigen of malignant B lymphocytes, which causes cell lysis and death; monitor for tumor lysis syndrome

        2) Stem cell transplant using client's own stem cells (autologous) to restore bone marrow function after chemotherapy or radiation

5. Priority nursing problems: potential for infection, inability to endure exercise or activity, fatigue, insufficient nutrients to meet bodily needs, body image alterations, loss of hope

6. Planning and implementation

    a. Institute nursing interventions for clients on chemotherapy or radiation therapy

    b. Assist in balancing activity with periods of rest

    c. Provide and assist in maintaining good nutritional state with liberal fluid intake to promote excretion of metabolic by-products

    d. Provide measures to diminish discomfort associated with pruritus

    e. Provide interventions to enable client to deal with body image changes such as alopecia, weight loss, and sterility

    f. Refer client and family to appropriate agencies for support such as American Cancer Society

    g. Plan interventions to prevent infection

    h. Offer counseling or referrals regarding sperm banking and family planning to help cope with treatment-induced sterility

7. Medication therapy: chemotherapeutic agents and biologic therapy agents

8. Client education

    a. Information about nature of disease, course of therapy, and associated interventions

    b. Medications prescribed, precautions, and side effects

    c. Symptoms requiring immediate medical intervention such as bleeding, infection, or fever

9. Evaluation: client is free of complications of bleeding or infection, regains normal weight, and verbalize absence of pain; client and family verbalize reasons for ongoing treatment and interventions

D. Multiple Myeloma

  1. Definition: a malignancy in which plasma cells (B-cell lymphocytes that produce antibodies) proliferate and infiltrate bone marrow, lymph nodes, spleen, and other tissues

  2. Etiology and pathophysiology

    a. Malignant cells produce abnormally large amounts of immunoglobulin M protein, which interferes with normal antibody production and impairs humoral immune response

    b. Increased blood viscosity from this protein may damage kidney tubules

    c. Proliferating myeloma cells replace bone marrow, progressively destroying bone

    d. Affected bones (usually vertebrae, pelvis, femur, clavicle, and scapula) are weakened and break without trauma (pathologic fracture)

    e. Disease progresses to invade other organs

    f. Incidence increases with age, rarely occurring before age 40; cause is unknown but may be related to genetic alterations, radiation, oncogenic virus, inflammatory stimuli, and chronic antigen stimulation

  3. Assessment

    a. Clinical manifestations related to effect on bones and impaired immune response

        1) Bone pain (most common presenting symptom)

        2) Hypercalcemia with neurologic dysfunction (lethargy, confusion, weakness)

    3) Recurrent infections
    4) Bence Jones proteins in the urine
    5) Progression to azotemia, renal failure, pancytopenia, and widespread organ infiltration
  b. Diagnostic and laboratory tests
    1) X-rays reveal fractures and lesions
    2) Bone marrow examination shows increased immature plasma cells
    3) CBC shows moderate to severe anemia and an elevation in ESR
    4) Bence Jones protein in urine
    5) Elevated serum calcium, creatinine, uric acid and BUN levels
    6) Spike of one type of antibody (usually IgG) on protein electrophoresis
    7) Biopsy of myeloma lesions confirms diagnosis
  4. Therapeutic management
    a. There is no cure
    b. Active observation indicated for some clients with a slowly progressive course of disease
    c. Chemotherapy followed by stem cell transplant and maintenance chemotherapy for clients with more rapid progression or in later stages
    d. Supportive care
      1) Hydration for hypercalcemia
      2) Bisphosphonate therapy to reduce bone loss
      3) Calcium, vitamin D, and fluoride supplements to support bone structure
      4) Plasmapheresis if acute renal failure to remove circulating M proteins
      5) Prompt treatment of infections
  5. Priority nursing problems: pain, reduced mobility, potential for injury
  6. Planning and implementation
    a. Pain management using pharmacological and nonpharmacological measures
    b. Gentle support of extremities during repositioning to reduce risk of pathologic fractures
    c. Safety measures
    d. Education about signs and symptoms of complications such as fractures or infection
    e. Referrals for home health and home maintenance services

Case Study

You are the nurse assigned to a client who was admitted 3 days ago with a diagnosis of septic shock. During your initial assessment, you note that the client's capillary refill on the left lower extremity is delayed. The dorsalis pedis and posterior tibial pulses on the left are significantly less (1+) than the right (2+). The extremity is cold, and the client claims to have pain on that side. On further examination, you notice that the client is oozing blood from previous IV and injection sites. His Foley catheter is draining pink-tinged urine. You suspect disseminated intravascular coagulopathy (DIC).

1. What factor(s) may have contributed to the development of DIC?

2. What immediate nursing interventions will you perform?

3. What laboratory tests do you anticipate the health care provider will recommend and why?

4. If your hunch was correct that the client is in DIC, what would you expect the laboratory results to be?

5. Identify 3 priority nursing problems for this client.

For suggested responses, see page 625.

POSTTEST

1 The nurse would assess a client who has undergone a small bowel resection of the ileum for development of which type of anemia?

1. Sickle cell anemia
2. Vitamin B_{12} deficiency anemia
3. Anemia of chronic disease
4. Aplastic anemia

2 The nurse is conducting a health screening at a local health fair. Which of the following factors should the nurse recognize as possibly increasing the risk for developing non-Hodgkin's lymphoma? Select all that apply.

1. Genetics
2. Epstein-Barr virus
3. High fat diet
4. Female gender
5. Age between 15 and 35 years

3 The nurse is assessing a group of clients and identifies which client as being at high risk for developing folic acid deficiency anemia?

1. Obese individual
2. A client with alcoholism
3. Person of African descent
4. An athlete

4 During nursing assessment, which question is important for the nurse to ask a client suspected of having a nutritional anemia?

1. "Do you have any pain?"
2. "What color are your stools?"
3. "Do you experience any tingling or numbness?"
4. "Have you noticed an increase in bruising?"

5 A couple seeks genetic counseling for sickle cell anemia. Both individuals have sickle cell traits. The nurse concludes that the couple has what chance with each pregnancy of having a child who develops sickle cell disease?

1. 0%
2. 25%
3. 50%
4. 100%

6 The nurse is preparing a teaching plan for a client with sickle cell disease about ways to prevent crisis episodes. Which of the following should be emphasized to prevent sickle cell crisis?

1. Eat nutritious foods that are high in iron.
2. Seek treatment for infections as soon as possible.
3. Take adequate amounts of supplemental vitamins and minerals.
4. Avoid any type of physical activity.

7 Which of the following nursing diagnoses should receive the highest priority in a client with sickle cell crisis?

1. Acute Pain
2. Self-Care Deficit
3. Activity Intolerance
4. Ineffective Health Maintenance

8 Which of the following statements made by a client with iron-deficiency anemia indicates the need for further teaching?

1. "I should stop taking the medicine if my stools turn black."
2. "I should dilute the liquid iron preparation and use a straw when taking it."
3. "I can prevent the constipation by increasing the intake of fluids and fiber."
4. "I should return to the clinic if my stomach upset worsens with this medication."

9 Which of the following statements made by a client with sickle cell trait indicates the need for further teaching?

1. "I don't have to worry about developing sickle cell crisis since I only have the trait."
2. "I will need to seek genetic counseling before I get married and plan children."
3. "I will need to plan my activities, avoiding those that decrease my oxygen levels."
4. "I need to avoid the use of recreational drugs and alcohol."

10 Which of the following nursing observations indicate that a positive outcome for a client with sickle cell crisis has been met?

1. Client has an intake of 3,000 mL per day.
2. Urinary output is 20 mL per hour.
3. Client reports persistent joint pain.
4. Client has a temperature of 100°F.

➤ *See pages 481–482 for Answers and Rationales.*

ANSWERS & RATIONALES

Pretest

1 **Answer: 3** **Rationale:** Vitamin B_{12} deficiency anemia prevents the transport of folic acid into the cell and DNA synthesis for RBC production. It also causes the production of abnormally large RBCs. There is an increase in the MCV and a decrease in the hemoglobin. Smaller size and reduced hemoglobin is characteristic of iron deficiency anemia. **Cognitive Level:** Applying **Client Need:** Physiological Adaptation **Integrated Process:** Nursing Process: Implementation **Content Area:** Adult Health **Strategy:** The critical word in the question is *vitamin B_{12}.* The core issue of the question is RBC reproduction and how abnormalities can affect health. Use specific nursing knowledge and the process of elimination to make a selection. **Reference:** LeMone, P., Burke, K., & Bauldoff, G. (2011). *Medical-surgical nursing: Critical thinking in patient care* (5th ed.). Upper Saddle River, NJ: Pearson Education, pp. 1071–1072.

2 **Answer: 2** **Rationale:** Hypoxia stimulates the release of the hormone erythropoietin from the kidney and increases bone marrow production of RBCs. The heme portion of the hemoglobin molecule carries iron to transport the oxygen. Reticulocytes mature in 24 to 48 hours, and their maturation or destruction is not influenced by hypoxia. **Cognitive Level:** Applying **Client Need:** Physiological Adaptation **Integrated Process:** Teaching and Learning **Content Area:** Adult Health **Strategy:** Understanding the role of the parts of the RBC molecule is helpful in answering this question as well as the body's feedback responses. **Reference:** LeMone, P., Burke, K., & Bauldoff, G. (2011). *Medical-surgical nursing: Critical thinking in patient care* (5th ed.). Upper Saddle River, NJ: Pearson Education, p. 882.

3 **Answer: 2, 1, 3, 4** **Rationale:** A bone marrow transplant requires healthy marrow from a donor with a close tissue match. The recipient will need high doses of chemotherapy and/or total body irradiations to destroy the leukemic cells. This leaves the recipient at high risk for infection and bleeding and should not be completed until a donor is found. The donor's marrow is aspirated and infused through a central venous line into the recipient. The recipient is monitored closely for graft-versus-host disease. **Cognitive Level:** Applying **Client Need:** Reduction of Risk Potential **Integrated Process:** Teaching and Learning **Content Area:** Adult Health **Strategy:** Consider what must happen before a subsequent step will apply. **Reference:** LeMone, P.,&Burke, K. (2008). *Medical-surgical nursing: Critical thinking in client care* (4th ed.). Upper Saddle River, NJ: Pearson Education, p. 1078.

4 **Answer: 1** **Rationale:** Lysis of red blood cells causes retention of iron and other substances including bilirubin to accumulate in plasma. The accumulation of bilirubin causes jaundice. Although hepatitis infection may be a reason for jaundice, there is no indication that this client has hepatitis. Loss of plasma proteins is more likely to cause ascites. Haptoglobin is a protein that binds free hemoglobin released by hemolysis. Haptoglobin levels decrease in clients with hemolytic anemia. **Cognitive Level:** Applying **Client Need:** Pharmacological and Parenteral Therapies **Integrated Process:** Nursing Process: Diagnosis **Content Area:** Adult Health **Strategy:** First recall what hemolysis is and determine its by-products. Then consider the pathophysiology of jaundice. Both of these content areas are necessary to select the correct response. **Reference:** LeMone, P., Burke, K., & Bauldoff, G. (2011). *Medical-surgical nursing: Critical thinking in patient care* (5th ed.). Upper Saddle River, NJ: Pearson

Education, p. 882. Kee, J. L. (2010). *Laboratory and diagnostic tests* (8th ed.). Upper Saddle River, NJ: Prentice Hall, pp. 216–217.

5 **Answer: 4** **Rationale:** The reticulocyte (immature RBC) count is an indicator that new RBCs are being produced by the bone marrow. An increase in the reticulocyte count in an anemic client indicates that the bone marrow is responding to the decrease in RBCs. The hematocrit count measures the percent of RBCs in the total blood volume. Hemoglobin is not directly linked to bone marrow activity. Serum ferritin levels reflect available iron stores. **Cognitive Level:** Applying **Client Need:** Physiological Adaptation **Integrated Process:** Nursing Process: Assessment **Content Area:** Adult Health **Strategy:** Defining each answer choice can help you in selecting the correct response. Alternatively, understanding that initially the bone marrow will produce immature cells known as reticulocytes could also lead to the correct response. **Reference:** LeMone, P., Burke, K., & Bauldoff, G. (2011). *Medical-surgical nursing: Critical thinking in patient care* (5th ed.). Upper Saddle River, NJ: Pearson Education, pp. 880–882, 1076.

6 **Answer: 3** **Rationale:** Because vitamin B$_{12}$ is important for neurologic function, paresthesias in the extremities and problems with proprioception develop. These manifestations are not present in other types of anemia. Shortness of breath is present with all types of anemia because it results from the decrease in tissue oxygenation. Pallor of the skin is common with all types of anemia because of the blood redistribution to vital organs and lack of hemoglobin. Tachycardia is common with all types of anemia because the decreased tissue oxygenation stimulates compensatory responses. **Cognitive Level:** Applying **Client Need:** Physiological Adaptation **Integrated Process:** Communication and Documentation **Content Area:** Adult Health **Strategy:** This question is actually asking for a sign of vitamin B$_{12}$ deficiency. Alternatively, define the terms in the answer choices to help eliminate incorrect distracters. **Reference:** LeMone, P., Burke, K., & Bauldoff, G. (2011). *Medical-surgical nursing: Critical thinking in patient care* (5th ed.). Upper Saddle River, NJ: Pearson Education, pp. 1069–1072.

7 **Answer: 2** **Rationale:** An acidic environment (such as in the presence of vitamin C) enhances the absorption of iron. Milk decreases absorption of iron. Administering the medication with meals or shortly after meals leads to iron binding with food and may interfere with its absorption. **Cognitive Level:** Applying **Client Need:** Pharmacological and Parenteral Therapies **Integrated Process:** Nursing Process: Planning **Content Area:** Pharmacology **Strategy:** Recall the mechanism of action of iron and recommended procedures for administration and use the process of elimination to select an option that is a true statement. **Reference:** LeMone, P., Burke, K., & Bauldoff, G. (2011). *Medical-surgical nursing: Critical*

thinking in patient care (5th ed.). Upper Saddle River, NJ: Pearson Education, p. 1078.

8 **Answer: 1, 2** **Rationale:** In disseminated intravascular coagulopathy (DIC), the deficiency of clotting factors causes clots to form in the microcirculation. Heparin is an anticoagulant that prevents further propagation of these clots. This maintains tissue perfusion by preventing arterial occlusion. Heparin does not act specifically to preserve the myocardium or to prevent DVT in a client with DIC, although heparin could have this effect in some clients. Heparin does not dissolve clots; this is the role of thrombolytic drugs. **Cognitive Level:** Applying **Client Need:** Pharmacological and Parenteral Therapies **Integrated Process:** Communication and Documentation **Content Area:** Adult Health **Strategy:** Compare the physiological process of disseminated intravascular coagulopathy (DIC) with the mechanism of action of heparin. Select the answer option that incorporates both content areas. **Reference:** LeMone, P., Burke, K., & Bauldoff, G. (2011). *Medical-surgical nursing: Critical thinking in patient care* (5th ed.). Upper Saddle River, NJ: Pearson Education, p. 1113.

9 **Answer: 4** **Rationale:** Liver and muscle meats are excellent sources of iron. Citrus fruits such as oranges and grapefruit are high in vitamin C, which may help absorb iron but do not supply iron themselves. Green leafy vegetables such as spinach and broccoli supply the B vitamins. Eggs and milk supply protein and calcium. **Cognitive Level:** Analyzing **Client Need:** Physiological Adaptation **Integrated Process:** Nursing Process: Evaluation **Content Area:** Foundational Sciences **Strategy:** This question is essentially asking for identification of foods high in iron. Associate anemia with the need for foods of animal origin that have a blood supply. Otherwise, use basic nutritional knowledge and the process of elimination to make a selection. **Reference:** LeMone, P., Burke, K., & Bauldoff, G. (2011). *Medical-surgical nursing: Critical thinking in patient care* (5th ed.). Upper Saddle River, NJ: Pearson Education, p. 1077.

10 **Answer: 1** **Rationale:** When administering an iron preparation intramuscularly, it should be given deep in the muscle. The site should be in the upper outer quadrant of the buttocks utilizing the Z track technique. A 22 gauge 2–3-inch needle should be used. It must be given into the dorsal gluteal muscle. The area should not be massaged after the injection. **Cognitive Level:** Applying **Client Need:** Pharmacological and Parenteral Therapies **Integrated Process:** Nursing Process: Implementation **Content Area:** Fundamentals **Strategy:** Recall the procedure for the administration of iron and the risk to soft tissue if not administered into a muscle. **Reference:** Wilson, B. A., Shannon, M. T., & Shields, K. M. (2012). *Pearson nurse's drug guide 2012.* Upper Saddle River, NJ: Pearson Education, pp. 807–810.

Posttest

1 **Answer: 2** **Rationale:** Resection of the distal ileum results in the impaired absorption of vitamin B_{12}. Sickle cell anemia is a genetic disorder. Aplastic anemia results from inadequate production of RBC from the bone marrow. The client is not identified as having a chronic disease with an inflammatory component and therefore anemia of chronic disease does not apply. **Cognitive Level:** Applying **Client Need:** Physiological Adaptation **Integrated Process:** Nursing Process: Assessment **Content Area:** Adult Health **Strategy:** Define each of the anemias in the answer choices. Compare these definitions to the situation in the question. **Reference:** LeMone, P., Burke, K., & Bauldoff, G. (2011). *Medical-surgical nursing: Critical thinking in patient care* (5th ed.). Upper Saddle River, NJ: Pearson Education, pp. 1069–1076.

2 **Answer: 1, 2** **Rationale:** The exact cause is unknown but genetic factors are believed to play a role. Viruses such as Epstein-Barr are believed to play a role in both Hodgkin's and non-Hodgkin's lymphoma. Diet has not been shown to play a role in development of lymphoma. Women are less likely to experience either Hodgkin's or non-Hodgkin's lymphoma. Age between 15 and 35 years is associated with Hodgkin's disease. Non-Hodgkin's lymphoma is more common in older adults. **Cognitive Level:** Applying **Client Need:** Health Promotion and Maintenance **Integrated Process:** Adult Health **Content Area:** Hematological **Strategy:** Apply knowledge of the physiology of the lymphatic system. **Reference:** LeMone, P., Burke, K., & Bauldoff, G. (2011). *Medical-surgical nursing: Critical thinking in patient care* (5th ed.). Upper Saddle River, NJ: Pearson Education, p. 1095.

3 **Answer: 2** **Rationale:** Individuals who are chronically undernourished including those with alcoholism, substance abuse, high metabolic requirements, on total parenteral nutrition and older adults are at risk for folic acid deficiency anemia. Obesity is a risk factor for cardiovascular diseases. People of African descent are at high risk for sickle cell anemia. Athletes are more inclined toward musculoskeletal injuries. **Cognitive Level:** Applying **Client Need:** Health Promotion and Maintenance **Integrated Process:** Nursing Process: Diagnosis **Content Area:** Adult Health **Strategy:** Note that each of the answer choices is a risk factor for specific diseases. Select the answer choice that is directly related to the deficiencies of malnutrition. **Reference:** LeMone, P., Burke, K., & Bauldoff, G. (2011). *Medical-surgical nursing: Critical thinking in patient care* (5th ed.). Upper Saddle River, NJ: Pearson Education, p. 1072.

4 **Answer: 3** **Rationale:** Vitamin B_{12} deficiency anemia causes neurologic symptoms such as numbness and paresthesia. Pain occurs during a sickle cell crisis in sickle cell anemia because the RBC sickling clogs vessels and causes ischemia. Blood loss as a cause of anemia can

cause black or tar-colored stools. Petechiae are an indication of the lack of production of platelets and indicate a bone marrow problem. **Cognitive Level:** Analyzing **Client Need:** Physiological Adaptation **Integrated Process:** Nursing Process: Assessment **Content Area:** Adult Health **Strategy:** Recall that a nutritional anemia is related to the type of food ingested and/or absorbed. Eliminate answer choices that are inconsistent with this type of anemia. **Reference:** LeMone, P., Burke, K., & Bauldoff, G. (2011). *Medical-surgical nursing: Critical thinking in patient care* (5th ed.). Upper Saddle River, NJ: Pearson Education, pp. 1069–1072.

5 **Answer: 2** **Rationale:** Sickle cell disease is an autosomal recessive genetic disorder that occurs when the individual acquires the abnormal gene from both parents. If both parents have sickle cell traits, there is a 25% chance that each pregnancy will produce a child with the disease. **Cognitive Level:** Analyzing **Client Need:** Health Promotion and Maintenance **Integrated Process:** Nursing Process: Diagnosis **Content Area:** Adult Health **Strategy:** This question is related to the transmission of a recessive gene when both parents are trait carriers. Recall that there are 4 scenarios: mother passes gene but father doesn't (trait); father passes gene and mother doesn't (trait); neither passes the gene; and both pass the gene (disease). Since there are 4 combinations, reason that the risk is therefore 25%. **Reference:** LeMone, P., Burke, K., & Bauldoff, G. (2011). *Medical-surgical nursing: Critical thinking in patient care* (5th ed.). Upper Saddle River, NJ: Pearson Education, p. 1073.

6 **Answer: 2** **Rationale:** Clients with sickle cell disease may have a scarred spleen resulting in decreased ability to fight off infection. The individual with sickle cell disease must seek early treatment of infections in order to avoid hypoxia that precipitates a sickling event. Foods and nutritional supplements are appropriate treatments for an anemia related to nutritional deficiency. Normal physical activity does not have to be restricted in any type of anemia and should be determined by symptoms, although anaerobic activities or activities that cause hypoxia should be avoided. **Cognitive Level:** Applying **Client Need:** Health Promotion and Maintenance **Integrated Process:** Nursing Process: Planning **Content Area:** Adult Health **Strategy:** Eliminate answer choices that are unrelated to sickle cell anemia. Select the answer choice that is related to the destruction of the tissue as a result of sickling. **Reference:** LeMone, P., Burke, K., & Bauldoff, G. (2011). *Medical-surgical nursing: Critical thinking in patient care* (5th ed.). Upper Saddle River, NJ: Pearson Education, pp. 1071–1073.

7 **Answer: 1** **Rationale:** The client in sickle cell crisis will have pain related to ischemic tissue injury resulting from obstruction of blood flow. The other diagnoses although important are of lesser priority than the nursing diagnosis of Acute Pain, especially since the others focus on activities of daily living and none of them significantly address threats to the airway, breathing, or circulation. **Cognitive Level:** Analyzing **Client Need:** Physiological Adaptation **Integrated Process:** Nursing Process: Diagnosis **Content Area:** Adult Health **Strategy:** The correct response is directly related to the lack of blood flow to the tissue beyond the area of sickling and occlusion. **Reference:** LeMone, P., Burke, K., & Bauldoff, G. (2011). *Medical-surgical nursing: Critical thinking in patient care* (5th ed.). Upper Saddle River, NJ: Pearson Education, pp. 1073–1074.

8 **Answer: 1** **Rationale:** The client taking an oral iron preparation should be taught to expect stools to be black because of the excessive iron that is eliminated. If the liquid oral form of iron is used, it should be placed on the back of the tongue with a dropper or be well diluted and taken with a straw to avoid staining the teeth. Iron can cause constipation, and fluids and fiber may prevent its development. If GI symptoms develop, an enteric-coated tablet can be prescribed. **Cognitive Level:** Analyzing **Client Need:** Pharmacological and Parenteral Therapies **Integrated Process:** Nursing Process: Evaluation **Content Area:** Pharmacology **Strategy:** Recall the mechanism of action of iron and recommended procedures for administration. Specific nursing knowledge is needed to answer this question. **Reference:** LeMone, P., Burke, K., & Bauldoff, G. (2011). *Medical-surgical nursing: Critical thinking in patient care* (5th ed.). Upper Saddle River, NJ: Pearson Education p. 1078.

9 **Answer: 1** **Rationale:** Clients with sickle cell trait may also develop sickle cell crisis, although their symptoms are often milder since only about 30% of their hemo-globin is abnormal. Since sickle cell is transmitted genetically, genetic counseling is advised. Vigorous exercise can create tissue hypoxia and cause a crisis. Recreational drugs and alcohol can induce a crisis. **Cognitive Level:** Applying **Client Need:** Health Promotion and Maintenance **Integrated Process:** Nursing Process: Evaluation **Content Area:** Adult Health **Strategy:** This item is asking for selection of the answer choice that does *not* indicate an understanding of sickle cell disease. Select the answer choice that is inconsistent with the disease. **Reference:** LeMone, P., Burke, K., & Bauldoff, G. (2011). *Medical-surgical nursing: Critical thinking in patient care* (5th ed.). Upper Saddle River, NJ: Pearson Education, pp. 1073, 1081.

10 **Answer: 1** **Rationale:** An observation for the client in sickle cell crisis that indicates a positive outcome includes an oral intake of 3,000 mL/day, which can help prevent a crisis by promoting blood flow. The normal urinary output is 30 mL/hour. A decrease may indicate the occurrence of renal insufficiency. Joint pain is indicative of a crisis. A temperature elevation increases the chance of hypoxia occurring and puts the client at risk for a crisis. **Cognitive Level:** Analyzing **Client Need:** Physiological Adaptation **Integrated Process:** Nursing Process: Evaluation **Content Area:** Adult Health **Strategy:** Eliminate the answer choices that are abnormal findings. Select the answer choice that indicates that the established goal is accomplished. **Reference:** LeMone, P., Burke, K., & Bauldoff, G. (2011). *Medical-surgical nursing: Critical thinking in patient care* (5th ed.). Upper Saddle River, NJ: Pearson Education, pp. 1073–1074.

References

Adams, M., & Holland, N. (2011). *Pharmacology for nurses: A pathophysiological approach* (3rd ed.). Upper Saddle River, NJ: Pearson Education.

Berman, A., & Snyder, S. (2012). *Kozier & Erb's fundamentals of nursing: Concepts, process, and practice* (9th ed.). Upper Saddle River, NJ: Pearson Education.

D'Amico, D., & Barbarito, C. (2012). *Health & physical assessment in nursing* (2nd ed.). Upper Saddle River, NJ: Pearson Education, Inc.

Ignatavicius, D. D., & Workman, M. L. (2013). *Medical-surgical nursing: Critical thinking for collaborative care* (7th ed.) Philadelphia: W. B. Saunders Company.

Kee, J. L. (2010). *Laboratory and diagnostic tests* (8th ed.). Upper Saddle River, NJ: Pearson Education.

Lehne, R. (2010). *Pharmacology for nursing care* (7th ed.). St. Louis, MO: Saunders.

LeMone, P., Burke, K., & Bauldoff, G. (2011). *Medical-surgical nursing: Critical thinking in patient care* (5th ed.). Upper Saddle River, NJ: Pearson Education.

Lewis, S., Dirksen, S., Heitkemper, M., Bucher, L., & Camera, I. (2011). *Medical surgical nursing: Assessment and management of clinical problems* (8th ed.) St. Louis, MO: Elsevier.

McCance, K. L., & Huether, S. E. (2010). *Pathophysiology: The biologic basis for disease in adults and children* (6th ed.). St. Louis, MO: Mosby, Inc.

Osborn, K. S., Wraa, C. E., & Watson, A. (2010). *Medical surgical nursing: Preparation for practice* (Vol. Combined). Upper Saddle River, NJ: Prentice Hall.

Smith, S. F., Duell, D. J., & Martin, B. C. (2012). *Clinical nursing skills: Basic to advanced skills* (8th ed.). Upper Saddle River, NJ: Pearson Education.

Reproductive Disorders

15

Chapter Outline

Overview of Anatomy and
Physiology
Diagnostic Tests and
Assessments
Common Nursing Techniques
and Procedures

Care of Postoperative
Client
Disorders of Male
Reproductive System
Sexually Transmitted
Infections (STIs)

Infertility
Disorders of Female
Reproductive System

Objectives

➤ Identify basic structures and functions of the reproductive system.
➤ Describe the pathophysiology and etiology of common reproductive
and sexual disorders.
➤ Discuss expected assessment data and diagnostic test findings for
selected reproductive and sexual disorders.
➤ Identify priority nursing problems for selected reproductive and
sexual disorders.
➤ Discuss therapeutic management of a client experiencing
reproductive and sexual disorders.
➤ Discuss nursing management of a client experiencing reproductive
and sexual disorders.
➤ Identify expected outcomes for the client experiencing
reproductive and sexual disorders.

NCLEX-RN® Test Prep

Use the accompanying online resource,
NursingReviewsandRationales, to test
yourself with hundreds of NCLEX®-style
practice questions.

Review at a Glance

amenorrhea absence of menstruation

colposcopy procedure for visualization of cervix

cystocele herniation of bladder into vagina

dysmenorrhea pain associated with menstruation

dyspareunia painful intercourse

gynecomastia abnormal enlargement of breasts in men

hydrocele abnormal fluid collection within layers of tunica vaginalis, surrounding testes

infertility inability to conceive after 1 year of regular intercourse with no contraceptive measures, or inability to

deliver a live fetus after 3 consecutive conceptions

impotence inability to achieve or maintain an erection

laparoscopy procedure to visualize internal pelvic organs, using scope inserted through incision in abdominal wall

menorrhagia excessive or prolonged menstrual bleeding

metrorrhagia bleeding between menstrual periods

oligomenorrhea scant menses, usually related to hormonal imbalance

orchitis infection or inflammation of testicles

phimosis constriction of foreskin so it can't be retracted over glans penis

priapism sustained, painful erection not associated with sexual arousal

rectocele herniation of rectum into vagina

testicular torsion twisting of testes and spermatic cord

uterine prolapse downward displacement of uterus into vaginal canal

varicocele cluster of dilated veins in spermatic cord

vulvitis inflammation or infection of vulva

PRETEST

❶ The nurse is caring for a client with suspected benign prostatic hyperplasia (BPH). In providing information about risk factors for the condition, what information should the nurse include?

1. Engaging in unprotected sex
2. Consuming a diet high in meats and fats
3. Exposure to chemical carcinogens
4. Use of corticosteroids

❷ A male client presents to the emergency department with priapism. The nurse understands that this client needs which of the following?

1. Immediate medical attention
2. A relaxing environment so his erection will recede
3. Warm soaks to the penis
4. Evaluation for sexual dysfunction

❸ The nurse is evaluating a client with erectile dysfunction (ED). Which medication currently used by the client could be an underlying cause?

1. Propranolol (Inderal)
2. Acetylsalicylic acid (aspirin)
3. Penicillin
4. Furosemide (Lasix)

❹ A 68-year-old female client presents to the gynecology clinic with complaints of painless vaginal bleeding. The nurse anticipates that the client will be tested for which condition?

1. Ovarian cyst
2. Cervical or uterine cancer
3. Polycystic ovarian syndrome
4. Endometriosis

❺ The nurse concludes that a client who undergoes nocturnal penile tumescence and rigidity (NPTR) monitoring is likely being evaluated for which disorder?

1. Prostate cancer
2. Infertility
3. Erectile dysfunction
4. Phimosis

❻ While the nurse is preparing a client for a Papanicolaou (Pap) test, the client asks why the Pap test needs to be done. Which reasons should the nurse include in a response? Select all that apply.

1. Diagnose uterine cancer
2. Detect the presence of sexually transmitted infections
3. Detect abnormal cells in the cervix
4. Diagnose cause of premenstrual syndrome (PMS)
5. Detect hormonal changes

❼ A client has just had a Papanicolaou (Pap) test to help confirm a diagnosis. The nurse completes the laboratory requisition indicating that the client has which possible diagnosis?

1. Vulvitis
2. Endometriosis
3. Human papilloma virus (HPV) infection
4. AIDS

❽ The nurse is evaluating a client for breast cancer. The nurse explains the risk factors for the development of the disease. Which information should the nurse include in the teaching? Select all that apply.

1. Menarche before age 12
2. Menopause beginning after age 55
3. Giving birth to first child after age 30
4. Being underweight
5. Breast feeding

❾ The nurse is teaching a 61-year-old female client to perform regular breast self-examination (BSE). At which time should the client perform the examination?

1. During menstrual flow
2. At the same time each month
3. At a random time each month
4. Every 2 months

10 When caring for a client with syphilis, the nurse instructs the client that syphilis may be transmitted by which type of contact?

1. Exposure to urinary contaminants
2. Engaging in sexual intercourse
3. Sharing of eating utensils
4. Contaminated hands from improper handwashing

➤ *See Pages 528–530 for Answers and Rationales.*

I. OVERVIEW OF ANATOMY AND PHYSIOLOGY

A. External male reproductive structures (see Figure 15-1)

1. Scrotum: skin-covered sac suspended from perineal region in front of anus; covers, protects, and regulates temperature of testes
2. Testes: male reproductive glands; paired organs suspended in scrotum by spermatic cord
   a. Develop in abdominal cavity of fetus and descend into scrotum
   b. Produce sperm and male hormone testosterone
3. Epididymis: a long, coiled tube attached to side and top of each testis; final area for storage and maturation of sperm; contracts to propel sperm through vas deferens to ampulla where they are stored until ejaculation
4. Ductus deferens (vas deferens): located between epididymis and ejaculatory duct; stores and transports sperm
5. Penis: attached to pubic area in front of scrotum; genital organ that encloses urethra; comparable to female clitoris
   a. Shaft: main part of penis; contains 3 columns of erectile tissue; 2 lateral columns are called corpora cavernosa, and central mass is called corpus spongiosum
   b. Glans: tip of penis
   c. Foreskin: double fold of skin covering glans

B. Internal male genitalia (refer again to Figure 15-1)

1. Urethra: begins at bladder and passes through prostate and penis; pathway for eliminating urine and semen

2. Prostate: encircles urethra just below urinary bladder; walnut-sized gland containing muscle tissue
   a. Secretes thin, milky alkaline fluid into excretory ducts that open into urethra
   b. Alkalinity helps protect sperm from acid present in male urethra and female vagina, thus increasing sperm mobility

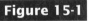

Figure 15-1

The male reproductive system

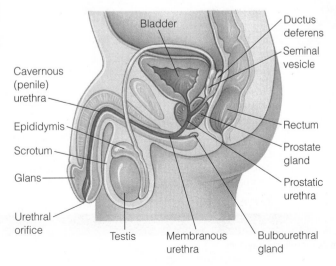

3. Seminal vesicles: located on posterior bladder wall in front of rectum; secrete alkaline fluid containing large amounts of fructose and prostaglandins to help nourish and activate sperm

4. Bulbourethral glands (Cowper's glands): 2 pea-sized structures located on each side of urethra, inferior to prostate; secrete alkaline fluid into urethra and neutralize traces of acidic urine in urethra

5. Semen (seminal fluid): milky, viscous liquid with pH of about 7.5; contains about 120 million sperm per milliliter (mL), plus glandular secretions

C. **Male reproductive physiology**

1. Hypothalamic-pituitary-testicular axis

a. Gonadotropin-releasing hormone from hypothalamus stimulates anterior pituitary to secrete interstitial cell-stimulating hormone

b. Interstitial cell-stimulating hormone in turn stimulates hyperplasia of interstitial cells of testes, leading to production of testosterone

2. Spermatogenesis: sperm produced at rate of 300 million per day; continues throughout male life cycle, but diminishes with age

3. Erection: enlargement and hardening of penis in response to physical or psychological stimuli; afferent input from stimuli are transmitted by pudendal nerve to cerebrum; efferent nerve fibers transmit impulses to sacral portion of parasympathetic nervous system, resulting in dilation of penis

4. Ejaculation: expulsion of semen from urethra to outside; reflex centered in lumbar section of spinal cord sends impulses to genital organs, carrying peristaltic contractions that propel sperm into urethra; ejaculation occurs when impulses reach pudendal nerves and stimulate skeletal muscles at base of penis

D. **Female reproductive structures (see Figure 15-2)**

1. Ovaries: flat, almond-shaped structures on each side of uterus; comparable to male testes; produce and discharge ova

a. Attached to uterus by a ligament

b. Store female germ cells and produce estrogen and progesterone, female hormones

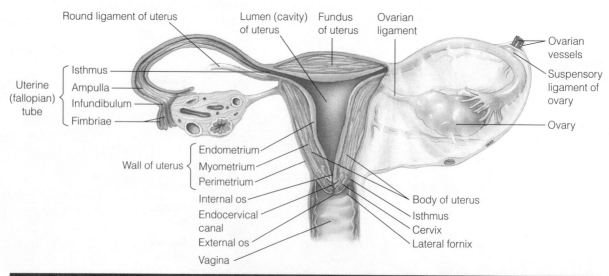

Figure 15-2

The internal organs of the female reproductive system

2. Uterus: pear-shaped, muscular organ with thick walls; located between bladder and rectum; contains 3 parts—fundus, body, and cervix
   a. Supported by 4 ligaments
   b. Receives fertilized ovum and provides site for growth and development of fetus
   c. Uterine wall has 3 layers: perimetrium (outer serous layer), myometrium (middle layer), and endometrium (inner lining)
3. Cervix: portion of uterus that forms pathway between uterus and vagina; softens in response to hormones during pregnancy
   a. Internal os: uterine opening of cervix
   b. External os: vaginal opening of cervix
   c. Endocervical canal: space between these 2 openings
4. Fallopian tubes: thin, cylindrical structures about 4 inches long, attached to uterus on 1 end and supported by broad ligament; propel ovum from ovaries to uterus
   a. Lateral ends are open and made of projections called fimbriae that drape over each ovary; fimbriae pick up ovum (egg) after discharge from ovary
   b. Tubes are lined with ciliated cells and muscle tissue that propel ovum toward uterus
   c. Fertilization of ovum usually occurs in outer portion of fallopian tube
5. Vagina: fibromuscular tube about 3–4 inches long located behind bladder and urethra, in front of rectum; upper end connects with cervix; is a route for excretion of menstrual fluid and is organ of sexual response
6. External genitalia
   a. Mons pubis: soft mound of adipose tissue located in front of symphysis pubis; protects and cushions symphysis pubis; enhances sexual sensations
   b. Labia majora: 2 longitudinal folds of tissue that begin at mons pubis and surround each side of vaginal opening; protect other structures and enhance sexual arousal
   c. Labia minora: smaller tissue folds enclosed by labia majora; protect clitoris, lubricate vulva, and enhance sexual arousal
   d. Vestibule: area enclosed by labia minora
   e. Bartholin's glands: located on each side of vaginal opening; secrete clear mucus during intercourse
   f. Skene's glands: open onto vestibule on each side of urethra; drain urethral glands and produce lubricating mucus
   g. Clitoris: small bud of erectile tissue just below joining of labia minora; stimulates and elevates sexual arousal
   h. Perineum: skin-covered muscular area between vaginal opening and anus; provides support for pelvic organs
7. Breasts: mammary glands located between third and seventh ribs on anterior chest wall; supply nourishment for an infant
   a. Areola: pigmented area containing sebaceous glands and a nipple
   b. Cooper's ligaments support breast and divide each into 15–25 lobes; each lobe contains alveolar glands connected by ducts that open to nipple

E. **Female reproductive physiology**
1. Female sex hormones produced by ovaries
   a. Estrogens: steroid hormones that occur in 3 forms (estradiol and estrone naturally produced by ovaries and estriol, their metabolic product); essential for development and maintenance of secondary sex characteristics and help stimulate female reproductive organs to prepare for growth of fetus; also serve other functions in body
   b. Progesterone: affects development of breast glandular tissue and endometrium
   c. Androgens: responsible for normal hair growth patterns at puberty and have metabolic effects

2. Menstruation cycle: periodic hormonal cycle involving hypothalamus, anterior pituitary gland, uterus, and ovaries; prepares body for pregnancy through release of a single mature ovum and prepares uterus for implantation; normal cycling begins at puberty (often ages 12–15) and ends with menopause (often in 40s or 50s); 28 days is average length of cycle

    a. Menstrual phase: from day 1 to 5; inner endometrial layer of uterus detaches and is expelled as menstrual fluid

    b. Proliferative phase: days 6 to 14; begins as maturing follicle begins to produce estrogen, which stimulates rapid growth of endometrium

    c. Secretory phase: days 14 to 28; corpus luteum produces progesterone, and rising levels increase vascularity of endometrium and change inner layer to secretory mucosa; these changes facilitate passage of sperm into uterus; if fertilization does not occur, hormone levels fall

    d. Ischemic phase: without fertilization, spasm of spiral arteries causes hypoxia of endometrial cells, which degenerate and slough off, leading to menstrual phase

F. Gestation

1. Natural fertilization occurs when ovum is penetrated by 1 sperm cell in fallopian tube; each reproductive cell (one gamete) carries 23 chromosomes; after fertilization, the fertilized egg descends to uterus

2. Embryo: fertilized ovum during first 2 months of development

    a. First 8 weeks, when major organs develop, is most vulnerable period for abnormality to occur

    b. Cells arrange themselves in 3 layers: ectoderm (outer layer), endoderm (inner layer), and mesoderm (middle layer)

3. Fetal membranes: membranes surrounding fetus; composed of 2 layers

    a. Amnion: glistening inner membrane; forms during second week of life; encloses the amniotic cavity

    b. Chorion: outer membrane

4. Amniotic fluid: forms within amniotic cavity and surrounds embryo; consists of 500–1,000 mL of fluid by end of pregnancy

5. Placenta: organ that provides for exchange of nutrients and waste products between mother and fetus; also acts as endocrine organ

    a. Develops by third month; formed by union of chorionic villi and decidua basalis

    b. Provides oxygen and removes carbon dioxide from fetal system

    c. Maintains fetal fluid and electrolyte and acid–base balance

    d. Exchange takes place through diffusion; nutrients pass through, along with drugs, antibodies to some diseases, and certain viruses

    e. Human chorionic gonadotropin (hCG): placental hormone detected in urine 6–9 days after fertilization; stimulates corpus luteum to maintain endometrium and is the basis of immunological test of pregnancy

    f. Human placental lactogen (hPL): similar effects to growth hormone

    g. Estrogen and progesterone: hormones produced by placenta

6. Umbilical cord: extends from fetus to center of fetal surface of placenta; contains blood vessels that supply nutrients and remove waste products

7. Fetal circulation

    a. Arteries carry deoxygenated blood while veins carry oxygenated blood

    b. Circulation bypass occurs because of nonfunctioning lungs: ductus arteriosus (between pulmonary artery and aorta) and foramen ovale (between right and left atrium)

    c. Ductus venosus bypass occurs because fetal liver is not used for waste exchange

    d. Bypasses should close after birth to permit blood to flow through lungs and liver

G. Lactation

1. Hormonal stimulation during pregnancy causes proliferation of glandular tissue within breasts
2. Breasts secrete colostrum for 2–3 days postpartum, a nutrient-rich fluid that also contains maternal antibodies and is a precursor to breast milk
3. Anterior pituitary: stimulates secretion of prolactin once placental hormones that inhibited pituitary gland are absent
4. Breasts become full, distended, tender, and warm within 3–4 days, indicating production of milk; milk usually produced with stimulus of sucking infant
5. Posterior pituitary discharges oxytocin, causing alveoli to contract and allow flow of milk in response to sucking—"let-down reflex"

H. Menopause: permanent cessation of menstruation from loss of ovarian follicular activity

1. Usually occurs at 40–50 years of age as ovaries stop producing progesterone and estrogen
2. Perimenopause: period just before, during, and after menopause
3. Physical changes
   a. Ovaries lose ability to respond to pituitary stimulation and normal ovarian function ceases
   b. Monthly flow becomes smaller, irregular, and gradually ceases
   c. Vagina becomes smaller and secretions diminish; vaginal wall thins and mucosal surface becomes fragile
   d. Uterus, bladder, rectum, and supporting structures lose tone, leading to uterine prolapse, rectocele, and cystocele
   e. Atherosclerosis and osteoporosis are more likely to develop
   f. Hot flashes occur, which are warm sensations that flow over body due to hormonal imbalance of estrogen, progesterone, and testosterone, and are typically accompanied by sweating; females may experience also psychological symptoms (such as irritability, mood swings, depression, anxiety), insomnia, weakness, headache, and dizziness, which are common during perimenopausal period
   g. Hormone replacement therapy (HRT) may be used to manage clients undergoing menopause, which includes estrogen and progestin (progesterone); estrogen given alone can lead to gynecological cancers and thromboembolic disorders; current evidence suggests that HRT accelerates pathogenesis of postmenopausal breast cancer

II. DIAGNOSTIC TESTS AND ASSESSMENTS

A. Laboratory tests

1. Androstenedione level: blood tests for androgen (male sex hormone) levels; normal results are lower in postmenopausal women than in men and adult premenopausal women
2. Estradiol, serum: may identify causes of infertility, menstrual irregularity, or precocious puberty; oral contraceptives lower estradiol levels
3. Estriol: measures fetal viability by measuring urine levels of placental estriol (predominant estrogen excreted in urine during pregnancy); a steady rise in estriol reflects a properly functioning placenta
4. Estrogen-progesterone receptor assay: estrogen and progesterone receptors are cellular proteins that bind hormones before they can elicit a cellular response
   a. Tissue samples in a client with breast cancer help predict client's response to therapy
   b. Clients with tumors positive for estrogen and progesterone receptors respond best to hormonal therapy

5. Estrogen, urine: measures quantity of estradiol, estrone, and estriol (major estrogen hormones) in urine; clinical indications include tumors of ovarian, adrenocortical, or testicular origin

6. Follicle stimulating hormone (FSH), serum: tests gonadal function by measuring plasma levels of FSH
   a. Aids diagnosis of infertility and disorders of menstruation, such as amenorrhea (lack of menstruation)
   b. Aids diagnosis of precocious puberty or hypogonadism

7. FTA-ABS: fluorescent treponemal antibody absorption test; detects antibodies to spirochete that causes syphilis; used to confirm primary or secondary syphilis and verify suspected false-positive results to VDRL

8. Gram stain: uses staining technique to identify infectious organisms in body fluid (for example, blood and urine)

9. Human chorionic gonadotropin (hCG), serum: measures glycoprotein hormone hCG, which should increase steadily during first trimester of pregnancy; levels then fall to less than 10% of peak
   a. Detects early pregnancy
   b. Determines adequacy of hormone production in high-risk pregnancies
   c. Aids diagnosis of certain tumors
   d. Monitors treatment for induction of ovulation and conception

10. Luteinizing hormone, plasma: part of infertility studies for women and men; helps detect ovulation, assess male or female infertility, evaluate amenorrhea, and monitor ovulation-inducing therapy

11. Pregnanetriol, urine: tiny amounts are normal; increased amounts help diagnose adrenogenital syndrome

12. Progesterone, plasma: provides information about corpus luteum function in infertility studies, or placental function in pregnancy; used in conjunction with basal body temperature readings to aid in confirming ovulation

13. Prolactin, serum: measures hormone needed to begin and maintain lactation; aids diagnosis of pituitary or hypothalamic dysfunction, and evaluates secondary amenorrhea

14. Prostate-specific antigen (PSA): helps track course of prostate cancer and response to treatment; is increasingly used as a screening procedure for prostate cancer in men over age 50, but should not be used alone without concurrent physical exam of prostate by digital rectal exam

15. Prostatic acid phosphatase: measures phosphatase enzymes found mostly in prostate; higher than normal levels are suspicious for prostate cancer

16. RPR (rapid plasma reagin): test that indicates whether non-specific antibodies are present in blood; if positive may indicate that organism (*Treponema pallidum*) that causes syphilis is present

17. Semen analysis: collected directly from client, from vagina of a sexual partner, or from vagina or skin of a victim of sexual assault; used to evaluate male fertility, substantiate effectiveness of a vasectomy, or to detect semen on body or clothing of a suspected sexual assault victim

18. Testosterone, serum: to evaluate male infertility or sexual dysfunction, diagnose male sexual precocity, and evaluate female hirsutism (excessive body hair) and virilization (male characteristics)

B. **Radiology studies**

1. Soft tissue mammography: low-dose x-ray examination of breast used to detect breast lesions; also allows comparison of current breast status with that shown by previous films

    2. Contrast mammography: magnetic resonance imaging (MRI) technique to evaluate breast for abnormal growth; uses a contrast medium that is picked up by vascular tumors; provides additional data after abnormal mammogram

    3. Ultrasonography: high-frequency sound waves are recorded as they strike tissues of different densities, providing an image of tissues; evaluates questionable areas detected by physical exam or mammogram

    4. Computed tomography (CT) scan: multiple x-rays are passed through tissues, providing computer-reconstructed images that offer cross-sectional views

C. Cytology

    1. Papanicolaou (Pap) smear: used to screen for cervical cancer, assess hormonal status, and identify presence of sexually transmitted infections, such as human papilloma virus infection; obtained during a pelvic exam by scraping tissue from cervical os

    2. Nipple discharge examination: uses a microscope to exam fluid; usually indicated when bloody or red-brown discharge is noted; may reveal presence of cancer cells

    3. Breast biopsy: tissue is removed from a breast lesion for histologic examination to determine whether cancer is present

        a. Aspiration biopsy: also called fine-needle aspiration biopsy; a fine needle is used to remove cells or fluid from breast lesion; mammography and a computer are used to guide needle

        b. Incisional biopsy: a larger piece of tissue is surgically removed from breast

        c. Excisional biopsy: entire breast lesion is surgically removed, along with surrounding tissue

        d. Tru-cut or core biopsy: a plug of tissue from a breast lesion is removed with a hollow-core needle

        e. Stereotactic needle biopsy: involves computer-guided breast tissue removal using mammographic images from nonpalpable breast lesions

        f. Sentinel node biopsy, used to detect presence of abnormal tissue in nodes, which signals metastases

D. *Colposcopy*: cervix is visualized and magnified using a colposcope (low power microscope) in bright light to identify abnormal areas; used when Pap tests indicate pathologic changes

E. *Laparoscopy*: procedure to visualize internal pelvic organs, using a laparoscope inserted through an incision in abdominal wall

    1. Diagnostic: for endometriosis, ectopic pregnancy, pelvic inflammatory disease, and signs of malignancy

    2. Therapeutic: most often used for tubal sterilization; also useful for removal of peritubal lesions and aspiration of ova for in vitro fertilization

F. Hysteroscopy: an endoscopic exam to visualize interior of uterus and cervical canal, remove intrauterine devices, and complement other diagnostic tests for unexplained bleeding and infertility

G. Nocturnal penile tumescence tests: measures penile tumescence or rigidity during sleep to document presence of sleep-associated erections; based on assumption that men with psychogenic impotence have normal erections during sleep, whereas men with organic impotence have impaired erections during sleep

H. Digital rectal examination: palpation of prostate gland; a gloved, lubricated index finger is inserted in rectum; normal prostate should be wide, nontender, and should feel smooth and rubbery

III. COMMON NURSING TECHNIQUES AND PROCEDURES

A. Breast self-examination (BSE): client education (see Figure 15-3)

    1. Teach client to observe breasts in front of a mirror in 4 positions: with arms relaxed down at side of body, with arms lifted overhead, with hands pressed against hips, and with hands pressed together at waist, leaning forward

Teaching Breast Self-Examination (BSE)

Step 1 Teach the client to observe her breasts in front of a mirror and in good lighting. Tell her to observe her breasts in 4 positions:

- With her arms relaxed and at her sides
- With her arms lifted over her head
- With her hands pressed against her hips
- With her hands pressed together at her waist, leaning forward

Instruct her to look at each breast individually, and then to compare them. She should observe for any visible abnormalities, such as lumps, dimpling, deviation, recent nipple retraction, irregular shape, edema, discharge, or asymmetry.

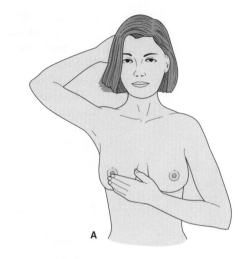

A

Step 2 Teach the client to palpate both breasts while standing or sitting, with one hand behind her head (Figure A). Tell her that many women palpate their breasts in the shower because water and soap make the skin slippery and easier to palpate. Show the woman how to use the pads of her fingers to palpate all areas of her breast, using the concentric circles technique (Figure B). Tell her to press the breast tissue gently against the chest wall, and to be sure to palpate the axillary tail.

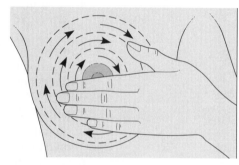

B

Step 3 Instruct the client to palpate her breasts again while lying down, as described in Step 2. Suggest that she place a folded towel under the shoulder and back on the side to be palpated. The arm on the examining side should be over the head, with the hand under the head (Figure C).

Step 4 Teach the client to palpate the areola and nipples next. Show her how to compress the nipple to check for discharge (Figure D).

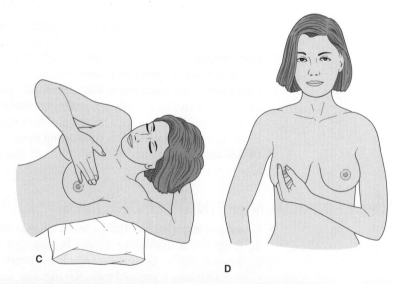

C

D

Step 5 Remind the client to use a calendar to keep a record of when she performs BSE. Teach her to perform BSE at the same time each month, usually 5 days after the onset of menses, when there is less hormonal influence on tissues.

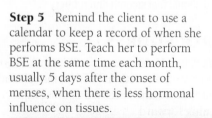

Figure 15-3

Teaching breast self-examination

2. Teach client to palpate both breasts while standing or sitting, holding one hand behind head (see Figure 15-3a); demonstrate using pads of fingers to palpate all areas, using concentric circles (Figure 15-3b)
3. Palpate breasts as described in step 2 while lying down (Figure 15-3c)
4. Teach client to palpate areola and nipples, compressing nipple to check for discharge (Figure 15-3d)
5. Remind client to perform BSE once a month at same time, usually 5 days after menstrual period begins, or same day of each month for postmenopausal women; men should also perform breast self-exam, especially below nipple (most common site of malignancy in men)

B. **Testicular self-examination**: client education
1. Self-examine testicles with soapy hands during a warm shower or bath
2. Gently roll each testicle between thumb and forefinger of each hand; if lumps are noted or one testicle feels significantly larger, notify health care provider
3. Check for any hard lump felt directly on testicle—this is abnormal
4. Perform exam on same day, at least once each month

IV. CARE OF POSTOPERATIVE CLIENT

A. **Nursing management of client undergoing prostate surgery**
1. Maintain usual postoperative assessment
2. If dressings are present, monitor for drainage and change as needed
3. Monitor vital signs (VS) closely for 24 hours, observing for occult and visible signs of hemorrhage (frank blood in urine, large blood clots, decreased hemoglobin and hematocrit, tachycardia, and hypotension)
4. In clients who have a urinary catheter following surgery, traction may be applied against prostatic fossa to prevent bleeding; balloon at tip of catheter exerts pressure to prevent hemorrhage; surgeon positions external end of catheter by anchoring it tightly to client's inner thigh to maintain traction; catheter should not be repositioned
5. A client with a large indwelling catheter may feel urge to void, which results from stimulation of micturition center; explain that this is a normal sensation; efforts by client to void or strain will increase risk of bleeding and worsen discomfort
6. Continuous bladder irrigation (CBI) may be prescribed for a client postoperatively
   a. Purpose of CBI is to prevent formation of blood clots
   b. If blood clots do form, urinary catheter will become blocked and prevent outflow of urine; obstruction will also cause bladder spasms and pain
   c. A key nursing intervention for client on CBI is to keep outflow from catheter light pink or clear; rate of administration of irrigating solution is titrated to keep color of outflow this color and prevent blood clots from forming; it is essential to subtract amount of irrigation intake from urinary catheter output to determine true urine output
   d. Indications that rate of irrigation is inadequate include decreased outflow from catheter, bladder spasms, and dark-colored or frank bloody drainage
7. Monitor mental status in older clients as this too could signal internal hemorrhage; more commonly seen with laparoscopic procedures
8. Irrigant used during and after surgery may be absorbed causing fluid overload and dilutional hyponatremia, referred to as TURP syndrome; monitor for signs of hyponatremia and bradycardia, nausea, and vomiting; monitor serum sodium levels, and hemoglobin and hematocrit (lowered with dilutional effect); in addition, other signs of volume excess will also be evident, including hypertension and confusion
9. If manual irrigations are ordered, maintain sterile technique
10. Medicate as needed for pain

Practice to Pass

A client who is receiving continuous bladder irrigation reports severe bladder spasms. What is your nursing action?

B. Nursing management of client undergoing a mastectomy
1. Maintain usual postoperative assessment
2. Begin emotional support before surgery and continue in postoperative period
3. Encourage client to turn, cough, and deep breathe to prevent respiratory complications; restrictive surgical dressing may decrease chest expansion
4. Position client on back or unaffected side with affected arm elevated to help prevent lymphedema
5. Jackson-Pratt drain or Hemovac may be in place to drain fluids that accumulate when lymph nodes are removed
6. Note signs of bleeding on dressing and reinforce pressure dressing as needed
7. Encourage early range of motion exercise to prevent contractures and lymphedema
8. Use unaffected arm only to provide IV fluids, obtain blood samples and take blood pressure
9. Discharge instructions
   a. Use caution when lifting heavy objects with arm on affected side
   b. Avoid injury and infection on affected side; wear rubber gloves when washing dishes and garden gloves when working outside
   c. Don't allow procedures, such as blood pressure, venipuncture, or intravenous lines, on affected side; elevate arm as recommended to prevent edema formation
   d. Teach care of Jackson Pratt drain if in place at discharge and signs and symptoms of incisional infection to report to surgeon
   e. Refer clients to support group for psychosocial support
   f. Follow-up for postsurgical care and surveillance as recommended

V. DISORDERS OF MALE REPRODUCTIVE SYSTEM

A. *Priapism*
1. Description: sustained, painful erection that lasts at least 4 hours and is not associated with sexual arousal
2. Etiology and pathophysiology
   a. High-flow, or arterial priapism may follow trauma to perineal area or injection of vasodilating drugs into penis to treat **impotence** (inability to achieve or maintain an erection)
   b. Veno-occlusive, or ischemic priapism, is caused by blood trapped within penis, possibly caused by clotting or failure of normal autonomic responses that cause detumescence
   c. Conditions such as sickle cell anemia, leukemia, multiple sclerosis, traumatic brain injury, and metastatic tumors may lead to priapism
   d. Requires medical attention as sustained pressure on tissue could lead to tissue fibrosis or impotence; requires surgical intervention if health care provider unable to successfully treat with medication
3. Assessment
   a. Clinical manifestations: sustained erection not associated with sexual arousal and that client reports is harder than normal, discoloration of penis and penile pain, and urinary retention and bladder distention
   b. Diagnostic and laboratory tests: none
4. Therapeutic management
   a. Analgesia and sedation
   b. Hydration
   c. Treatment of the underlying condition
   d. Aspiration and irrigation of corpus cavernosum and injection of dilute vasoconstrictive agents are possible treatments

e. Surgery may be required if other treatments fail; under local anesthesia, a large needle is passed through glans penis down to distal shaft, and a core of tissue is removed; this is repeated to create fistulas from which blood can drain into corpus spongiosum

5. Priority nursing problems: pain, potential for retained urine, potential for alteration in sexual function

6. Planning and implementation

a. Administer analgesics and sedative promptly, before pain becomes severe and difficult to control

b. Apply ice packs to penis as ordered for pain relief and edema control

c. Facilitate voiding by helping client to a standing position, offering fluids, and running water in sink

d. Report signs of urinary retention: inability to void or voiding in small amounts, may require bladder scan to determine residual volumes

e. Encourage client to verbalize concerns and answer questions pertaining to sexuality and procreation

7. Medication therapy: analgesics and sedation for pain relief; alpha-adrenergic drugs injected into corpora cavernosa to reverse effects of vasodilating drugs when priapism is caused by intracavernosal injection; and intracavernosal injection of alpha-adrenergic drug (epinephrine or phenylephrine) for decompression and detumescence

8. Client education

a. Causes of condition and treatment measures

b. Seek medical attention early if priapism recurs

c. Sexual potency is usually maintained after shunting procedure

d. Report difficulty voiding or painful urination

e. How to care for sutures (if surgery is performed)

9. Evaluation: client reports diminished pain; initiates voiding with output of at least 120 mL; discusses concerns and prognosis with his sexual partner

B. *Phimosis*

1. Description: constriction of foreskin so that it cannot be retracted over glans penis

2. Etiology and pathophysiology

a. May be congenital or related to chronic infections under foreskin (balanoposthitis), leading to adhesions

b. Phimosis prevents adequate hygiene, which may lead to malignant changes and stenosis of meatus

c. Phimosis interferes with erection; penile edema may cause severe pain

3. Assessment

a. Clinical manifestations: nonretractable foreskin, signs of infection (swelling, redness, purulent discharge, and pain), painful erections, and decreased urinary flow, painful urination, and straining to void

b. Diagnostic and laboratory tests: none

4. Therapeutic management

a. A dorsal slit of foreskin may be necessary as an emergency measure

b. Stretching of foreskin by repeated retraction behind glans

c. Circumcision

5. Priority nursing problems: pain, potential for infection or retained urine

6. Planning and implementation

a. Administer antibiotics and apply warms soaks

b. Monitor client's urinary status, including ability to void

c. Encourage fluids to increase urine output

d. Apply cool packs to area for pain relief and to decrease edema

      e. Be aware that circumcision is usually indicated after obstruction and infection are resolved

  7. Medication therapy: antibiotics to treat infection; analgesics for pain relief

  8. Client education

      a. If circumcision or dorsal slit is performed, teach client how to care for incisions; a dry dressing may cover petrolatum gauze dressing and may need to be changed with each voiding; sutures will be absorbed

      b. Sexual intercourse is usually permitted 1 week after surgery

      c. Instruct in personal hygiene measures, especially if circumcision is not performed

      d. Instruct client to report purulent drainage, redness, or edema of penis

  9. Evaluation: client reports that pain is decreased or resolved; voids at least 200 mL of urine within 8 hours after treatment or surgery; foul-smelling or purulent drainage is absent; client describes proper hygiene and wound care; client describes signs of infection

C. Erectile dysfunction (ED)

  1. Description

      a. Inability to attain and maintain an erection sufficient to perform satisfactory sexual intercourse

      b. The term *impotence* is synonymous with ED; may describe total inability to achieve erection, or inconsistent erections, or ability to sustain only brief erections

  2. Etiology and pathophysiology

      a. Age-related changes involve cellular and tissue changes in penis, decreased sensory activity, decreased testosterone levels, and effects of chronic illness such as diabetes mellitus

      b. Veno-occlusive mechanism prevents blood from leaving penis; problems with this mechanism cause incomplete erections

      c. Damage to arteries, smooth muscles, and fibrous tissues by disease is most common cause of ED (diabetes, kidney disease, chronic alcoholism, atherosclerosis, and vascular disease cause 70% of cases)

      d. Prostate surgery may damage innervation and blood flow to penis

      e. Many medications, such as antihypertensive agents or psychotropic agents (haloperidol [Haldol], chlorpromazine [Thorazine]), can lead to impotence

      f. Psychogenic causes include depression, stress, fatigue, and fear of failure

      g. Substance abuse often causes erectile dysfunction

  3. Assessment

      a. Clinical manifestations: inability to have or maintain an erection or inability to penetrate for intercourse

      b. Diagnostic and laboratory tests

         1) Blood profiles

         2) Nocturnal penile tumescence and rigidity (NPTR)

         3) Cavernosometry (evaluates arterial inflow and venous outflow of penis)

         4) Intracavernous injections to differentiate between physical and psychological causes of erectile dysfunction

         5) Psychological evaluation

  4. Therapeutic management: external mechanical devices such as vacuum constriction device (VCD), counseling and sex therapy, implantation of prosthetic devices, and vascular reconstructive surgery

  5. Priority nursing problems: possible altered sexual function, reduced self-esteem, reduced ability to perform roles, reduced coping

  6. Planning and implementation

      a. Be aware that some clients feel shame and have difficulty discussing ED

      b. Vacuum devices may be used, but they are clumsy and reduce spontaneity

7. Medication therapy
   a. Phosphodiesterase type 5 inhibitors such as sildenafil (Viagra), tadalafil (Cialis), and vardenafil (Levitra) may relax smooth muscle in corpus cavernosum, increasing ability to maintain an erection; assess medication history (contraindicated for men taking nitrates because of risk of hypotension); assess risk of priapism (men with sickle cell disease, leukemia, or physical abnormality of penis)
   b. Self-administered intracavernous injections of papaverine or prostaglandin E may be used
   c. Transdermal nitroglycerin paste may occasionally restore erectile function caused by arteriolar dilation
   d. Alprostadil (Muse), a single use urethral suppository with applicator, leads to erection within approximately 10 minutes, but reduces spontaneity and can cause burning of urethra
8. Client education
   a. For clients who take phosphodiesterase inhibitors: take drug at times recommended before sexual activity; do not use drug more than once a day; discontinue drug and notify health care provider if chest pain or shortness of breath occur with use
   b. Technique of intracavernous injection and use of any prescribed topical drugs
   c. Use of mechanical devices, such as vacuum constriction device
   d. Causes of sexual dysfunction that can be controlled include smoking, alcohol use, and drug abuse
   e. Provide list of support services for client and sexual partner
   f. Encourage discussion of alternate sexual practices
9. Evaluation: demonstrates use of mechanical device; verbalizes actions and use of medication; states satisfaction with and acceptance of alternative sexual practices; understands cause of sexual dysfunction and verbalizes appropriate treatment

D. **Orchitis**
   1. Description: infection or inflammation of one or both of testicles
   2. Etiology and pathophysiology
      a. Rarely a primary infection; usually caused by ascending infection from epididymis, or spread from elsewhere in body by lymph nodes
      b. Many different organisms lead to infection, including bacteria, viruses, parasites, and fungi
      c. Trauma or surgery may cause inflammation of testes
      d. Orchitis related to mumps usually occurs 4–6 days after inflammation of parotid glands
      e. Testicular abscesses, atrophy, fibrosis, and infertility may result from orchitis
   3. Assessment
      a. Clinical manifestations
         1) Fever, chills, and sudden pain that involves testes, radiating to groin
         2) Nausea and vomiting may accompany pain
         3) Tenderness, redness, and warmth; scrotal skin may also be red and edematous
         4) Some men experience few symptoms and may report only scrotal edema
         5) Presence of other infections, including mumps, urinary tract infection (UTI), or epididymitis
      b. Diagnostic and laboratory tests: urine culture to determine presence of infection, and sensitivity test to determine appropriate antibiotic treatment
   4. Therapeutic management
      a. Antibiotics
      b. Aspiration of fluid if hydrocele is present to be sent for pathology testing
   5. Priority nursing problems: scrotal pain, potential for infection, fever, fear

6. Planning and implementation
   a. Bed rest, scrotal elevation, and cold applications to decrease inflammation of testes
   b. Administer antibiotic therapy based on causative organism
   c. Monitor symptoms, including fever, pain, nausea, and vomiting
7. Medication therapy: antibiotics to treat infection, analgesics for discomfort, anti-emetics for nausea, anti-inflammatory agents for inflammation, and corticosteroids to reduce symptoms
8. Client education
   a. How to use medications and importance of finishing antibiotic regime, even after symptoms resolve
   b. How to change dressing (if incision and drainage done); observe wound for redness and drainage; cleanse site gently with sterile water or saline
   c. How to apply a scrotal support to provide elevation and secure dressing
   d. Exposure to mumps can result in sterility because of orchitis
9. Evaluation: client verbalizes purpose and correct use of medications, demonstrates dressing change procedure and use of scrotal support, states that pain is diminished or absent, temperature is reduced or normal, and describes measures to prevent recurrences

E. **Epididymitis**
   1. Description: infection or inflammation of epididymis, a small structure that rests on testes
   2. Etiology and pathophysiology
      a. Most common intrascrotal infection, but causes differ among younger and older men
      b. In younger men, most often caused by sexually transmitted urethritis caused by *Chlamydia trachomatis* or *Neisseria gonorrhoeae*, or by physical trauma
      c. In older men, usually associated with UTI or prostatitis
      d. Usually is unilateral and caused by infection; may be a complication of invasive urinary tract procedures, such as catheterization or cystoscopy; bilateral orchitis (rarer) is typically associated with tuberculosis
   3. Assessment
      a. Clinical manifestations: red and swollen scrotum; possible urethral discharge; severe pain and tenderness in groin and scrotum on affected side; fever; nausea and vomiting; burning, frequency, and urgency with urination; possible "duck waddle" walk to avoid pressure on groin and scrotum
      b. Diagnostic and laboratory tests
         1) White blood cell count may be elevated (between 20,000 and 30,000/mm^3)
         2) Urinalysis shows increased WBC and presence of bacteria and urine culture to identify organism
         3) Scrotal ultrasound
         4) Radionuclide scan
         5) Aspiration of fluid from the epididymis
         6) Cytologic examination of semen
   4. Therapeutic management: antibiotic therapy and anti-inflammatory drugs
   5. Priority nursing problems: pain, fever, fear
   6. Planning and implementation
      a. Encourage bedrest for 5–7 days or until pain free
      b. Elevate client's scrotum and provide cold packs to control pain and edema
      c. Administer antibiotics as ordered; severe cases require IV antibiotics
      d. Inspect scrotal area for changes
      e. Monitor temperature and provide antipyretics as prescribed; offer fluids to replace fluid lost through diaphoresis and increased metabolism
      f. Check results of any STI test done to ensure adequate treatment has been started

7. Medication therapy: antibiotics to treat infection, antipyretics for fever, analgesics for pain relief, antiemetics to treat nausea

8. Client education

   a. Elevate scrotum with a towel or scrotal support to reduce pain and edema; scrotal support may be worn up to 6 weeks as necessary

   b. Application of intermittent cold compresses to scrotum or taking sitz baths

   c. Purpose, use, and potential adverse effects of antibiotics; take all medication, even if symptoms resolve

   d. Client should ask questions about effects of infection on fertility; sterility is usually a complication of bilateral epididymitis and may develop with recurrences of infection; erectile dysfunction is not a concern

   e. Cause of epididymitis and reasons for treatment; how to prevent recurrence of infection (drink 3,000 mL of fluid daily to prevent UTI) and other measures to decrease risk of reinfection

   f. If caused by a sexually transmitted organism, advise client to avoid sexual intercourse until partner has been examined and efficiently treated

9. Evaluation: client states that pain is diminished or absent; temperature is reduced or returned to normal; discusses concerns about sterility and sexual function; states cause of infection; correctly describes self-care activities; describes measures to prevent recurrences

F. **Hydrocele**

1. Description: abnormal fluid collection within layers of tunica vaginalis, which surrounds testis

2. Etiology and pathophysiology

   a. May be unilateral or bilateral

   b. In adults, may be secondary to epididymo-orchitis, scrotal trauma, testicular cancer, or hypoalbuminemia

   c. Caused by increased production of fluid within scrotum, or decreased reabsorption of fluid; size of hydrocele depends on extent of imbalance between fluid production and reabsorption

   d. Large hydrocele can impair physical activity and compromise blood supply to testis

   e. Fluid characteristics depend on cause; fluid associated with infection may be cloudy and contain bacteria

3. Assessment

   a. Clinical manifestations: swelling, pain and tenderness of testes; discrepancies in size of testes

   b. Diagnostic and laboratory tests: transillumination with a bright light shows fluid collection in mass

4. Therapeutic management: no treatment is needed unless mass enlarges and causes discomfort; treatment may include aspiration via a needle and syringe or hydrocelectomy (removal of fluid-filled sac)

5. Priority nursing problems: potential for altered sexual function or infection

6. Planning and implementation

   a. Observe and monitor degree of scrotal edema

   b. Treatment may be unnecessary, but provide supportive care for client

   c. Fluid aspiration is most conservative treatment; provide information as needed and allow client to verbalize concerns and questions

   d. Provide medication for pain control as needed

   e. If hydrocelectomy is performed, make standard postoperative assessments, note color and amount of wound drainage; provide scrotal support, cold packs, and pain medication

Practice to Pass

What advice would you give a client who contracted epididymitis from a sexual partner?

7. Medication therapy: analgesics for pain control; sclerosing drug, such as 5% tetracycline, may be injected into scrotal sac after aspiration of fluid
8. Client education instructions after hydrocelectomy
   a. Apply ice packs to scrotum as instructed
   b. Change dressing daily and as needed; cleanse wound with soap and water
   c. Reapply clean scrotal support
   d. Keep scrotum elevated until edema resolves
   e. Remind client that scrotal edema will disappear in 2–4 weeks
   f. Avoid intercourse and strenuous activity until directed by care provider
   g. Sutures are absorbable
9. Evaluation: client describes procedure for applying cold packs to scrotum; demonstrates changing scrotal wound dressing; verbalizes reason for elevating scrotum; lists symptoms to be reported; reports that symptoms are relieved

G. Varicocele

1. Description: a cluster of dilated veins from pampiniform venous complex on spermatic cord that form a soft mass that can cause pain
2. Etiology and pathophysiology
   a. Usually occurs in men between ages 15 and 40, with no known cause
   b. Occasionally caused by defect in valves of internal spermatic veins
   c. Commonly associated with infertility, for unclear reasons; venous enlargement may increase scrotal temperature (impairing sperm production and motility)
3. Assessment
   a. Clinical manifestations
      1) Often asymptomatic; dull ache or heavy feeling in scrotum on affected side
      2) Dilated, tortuous veins may be palpated posterior to and above affected testis when standing; mass usually disappears when client lies down
      3) Rush of blood can be felt in scrotum when client performs Valsalva maneuver
   b. Diagnostic and laboratory tests: Doppler ultrasonogram or venogram may confirm diagnosis
4. Therapeutic management
   a. Surgical repair of varicocele (varicocelectomy)
   b. Embolization (occluding internal spermatic vein on affected side, using a balloon-tipped catheter, coil, or sclerosing agent) may be performed in conjunction with venography
   c. Ligation of spermatic vein
5. Priority nursing problems: pain, potential for infection
6. Planning and implementation: apply scrotal support to relieve discomfort; prepare client for surgery as indicated (client often returns home within a few hours of surgery)
7. Medication therapy: sclerosing agent injected into internal spermatic vein; analgesic medications for discomfort
8. Client education after varicocelectomy
   a. Remain at home for about 5 days and avoid driving for 1 week
   b. Avoid strenuous physical activity for 3 weeks
   c. Follow health care provider's instructions for resuming sexual activity
   d. Fertility may not be restored by procedure, and effects won't be known for several months
   e. Remove soiled dressing and cleanse wound gently with soap and water
   f. Wear scrotal support to decrease edema
9. Evaluation: client describes importance of wearing scrotal support; demonstrates changing wound dressing; verbalizes reason for elevating scrotum; lists symptoms to be reported

Practice to Pass

At what ages are male clients most likely to develop a varicocele?

H. *Testicular torsion*

1. Description: twisting of spermatic cord
2. Etiology and pathophysiology
   - **a.** Is considered a urological surgical emergency; twisting cuts off blood flow to testes and may lead to testicular ischemia and necrosis on affected side, depending on degree of torsion and length of time blood flow is compromised
   - **b.** Almost always occurs between birth and age 20
   - **c.** Cause is not well understood; possibly related to elevated hormone levels and abnormal attachment of testicles to scrotum; is more common in men who had prolonged undescended testes
   - **d.** Three types of testicular torsion: intravaginal (twisting of testicle within its outer coat), extravaginal (strangulation of spermatic cord at external inguinal ring), and torsion of appendix teste (twisting of 1 of 4 testicular appendages)
3. Assessment
   - **a.** Clinical manifestations (see Box 15-1 for clinical signs of testicular torsion)
   - **b.** Diagnostic and laboratory tests: urinalysis usually is normal; orchiogram, testicular scan, and Doppler study shows diminished or obstructed blood flow
4. Therapeutic management: detorsion (surgical untwisting of spermatic cord), orchiopexy (surgical fixation of testis to scrotal wall), or orchiectomy (surgical excision of testicle)
5. Priority nursing problems: pain, anxiety, alteration in body image, inadequate knowledge
6. Medication therapy: analgesics for pain relief
7. Planning and implementation
   - **a.** Prepare client for diagnostic studies; once diagnosis is confirmed or likely, prepare client for emergency surgery
   - **b.** After surgery for detorsion of testicle and fixation of scrotum, which usually requires a small, midline incision in scrotum: apply cold packs and scrotal support to minimize pain; observe incision for redness or purulent drainage; provide analgesics as needed

---

Box 15-1	**Intravaginal Torsion**: caused by twisting of testicle within its outer coat
Clinical Signs of Testicular Torsion	• Sudden onset of scrotal pain, sometimes related to trauma, may radiate to lower abdomen and groin; acute on-and-off pain suggests intermittent torsion; swollen, reddened and tender testis; the affected side is usually elevated

Intravaginal Torsion: caused by twisting of testicle within its outer coat

- Sudden onset of scrotal pain, sometimes related to trauma, may radiate to lower abdomen and groin; acute on-and-off pain suggests intermittent torsion; swollen, reddened and tender testis; the affected side is usually elevated
- Tender epididymis
- Nausea and vomiting
- Cremasteric reflex depressed or absent on same side of torsion (elicited by stroking or gently pinching skin of upper inner thigh while observing scrotum; a normal response is contraction of cremasteric muscles of scrotum, with elevation of testis)

Extravaginal Torsion: caused by strangulation of spermatic cord at external inguinal ring

- Symptoms similar to those of intravaginal torsion

Torsion of Appendix Teste: caused by twisting of 1 of 4 testicular appendages

- Less severe symptoms
- Cremasteric reflex present

Practice to Pass

Why is testicular torsion considered a medical emergency?

   8. Client education
      a. Reinforce knowledge concerning effect of surgery on sexuality
      b. Signs and symptoms of complications; bleeding, gaping incision, purulent drainage from incision
      c. Methods to control pain, such as ice packs and scrotal support
      d. Remain at home for about 5 days and avoid driving for 1 week
      e. Avoid strenuous physical activity for 3 weeks
      f. Follow health care provider's instructions for resuming sexual activity
   9. Evaluation: client describes importance of wearing scrotal support; demonstrates changing wound dressing; verbalizes reason for elevating scrotum; and lists symptoms to be reported

I. Testicular cancer

   1. Description: unregulated growth of abnormal cells within testicles
   2. Etiology and pathophysiology
      a. Exact cause is unknown, but risk factors include cryptorchidism (undescended testicles at birth), maternal treatment with diethylstilbestrol (DES) during pregnancy, mumps orchitis, trauma, environmental factors, and age or treatment with DES for prostate cancer
      b. Testicular cancer is most common cancer among males age 15–35
      c. 90% of cancers arise from germ cell epithelium of testes
      d. Testicular cancer is usually slow-growing and localized with a good prognosis
   3. Assessment
      a. Clinical manifestations
         1) Presenting sign is most often a painless, hardened area or lump found during self-exam
         2) Dull ache in pelvis or scrotum
         3) Testicular pain may occur with associated infection, necrosis, or hemorrhage
         4) Weight loss and fatigue
         5) Metastatic signs such as respiratory symptoms, GI disturbances, lumbar back pain, lymphadenopathy, and **gynecomastia** (abnormal enlargement of breasts in men)
      b. Diagnostic and laboratory tests
         1) Scrotal ultrasound; CT scan or MRI of chest, abdomen, and pelvis to rule out metastasis
         2) Intravenous pyelogram
         3) Alpha fetoprotein (AFP) and beta unit of human chorionic gonadotropin (hCG) are markers used to monitor therapeutic responses; elevated levels provide strong evidence of testicular cancer; markers are measured after surgery to help determine presence of residual disease, possibly in lymph nodes
         4) Serum lactic acid dehydrogenase (LDH) is elevated with testicular cancer
   4. Therapeutic management
      a. Orchiectomy and exploration of adjacent area to identify cancer cell type and stage disease (see Box 15-2)

Box 15-2	• **Stage A (I)** Tumor confined to the testis
Staging of Testicular Cancer	• **Stage B1 (IIa)** A few lymph nodes affected in the retroperitoneum, usually detected at time of node dissection
	• **Stage B2 (IIb)** Nodes greater than 2 cm to 6 cm
	• **Stage B3 (IIc)** Nodes greater than 6 cm
	• **Stage C (III)** Spread above the diaphragm, especially to the lungs or abdominal solid organs

     b. Nonsurgical therapies include radiation therapy and chemotherapy

     c. Lymphadenectomy

  5. Priority nursing diagnosis: Risk for Disturbed Body Image, Risk for Ineffective Health Maintenance, Deficient Knowledge, Ineffective Coping

  6. Planning and implementation

     a. Prepare client for screening tests to determine type of cancer and stage

     b. Provide emotional support for client and family; respond to questions and encourage client to express his feelings

     c. Prepare client for surgery if indicated

     d. Prepare client for chemotherapy after surgery and possible radiation therapy, if cancer has spread to lymph nodes

     e. After surgery: provide analgesics, ice packs, and scrotal support to control; monitor for complications, such as bleeding or infection

     f. Refer for education and counseling related to sperm banking pretreatment

  7. Medication therapy: chemotherapy with combination of drugs

  8. Client education

     a. Type of cancer found, extent of disease, and plans for treatment

     b. Importance of monthly testicular examination, because malignancy may develop in remaining testis

     c. Possibility of preserving sperm in a bank before surgery to help relieve client's fears about infertility

     d. Orchiectomy should have no lasting effects on client's sexual or reproductive function

     e. Signs of complications: bleeding, gaping incision, or purulent drainage from incision

     f. Methods to control pain, such as ice packs and scrotal support

     g. Remain at home for about 5 days and avoid driving for 1 week

     h. Avoid strenuous physical activity for 3 weeks

     i. Follow health care provider's instructions for resuming sexual activity

     j. Importance of follow-up, especially if retroperitoneal lymph nodes were not surgically explored; client will need periodic physical examinations, tumor markers, and CT scans of retroperitoneal nodes for 5–10 years after surgery

  9. Evaluation: client reports that postoperative pain is decreased or absent; describes realistically effects of surgery on appearance and function; resumes self-care activities; describes treatment plan; demonstrates care of incision; describes importance of monthly self-exam; demonstrates testicular self-exam; states date and time of first postoperative follow-up visit and importance of frequent appointments

J. Prostatitis

  1. Definition: inflammation of prostate gland caused by an infectious agent

  2. Etiology and pathophysiology

     a. Bacterial infection usually ascends from urinary tract or comes from blood or lymph nodes; *Escherichia coli* most common organism

     b. Chronic bacterial prostatitis may follow an acute episode of illness

     c. Nonbacterial prostatitis is most common type; cause is unknown

     d. Prostatodynia: symptoms of prostatitis without physical findings; possibly caused by muscle spasms of urethral sphincter; also referred to as nonbacterial prostatitis (NBP)

  3. Assessment

     a. Clinical manifestations

        1) Client reports urinary burning, urgency, frequency

        2) Urethral discharge

        3) Low back pain or perineal pain

        4) Generalized pain or pain associated with ejaculation or voiding

        5) If acute, client may have sudden onset of fever, chills, and pain

        6) Symptoms of acute cystitis including cloudy and malodorous urine, and possibly blood in urine

        7) Tender, swollen prostate; in chronic prostatitis, prostate may be irregular, firm, and tender on manual examination

    b. Diagnostic and laboratory tests

        1) WBC elevated

        2) Urine positive for WBCs and bacteria

        3) Culture of prostatic secretions for blood cells and bacteria; typically WBCs are present in prostatic secretions

        4) Note PSA levels (though typically associated with cancer) are often elevated with both bacterial and NBP

4. Therapeutic management: antibiotic therapy; anti-inflammatory agents in nonbacterial prostatitis; prostatic massage

5. Priority nursing problems: pain, potential for infection, potential for retained urine, potential alteration in body image, inadequate knowledge

6. Planning and implementation

    a. Administer antibiotic therapy as prescribed

    b. Maintain bed rest to decrease prostate swelling and pain until symptoms subside

    c. Promote comfort with analgesics, antispasmodics, sedatives

    d. Offer warm sitz baths and rectal irrigation for pain relief

    e. Reassure client that sexual and reproductive functions are not damaged

7. Medication therapy: antibiotics to treat infection; analgesics for discomfort; nonsteroidal anti-inflammatory drugs (NSAIDs) for inflammation; anticholinergic drugs to facilitate voiding; alpha-blocking agents for prostatodynia to relax perineal muscles; and stool softeners to promote comfort during bowel elimination

8. Client education

    a. Instruct in purpose, use, and potential adverse effects of medications

    b. Encourage normal sexual activity during prostatodynia unless ejaculation is painful or there is increasing discomfort during this activity

    c. Provide instructions on use of sitz baths to control pain and spasms

    d. Encourage client to drink 2,000–3,000 mL of water daily to dilute urine and keep feces soft; high-fiber diet helps soften stools, but consider low residue diet to decrease bulking in rectum

    e. Instruct clients with chronic bacterial prostatitis that periodic prostate massage may be helpful to release pus cells and bacteria

    f. Instruct that alcohol, caffeine, and foods containing hot spices may increase symptoms

9. Evaluation: client states that pain and urinary symptoms have decreased or are gone; verbalizes need to restrict certain foods and beverages; describes measures to prevent recurrence; and verbalizes correct use of medications

K. Benign prostatic hyperplasia (BPH)

1. Definition: overgrowth of cells in prostate gland

2. Etiology and pathophysiology

    a. Appears to be a normal part of aging, but exact cause is unknown; occurs in aging men with normal testicular function

    b. Usually occurs as nodules in lateral or middle lobes of prostate; nodules grow and compress normal prostatic tissue

        c. Nodular enlargement also presses against urethra and narrows it

            1) Bladder muscles hypertrophy (enlarge) to compensate for resistance to urination; fibromuscular bands or cords form, along with bladder diverticula; client has increased risk for bladder calculi and urinary retention

            2) Ureters may dilate because of increased voiding pressure

            3) Kidneys may become distended, leading to renal insufficiency

3. Assessment

    a. Clinical manifestations

        1) Many men have no symptoms

        2) Classic symptoms: urinary frequency, nocturia, difficulty starting and stopping urine stream, a weak stream, overflow dribbling, and feeling of being unable to completely empty bladder

        3) Signs of cystitis, which may develop due to retained urine: painful urination, pyuria, and fever

        4) Digital rectal exam will reveal an enlarged prostate gland

    b. Diagnostic and laboratory tests

        1) Routine urinalysis and culture

        2) Acid phosphatase and PSA to rule out prostatic cancer

        3) Urodynamic studies to determine degree of urinary obstruction

        4) Post-voiding catheterization; residual urine of more than 100 mL is considered high

        5) Diagnostic studies include ultrasound and cystoscopy

4. Therapeutic management

    a. Pharmacologic (see section to follow)

    b. Nonsurgical invasive management

        1) Application of heat

        2) Balloon dilation: balloon-tipped catheter is inserted through urethra and then is inflated to stretch urethra where it is narrowed by prostate

        3) Laser ablation

        4) Application of stents or coils in prostatic urethra

    c. Surgical intervention

        1) Transurethral resection of the prostate (TURP): most common approach for partial removal of prostate; no surgical incision is made; approach is through a resectoscope inserted through urethra

        2) Transurethral incision of prostate (TUIP): incision is made through bladder neck

        3) Suprapubic resection: surgical approach involves an abdominal incision and cutting through bladder to anterior aspect of prostate

        4) Retropubic resection: a low midline abdominal incision is made to approach prostate

        5) Perineal resection: this is used commonly in cases of prostatic cancer; incision to approach prostate is made between anus and scrotum

5. Priority nursing problems: potential for retained urine or infection, potential alteration in body image, inadequate knowledge

6. Planning and implementation

    a. Client's treatment is based on severity of symptoms, degree of prostate enlargement, and presence of complications (urinary retention leading to UTIs, pyelonephritis, and sepsis)

    b. Monitor medication therapy if indicated

    c. Encourage fluids (2,000–3,000 mL per day) to reduce risk of infection

    d. Suggest diet high in minerals: calcium, magnesium, zinc, and manganese

e. Avoid drugs that could cause urinary retention (anticholinergics)

f. Provide postoperative care following prostatectomy

g. The client who undergoes a TURP will have a 3-way urinary catheter and CBI (refer back to CBI discussion earlier in chapter)

h. After retropubic prostatectomy, assess abdominal incision for signs of infection; urine in dressing is not a normal finding since bladder is not accessed in this type of surgery

i. After suprapubic prostatectomy, monitor outputs from both suprapubic and urethral catheters

j. After perineal prostatectomy, preventing infection is vital since incision is near to anus; avoid rectal temperatures or enemas

k. Monitor urine character following prostatectomy
   1) Clear to pale pink: normal during entire hospital course
   2) Light red to red: normal or expected on day of surgery and first postoperative day
   3) Very dark red: could indicate venous bleeding or inadequate CBI flow; check flow rate and VS and tell surgeon
   4) Bright red: could indicate arterial bleeding; check CBI flow rate, check VS, and notify surgeon
   5) Blood clots: are normal if they are only occasional, but increase CBI flow rate to prevent catheter obstruction

7. Medication therapy: finasteride (Proscar) reduces hypertrophy but has severe side effects (impotence); alpha blockers inhibit alpha-adrenergic mediated contraction of prostatic smooth muscle to decrease straining on urination

8. Client education
   a. Engaging in regular prostatic massage and sexual intercourse helps decrease prostatic congestion
   b. Limit amount of fluids taken at one time to avoid bladder distention
   c. Increase fluid intake to 2,000–3,000 mL daily to decrease risk for bladder infection
   d. Do not ignore urge to void; urinate when sensation of bladder fullness occurs
   e. Avoid drugs that can cause urinary retention, such as anticholinergics, antidepressants, decongestants, and tranquilizers

9. Evaluation: client voids without difficulty and reports steady stream of urine; free of signs of UTI; verbalizes use, purpose, and potential adverse effects of medications; verbalizes usefulness of regular prostatic massage; increases fluid intake to 2,000–3,000 mL per day; and lists drug classes that cause urinary retention

L. Prostate cancer

1. Description: unregulated growth of abnormal cells in prostate gland

2. Etiology and pathophysiology
   a. Adenocarcinoma is most common type; high levels of testosterone may play a role
   b. Usually begins in peripheral tissue on back and sides of gland
   c. Metastasis via lymph and venous channels is common; bony tissue is major site of distant metastasis—especially pelvic bones and spine
   d. Is seen predominantly over 40 years of age

3. Assessment
   a. Clinical manifestations
      1) Clients in early stages often show no symptoms; tumor may be found during digital prostate exam

Practice to Pass

What symptoms would alert you to a possible enlarged prostate gland?

2) Genitourinary (GU): dysuria, frequency, reduced force of stream, hematuria, nocturia, abnormal prostate found on digital rectal exam

3) Musculoskeletal: back pain, migratory bone pain, bone or joint pain

4) Neurological: nerve pain, muscle spasms, bowel or bladder dysfunction, bilateral weakness of lower extremities

5) Systemic: fatigue and weight loss

    b. Diagnostic and laboratory tests: PSA levels, transrectal ultrasonography (obtained if PSA results are abnormal), tissue biopsy, bone scan; MRI, or CT scans to detect metastasis

4. Therapeutic management

    a. Hormone therapy

    b. Radiation therapy; brachytherapy (radioactive seeds implanted in prostate)

    c. Prostatic cryosurgery

    d. Surgery

        1) Orchiectomy decreases androgen production

        2) Radical procedures include removal of gland, capsule, ampulla, vas deferens, seminal vesicles, adjacent lymph nodes, and cuff of bladder neck

        3) Suprapubic prostatectomy: abdominal and bladder incisions to remove prostate tissue

        4) Retropubic prostatectomy: low abdominal incision without opening bladder

        5) Perineal prostatectomy: incision between scrotum and anus (perineal area)

        6) Homium laser: laser treatment; less bleeding, fewer complications, and shorter hospital stay

5. Priority nursing problems: alteration in urinary elimination, altered sexual function, pain, reduced self-esteem, alteration in body image

6. Planning and implementation

    a. Treatment is complex and depends on stage of cancer, client's age, and general health

    b. Encourage annual prostate exam for men 40 years old and above

    c. Complete preoperative and postoperative care of client undergoing prostate surgery (discussed earlier in chapter)

7. Medication therapy: estrogen therapy or luteinizing hormone antagonist (Lupron) given to slow rate of growth and extension of tumor

8. Client education

    a. Nature of health problem and treatment plan; reinforce knowledge and option questions

    b. Methods to deal with urinary incontinence, which occurs temporarily after surgery, but could be permanent if bladder sphincters have been permanently damaged

    c. Care of urinary catheter

    d. Methods of pain control

    e. Impact of therapy on sexual function (temporary or permanent impotence, permanent infertility after radical prostatectomy)

    f. Importance of follow-up tests for recurrence of disease

    g. Signs of spinal cord compression (back pain and lower extremity weakness), because of high incidence of metastasis to spinal cord

    h. Maintain activity levels as prescribed

    i. Refer client to support groups, such as the American Cancer Society

9. Evaluation: client verbalizes knowledge of disease and treatment plan, importance of follow-up visits, signs of spinal cord compression, and activity limitations following surgery

VI. SEXUALLY TRANSMITTED INFECTIONS (STI)

A. Pelvic inflammatory disease (PID)

1. Description: inflammatory condition of pelvic cavity that may involve ovaries, fallopian tubes, vascular system, or pelvic peritoneum
2. Etiology and pathophysiology
   a. Usually caused by more than one microbe (polymicrobial)
   b. Microorganisms enter vagina and travel to uterus during sexual activity, childbirth, abortion, or surgery
   c. Infection spreads to uterine tubes and obstructs them with scar tissue; may cause abscesses on ovaries and spread to blood stream through lymphatic system
   d. PID is a major cause of female infertility
   e. Prognosis depends on number of episodes, prompt treatment, and modification of risk factors by client
3. Assessment
   a. Clinical manifestations: fever and malaise; nausea and vomiting; purulent foul-smelling vaginal discharge, dysuria and **dyspareunia** (painful intercourse); tenderness to severe lower abdominal pain; moving or walking may aggravate pain
   b. Diagnostic and laboratory tests: vaginal examination, elevated leukocytes and erythrocyte sedimentation rate (ESR), cultures from the vagina or cervix, and ultrasound to detect abscess
4. Therapeutic management: antibiotic therapy, application of heat to relieve pain, and surgical excision of abscess if present
5. Priority nursing problems: pain, potential for nonadherence to treatment plan, alteration in sexual function
6. Planning and implementation
   a. Place client in semi-Fowler's position to facilitate drainage
   b. Apply warmth to abdomen for comfort
   c. Administer warm douches to improve circulation
   d. Monitor VS, especially temperature
   e. Administer antibiotics as prescribed
   f. Note nature and amount of vaginal discharge
   g. Use infection control techniques (standard precautions)
7. Medication therapy: broad-spectrum antibiotics to treat infection; analgesics for discomfort; and antipyretics for fever
8. Client education
   a. Risk factors for PID: use of IUDs, history of STI, multiple sexual partners, and previous PID
   b. Importance of completing treatment regime and keeping follow-up appointments, even if symptoms resolve (noncompliance is common)
   c. Proper perineal care, especially wiping from front to back
   d. Use tampons cautiously; change tampons at least every 4 hours
   e. Information about safe sexual practices and family planning
   f. Report unusual vaginal discharge or odor
9. Evaluation: client reports abdominal pain and abnormal vaginal discharge resolved; body temperature returns to normal limits; lists causes and risk factors for PID; states importance of completing treatment regime and follow-up visits; and verbalizes proper perineal care

B. Syphilis

1. Description: a systemic STI caused by a spirochete, which may infect almost any body tissue or organ
2. Etiology and pathophysiology

a. Caused by spirochete *Treponema pallidum*, transmitted from open lesions during any type of sexual contact (oral–genital, anal–genital, or genital–genital)

b. Organism can survive for days in fluids; average incubation period is 10–90 days

c. Course of disease varies and is prolonged; 30–40 years may pass between initial infection and late clinical signs; many clients experience a latency period when no symptoms are present (see Table 15-1)

d. Primary syphilis: stage 1, occurs 3–4 weeks after infection; disease is highly infectious at this stage, but often goes unrecognized; chancres (painless indurated lesions) are seen in this stage

e. Secondary syphilis: stage 2, occurs 2 weeks to 6 months after initial chancre appears; signs disappear within 2–6 weeks and latency period begins; highly infectious (latent syphilis: begins 2 or more years after initial infection and can last up to 50 years; disease not transmitted by sexual contact during this stage)

f. Tertiary syphilis: spirochetes enter internal organs and cause irreversible damage, especially to cardiovascular system (aorta and aortic valve) and central nervous system (meningitis, general paresis, progressive mental deterioration leading to insanity)

3. Assessment

   a. Clinical manifestations: refer again to Table 15-1

   b. Diagnostic and laboratory tests: RPR titers become positive (if VDRL done) 4–6 weeks after infection, but is nonspecific; FTA-ABS is specific for syphilis and can confirm diagnosis; once a client has positive serology test, it will remain positive indefinitely

4. Therapeutic management: parenteral penicillin G

5. Priority nursing problems: potential inability to maintain health, nonadherence, altered sexual function, reduced social interaction, reduced coping, inadequate knowledge

6. Planning and implementation

   a. Education is primary nursing intervention for syphilis (see client education section that follows)

   b. Administer penicillin as prescribed and monitor client periodically to see that adequate treatment has occurred; treatment is based on length of illness and stage of disease

   c. Create an environment where client feels safe to discuss questions and concerns

   d. Encourage all clients with syphilis to be tested for HIV

   e. Encourage client to refer sexual partners for evaluation and treatment

   f. Report all cases of syphilis to health authorities for treatment of contacts

Table 15-1 Stages and Clinical Signs of Syphilis

Primary Syphilis	Secondary Syphilis	Latent Syphilis	Tertiary Syphilis
Appearance of chancre: at site of inoculation	Skin rash, especially on palms of hands or soles of feet	No apparent symptoms Disease not transmitted by sexual contact	Benign late syphilis: localized tumors in skin, bones, liver
Lymphadenopathy	Mucous patches in oral cavity, sore throat, general lymphadenopathy	Occurs 2 or more years after initial infection; may last for 50 years	Diffuse inflammatory syphilis: involves CNS and cardiovascular system
Highly infectious but onset often goes unnoticed	Onset any time from 2 weeks to 6 months after original chancre appears; highly infectious		

7. Medication therapy: penicillin G, given intramuscularly
8. Client education
   a. How to recognize signs of syphilis
   b. Seek immediate treatment if exposure occurs
   c. Abstain from sex for 1 month after treatment
   d. Need for simultaneous treatment of partner
   e. Need for follow-up testing in 3 and 6 months; client should expect a 4-fold decrease in RPR titer in 12 months after treatment begun, soon after serologic tests should be negative.
9. Evaluation: client states cause, symptoms, primary mode of transmission of and treatment regime for syphilis; takes medications as prescribed; returns for follow-up visits; identifies ways to prevent reinfection

Practice to Pass

List two reasons why client education is so important in treating syphilis.

C. **Gonorrhea**
   1. Description: infection caused by *Neisseria gonorrhoeae*, leading to inflammation of mucous membranes of GU tract
   2. Etiology and pathophysiology
      a. *Neisseria gonorrhoeae* is a gram-negative diplococcus; resistance to antibiotics is a rising concern
      b. Incidence is of epidemic proportion in United States
      c. Incubation period is 2–8 days after exposure
      d. Transmitted by direct sexual contact; organism targets cervix and male urethra, spreads to other organs (such as rectum, joints, oral mucosa) unless treated
      e. May lead to sterility in males, PID and other infections in women, and blindness and other serious problems for neonates exposed in birth canal
   3. Assessment
      a. Clinical manifestations
         1) Male clients: dysuria; signs of urethritis, serous, milky, or purulent urethral discharge, and lymphadenopathy; may be asymptomatic
         2) Female clients: dysuria, abnormal vaginal discharge, and urinary frequency; many women have no symptoms
         3) Proctitis (transmitted through anal intercourse or contamination)
         4) Pharyngitis (transmitted through orogenital sex)
      b. Diagnostic and laboratory tests: culture (urethra, throat, and rectum) isolates organism; gram stain smear of urethral discharge; polymerase chain reaction (PCR)
   4. Therapeutic management: medication therapy (see below)
   5. Priority nursing problems: potential inability to maintain health, nonadherence, altered sexual function, reduced social interaction
   6. Planning and implementation
      a. Teaching is an important nursing intervention (see client education section that follows)
      b. Administer antibiotics as prescribed
      c. Arrange treatment for sexual partner
      d. Evaluate client's response to treatment and allow time to discuss concerns
   7. Medication therapy: broad-spectrum antibiotic therapy; many strains of *N. gonorrhoeae* are now penicillin resistant; ceftriaxone (Rocephin) single dose intramuscularly and doxycycline for uncomplicated cases
   8. Client education
      a. Signs of gonorrhea
      b. Seek immediate treatment if exposure occurs
      c. Abstain from sex until cure is achieved; sexual intercourse can spread disease and also delays healing because of vascular congestion resulting from this activity

!   **d.** Refrain from alcohol for 2–4 weeks; it interrupts healing of urethral walls

   e. Need for simultaneous treatment of partner

!   **f.** Need for follow-up visit 4–7 days after completing treatment

   g. Importance of taking medication exactly as prescribed

!   **h.** Report all cases of gonorrhea to health authorities for treatment of contacts

   9. Evaluation: client states causes, symptoms, primary mode of transmission, and treatment regime for gonorrhea; takes medications as prescribed; returns for follow-up visits; follow-up tests are negative; and identifies ways to prevent reinfection

D. Genital herpes

   1. Description: infection with herpes simplex virus (HSV), usually type 2

   2. Etiology and pathophysiology

   a. Spread by oral–genital, vaginal, or anal contact; incubation period is 3–7 days; virus enters body through mucous membranes or small breaks in skin

!   **b.** Lesions are small, painful blisters in genital area; blisters contain virus particles, which can spread to other parts of body

   c. A chronic, often asymptomatic, disease; may cause periodic recurrences

   d. First episode lasts about 12 days; recurrent infections lasts 4–5 days; period between outbreaks is called latency (virus is dormant)

   e. 45 million diagnosed cases in United States

!   **f.** May be lethal to fetus if exposed during delivery

   3. Assessment

   a. Clinical manifestations

!   **1)** Localized: herpetic lesions, tender swollen regional lymph nodes, dysuria, urinary retention, vaginal discharge (females), urethral discharge (males)

   2) Systemic: general malaise, fever, headache

!   **3)** Factors that may trigger a recurrent outbreak: heat, intercourse, stress, anxiety, emotional upset, menstruation, or ovulation

   b. Diagnostic and laboratory tests

   1) Tissue culture isolates virus

   2) Anti-HSV antibodies; is unreliable for differentiating HSV1 from HSV2 antibodies

   4. Therapeutic management: symptomatic treatment, pain management of lesions, and antiviral medication therapy

   5. Priority nursing problems: pain, potential for altered sexual function or infection, anxiety, possible inability to self-manage treatment plan

!   **6.** Medication therapy: anti-viral drug acyclovir (Zovirax) to reduce length and severity of first episode and recurrences; some strains becoming resistant to acyclovir, so foscarnet (Foscavir) is used; and acetylsalicylic acid (aspirin) or acetaminophen (Tylenol) for pain; valacyclovir (Valtrex) is also used

   7. Planning and implementation

!   **a.** Cleanse genital area with warm water several times daily; dry with hair dryer or air dry

   b. Avoid lubricants and cream, which can prolong healing time

   c. Apply drying agents to relieve pain and itching

   d. Use soaks and compresses to promote drying and comfort

   e. Provide supportive, nonjudgmental environment; encourage client to ask questions and express feelings

Practice to Pass

How would you reply to a client who asks how you plan to cure her genital herpes?

   8. Client education

   a. Female clients should pour water over genitals while voiding to dilute acidity of urine during outbreak

   b. Wear loose clothing and cotton underwear to promote drying and reduce pressure

   c. Keep lesions and surrounding areas clean and dry

  d. Symptoms and factors that trigger recurrences
  e. Abstain from sexual activity from time prodromal symptoms appear until 10 days after all lesions are healed
  f. Avoid touching or scratching lesions
  g. Need to inform sexual partners about disease, in order to plan prevention of transmission
  h. Need for special precautions with pregnancy
  i. Support groups and other resources
9. Evaluation: client describes prodromal symptoms and potential causes of recurrences; states that pain is diminished or absent; carries out normal daily activities; signs of secondary infection are absent; performs skin care as instructed; and describes health practices to reduce risk of infection and transmission

E. Genital warts
  1. Description: warts that appear in anogenital area, caused by human papillomavirus (HPV); note HPV may be present without obvious warty growths
  2. Etiology and pathophysiology
    a. Also called condyloma acuminatum, or venereal warts; more than 20 subtypes
    b. Virus infects nuclei of epithelial cells, causing them to proliferate
    c. May occur anywhere in genital area: cervix, vagina, vulva, penis, urethra, scrotum, or anus
    d. Transmitted by direct skin-to-skin contact, usually through sexual activity; nonsexual transmission is possible
    e. Incubation period ranges from 6 weeks to 8 months, with an average of 3 months
    f. Warts may resolve spontaneously within 1–2 years
  3. Assessment
    a. Clinical manifestations
      1) Small to large wartlike growths on genitals (only symptom); warts are usually multiple and may form large masses; may spread internally to vagina and anus
      2) Bleeding and infection of warts may occur
    b. Diagnostic and laboratory tests: Pap smear to assess for cervical cell changes—cervical cancer is often associated with genital warts
  4. Therapeutic management
    a. Medication therapy
    b. Cryotherapy, electrocautery, or surgical excision
  5. Priority nursing problems: potential for altered sexual function or infection, anxiety or fear, reduced tissue integrity, inadequate knowledge
  6. Planning and implementation
    a. Suggest annual Pap test for female clients to detect cancer
    b. Administer antibiotics to treat infection
    c. Apply podophyllin (a cytotoxic agent), as ordered, to surfaces of warts, avoiding normal skin surfaces; treatment repeated every 7 days for up to 4 weeks
    d. Provide emotional support and education for client
    e. Recommend HPV vaccinations if in recommended age group for both males and females
  7. Medication therapy: podophyllin (cytotoxic agent) applied topically; trichloroacetic and dichloroacetic acids applied topically to external warts
  8. Client education
    a. Increased risk for genital malignancy and need for annual gynecologic exams for females
    b. Keep lesions and surrounding areas clean and dry; recognize signs of infection (pain, drainage, tenderness)
    c. Use condoms to help prevent spread of genital warts

        d. Avoid touching or scratching lesions

        e. Notify sexual partners to plan for prevention of transmission

    9. Evaluation: client states cause, symptoms, and mode of transmission of genital warts; identifies ways to decrease risk of infection; uses medications as prescribed; performs skin care techniques as instructed; and verbalizes need for annual gynecologic exams

F. Trichomoniasis

    1. Description: vaginal protozoan infection caused by *Trichomonas vaginalis*

    2. Etiology and pathophysiology

        a. One of most common STIs; often found with other STIs

        b. Overgrowth of protozoan normally present in vaginal tract

        c. May be carried by asymptomatic male partners, but is difficult to isolate in men

    3. Assessment

        a. Clinical manifestations

            1) Malodorous and profuse vaginal discharge that may cause discomfort; discharge is greenish gray and watery, may appear frothy

            2) Burning with urination and itching; red and inflamed genitals

            3) Hemorrhagic spots on cervix or vaginal walls

        b. Diagnostic and laboratory tests: saline microscopic examination

    4. Therapeutic management: medication therapy (see below)

    5. Priority nursing problems: pain, anxiety, possible inability to maintain health

    6. Planning and implementation

        a. Administer metronidazole (Flagyl) as prescribed

        b. Give soothing compresses, colloidal baths

        c. Apply medicated creams

        d. Treat sexual partners concurrently

    7. Medication therapy: metronidazole (Flagyl), single dose

    8. Client education

        a. Abstain from sexual intercourse during active infection, or use condoms

        b. How infection is transmitted, including by towels and other personal items

        c. Use cool compresses, sitz baths, and vinegar–water douches to relieve discomfort and itching

        d. Pour water over genitals while voiding to ease dysuria

        e. Genital hygiene practices and need to maintain normal vaginal flora

    9. Evaluation: client states itching and pain are diminished or absent; able to carry out normal daily activities and recommended hygiene practices; signs of secondary infection are absent; recognizes cause and symptoms of trichomoniasis

G. Chlamydia

    1. Description: bacterial infection of vulva or vagina caused by *Chlamydia trachomatis*

    2. Etiology and pathophysiology

        a. Most common STI; contracted by 3–4 million Americans each year; leading cause of pelvic inflammatory disease (PID)

        b. Incubation period is 1–2 weeks after initial exposure

        c. *Chlamydia trachomatis* is a bacterium, but behaves like a virus because it reproduces only within host cell; takes over a cell and uses its energy

        d. *Chlamydia trachomatis* conjunctivitis causes blindness; common cause of blindness in undeveloped countries; may also cause blindness or pneumonia in newborns exposed during birth

        e. Asymptomatic infection is common; symptoms usually don't occur until infection invades uterus and uterine tubes

        f. Spread by any form of sexual contact

g. Risk factors: personal or partner history of STI, pregnancy, adolescent sexual activity, oral contraceptive use, unprotected sex, and multiple sexual partners

3. Assessment

a. Clinical manifestations

1) Vaginal or urethral discharge, white or mucous in males, purulent yellow or green cervical discharge in females

2) Signs and symptoms of urethritis (dysuria, urethral discharge), epididymitis (fever, scrotal pain), proctitis (rectal discharge and pain) in men

3) Signs and symptoms of PID may be first symptom a female client notices (refer back to earlier discussion of PID)

b. Diagnostic and laboratory tests

1) A tissue sample for direct-slide monoclonal antibody test is fastest and least expensive diagnostic test

2) For definitive diagnosis, tissue samples for culture are obtained, which may take up to 7 days; treatment often begun on a presumptive basis

4. Therapeutic management: antibiotic therapy

5. Priority nursing problems: pain, alteration in body image, potential for infection or reinfection, potential nonadherence, anxiety

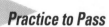

Practice to Pass

Why is chlamydia difficult to diagnose based on physical examination findings alone?

6. Planning and implementation

a. Administer antibiotics as prescribed and treat client's sexual partner

b. Provide privacy and confidentiality

7. Medication therapy: antibiotics such as doxycycline and azithromycin

8. Client education

a. Importance of taking all prescribed medication

b. Symptoms, cause, and potential complications of chlamydia

c. Refer sexual partners for evaluation and treatment

d. Abstain from sexual activity for 1 month after treatment

e. Need to use condoms to prevent future infections

9. Evaluation: client states symptoms and complications of chlamydial infections; lists ways to reduce risk of reinfection or transmission; states risk factors; takes medications as ordered and verbalizes actions, schedule, and adverse effects; and sexual contacts seek medical consultation and evaluation

VII. INFERTILITY

A. **Description: infertility** is an inability to conceive after 1 year of regular intercourse with no contraceptive measures, or inability to deliver a live fetus after 3 consecutive conceptions

B. **Etiology and pathophysiology**

1. Approximately 8–10% of couples in United States are infertile; 10–20% of these have no physical basis for infertility

2. Approximately 40–50% of infertility is attributed to female disorders

3. Female causes of infertility

a. Hormonal dysfunction leading to insufficient gonadotropin secretions

b. Ovarian, uterine, tubal, peritoneal, or cervical abnormalities

c. Psychological problems

d. Immunologic reaction to partner's sperm

4. Male causes of infertility

a. Semen disorders: volume, motility, density; abnormal or immature sperms

b. Systemic disorders, such as diabetes mellitus, and autoimmune disorders, such as antiphospholipid syndrome (APS)

c. Genital infection

d. Disorders of testes, other structural abnormalities, or genetic defects

e. Immunologic disorders

        f. Chemicals, drugs, and environmental factors

        g. Psychological or sexual problems

C. Assessment

  1. A complete medical history and physical assessment for both partners; there must be a notable report of inability to conceive or carry a fetus to term

  2. Diagnostic and laboratory tests

    a. Female clients: basal body temperature graph, endometrial biopsy, progesterone blood levels, and tests to determine structural integrity of tubes, ovaries, and uterus

    b. Male clients: semen analysis (most conclusive test), testicular biopsy, other laboratory tests such as gonadotropin assay, serum testosterone levels, and urine 17-ketosteroid levels

D. Therapeutic management

  1. Female clients: identify and correct underlying abnormalities or problems; hormone therapy; surgical restoration

  2. Male clients: identify and correct underlying abnormalities or problems; counseling for sexual dysfunction; hormone supplements

E. Priority nursing problems: anxiety, inadequate knowledge, reduced self-esteem

F. Planning and implementation

  1. Assist in improving general health of couple

  2. Teach stress reduction techniques; treatment can be stressful to both partners

  3. Discuss intrauterine insemination

  4. Discuss and assist with in-vitro fertilization

  5. Provide emotional support and refer couple to a support group prn

G. Medication therapy: testosterone or chorionic gonadotropin hormone therapy for male clients; female hormones for female clients

H. Client education

  1. Diagnostic and treatment techniques

  2. Reproductive and sexual function and factors that may interfere with fertility

  3. Encourage questions; encourage couple to discuss their frustrations and other feelings

  4. Explore alternatives, such as adoption

I. Evaluation: clients identify feelings and concerns about infertility; state reproductive functions and factors that interfere with fertility; state purpose of diagnostic tests; identify reason for infertility and possible treatments; and discuss alternatives, such as adoption

VIII. DISORDERS OF FEMALE REPRODUCTIVE SYSTEM

A. Premenstrual syndrome (PMS)

  1. Definition: group of symptoms preceding monthly menses that regress or disappear during menstruation

  2. Etiology and pathophysiology

    a. Affects women of all ages, races, and cultures

    b. Believed to be related to hormonal changes such as altered estrogen–progesterone ratios, increased prolactin levels, and rising aldosterone levels during luteal phase of menstrual cycle (7–10 days before onset of flow)

    c. Increased aldosterone causes sodium retention and edema

    d. Decreased monamine oxidase in brain causes depression

    e. Decreased serotonin causes mood swings

    f. Produces multisystem effects that vary with each client and from month to month

  3. Assessment

    a. Clinical manifestations

      1) See Figure 15-4 for multisystem effects of premenstrual syndrome

      2) Clinical manifestations appear only during luteal phase of menstrual cycle (7–10 days before menstrual flow)

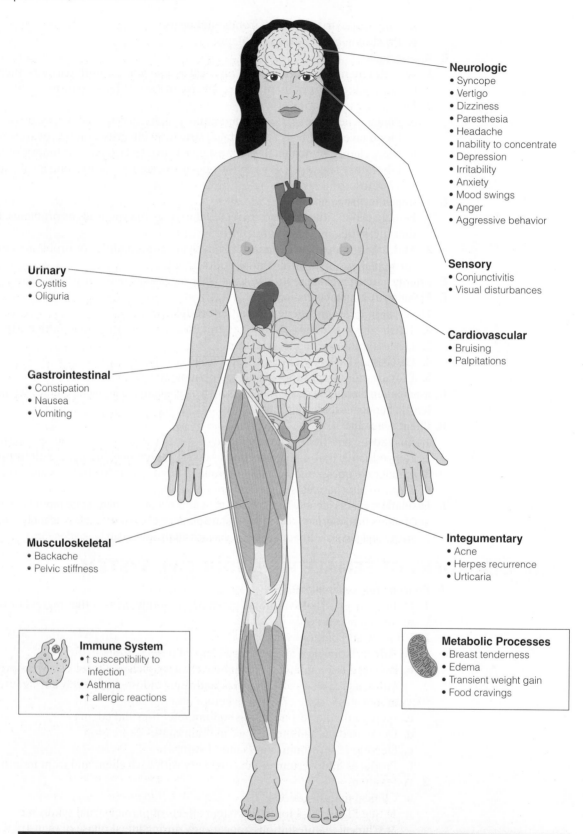

Neurologic
- Syncope
- Vertigo
- Dizziness
- Paresthesia
- Headache
- Inability to concentrate
- Depression
- Irritability
- Anxiety
- Mood swings
- Anger
- Aggressive behavior

Sensory
- Conjunctivitis
- Visual disturbances

Cardiovascular
- Bruising
- Palpitations

Integumentary
- Acne
- Herpes recurrence
- Urticaria

Urinary
- Cystitis
- Oliguria

Gastrointestinal
- Constipation
- Nausea
- Vomiting

Musculoskeletal
- Backache
- Pelvic stiffness

Immune System
- ↑ susceptibility to infection
- Asthma
- ↑ allergic reactions

Metabolic Processes
- Breast tenderness
- Edema
- Transient weight gain
- Food cravings

Figure 15-4

Manifestations of premenstrual syndrome

    b. Diagnostic and laboratory tests: organic causes are ruled out first; there are no definitive diagnostic tests for PMS

4. Therapeutic management

    a. Pharmacologic management

    b. Nonpharmacological management includes modifications in diet (see section that follows), establishing an exercise plan, and stress management

5. Priority nursing problems: pain, reduced ability to cope

6. Planning and implementation

    a. Nursing care focuses on teaching self-care and relieving symptoms

    b. Ask client to keep menstrual log on a daily basis for 1–4 months, recording symptoms and their relationship to the menstrual cycle

    c. Evaluate severity of symptoms and their effects on client's life

    d. Reduce sodium intake to minimize fluid retention

    e. Diet should be high in complex carbohydrates with limited simple sugars and alcohol to minimize reactive hypoglycemia

    f. Restrict caffeine to reduce irritability

    g. Increase intake of calcium, magnesium, and vitamin B_6

7. Medication therapy: oral contraceptives to suppress ovulation in severe cases; NSAIDs to relieve cramping; diuretics to relieve bloating; and selective serotonin reuptake inhibitors, such as fluoxetine (Prozac), sertraline (Zoloft), paroxetine (Paxil) to manage mood swings

8. Client education

    a. Measures to relieve pain

    b. Use relaxation techniques, get regular physical exercise, and eat a well-balanced diet

    c. Keep a diary of PMS symptoms and methods that produce relief

    d. Self-care measures to help with mood alterations, including stress identification

9. Evaluation: client identifies personal symptoms of PMS and ways to cope with each symptom; demonstrates use of menstrual log; identifies sources of stress and ways to reduce stress; states need for adequate rest and exercise and dietary interventions to prevent PMS symptoms

B. *Dysmenorrhea*

1. Description: pain associated with menstruation

2. Etiology and pathophysiology

    a. In primary dysmenorrhea, excess prostaglandins cause uterine muscle fibers to contract, producing uterine ischemia and painful cramps

    b. Onset is just before or at beginning of first menstrual flow—lasts from a few hours to several days

    c. Childbirth tends to reduce severity

    d. Secondary dysmenorrhea is related to underlying conditions that cause scarring or injury to reproductive tract (endometriosis, fibroid tumors, PID, and ovarian cancer)

3. Assessment

    a. Clinical manifestations

      1) Sharp pain located in lower abdomen, radiating to lower back, groin, or thighs

      2) Headache, nausea, anorexia, bloating, diarrhea, faintness, or fatigue

    b. Diagnostic and laboratory tests

      1) Pelvic examination to determine structural abnormalities

      2) FSH and LH levels to assess pituitary gland function

      3) Progesterone and estradiol levels to assess ovarian function

      4) Thyroid function tests

      5) CT or MRI

        6) Laparoscopy

        7) Dilation and curettage (D&C) to obtain tissue samples for analysis

    4. Therapeutic management: pharmacologic management, stress reduction, exercise, and dietary counseling

    5. Priority nursing problems: pain, reduced ability to cope, alteration in sleep pattern, reduced ability to perform roles

    6. Planning and implementation

        a. Provide information on use of relief measures, including medication, heat, relaxation, and exercise

        b. Recommend reducing intake of sodium, sugar, caffeine, and alcohol

        c. Ask client to describe type, degree, time of onset, and duration of pain

        d. Assess characteristics of menstrual cycle, such as length of cycle, age at onset, type of flow usually experienced

        e. Assess for presence of underlying problems, such as STIs, PID, fibroid tumors, and ovarian cancer

        f. Ask client about relief measures she has tried

        g. Note physical factors that may contribute: poor posture, poor hygiene, and lack of exercise

    7. Medication therapy: either nonprescription prostaglandin inhibitors or NSAIDs for pain relief; oral contraceptives in severe cases to inhibit ovulation

    8. Client education

        a. In most cases, disorder is benign in nature

        b. Use relief measures, such as regular exercise, good posture, balanced diet and good hygiene; waist-bending exercises before onset of menstruation can help

        c. Avoid constipation, which creates abdominal pressure

        d. Use a heating pad to help reduce pain

        e. Increased intake of protein, calcium, magnesium, and vitamin B_6 may help relieve symptoms

    9. Evaluation: client describes use of nonpharmacologic interventions; identifies and complies with taking prescribed medications; explains relationship of good posture, exercise, balanced diet, and good hygiene in preventing dysmenorrhea

C. Abnormal uterine bleeding

    1. Description: vaginal bleeding that is painless but abnormal in amount, duration, or time of occurrence

    2. Etiology and pathophysiology

        a. Primary **amenorrhea**: absence of menstruation; caused by structural abnormalities, hormonal imbalances, polycystic ovary disease, or imperforate hymen

        b. Secondary amenorrhea: absence of menstruation in a previously menstruating client; caused by anorexia nervosa, excessive athletic activity, hormonal imbalance, or ovarian tumors

        c. **Oligomenorrhea**: scant menses; usually related to hormonal imbalance

        d. **Menorrhagia**: excessive or prolonged menstruation; related to thyroid disorders, endometriosis, PID, ovarian cysts, or uterine fibroids

        e. **Metrorrhagia**: bleeding between menstrual periods; caused by hormonal imbalance, PID, cervical or uterine polyps or cancer; early evaluation for cancer is important with metrorrhagia

        f. Postmenopausal bleeding: caused by endometrial polyps, endometrial hyperplasia, or uterine cancer; early evaluation for cancer is important

    3. Assessment

        a. Clinical manifestations: abnormal amount of vaginal bleeding

        b. Diagnostic and laboratory tests

            1) CBC to rule out other causes

            2) Endocrine studies, including thyroid hormones, to rule out cause

      3) hCG levels

      4) Pelvic ultrasound

      5) Hysteroscopy to detect uterine abnormalities

      6) Endometrial biopsy

    4. Therapeutic management

      a. Hormonal therapy

      b. Therapeutic dilation and curettage or scraping uterine wall to correct excessive bleeding

      c. Endometrial ablation, destroying endometrial layer of uterus with laser surgery, which ends menstruation and reproduction

      d. Hysterectomy or removal of uterus

    5. Priority nursing problems: reduced ability to cope, alteration in sexual function, reduced self-esteem

    6. Planning and implementation

      a. Assess characteristics of client's menstrual cycle

      b. Evaluate symptoms, including type and duration of menstrual bleeding, absence of bleeding, pain, mood changes, breast tenderness, nausea, headache, and bloating

      c. Assess client's coping strategies and psychosocial support system

      d. Assist client in dealing with self-esteem disturbances and anxiety

      e. Assist client through diagnostic and treatment processes

    7. Medication therapy: hormonal agents used to correct many menstrual irregularities; oral iron supplements to replace iron lost through excessive bleeding

    8. Client education

      a. Physiology of normal menstruation; answer questions about myths and cultural beliefs

      b. Purpose, benefits, and risks of diagnostic tests and treatments

      c. Results of all tests and examination; encourage questions

      d. Normal hygiene during menstruation (use of tampons, importance of cleanliness, and normal activities)

      e. Measures to reduce discomfort associated with menstruation or treatments (see section on Dysmenorrhea)

      f. Need to report episodes of excessive bleeding or postmenopausal bleeding due to the risk for cancer

    9. Evaluation: client states understanding of diagnosis and treatment plan; identifies prescribed medications and their correct use; states importance of follow-up visits to evaluate progress, and reports normal menstrual cycle at follow-up visit

  D. *Uterine prolapse*

    1. Description: downward displacement of uterus into vaginal canal

      a. First-degree prolapse: less than half of uterus extends into vagina

      b. Second-degree prolapse: descent of entire uterus into vaginal canal

      c. Third-degree prolapse (procidentia): complete prolapse of uterus outside body, with inversion of vaginal canal

    2. Etiology and pathophysiology

      a. May be congenital or acquired

      b. Usually related to weakened pelvic musculature caused by stretching of supporting ligaments during pregnancy and childbirth; more common in women with multiple vaginal births

      c. Risk factors: unrepaired lacerations from childbirth, rapid deliveries, multiple pregnancies, congenital weakness, loss of elasticity and muscle tone with aging, and chronic coughing

      d. Prolapse is often accompanied by cystocele or rectocele

    3. Assessment

      a. Clinical manifestations

        1) Lump protruding from vagina; typically painless and has increased in size for months or years; usually worse with standing or straining

        2) Discomfort in lower abdomen, or pressure and heaviness in vaginal area; client may complain of low backache with standing

        3) Difficulty in defecation due to rectocele

        4) Difficulty urinating due to cystocele

        5) Urinary incontinence

        6) Pain with intercourse

        7) Signs of infection, chafing, ulceration, and bleeding from exposed uterus in third-degree prolapse

      b. Diagnostic and laboratory tests: pelvic examination

    4. Therapeutic management

      a. Kegel exercises

      b. Insertion of a vaginal pessary, a donut-shaped ring placed in vagina to provide uterine support

      c. Vaginal hysterectomy

    5. Priority nursing problems: alteration in body image, potential for infection, anxiety, potential for stress incontinence

    6. Planning and implementation

      a. Advise client about nonsurgical techniques to manage prolapse, such as Kegel exercises to strengthen pelvic muscles

      b. Discuss use of pessary, device inserted into vagina to provide temporary support

      c. Most women can be treated without surgery if symptoms are severe and there is minimal change with noninvasive treatment, encourage client to discuss surgical options with the surgeon

      d. Teach ways to deal with stress incontinence, which may accompany uterine prolapse

    7. Medication therapy: none

    8. Client education

      a. Kegel exercises to strengthen pelvic muscles

      b. Use of pessary: insertion and cleaning

      c. Perineal care and importance of good hygiene to prevent infection

      d. Dietary counseling if obesity is a factor

      e. Encourage questions from client and explain treatment options

    9. Evaluation: client states purpose and technique of Kegel exercises, importance of good hygiene to prevent infection, and understanding of treatment options

E. Cystocele and rectocele

    1. Description

      a. Cystocele: herniation of bladder into vagina

      b. Rectocele: herniation of rectum into vagina

    2. Etiology and pathophysiology

      a. Both conditions are usually related to weakened pelvic musculature caused by stretching of supporting ligaments during pregnancy and childbirth

      b. With cystocele, client may experience stress incontinence and difficulty emptying bladder, leading to retention and infection

      c. Risk factors: unrepaired lacerations from childbirth, rapid deliveries, multiple pregnancies, congenital weakness, loss of elasticity and muscle tone with aging, chronic coughing

    3. Assessment

      a. Clinical manifestations

1) Bearing-down sensation in pelvic area, constipation, hemorrhoids, urinary incontinence, and fecal incontinence
2) With rectocele, client reports she has to press on rectocele from inside of vagina in order to defecate
3) With cystocele, signs of UTI, urinary retention, and stress incontinence
4) Cystocele and rectocele can sometimes be seen on inspection, but usually recede when client is lying down; diagnosis is made by asking client to bear down
5) Bulging just below urethral orifice

   b. Diagnostic and laboratory tests: cystography to determine bladder herniation, measurement of residual urine, and urinalysis and culture

4. Therapeutic management
   a. Kegel exercises
   b. Surgical correction
      1) Posterior colporrhaphy for rectocele, to shorten pelvic muscles and provide tighter support for rectum
      2) Anterior colporrhaphy for cystocele, to shorten pelvic muscles and provide tighter support for bladder
      3) Marshall-Marchetti-Krantz procedure suspends bladder in correct anatomic position to help correct cystocele

5. Priority nursing problems: stress incontinence, alteration in body image, potential for infection, reduced self-esteem, possible altered sexual function

6. Planning and implementation
   a. Advise client about available treatments, which often involve surgery
   b. Provide emotional support
   c. Pre- and postoperative care of client undergoing surgery

7. Medication therapy: none

8. Client education
   a. Kegel exercises to reduce stress incontinence
   b. Treatment options and prepare client for surgery, which is main treatment for rectocele and cystocele
   c. What to expect during postoperative period
   d. Both colporrhaphy procedures shorten overall length of vagina and may result in discomfort during sexual intercourse

9. Evaluation: client states understanding of diagnosis and treatment plan, procedure for Kegel exercises to strengthen pelvic muscles, and importance of follow-up visits to evaluate progress; reports normal voiding and defecation at follow-up

F. *Vulvitis*

1. Definition: inflammation or infection of vulva

2. Etiology and pathophysiology
   a. Skin of vulva is prone to inflammation from mechanical or chemical irritation, due to its location
   b. Causes: tight-fitting clothes; exposure to urine, fecal material, vaginal discharge, and glandular secretions; chemical irritants, such as soap, feminine hygiene spray, powder, vaginal lubricants, etc.

3. Assessment
   a. Clinical manifestations: itching (cardinal symptom), burning sensation aggravated by urination or defecation; red and swollen tissues with possible abrasions where client has scratched; vaginal discharge may be present with vaginitis
   b. Diagnostic and laboratory tests: culture of discharge; KOH analysis, wet smear analysis, and gram stain; urinalysis and urine culture; serologic testing

4. Priority nursing problems: pain, possible inability to maintain health

5. Planning and implementation

    a. Assess personal habits that could contribute to inflammatory process: type of undergarments, allergies, use of perfumed soap and powder, overuse of feminine hygiene products such as sprays or douches

    b. Identify type of infection through observation or cultures

    c. Provide appropriate pharmacologic treatment for infection and inflammation

    d. Give soothing compresses or colloidal baths

    e. Apply medicated creams

6. Medication therapy: topical creams to relieve inflammation and antibiotics if infection is present

7. Client education

    a. How to properly clean vulva: don't use soap between labia, rinse thoroughly to remove soap residue, dry area completely

    b. Avoid tight-fitting clothes, wear 100% cotton underpants, and wear knee-high or thigh-high stockings instead of pantyhose when possible

    c. Avoid strong laundry soaps, talcum powder, perfumed soap, scented toilet paper, and deodorant sprays (to protect vaginal flora)

    d. To kill yeast in underwear, soak in half-strength bleach for 20 minutes before washing

    e. Use comfort measures, such as sitz baths, cool or warm compresses, and topical creams

8. Evaluation: client lists ways to prevent vulvitis and describes proper techniques for cleaning vulva; reports that pruritus is relieved; vulvar tissue free of redness and edema

G. Candidiasis

1. Definition: fungal vaginal infection caused by *Candida albicans* (yeast)

2. Etiology and pathophysiology

    a. Very common—is usually seen in women

    b. Widespread use of antibiotics increases incidence, because they destroy normal vaginal flora

    c. Vaginal flora is normally acidic; changes in flora allow yeast to proliferate

    d. Candida thrives on sugar-carbohydrate rich environment

    e. Risk factors: tampons; sexual intercourse; chemical irritation; fecal contamination; infestation with parasites, such as pinworms; sexually transmitted organisms, frequent or prolonged use of antibiotics

3. Assessment

    a. Clinical manifestations

        1) Scant white cottage cheeselike vaginal drainage

        2) Itching of vulva and burning with urination

        3) Vulva and vaginal area red and swollen

        4) Inflamed cervix

        5) If present in men typically seen as a pink papular rash; also known as "jock itch"; recurrent candidiasis is associated with immune deficiency and HIV infections

    b. Diagnostic and laboratory tests: wet mounts (direct microscopic examination of vaginal discharge); vaginal, urethral, or cervical cultures and gram stain; recommend HIV screen if status unknown when infection is recurrent

4. Therapeutic management: medication therapy (see below)

5. Priority nursing problems: pain, inadequate knowledge, potential inability to maintain health

6. Planning and implementation

    a. Identify type of infection through observation or cultures

    b. Provide appropriate pharmacologic treatment for infection and inflammation

        c. Give soothing compresses or colloidal baths

        d. Apply medicated creams or powder as recommended

    7. Medication therapy: miconazole (Monistat), clotrimazole (Lotrimin), or terconazole (Terazol 7 or Terazol 3) creams or suppositories; povidone-iodine or vinegar douches if prescribed

    8. Client education

        a. How to properly clean vulva: don't use soap between labia; rinse thoroughly to remove soap residue; dry area completely

        b. Avoid tight-fitting clothes, wear 100% cotton underpants, and wear knee-high or thigh-high stockings instead of pantyhose when possible; change out of damp clothing soon after exercise

        c. To protect vaginal flora, avoid strong laundry soaps, talcum powder, perfumed soap, scented toilet paper, and deodorant sprays

        d. To kill yeast in underwear, soak in half-strength bleach for 20 minutes before washing

        e. Use comfort measures, such as sitz baths, cool or warm compresses, and topical creams

        f. Consume 8 ounces of yogurt containing live active cultures daily to help restore normal vaginal flora

        g. How infection is transmitted; sexual partner will also need treatment; infection may be asymptomatic in one partner

    9. Evaluation: pruritus and discharge have resolved; vaginal tissue is free of redness and edema; client states ways to prevent candidiasis and proper techniques for cleaning vulva; sexual partner presents for treatment and verbalizes need for safe-sex practices

H. Cervical cancer

    1. Description: unregulated growth of abnormal cells in cervix

    2. Etiology and pathophysiology

        a. Most common cancer of reproductive system

        b. Usually seen in clients ages 30–50

        c. May become invasive and spread to tissue outside cervix, fundus of uterus, and lymph glands

        d. Treatment depends on extent of disease

        e. Squamous cell carcinoma accounts for 90% of cervical cancers; they have gradual onset; spread by direct invasion of accessory structures

    3. Assessment

        a. Clinical manifestations

            1) Thin, watery, blood-tinged vaginal discharge, which may go unnoticed by client

            2) Painless bleeding between periods, often seen after intercourse, douching, or other contact

            3) Late symptoms occur as cancer progresses to other organs, including referred pain in back and thighs, hematuria, bloody stools, anemia, and weight loss

            4) Early diagnosis is critical, because cervical cancer can be cured in early stages

        b. Diagnostic and laboratory tests: cervical Pap test; abnormal results call for repeat test, colposcopic exam of cervix, and tissue biopsy; diagnosis is based on biopsy results

    4. Therapeutic management: chemotherapy, radiation therapy, and surgery

    5. Priority nursing problems: fear, anxiety, inadequate knowledge, potential for reduced tissue integrity, reduced coping

    6. Planning and implementation

        a. Assist client in dealing with psychological effects of illness; provide information and emotional support

       b. Explore treatment options with client and family

       c. Develop strategies for pain control

       d. Maintain skin and tissue integrity during radiation treatment and following surgery

       e. Observe for fistula formation between vagina and bladder or rectum, a possible complication of radiation therapy

       f. Recommend a high-carbohydrate, high-protein diet

  7. Medication therapy: chemotherapy for tumors not responsive to other therapy, tumors that cannot be removed, or as adjunct therapy for metastasis; and analgesics for pain control

  8. Client education

       a. Diagnostic tests and treatments; allow client time to express feelings and ask questions

       b. Wound and skin care if surgery or radiation therapy is performed

       c. Importance of regular screening exams and follow-up after treatment is completed

  9. Evaluation: client makes informed decisions about treatment options; develops strategies for pain control; expresses feelings about fear of cancer and death; and maintains skin and tissue integrity during treatment

I. Ovarian cancer

  1. Description: unregulated growth of abnormal cells in ovaries

  2. Etiology and pathophysiology

       a. Is most lethal of gynecologic cancers; etiology not understood

       b. Symptoms are often vague and can be misdiagnoses as other common female ailments, leading to a true late diagnosis; usually detected by chance, not through screening

       c. Risk increases after age 40

       d. May involve one or both ovaries; staged according to tissue involvement

       e. Four stages of ovarian cancers: Stages: I—limited to ovaries; II—pelvic extension; III—metastasis outside pelvis or positive lymph nodes, and IV—distant metastasis

  3. Assessment

       a. Clinical manifestations

          1) Symptoms are rare until extensive tumor growth is present

          2) Feeling of pelvic pressure or heaviness, vague abdominal discomfort, dyspepsia, bloating, constipation, urinary frequency, and increased abdominal size

          3) Palpable hard, fixed, firm mass in area of ovaries during pelvic exam

       b. Diagnostic and laboratory tests

          1) No definitive diagnostic study is available; diagnosis is made during surgery (exploratory laparotomy)

          2) CA125 antigen level is sometimes useful in detecting ovarian cancer; CA125 is a laboratory tumor marker

  4. Therapeutic management: surgery, radiation therapy, and chemotherapy

  5. Priority nursing problems: fear or anxiety, interrupted skin integrity, constipation or diarrhea, reduced coping

  6. Planning and implementation

       a. Explore treatment options with client and family; surgery is treatment of choice, radiation is used for palliative purposes to shrink tumor

       b. Assist client in dealing with psychological effects of illness; provide information and emotional support

       c. Develop strategies for pain control

       d. Maintain skin and tissue integrity during radiation treatment and following surgery

       7. Medication therapy: chemotherapy may be used to achieve remission, but is not a cure

       8. Client education

         a. Diagnostic tests and treatments; allow client time to express feelings and ask questions

         b. Wound and skin care if surgery or radiation therapy is performed

         c. Importance of regular screening exams and follow-up after treatment is completed

         d. Do not ignore vague symptoms, such as indigestion, nausea, or urinary frequency

       9. Evaluation: client makes informed decisions about treatment options; develops strategies for pain control; expresses feelings about fear of cancer and death; maintains skin and tissue integrity during treatment; and verbalizes need for follow-up visits after treatment

J. Breast cancer

       1. Definition: unregulated growth of abnormal cells in breast tissue

       2. Etiology and pathophysiology

         a. Cause unknown, but many risk factors influence development

           1) Female gender and white/Caucasian race

           2) Family history of mother or sister with breast cancer

           3) Medical history of cancer of other breast, endometrial cancer, or atypical hyperplasia

           4) Menarche before age 12 (early) or menopause after age 50 (late)

           5) First birth after 30 years of age, oral contraceptive use (early or prolonged), prolonged use of estrogen replacement therapy

           6) Lifestyle factors: high-fat diet, obesity, high socioeconomic status, breast trauma, smoking, ingesting more than 2 alcoholic drinks daily

           7) Exposure to radiation through chest x-ray, fluoroscopy

         b. Begins as a single transformed cell and is hormone-dependent; does not develop in women without functioning ovaries who never received hormone replacement therapy

         c. Most often occurs in ductal areas of breasts

         d. Noninvasive: does not penetrate surrounding tissues; may be ductal or lobular; usually diagnosed through mammogram or nipple discharge

         e. Invasive: penetration of tumor into surrounding tissue; 5 types of invasive cancers, with only slight differences in prognosis

         f. Staging depends on size of tumor, lymph node involvement, and metastasis to distant sites

         g. About 70% of clients with Stage I tumors survive for 10 years with therapy

       3. Assessment

         a. Clinical manifestations

           1) Lump usually in upper outer quadrant of breast, usually nontender, but may be tender

           2) Dimpling of breast tissue surrounding nipple, or bleeding from nipple or changes in thickness of skin (latter seen more often in inflammatory breast cancer)

           3) Asymmetry, with affected breast being higher

           4) Regional lymph nodes swollen and tender

         b. Diagnostic and laboratory tests: mammography, ultrasonography, MRI, PET, tissue biopsy, sentinel node biopsy (uses radionuclides to locate sentinel node for removal and analysis rather than a chain of nodes)

    4. Therapeutic management: surgery, radiation therapy, chemotherapy, and hormonal therapy

    5. Priority nursing problems: anxiety or fear, anticipatory grief, potential for infection or injury, potential for body image alteration

    6. Planning and implementation

        a. Explore treatment options with client and family; prepare client for treatment, which is based on stage of disease

        b. Radiation therapy is used to destroy remaining cancer cells after surgery, or to shrink tumor prior to surgery

        c. Various types of mastectomy may be performed

            1) Segmental mastectomy or lumpectomy: removes tumor and a margin of breast tissue surrounding tumor

            2) Simple mastectomy: removal of complete breast but no other structures

            3) Modified radical mastectomy: removal of breast and axillary lymph nodes, but chest wall muscles are not resected

            4) Radical mastectomy: removal of breast, axillary lymph nodes, and underlying chest wall muscles

            5) Breast reconstruction: may be performed at time of mastectomy or at a later time; can be accomplished through submuscular breast implant, placing an implant after using a tissue expander, using muscles with intact blood supply from back or abdomen, or creating a free muscle flap with gluteus maximus muscle

        d. Assist client in dealing with psychological effects of illness; provide information and emotional support, including information about breast reconstruction surgery

        e. Maintain skin and tissue integrity during radiation treatment and following surgery

    7. Medication therapy: tamoxifen (Nolvadex) interferes with estrogen activity for treating advanced breast cancer, and chemotherapy when axillary nodes are involved

    8. Client education

        a. Diagnostic tests and treatments; allow client time to express feelings and ask questions

        b. Information about mastectomy surgery and what to expect afterward

        c. Wound care if surgery is performed, including care of short-term wound drains

        d. Techniques for proper skin care if radiation therapy is performed

        e. How to protect affected arm and hand from infection and injury if lymph nodes are removed during mastectomy (refer back to client care following mastectomy earlier in chapter)

        f. Postoperative exercises and self-breast examination

        g. Self-care during radiation and chemotherapy treatments

        h. Importance of regular screening exams and follow-up after treatment is completed

        i. Encourage client to meet other women who have undergone treatment, if appropriate

    9. Evaluation: client makes informed decisions about treatment options; develops strategies for pain control; expresses feelings about fear of cancer and death; maintains skin and tissue integrity during treatment; verbalizes need for follow-up visits and breast self-exam after treatment; demonstrates care of affected arm and hand; and demonstrates postoperative exercises

Case Study

A 48-year-old female client is scheduled for an incisional biopsy to evaluate a lump in her left breast. You are the nurse in the ambulatory care center where the procedure will take place.

1. How will you describe the surgery to the client when she arrives at the clinic?

2. If the biopsy is malignant, list 3 nursing diagnoses for this client.

3. How could breast cancer treatment affect sex and intimacy for the client?

4. What steps would you take when helping the client decide what treatment to undergo for breast cancer?

5. How would you describe a modified radical mastectomy to the client?

For suggested responses, see pages 625–626.

POSTTEST

POSTTEST

1 The nurse is preparing a health education class for a group of high school students. Which disease prevention and health promotion strategies should be included to support reproductive health in this population? Select all that apply.

1. Perform breast self-exam annually.
2. Perform monthly testicular self-exam.
3. Use condoms when sexually active.
4. Have annual Papanicolaou (Pap) test if sexually active.
5. Change tampons every 3 to 6 hours.

2 A client with syphilis exhibits flulike symptoms, a skin rash on the palms of the hands, and hair loss. The nurse develops a plan of care based on which stage of the disease?

1. Primary syphilis
2. Secondary syphilis
3. Tertiary syphilis
4. Latent syphilis

3 A client with an initial outbreak of genital herpes visits the clinic. In planning care for the client, what should the nurse administer initially?

1. Analgesics to decrease pain
2. Antibacterials to prevent further outbreaks
3. Anxiolytics to alleviate anxiety
4. Antibiotics for a secondary infection

4 The nurse is conducting a teaching session on testicular cancer. Which information should the nurse include in the discussion about the disease? Select all that apply.

1. It may present as painless swelling in one testicle.
2. Elevated levels of human chorionic gonadotropin (HCG) may be present.
3. Testicular self-examination monthly may aid in early detection.
4. It rarely affects younger men.
5. A history of cryptorchidism increases the risk.

5 The nurse in an urgent care center is admitting a 10-year-old boy who reports sudden severe testicular pain while playing tackle football. What should be the nurse's initial intervention?

1. Apply ice because the symptoms suggest priapism.
2. Observe the client hourly because the client may have cryptorchidism.
3. Notify the primary care provider as the client may have testicular torsion.
4. Question the parents about the circumstances that caused the injury.

6 When examining an adult female client, the nurse observes tissue protruding from the vaginal opening. The nurse reviews the medical record for a documented history what disorder?

1. Endometriosis
2. Leiomyoma
3. Pelvic infection
4. Uterine prolapse

7 The nurse anticipates that a client being evaluated for erectile dysfunction (ED) may receive a prescription for which of the following medications?

1. Propranolol (Inderal)
2. Diazepam (Valium)
3. Tadalafil (Cialis)
4. Progesterone (generic)

8 The nurse is teaching a group of clients about sexually transmitted infections (STIs). What is the greatest concern about a chlamydial infection that the nurse should emphasize?

1. It is resistant to azithromycin (Zithromax).
2. There may be lack of symptoms until the infection invades the uterus.
3. It is caused by yeast infection that spreads easily.
4. Older women are at highest risk in contracting the disease.

9 The nurse is conducting a teaching session on prostate cancer. What information should the nurse include in the discussion?

1. Oral medications may be used to treat the cancer.
2. Metastasis to the bowel is common if left untreated.
3. The disease is less common in older adults.
4. Asians and Native Americans having the highest risk for developing the cancer.

10 The nurse is interviewing a 79-year-old male client who has come to the clinic for a routine examination. The nurse should question the client about symptoms of what condition common in older men?

1. Testicular cancer
2. Benign prostatic hyperplasia
3. Testicular torsion
4. Gonorrhea

➤ *See pages 530–531 for Answers and Rationales.*

ANSWERS & RATIONALES

Pretest

1 **Answer: 2 Rationale:** Engaging in unprotected sex is associated with sexually transmitted infections (STI) and not benign prostatic hyperplasia (BPH). Consuming a diet high in meats and fats has been associated with BPH. Exposure to chemical carcinogens is more likely to be associated with the development of cancer, not BPH. The use of corticosteroids has not been associated with the development of BPH. **Cognitive Level:** Applying **Client Need:** Physiological Adaptation **Integrated Process:** Teaching and Learning **Content Area:** Adult Health **Strategy:** This question requires you to make the distinction between an association and a causal link. **Reference:** LeMone, P., Burke, K., & Bauldoff, G. (2011). *Medical-surgical nursing: Critical thinking in patient care* (5th ed.). Upper Saddle River, NJ: Pearson Education, pp. 1660–1662.

2 **Answer: 1** **Rationale:** Priapism is considered a medical emergency, because continued erection may lead to ischemia. Immediate treatment involves iced saline enema or anesthesia. A relaxing environment will not correct the condition, and the client does not require an evaluation for sexual dysfunction. **Cognitive Level:** Applying **Client Need:** Reduction of Risk Potential **Integrated Process:** Nursing Process: Implementation **Content Area:** Adult Health **Strategy:** Understanding of priapism is needed to determine that the treatment is aimed at relieving the congestion and preserving organ function. **Reference:** LeMone, P., Burke, K., & Bauldoff, G. (2011). *Medical-surgical nursing: Critical thinking in patient care* (5th ed.). Upper Saddle River, NJ: Pearson Education, pp. 1654–1656.

3 **Answer: 1** **Rationale:** Propranolol (Inderal), a beta adrenergic blocker, and many other antihypertensive medications can contribute to erectile dysfunction (ED). Other examples include clonidine (Catapres) and benazepril (Lotensin). Acetylsalicylic acid (aspirin), penicillin, and furosemide (Lasix) aren't known to have this effect. **Cognitive Level:** Applying **Client Need:** Pharmacological and Parenteral Therapies **Integrated Process:** Nursing Process: Diagnosis **Content Area:** Pharmacology **Strategy:** Identify the side effects for the drug in each answer option. Alternatively, understanding that the loss of sympathetic innervation from a beta blocker can prevent sexual arousal enables selection of the correct answer. **Reference:** LeMone, P., Burke, K., & Bauldoff, G. (2011). *Medical-surgical nursing: Critical thinking in patient care* (5th ed.). Upper Saddle River, NJ: Pearson Education, pp. 1650–1651.

4 **Answer: 2** **Rationale:** Because painless vaginal bleeding is often the only symptom of cervical or uterine cancer, this client should be tested for cancer. Ovarian cyst and endometriosis are not probable given the client's age. Polycystic ovarian syndrome is associated with amenorrhea or irregular menses and is usually diagnosed in young women of child-bearing age. **Cognitive Level:** Applying **Client Need:** Reduction of Risk Potential **Integrated Process:** Nursing Process: Planning **Content Area:** Adult Health **Strategy:** Vaginal bleeding in a woman past menopause is always an indication of pathology. Considering the age of the client helps to narrow the most probable cause. **Reference:** LeMone, P., Burke, K., & Bauldoff, G. (2011). *Medical-surgical nursing: Critical thinking in patient care* (5th ed.). Upper Saddle River, NJ: Pearson Education, p. 1685.

5 **Answer: 3** **Rationale:** Nocturnal penile tumescence and rigidity (NPTR) monitoring helps differentiate between psychogenic and organic causes of erectile dysfunction. Prostate cancer, infertility and phimosis are not assessed using NPTR monitoring. **Cognitive Level:** Applying **Client Need:** Physiological Adaptation **Integrated Process:** Nursing Process: Diagnosis **Content Area:** Adult Health **Strategy:** Understanding how the test is done and what it determines will enable identification of the correct response. **Reference:** LeMone, P., Burke, K., & Bauldoff, G. (2011). *Medical-surgical nursing: Critical thinking in patient care* (5th ed.). Upper Saddle River, NJ: Pearson Education, p. 1652.

6 **Answer: 2, 3, 5** **Rationale:** A Papanicolaou (Pap) test is done by scraping cells from the cervical os. The specimen is then examined for the presence of infections or precancerous or cancerous lesions of the cervix. In addition, a Pap test can detect hormonal changes and the effects of hormone replacement. The Pap test does not diagnose premenstrual syndrome or uterine cancer (because the scraping comes from the cervix only). **Cognitive Level:** Applying **Client Need:** Reduction of Risk Potential **Integrated Process:** Nursing Process: Implementation **Content Area:** Adult Health **Strategy:** Review the indications for a Papanicolaou (Pap) test. Recall that most disease processes that affect the cervix can be detected by the Pap test. **Reference:** LeMone, P., Burke, K., & Bauldoff, G. (2011). *Medical-surgical nursing: Critical thinking in patient care* (5th ed.). Upper Saddle River, NJ: Pearson Education, p. 1640.

7 **Answer: 3** **Rationale:** The Papanicolaou (Pap) smear test is used to screen women for cervical cancer, assess hormonal status, and identify the presence of sexually transmitted diseases, such as human papilloma virus (HPV) infection. AIDS is diagnosed using a CD 4 cell count. Endometriosis may be diagnosed using ultrasound. Vulvitis is recognized by visual inspection of the vulva. **Cognitive Level:** Applying **Client Need:** Reduction of Risk Potential **Integrated Process:** Nursing Process: Assessment **Content Area:** Adult Health **Strategy:** Determine the purpose of the Papanicolaou (Pap) test and then compare this with each answer option. Eliminate any answer options unrelated to the cervix and cellular changes. **Reference:** LeMone, P., Burke, K., & Bauldoff, G. (2011). *Medical-surgical nursing: Critical thinking in patient care* (5th ed.). Upper Saddle River, NJ: Pearson Education, p. 1694.

8 **Answer: 1, 2, 3** **Rationale:** Menarche before age 12, menopause beginning after age 55, and giving birth to first child after age 30 are risk factors for the development of breast cancer. Being overweight, not underweight, is a risk factor for the development of breast cancer. Breast feeding has been associated with a lower, not a higher risk of developing breast cancer. **Cognitive Level:** Applying **Client Need:** Physiological Adaptation **Integrated Process:** Teaching and Learning **Content Area:** Adult Health

ANSWERS & RATIONALES

Strategy: Review the risk factors for breast cancer and compare this list to each answer option. Eliminate each answer option that does not reflect the risk factors. **Reference:** LeMone, P., Burke, K., & Bauldoff, G. (2011). *Medical-surgical nursing: Critical thinking in patient care* (5th ed.). Upper Saddle River, NJ: Pearson Education, pp. 1703–1704.

9 Answer: 2 Rationale: Breast examinations should be done monthly at the same time of the month, not every other month or randomly. A postmenopausal woman would select the same date each month, while premenopausal women should do breast self-examination (BSE) at completion of the menstrual cycle because fluid retention and breast tenderness are less likely to be present. Breast examination during menstrual flow is not the best time, because of hormonal influences on the breasts. **Cognitive Level:** Applying **Client Need:** Health Promotion and Maintenance **Integrated Process:** Nursing Process: Implementation **Content Area:** Adult Health **Strategy:** Density of breast tissue is influenced by hormone levels. Doing the breast self-examination (BSE) when the hormones are most stable gives the person the best chance of feeling abnormalities in the breast tissue. **Reference:** LeMone, P., Burke, K., & Bauldoff, G. (2011). *Medical-surgical nursing: Critical thinking in patient care* (5th ed.). Upper Saddle River, NJ: Pearson Education, p. 1709.

10 Answer: 2 Rationale: Syphilis is transmitted from open lesions during any sexual contact: genital, oral-genital, or anal-genital. Exposure to urinary contaminants, sharing eating utensils, and improper handwashing do not transmit the disease. **Cognitive Level:** Applying **Client Need:** Health Promotion and Maintenance **Integrated Process:** Nursing Process: Diagnosis **Content Area:** Adult Health **Strategy:** Transmission of sexually transmitted infections is directly related to the level of physical intimacy between partners. Select the most physically intimate distracter. **Reference:** LeMone, P., Burke, K., & Bauldoff, G. (2011). *Medical-surgical nursing: Critical thinking in patient care* (5th ed.). Upper Saddle River, NJ: Pearson Education, pp. 1729–1732.

Posttest

1 Answer: 2, 3, 4, 5 Rationale: Breast self-exams are done monthly to detect early breast cancer. Testicular exams should also be done monthly to detect testicular cancer. The use of condoms prevents the transmission of sexually transmitted infections (STIs), HIV, and prevents pregnancy. An annual Papanicolaou (Pap) test is required once sexual activity begins to diagnose human papilloma virus, cervical cancer, and sexually transmitted infections. Changing tampons every 3 to 6 hours has been demonstrated to prevent toxic shock syndrome. **Cognitive Level:** Applying **Client Need:** Health Promotion

and Maintenance **Integrated Process:** Nursing Process: Implementation **Content Area:** Adult Health **Strategy:** Select answer options that can prevent or detect diseases that could occur in the teenage population. **Reference:** LeMone, P., Burke, K., & Bauldoff, G. (2011). *Medical-surgical nursing: Critical thinking in patient care* (5th ed.). Upper Saddle River, NJ: Pearson Education, pp. 259, 1641, 1657–1659, 1702–1703, 1709.

2 Answer: 2 Rationale: The client's symptoms are consistent with secondary syphilis, which occurs 2 weeks to 6 months after the initial chancre disappears. Primary syphilis is indicated by the presence of a chancre and enlarged lymph nodes. Latent syphilis produces no symptoms. Tertiary syphilis is the final stage of the illness and is characterized by the development of infiltrating tumors and involvement of the central, nervous, and cardiovascular systems. **Cognitive Level:** Analyzing **Client Need:** Physiological Adaptation **Integrated Process:** Nursing Process: Planning **Content Area:** Adult Health **Strategy:** Differentiate the presentation of primary, secondary, and tertiary syphilis. **Reference:** LeMone, P., Burke, K., & Bauldoff, G. (2011). *Medical-surgical nursing: Critical thinking in patient care* (5th ed.). Upper Saddle River, NJ: Pearson Education, pp. 1729–1732.

3 Answer: 1 Rationale: Herpetic lesions are painful, so the first priority is to provide comfort measures for the client. Antivirals, not antibacterials, are used to control the extent of the outbreak. Anxiolytics may be appropriate but are not a priority. There is no evidence of a secondary infection in the client. **Cognitive Level:** Analyzing **Client Need:** Physiological Adaptation **Integrated Process:** Nursing Process: Planning **Content Area:** Adult Health **Strategy:** Eliminate untrue or nonpriority answer options. Select the answer option that reflects the pathology of the herpes virus. **Reference:** LeMone, P., Burke, K., & Bauldoff, G. (2011). *Medical-surgical nursing: Critical thinking in patient care* (5th ed.). Upper Saddle River, NJ: Pearson Education, pp. 1719–1721.

4 Answer: 1, 2, 3, 5 Rationale: Painless swelling in one testicle is a common symptom of testicular cancer. Elevated levels of human chorionic gonadotropin (HCG) provide strong evidence of testicular cancer. Testicular self-examination should be performed monthly for early detection. Testicular cancer is the most common cancer in men between the ages of 15 and 40. A history of cryptorchidism (undescended testicle) increases the risk of developing testicular cancer. **Cognitive Level:** Applying **Client Need:** Health Promotion and Maintenance **Integrated Process:** Nursing Process: Implementation **Content Area:** Adult Health **Strategy:** This question is aimed at engaging men in early detection. Eliminate untrue statements and select answer options that would achieve the goal of getting men to participate in health screening. **Reference:** LeMone, P., Burke, K., & Bauldoff, G. (2011). *Medical-surgical nursing: Critical thinking in patient care* (5th ed.). Upper Saddle River, NJ: Pearson Education, pp. 1657–1659.

5 **Answer: 3** **Rationale:** Testicular torsion, or twisting of the testes and spermatic cord, is a potential emergency, because compromised blood flow to the testicle may lead to ischemia and necrosis. Priapism is a sustained erection that is treated with ice, but there is no indication that this is the boy's problem. Cryptorchidism is an undetected testicle that usually descends in infancy. The priority for the client is to rule out testicular torsion. The circumstances surrounding the injury are not as important as notifying the health care provider for treatment. **Cognitive Level:** Analyzing **Client Need:** Physiological Adaptation **Integrated Process:** Nursing Process: Planning **Content Area:** Child Health **Strategy:** Define each disorder in the answer options. Eliminate answer options that are inconsistent with the client's presentation. Conversely, select the answer option that is consistent with the clinical presentation. **Reference:** LeMone, P., Burke, K., & Bauldoff, G. (2011). *Medical-surgical nursing: Critical thinking in patient care* (5th ed.). Upper Saddle River, NJ: Pearson Education, p. 1657.

6 **Answer: 4** **Rationale:** Third-degree uterine prolapse is visible outside the body as the uterus protrudes through the opening of the vaginal canal. A pelvic infection would not cause tissue protrusion from the vagina, although the vaginal tissues would be reddened and/or edematous. Endometriosis is the implantation of endometrial tissue in the pelvic cavity. It does not present as tissue protruding from the vagina. A leiomyoma is a benign tumor of the uterus. It does not present as tissue protruding from the vagina. **Cognitive Level:** Applying **Client Need:** Physiological Adaptation **Integrated Process:** Nursing Process: Assessment **Content Area:** Adult Health **Strategy:** Define each answer option. When taken in the context of normal anatomy, the correct response is identifiable. **Reference:** LeMone, P., Burke, K., & Bauldoff, G. (2011). *Medical-surgical nursing: Critical thinking in patient care* (5th ed.). Upper Saddle River, NJ: Pearson Education, pp. 1687–1693.

7 **Answer: 3** **Rationale:** Tadalafil (Cialis) is an oral medication used to treat erectile dysfunction in men. Propranolol (Inderal) is a beta-adrenergic blocker used for cardiovascular conditions. Diazepam (Valium) is used as an antianxiety, antiseizure medication. Progesterone is a female hormone. **Cognitive Level:** Applying **Client Need:** Pharmacological and Parenteral Therapies **Integrated Process:** Nursing Process: Planning **Content Area:** Adult Health **Strategy:** Review the mechanism of action for each of the drugs listed. Eliminate any answer option that may depress sexual function. **Reference:** LeMone, P.,

Burke, K., & Bauldoff, G. (2011). *Medical-surgical nursing: Critical thinking in patient care* (5th ed.). Upper Saddle River, NJ: Pearson Education, pp. 1650–1654.

8 **Answer: 2** **Rationale:** Chlamydial infection may be present for months or years without producing symptoms in women, and if untreated can ascend into the uterus and cause pelvic inflammatory disease or PID. It is caused by *Chlamydia trachomatis*, a bacterium that behaves like a virus and is treated with azithromycin (Zithromax). Young women who are sexually active and not using a condom are at the highest risk. **Cognitive Level:** Applying **Client Need:** Safety and Infection Control **Integrated Process:** Nursing Process: Implementation **Content Area:** Adult Health **Strategy:** Review the clinical presentation of sexually transmitted infections (STIs). Eliminate answer options that are inconsistent with chlamydia. Select the answer option that indicates the greatest risk with chlamydia. **Reference:** LeMone, P., Burke, K., & Bauldoff, G. (2011). *Medical-surgical nursing: Critical thinking in patient care* (5th ed.). Upper Saddle River, NJ: Pearson Education, pp. 1844–1845.

9 **Answer: 1** **Rationale:** Oral hormonal medications may be used to treat prostate cancer. Metastasis to the bowel is uncommon because a tough sheet of fascia separates the two organs. The disease is more common in the elderly. The disease may affect 70% of men in their 80s. Asians and Native Americans have the lowest risk for developing prostate cancer. **Cognitive Level:** Applying **Client Need:** Health Promotion and Maintenance **Integrated Process:** Nursing Process: Implementation **Content Area:** Adult Health **Strategy:** This question is testing knowledge of the principle for early detection of cancer increasing the rate of cure. Select the answer option that is consistent with this principle. **Reference:** LeMone, P., Burke, K., & Bauldoff, G. (2011). *Medical-surgical nursing: Critical thinking in patient care* (5th ed.). Upper Saddle River, NJ: Pearson Education, pp. 1666–1668.

10 **Answer: 2** **Rationale:** Benign prostatic hyperplasia (BPH) is the most common disorder of the aging male client. Testicular cancer is the most common cancer in men between the ages of 15 and 35. Testicular torsion occurs most often between birth and age 20. Gonorrhea is highest in occurrence during the sexually active years; women ages 15 to 19 and men ages 20 to 24 have the highest rate. **Cognitive Level:** Applying **Client Need:** Reduction of Risk Potential **Integrated Process:** Nursing Process: Assessment **Content Area:** Adult Health **Strategy:** Each of the options is related strictly to males. Occurrence is directly related to the age of the client. Select the option most likely to occur in the older adult population. **Reference:** LeMone, P., Burke, K., & Bauldoff, G. (2011). *Medical-surgical nursing: Critical thinking in patient care* (5th ed.). Upper Saddle River, NJ: Pearson Education, pp. 1660–1666.

ANSWERS & RATIONALES

References

Adams, M., & Koch, R. (2010). *Pharmacology: Connections to nursing practice.* Upper Saddle River, NJ: Prentice Hall.

Berman, A., & Snyder, S. (2012). *Kozier & Erb's fundamentals of nursing: Concepts, process, and practice* (9th ed.). Upper Saddle River, NJ: Pearson Education.

D'Amico, D., & Barbarito, C. (2012). *Health & physical assessment in nursing* (2nd ed.). Upper Saddle River, NJ: Pearson Education, Inc.

Ignatavicius, D. D., & Workman, M. L. (2013). *Medical-surgical nursing: Critical thinking for collaborative care* (7th ed.) Philadelphia: W. B. Saunders Company.

Kee, J. L. (2010). *Laboratory and diagnostic tests* (8th ed.). Upper Saddle River, NJ: Pearson Education.

Lehne, R. (2010). *Pharmacology for nursing care* (7th ed.). St. Louis, MO: Saunders.

LeMone, P., Burke, K., & Bauldoff, G. (2011). *Medical- surgical nursing: Critical thinking in patient care* (5th ed.). Upper Saddle River, NJ: Pearson Education.

Lewis, S., Dirksen, S., Heitkemper, M., Bucher, L., & Camera, I. (2011). *Medical surgical nursing: Assessment and management of clinical problems* (8th ed.). St. Louis, MO: Elsevier.

McCance, K. L., & Huether, S. E. (2010). *Pathophysiology: The biologic basis for disease in adults and children* (6th ed.). St. Louis, MO: Mosby, Inc.

Murray, R. B., Zentner, J. P., & Yakimo, R. (2009). *Health promotion strategies through the life span* (8th ed.). Upper Saddle River, NJ: Pearson Education.

Osborn, K. S., Wraa, C. E., & Watson, A. (2010). *Medical surgical nursing: Preparation for practice* (Vol. Combined). Upper Saddle River, NJ: Pearson Education.

Smith, S. F., Duell, D. J., & Martin, B. C. (2012). *Clinical nursing skills: Basic to advanced skills* (8th ed.). Upper Saddle River, NJ: Pearson Education.

Wilson, B. A., Shannon, M. T., & Shields, K. M. (2012). *Pearson nurse's drug guide 2012*. Upper Saddle River, NJ: Pearson Education.

Eye and Ear Disorders

16

Chapter Outline

Overview of Anatomy and
  Physiology of Eye and Ear
Diagnostic Tests and
  Assessments of Eye
Diagnostic Tests and
  Assessments of Ear
Common Nursing Techniques
  and Procedures for Eyes
  and Ears

Nursing Management of Client
  Having Eye Surgery
Nursing Management of Client
  Having Ear Surgery
Glaucoma
Cataracts
Detached Retina
Macular Degeneration
Diabetic Retinopathy

Eye Infections or
  Inflammations
Eye Injury
Legal Blindness
Ear Infections
Otosclerosis
Ménière's Disease

Objectives

➤ Identify basic structures and functions of the eye and ear.
➤ Describe the pathophysiology and etiology of common eye and
  ear disorders.
➤ Discuss expected assessment data and diagnostic test findings for
  selected eye and ear disorders.
➤ Identify priority nursing problems for selected eye and ear disorders.
➤ Discuss therapeutic management of selected eye and ear disorders.
➤ Discuss nursing management of a client experiencing an eye or
  ear disorder.
➤ Identify expected outcomes for the client experiencing an eye or
  ear disorder.

NCLEX-RN® Test Prep

Use the accompanying online resource,
NursingReviewsandRationales, to test
yourself with hundreds of NCLEX®-style
practice questions.

Review at a Glance

cataract a progressive and gradual
development of opacity in lens or lens
capsule that results in loss of vision
conjunctivitis inflammation of
conjunctiva of eye caused by infection,
allergen, toxin, or other irritant
cycloplegic referring to an ability to
paralyze ciliary muscle of eye
glaucoma an eye disorder characterized by an imbalance between aqueous
humor production and drainage, leading
to increased intraocular pressure
gonioscopy measurement of angle
of anterior chamber of eye
labyrinthectomy complete removal
of labyrinth that destroys cochlear function,

relieving vertigo but causing loss of any
minimal remaining hearing as well
Ménière's disease an inner ear
disorder in which there is
excessive accumulation of
endolymphatic fluid in membranous
labyrinth
miotic ability to constrict pupil of eye
mydriatic ability to dilate pupil of eye
myringotomy surgically performed
perforation of tympanic membrane to
allow drainage of middle ear secretions and relieve pain and pressure of
otitis media
nystagmus involuntary rhythmic,
oscillating movement of eyes that

can be horizontal, vertical, rotary, or a
mixture of these
otosclerosis hereditary disorder
of labyrinthine capsule in which
abnormal bone growth occurs
around ossicles and causes fixation
of stapes, leading to conductive
hearing loss
presbycusis an age-related
change in ear that results in a
decreased ability to hear high-
frequency sounds
presbyopia an age-related decrease
in elasticity of lens of eye, making it more
difficult to focus on objects at a
short distance

533

proprioception sensation about body's position in space that is transferred to brain after changes in body position trigger fluid movement and bending of hair cells in vestibular structures

tonometry a diagnostic test for glaucoma that measures intraocular pressure by determining resistance of eyeball to an applied force

tympanoplasty surgical reconstruction of ossicles and tympanic membrane of middle ear to help restore hearing

PRETEST

1 The nurse is admitting to the emergency department a client who is holding his hand over his eye. The client reports being a sheet metal worker who was injured at work. For which of the following diagnostics should the nurse prepare the client prior to seeing the health care provider?

1. Instillation of fluorescein into the eye
2. Gonioscopy
3. Tonometry examination
4. Fundoscopy

2 A client has been prescribed brimonidine (Alphagan) for newly diagnosed glaucoma. What should the nurse remember to include in the teaching plan for this client?

1. Brimonidine increases visual acuity.
2. Brimonidine eye drops do not produce systemic side effects.
3. There is no effect on vision after instillation.
4. Place pressure on inner canthus of the eye after administration.

3 A client has just been diagnosed with glaucoma. The nurse should place highest priority on teaching the client which piece of information?

1. Fluid restriction is needed to reduce intraocular pressure.
2. Disorder often has no symptoms.
3. Adherence to medication therapy is essential to reduce risk of vision loss.
4. Disorder is typically diagnosed after an episode of eye infection.

4 After noting a slight cloudy appearance to the lens of a 64-year-old client's eye, the nurse should question the client about which symptom?

1. Seeing bright flashes of light
2. Blurring of vision
3. Night blindness
4. Photophobia

5 A client admitted to the hospital has impaired vision from glaucoma. To assist the client's compensation, the nurse instructs the nursing assistant to arrange the client's room in which way?

1. Place objects that he may need so they are directly in front of him.
2. Move the overbed table so there is direct light on it.
3. Arrange furniture and objects so he can use his peripheral vision.
4. Ensure that there are no obstructions between the bed and bathroom.

6 A client with a suspected impaction of cerumen has an order for an otic irrigation. The nurse should take which essential action before beginning the irrigation?

1. Draw up no more than 120 mL of solution for use at one time.
2. Make sure client is seated comfortably in bathroom.
3. Make sure irrigant is at room temperature.
4. Examine tympanic membrane to be sure it is intact.

7 A client has been treated for acute otitis media. To evaluate the effectiveness of therapy, the nurse questions whether the client obtained relief from which primary symptom associated with this disorder?

1. Purulent drainage from the ear
2. Loss of balance
3. Ear pain
4. Tinnitus

8 The nurse is caring for a client who receives pilocarpine (Pilocar) eye drops for glaucoma. What information must the nurse include in a teaching plan so the client can self-administer the eye drops? Select all that apply.

1. Instill drops into the inner canthus.
2. Wash hands prior to administering the eye drops.
3. Use aseptic technique.
4. Expect pupillary dilation to occur.
5. Instill drops into lower conjunctival sac.

9 The nurse is demonstrating to a client how to administer ear drops. Place the steps of the procedure in the proper order.

1. Clean the pinna of the ear and the meatus of the ear canal.
2. Administer the ear drops.
3. Pull the pinna upward and backward.
4. Position the client with the ear being treated uppermost.
5. Press gently but firmly a few times on the tragus of the ear.

10 The nurse has conducted discharge teaching for a client diagnosed with Ménière's disease. The nurse evaluates that the client understood the instructions given if the client states to refrain from eating which favorite food?

1. Granola bars
2. Baked eggplant
3. Sugar-free cookies
4. Salted cashews

➤ *See pages 561–562 for Answers and Rationales.*

I. OVERVIEW OF ANATOMY AND PHYSIOLOGY OF EYE AND EAR

A. Eye structures
1. Outer protective layer, also referred to as fibrous coat
   a. Sclera: white and opaque in color, made of fibrous connective tissue
   b. Cornea: clear fibrous covering that continues anteriorly from sclera; is avascular, and is part of refractive media of eye
2. Middle vascular layer, also referred to as uveal tract
   a. Iris: thin, pigmented muscle with a central aperture called a pupil; responsible for constricting and dilating pupil to regulate amount of light entering eye
   b. Ciliary body: circular structure that surrounds lens and connects anteriorly to iris and posteriorly to choroids; maintains intraocular pressure by producing aqueous humor (a watery refractive medium) that flows from posterior to anterior chamber before draining through trabecular meshwork into Canal of Schlemm
   c. Choroid: thin membrane that contains blood vessels to supply eye tissues, attaches to both ciliary body and optic nerve
3. Inner layer, the retina: thin, semitransparent layer containing rods and cones, responsible for vision in dim light and for perception of fine details, respectively

B. Eye functions
1. Eye receives light waves through cornea; waves are refracted by aqueous humor, the lens, and vitreous humor as they are transmitted to retina; retinal images formed by light rays are inverted and reversed by the biconvex lens
2. Rods and cones of retina translate light waves into neural impulses for relay to optic nerve, and then to brain's occipital lobes for interpretation as vision
3. Fusion of images from each eye into a single image in brain is called binocular vision

! ▶ **C. Age-related changes of eyes that affect vision**
1. Decreased ability of pupil to dilate, which reduces night vision and increases light needed for reading and small motor tasks, such as sewing
2. Development of **presbyopia**, a decreased elasticity of lens that makes focusing for near vision more difficult and results in farsightedness
3. Lens becomes discolored and opacified, which reduces color perception (especially green, blue, and violet), interferes with night vision, and increases sensitivity to glare
4. Decreased eye motility and senile enophthalmos (sinking in) of eyes, limits peripheral vision upward, downward, and to sides
5. Degenerative changes to choroid, retina, and optic nerve reduce depth perception and ability to see lines of demarcation (stair edges, doorframes)
6. Lipid deposits, collection of debris and pulling away of vitreous body from retina causes blurred vision and "floaters"
7. Decreased corneal sensitivity increases risk for injury

D. Ear structures
1. External ear: outer visible ear or auricle, external auditory canal, and tympanic membrane
2. Middle ear: malleus, incus, and stapes bones; and window membranes; posterior wall contains mastoid antrum which communicates with mastoid sinuses and Eustachian tube, allowing middle ear to adjust to changes in pressure and equalize air pressure; mucous membrane lining middle ear is continuous with mucous membrane lining throat
3. Inner ear: semicircular canals, cochlea, distal portion of cranial nerve VIII (vestibulocochlear nerve)

E. Ear functions
1. Hearing: sound is transferred from tympanic membrane to malleus, incus, and stapes and through cochlea; vibrations are changed by transduction into action potentials that are sent to brain as neural impulses
2. **Proprioception** (balance): sensation about body's position in space that is transferred to brain after changes in body position trigger fluid movement and bending of hair cells in vestibular structures

F. Age-related changes of ears that affect hearing
1. External auditory canal narrows; cerumen glands atrophy and produce thicker, drier cerumen
2. Tympanic membrane is less flexible, and ossicle joints calcify; degeneration and atrophy of inner ear structures affect balance and increase risk for falls
3. Cochlear hair cell degeneration and loss of auditory neurons in organ of Corti lead to **presbycusis**, an age-related sensorineural hearing loss, characterized by decreased ability to hear high-frequency sounds and resulting in difficulty hearing and localizing normal speech

II. DIAGNOSTIC TESTS AND ASSESSMENTS OF EYE

A. Fluorescein angiography: injection of sodium fluorescein into arm vessel, followed by serial imaging and recording to detect disorders in retinal vessels, such as with diabetic retinopathy and eye tumors
1. Preprocedure care
   a. Assess for allergies and/or history of reactions to dye
   b. Ensure client has given informed consent
   ! ▶ c. Give prescribed mydriatic medication 1 hour prior to test to dilate pupil
2. Postprocedure care
   a. Encourage rest and increased fluid intake (fluids aid in dye excretion)

      b. Teach client that dye causes temporary skin discoloration in injected area and temporary green discoloration of urine

      c. Teach client to avoid sunlight or other bright light sources for some hours until pupil dilation returns to normal

B. Corneal staining: instillation of dye into conjunctival sac to highlight irregularities caused by trauma, abrasions, or ulcers; damaged corneal epithelium appears green when viewed through a blue filter

    1. Ensure that contact lenses are removed prior to procedure, if worn

    2. Tell client to blink to distribute dye evenly over cornea

    3. Wipe excess dye from cheeks and instruct client not to rub eyes

C. *Tonometry*: measurement of intraocular pressure (IOP) to detect glaucoma, by determining resistance of the eyeball to an applied force

    1. Normal IOP ranges from 10–21 mmHg; routine screening is recommended for all clients over age 60 years

    2. Eye may be anesthetized, and client stares forward

    3. Applanation: most accurate method, measures force needed to flatten a small area of cornea; eye is anesthetized

    4. Indentation: measures change in form of globe after standard weight (Schiøtz tonometer) is applied to cornea; eye is anesthetized

    5. Noncontact: calculates IOP by measuring deflection of a puff of air applied to cornea; no anesthetic needed

    6. Tell client not to rub eyes after test if anesthetic was used to avoid possible corneal scratches or injury

D. Physical assessment of eye and vision

    1. Acuity of distance vision: measures vision using Snellen chart hung 20 feet away

      a. Client reads chart lines with one eye covered, moving downward from row that is most clear, until unable to cite more than one-half of characters in a line

      b. Record findings as a fraction: the numerator being the client's distance from chart (20 feet), and the denominator being the number identified at end of smallest line read, which corresponds to distance at which a normal eye can read that line; normal vision is 20/20; a larger denominator indicates myopia (nearsightedness)

      c. Repeat process for other eye

      d. Test eyes of clients with corrective lenses both with and without correction, noting *sc* (sine correctio, without correction) and *cc* (cum correctio, with correction)

    2. Acuity of near vision: measures vision using a Rosenbaum chart or a card with newsprint 12–14 inches from client's eyes; impairment indicates hyperopia (farsightedness) in a young client, or presbyopia in an adult after approximately 45 years of age

    3. Refraction test

      a. Uses Snellen chart to assess visual acuity while client reads through various strengths of corrective lenses

      b. Used to measure and prescribe correction for errors in visual focus with *myopia* (nearsightedness), *hyperopia* (farsightedness), and *astigmatism* (irregularity or indentation of corneal surface that inhibits light rays from focusing clearly on retina)

    4. Visual fields: measures peripheral vision, often called confrontation test

      a. Client and examiner sit facing each other with client looking into examiner's eyes

      b. Client covers right eye and examiner covers left eye

      c. Examiner raises a finger or other small object at arm's length midway between client and examiner and brings it in from periphery into line of vision; procedure is repeated from above and below on same side

      d. Client states "now" when able to see object; examiner should see object at about same time (test assumes examiner has normal peripheral vision)

      e. Test is repeated on the other eye

5. Color vision
   a. Tested for driver's license, employment requiring color discrimination, or with history of difficulty distinguishing colors; sensitive for red/green blindness, but not for blue
   b. Involves picking colored numbers or letters out of plates with multiple colors in background (such as an Ishihara chart)
   c. Results recorded as a fraction of number of plates identified correctly and total number shown
6. Extraocular muscle movements (cardinal fields of vision)
   a. Client holds head still and follows a small object with the eyes through 6 cardinal positions of gaze: to right (lateral), upward and right (temporal), down and right, left (lateral), upward and left (lateral), and down and left
   b. Client should have parallel eye movement and absence of *nystagmus*, involuntary rhythmic oscillating eye movements (vertical, horizontal, rotary, or mixed)
   c. As last step, client follows finger as it moves in to bridge of nose; eyes should sustain convergence to within 5–8 centimeters
7. Outer eye structures
   a. Sclera white in color, although in dark-skinned client may appear to have slight yellow cast or pigmented dots; yellow discoloration (or heightened yellow) can indicate jaundice
   b. Cornea normally transparent, smooth, and shiny; opacities (cloudy areas) or specks may indicate prior injury
   c. Pupils should be round, equal in size, and constrict in response to direct light or to light shone in opposite pupil (consensual response); pupils should constrict and converge when looking at object over examiner's shoulder and then shifting gaze to an object 4–6 inches from own nose (accommodation)
8. Ophthalmoscopy
   a. Used to examine retina, optic disk, optic blood vessels, fundus, and macula
   b. Client sits in darkened room to heighten pupil dilation, stares straight ahead
   c. Examiner holds ophthalmoscope in right hand and uses own right eye when examining client's right eye and vice versa
   d. Examiner approaches client from 12–15 inches away and 15 degrees lateral to client's line of vision
   e. As light shines on pupil, reflection of light on retina causes a red glare (red reflex); absence of red reflex may indicate lens opacity; a *cataract* is an opacity of lens that may be due to trauma, aging, diabetes mellitus, or a congenital defect

III. DIAGNOSTIC TESTS AND ASSESSMENTS OF EAR

A. Otoscopic examination

1. Use largest speculum that will fit into client's auditory canal without discomfort; hold speculum with handle downward if client is cooperative, or with handle upward if uncooperative; rest hand holding otoscope against client's head for support if needed while handle is upward
2. Tilt client's head slightly away, pull pinna up and back in an adult (down and back in a child) to straighten external auditory canal, and insert speculum while visualizing the canal
3. Normal findings
   a. Pink, intact external canal with no lesions and variable amount of cerumen and fine hairs; absence of inflammation, deviations, or foreign bodies
   b. Tympanic membrane that is transparent, opaque, pearly gray, slightly concave, intact, and free of lesions or perforations; a triangular light reflex should be seen and membrane should move in and out when client performs Valsalva maneuver

    4. Abnormal findings: tympanic membrane

       a. White opaque areas are often scars

       b. Bulging may be caused by otitis media or malfunctioning auditory tubes

       c. Retractions may be due to an obstructed auditory tube

       d. Bluish tinge may indicate presence of blood in middle ear caused by head trauma

       e. Absent light reflex may indicate otitis media

       f. Dark spot on eardrum may indicate perforation

B. Whisper test

    1. Have client occlude one ear at a time with a finger, and stand 1–2 feet away from client on side of unoccluded ear

    2. Whisper numbers or a statement and ask client to repeat; repeat for other ear

    3. Note whether it is necessary to stand closer or speak louder to be heard

    4. A similar test is the watch test, in which a ticking watch is held 5 inches from each ear and hearing is assessed

C. Rinne test

    1. Hold a tuning fork by the stem and strike tines softly on back of hand to activate it; place stem on mastoid bone and ask client to signal when sound is no longer heard

    2. Quickly place vibrating end of tuning fork in front of ear close to ear canal; ask client if the sound is heard; if yes, have client indicate when sound is no longer heard

    3. With no conductive hearing loss, sound is heard twice as long by air conduction as by bone conduction

    4. With conductive hearing loss, bone conduction is greater than air conduction in affected ear

D. Weber test

    1. Is especially valuable when hearing in one ear is reported as better than in the other

    2. Place stem of vibrating tuning fork on midline of forehead or vertex of head (skull) and ask whether sound is heard equally in both ears or if one side is better than the other

    3. Sound that lateralizes to one ear indicates conductive hearing loss in that ear or sensorineural hearing loss in opposite ear

E. Audiometry: quantifies hearing deficits by presenting various sound frequencies to each ear by either sound or bone conduction; client sits in soundproof room wearing earphones, and is asked to signal when tones are heard

F. Speech audiometry: identifies intensity at which speech is identifiable

G. Tympanometry: indirectly monitors compliance and impedance of middle ear to sound transmission after neutral, positive, and negative air pressure is applied to external auditory meatus

H. Tests of vestibular function

    1. Test for falling: assure client that a fall will be prevented; then ask client to close eyes while feet are together and arms are hanging at sides; observe for a normal slight sway; significant sway is called a positive Romberg test

    2. Caloric test

       a. Cold or warm water is used to irrigate ear canals one at a time; test is contraindicated if tympanic membrane is perforated

       b. Normally nystagmus will occur in eye opposite to ear being irrigated; if no nystagmus occurs, client needs further testing for brain lesions

       c. Use of alcohol, CNS depressants, and barbiturates may alter test results

    3. Past pointing test

       a. Have client sit facing examiner, close eyes, and point both index fingers at examiner

       b. Place own index fingers under client's to provide a reference point, then ask client to raise both arms and then lower them to original location with eyes closed

       c. With normal response, client can return to reference point easily; with vestibular dysfunction, fingers deviate to left or right

4. Gaze nystagmus test: observe client's eyes as they look straight ahead, 30 degrees to each side, upward, and downward; with vestibular problems the eyeballs exhibit nystagmus, an involuntary, constant, and cyclical movement of eyeballs in any direction

5. Hallpike maneuver: have client lie supine and rotate head to side for one minute; the test is positive for positional vertigo or induced dizziness if nystagmus occurs

IV. COMMON NURSING TECHNIQUES AND PROCEDURES FOR EYES AND EARS

A. Ocular medications

1. Eye drops
   a. Ensure that medication is sterile and treat each eye separately, if both being medicated, to prevent cross-contamination; always use aseptic technique during administration of eye drops
   b. Tilt client's head back slightly, having client look up with eyes open
   c. Expose lower conjunctival sac by gently pulling down skin of cheekbone with gloved hand
   d. Hold bottle like a pencil and rest wrist on client's forehead or cheek for stability to prevent bottle from touching eye and causing injury
   e. Instill correct number of drops into outer third of conjunctival sac
   f. Have client close eye gently (not squeezing) and move eye inside closed lid to evenly distribute medication; apply pressure to nasolacrimal duct (tear duct, at inner canthus) with tissue or cotton ball to prevent systemic drug absorption
   g. Wipe away excess from cheek with tissue or cotton ball if needed
   h. Wait 2–5 minutes between drops as per manufacturer's directions

2. Eye ointments
   a. Use same client positioning as for eye drops
   b. Squeeze a thin bead of ointment along inside of outer third of conjunctival sac or from inner to outer canthus
   c. Have client close eye gently and move eyeball to evenly distribute ointment
   d. Instruct client that the ointment may blur the vision temporarily

3. Medicated eye disk
   a. Open package and press tip of index finger of gloved hand against convex part of disk
   b. Position client as for eye drops or ointment and expose lower conjunctival sac
   c. Place disk horizontally in sac between iris and lower eyelid
   d. Pull lower eyelid out and up over disk and ask client to blink a few times until disk is not visible
   e. Have client press fingers against closed lids without moving eyes or disk to secure disk in position
   f. To remove disk, expose lower conjunctival sac and use thumb and index finger to pinch and lift disk from sac; if positioned in upper eye, stroke closed eyelid gently in long circular motions; once disk moves to corner of eye, slide to lower lid and remove as described

B. Ocular irrigation

1. Position client with head tilted toward side to be irrigated and place waterproof pad and curved basin under affected side
2. Cleanse eyelids and lashes with gloved hand and moistened cotton ball, discarding each cotton ball after one wipe
3. Draw up ordered irrigant into sterile irrigation set or bulb syringe
4. Use nondominant hand to hold eyelids open
5. Hold syringe 1 inch above eye and push fluid gently into conjunctival sac (fluid flows across eye from inner to outer canthus)

6. Avoid flushing directly onto eyeball to avoid damage to cornea
7. Eyelid speculum or irrigating contact lens may be used if ordered; in special circumstances, topical anesthetic may be used

C. **Eye patches and shields**
   1. Have client close both eyes during application of patch or shield
   2. Position patch and secure with two strips of tape extending from midforehead to lateral cheekbone (medial top to lateral bottom) on same side
   3. Do not use pressure unless specifically ordered, and then use 2–3 pads and extra tape
   4. Change only with physician order
   5. Apply shield alone or over an eye patch to protect eye from pressure or other type of irritation
   6. Place shield on bony prominences of cheek, nose, and brow; secure with transparent tape in same manner as for eye patch

D. **Eye prosthesis (artificial eye) care**
   1. Allow client to perform own artificial eye care if preferred; some prostheses are permanently implanted while others are removable
   2. Remove prosthesis by retracting lower eyelid and exerting pressure just below eye to break suction and lift it from socket; can also use rubber bulb syringe or medicine dropper bulb to create suction effect
   3. Cleanse with normal saline, mild soap and water, or tap water according to client's routine; do not use abrasives or chemicals
   4. Irrigate eye socket with normal saline or clean warm water using aseptic technique if ordered (such as for infection)
   5. Cleanse edges of eye socket and surrounding area with moistened gauze
   6. Reinsert by retracting upper and lower eyelids and slipping prosthesis into eye socket comfortably under upper eyelid
   7. When prosthesis is stored, place in labeled container with saline or tap water

E. **Otic medications**
   1. Use clean technique unless tympanic membrane is damaged, then use sterile technique
   2. Assist client to a side-lying position with ear being medicated uppermost
   3. Clean pinna of ear and opening of external ear canal with solution and cotton-tipped applicators as needed; ensure that applicators are not inserted into ear canal to avoid damage to tympanic membrane or wax becoming impacted within canal
   4. Warm medication container in hand or warm water for comfort; partially fill ear dropper with medication
   5. Straighten auditory canal by pulling pinna up and back in an adult or older child, or down and back in an infant or child age 3 years or younger
   6. Hold bottle or dropper 1/2-inch above ear canal and instill correct number of drops along side of ear canal
   7. Apply gentle pressure with finger to tragus of ear to enhance flow of medication into ear canal
   8. Have client maintain a side-lying position for 5 minutes for even medication dispersion
   9. Before client arises, loosely place a cotton ball at meatus and leave in place for 20–30 minutes to prevent medication loss

F. **Otic irrigation**
   1. Assist client to a sitting or lying position with head tilted toward affected ear; place a waterproof pad and drainage receptacle under affected ear
   2. Check that temperature of irrigant is 37°C or 98°F
   3. Determine that tympanic membrane is intact before beginning an otic irrigation
   4. Straighten ear canal and gently insert syringe tip into auditory meatus; direct solution slowly and steadily along wall of canal (not center, which could damage tympanic membrane); use no more than 50–70 mL at one time

5. After solution drains, dry outside of ear with cotton balls and place a dry one in auditory meatus lightly to absorb remaining excess fluid

6. Assist client to a side-lying position on affected side for further drainage, and assess client for discomfort

G. **Hearing aid prosthesis care**

1. There are several types of hearing aids: behind-the-ear (BTE, postaural), in-the-ear (ITE, intra-aural), in-the-canal (ITC), eyeglasses aid, and body hearing aid; hearing aids are useful to improve quality of hearing with conductive hearing loss but only intensify distortions heard with sensorineural hearing loss (they may be useful in signaling client of danger, for example, able to hear alarms)

2. Wash hands before handling an external hearing aid

3. Make sure battery is working properly and is inserted correctly; keep an extra battery on hand

4. Do not drop hearing aid or twist the cord

5. To insert a hearing aid: inspect to ensure it is intact, turn off hearing aid and turn down volume, insert ear mold first into ear canal, then secure rest of device according to its design; once in place, turn on hearing aid and turn up volume slowly until comfortable, and check for structural problems or placement problems if feedback occurs

6. Remove a hearing aid after turning it off and lowering volume; remove earmold by rotating it forward slightly and pulling outward

7. After removal of a hearing aid, clean a detachable earmold with mild soap and water, rinse and dry well, and avoid excessive wetting or use of alcohol, which can damage the aid; wipe nondetachable earmolds with a damp cloth

8. Avoid using aerosol sprays, oils, or cosmetic products near hearing aid, because earmold opening could become clogged

9. Remove battery to prevent battery corrosion and leakage if aid will not be used for more than 24 hours; store in a safe place away from moisture and heat

H. **Cochlear implant**: for sensorineural hearing loss 2 types of procedures are available depending on whether there are remaining auditory neurons capable of being excited

1. A device is implanted in ear for use in receiving and transmitting sound; 2 types of devices are available

   a. An electrode that is implanted in cochlea receives stimuli from a processor worn on body; used for a client with intact neurons capable of stimulation (see Figure 16-1)

   b. A second type of device, used for clients with no excitable auditory fibers, amplifies and transmits a signal to a receiver implanted in brainstem

2. Devices do not restore normal hearing but allow perception of sound to alert a client to conversation or dangers in environment

3. Complications of all inner ear surgical procedures include infection and cerebrospinal fluid leakage

V. NURSING MANAGEMENT OF CLIENT HAVING EYE SURGERY

A. **Preoperative period**

1. Reduce anxiety through preoperative teaching about procedure and postoperative course and care

2. Assess client's support systems and ability to care for self after surgery, including assessment of environmental safety (such as handrails, absence of throw rugs)

3. Complete shampoo or scrub around eyes if ordered; remove eye makeup; store contact lens or eyeglasses (needed to aid vision in other eye) so they are available upon completion of surgery

4. Administer preanesthetic medications and eyedrops as ordered, which commonly include **mydriatic** eye drops (to dilate pupils) and **cycloplegic** eye drops (to paralyze ciliary muscles); see Table 16-1 for overview of commonly ordered eye medications

Figure 16-1

Cochlear implant used in sensorineural hearing loss in which excitable auditory neurons remain

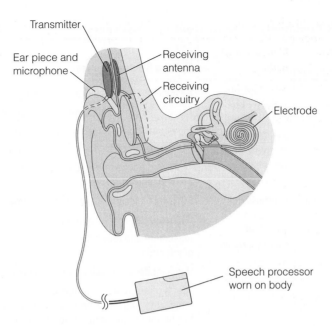

Transmitter

Ear piece and microphone

Receiving antenna

Receiving circuitry

Electrode

Speech processor worn on body

B. **Postoperative period**
1. Perform baseline assessments as for all postoperative clients (vital signs, level of consciousness, status of dressing); changes may be minimal if surgery done under local anesthesia
2. Maintain eye patch or eye shield in place to prevent injury to eye, and instruct client not to rub or touch the area
3. Elevate head to 30–45 degrees and have client lie on back or unaffected side (to reduce intraocular pressure) after surgery done to treat cataracts or glaucoma; use small pillows at sides of head to immobilize head when lying on back
4. Position client with repair of detached retina as prescribed so that area of detachment is dependent/inferior (to maintain pressure on repaired retinal area and improve its contact with choroid)
5. Instruct and assist client to avoid activities that increase IOP, such as coughing, sneezing, vomiting, or straining at stool; if it is necessary to cough or sneeze, client should do so with mouth open
6. Maintain client safety: orient to environment, keep articles and call bell on unaffected side, use side rails with bed in low position, and assist with ambulation
7. Give antibiotic, anti-inflammatory, and other prescribed topical (eye) or systemic medications
8. Give analgesics as ordered, avoiding or using caution with opioids to prevent postoperative nausea, vomiting, and constipation; discomfort may be described as achy or scratching; avoid morphine, which can cause miosis
9. Assess for possible surgical complications that should be reported immediately to preserve sight:
   a. Sudden sharp eye pain, possibly indicating hemorrhage, sudden rise in intraocular pressure, or other ocular emergency
   b. Hemorrhage, with blood noted in anterior chamber of eye
   c. Retinal detachment, noted by client sensations of flashes of light, floaters, or a curtain being drawn over the eye
   d. Corneal edema, noted by a cloudy appearance to cornea
10. Teach client and family about postdischarge care (see Box 16-1, p. 546)
11. Refer to community health agency for assistance with postdischarge home care if needed

Table 16-1		Medications Commonly Used to Treat Eye Disorders	
Drug Class and Name: Generic (Trade)	**Therapeutic Use(s)**	**Mechanism of Action**	**Nursing Responsibilities**
Ophthalmic Anesthetics Proparacaine (Ophthetic) Tetracaine (Pontocaine)	Numb cornea before measuring intraocular pressure (IOP) or before minor procedures	Anesthetizes corneal nerves and surrounding tissue; partial or complete loss of sensation	Assess for signs of allergic reaction Explain that blink reflex will be temporarily eliminated May need to patch eye following procedure for protection Teach not to rub or touch eyes for several minutes Tears and edges of eyelids and lashes will be yellow temporarily; color washes out with tears
Ophthalmic Anti-infectives Idoxuridine (Herplex) Natamycin (Natacyn) Sulfacetamide (AK-Sulf, Cetamide) Trifluridine (Viroptic)	Local treatment of bacterial or viral infections	Interfere with reproduction or growth of microorganisms	Assess eye lesions daily during therapy Assess for allergy to sulfonamides prior to use (sulfacetamide) Implement and teach careful handwashing to prevent spread of infection Use aseptic technique during administration Teach client to use caution with activities if drug causes temporary blurred vision, wear sunglasses, and avoid bright light to prevent photophobic reactions, use exactly as prescribed
Ophthalmic Beta-adrenergic Blocking Agents Betaxolol (Betoptic) Carteolol (Ocupress) Levobunolol (Betagan) Metipranolol (OptiPranolol) Timolol (Timoptic)	Treatment of glaucoma	Decrease formation of aqueous humor to lower intraocular pressure	Use cautiously in clients with asthma or bronchospasm, heart failure, other cardiovascular disease, or diabetes mellitus Monitor intake and output, daily weight, lung crackles, peripheral edema, pulse, and blood pressure Teach diabetic client that tachycardia and increased blood pressure that accompany hypoglycemia may be masked by this drug Teach client to use exactly as prescribed; follow instructions precisely if changing from one drug to another; expect transient stinging or burning with instillation, but report if severe; wear sunglasses to minimize risk of photophobia; keep appointments for follow-up eye exams
Ophthalmic and Non-ophthalmic Carbonic Anhydrase Inhibitors Acetazolamide (Diamox) Brinzolamide (Azopt) Dichlorphenamide (Daranide) Dorzolamide (Trusopt) Methazolamide (Neptazane)	Treatment of glaucoma	Inhibits carbonic anhydrase to reduce secretion of aqueous humor in eye, causes self-limiting excretion of sodium, potassium, bicarbonate, and water; therefore lowering IOP	May be given PO, IM, IV, or topically to eye to lower IOP Assess for contraindications to therapy: allergy to sulfa drugs, severe liver or kidney disease, existing electrolyte or acid-base imbalances Assess for eye discomfort, reduced visual acuity, or local adverse effects such as conjunctivitis or lid reactions Assess for anorexia, malaise, metallic or bitter taste, paresthesias, electrolyte or acid–base imbalances, nephrolithiasis Monitor intake and output, daily weight, vital signs for possible fluid volume deficit Give in a.m. to prevent diuresis from disrupting sleep Teach client to avoid driving or other activities requiring alertness if drowsiness occurs, use sunscreen to avoid photosensitivity reactions, and keep appointments for follow-up eye exams

(continued)

Table 16-1   **Medications Commonly Used to Treat Eye Disorders (Continued)**

Drug Class and Name: Generic (Trade)	Therapeutic Use(s)	Mechanism of Action	Nursing Responsibilities
Ophthalmic Cholinergic Agents *Prostaglandin* Latanoprost (Xalatan) *Direct-Acting Cholinergics* Carbachol (Carboptic) Pilocarpine (Pilocar, Ocusert-Pilo, others) *Cholinesterase Inhibitors* Demecarium (Humorsol) Echothiophate (Phospholine Iodide) Isoflurophate (Floropryl) Physostigmine (Isopto Eserine)	Miotics used in treatment of glaucoma	Facilitate the outflow of aqueous humor to lower intraocular pressure	Latanoprost can cause or increase brown pigmentation to eye and increase eyelash growth; do not use latanoprost with thimerosal Avoid concurrent use of anticholinergic drugs, such as atropine, that block drug action Monitor blood pressure, pulse, and lung sounds; report hypotension, bradycardia, bronchospasm Assess for and report symptoms of systemic absorption: shortness of breath, increased sweating or salivation, nausea, vomiting, diarrhea, abdominal cramps, increased urge to urinate Avoid concurrent use of drugs that block drug effects, including many OTC sleep and cough preparations Teach client that pupil size will decrease (miosis); blurred vision, eye or brow ache, and reduced night vision can occur; use safety precautions such as nightlights and avoid night driving; it is important to keep follow-up eye appointments
Ophthalmic Cycloplegic Cyclopentolate (Cyclogyl, others) Homatropine (Isopto Homatropine) Tropicamide (Opticyl, others) Atropine (Ocutropine)	Local therapy before eye surgery or ophthalmic examination, treatment of inflammatory disorders of the iris	Paralyzes iris sphincter (blocking constriction) and paralyzes ciliary muscle for accommodation (cycloplegic effect)	These drugs are contraindicated with sensitivity to belladonna alkaloids and are either contraindicated or must be used cautiously in clients with glaucoma Assess for and report signs of systemic absorption: drowsiness, confusion, tachycardia, dry mouth, flushed face Assess for hallucinations and psychotic reactions as adverse CNS effects Teach client to use caution because drug may temporarily impair ability to judge distances, and to wear dark glasses because pupil(s) cannot constrict in bright light
Ophthalmic Mydriatics Phenylephrine (Neo-Synephrine)	Pupil dilation for diagnostic procedures, laser therapy, etc.	Produces pupillary dilation by stimulating iris dilator muscle and paralyzing iris sphincter and ciliary muscle	Contraindicated in clients with narrow-angle glaucoma May cause adverse effects if used with monoamine oxidase inhibitor (MAOI) or tricyclic antidepressants Advise to wear sunglasses to block ultraviolet light exposure and that driving with eyes dilated may cause difficulty
Ophthalmic Sympathomimetics (Alpha$_2$ Agonists) Apraclonidine (Iopidine) Brimonidine (Alphagan P) Dipivefrin (Propine) Epinephrine (generic)	Reduction of intraocular pressure during laser eye surgery (apraclonidine) or due to open-angle glaucoma	Decreases aqueous humor formation (apraclonidine, brimonidine) or increases aqueous outflow (epinephrine, dipivefrin)	Use aseptic technique during administration Monitor for increased pulse and BP, and CNS effects such as nervousness, muscle tremors, and anxiety Teach client to wear dark glasses and use caution in bright light because pupillary dilation will occur; keep appointments for follow-up eye exams; report signs of hypersensitivity reaction: itching, lid edema, and eye discharge; report changes in visual acuity or eye pain; eye pain could indicate an attack of angle-closure glaucoma; avoid OTC sinus and cold medications that contain sympathomimetics (pseudoephedrine, phenylephrine) and could increase side effects

(continued)

Table 16-1	Medications Commonly Used to Treat Eye Disorders (Continued)		
Drug Class and Name: Generic (Trade)	**Therapeutic Use(s)**	**Mechanism of Action**	**Nursing Responsibilities**
Osmotic Diuretics Glycerin (Ophthalgan) Mannitol (Osmitrol) Urea	Short-term reduction of corneal edema before ophthalmic exam or surgery (glycerin) and short-term reduction of intraocular pressure (all)	Increases osmotic pressure of glomerular filtrate, thus inhibiting reabsorption of electrolytes and water	Administer 60 to 90 minutes before surgery as ordered Ophthalmic solution of glycerin may cause eye pain and irritation; precede with local anesthetic as ordered Monitor intake and output, assess for signs of dehydration Avoid infusing hypotonic fluids following administration, because this will offset the osmotic effect of glycerin

Box 16-1	Include the following points in client and family discharge instructions after eye surgery:
Client Education Following Eye Surgery	• Leave eye shield in place until the surgeon's office visit on the day after surgery, then use eye shield at night during sleep for eye protection as prescribed • Avoid rubbing, scratching, touching, squeezing, or putting pressure on surgical eye • Avoid activities that increase intraocular pressure, such as sneezing, coughing, vomiting, straining, moving rapidly, bending, or lifting more than 5 pounds • Maintain sedentary lifestyle for approximately 2 weeks or as prescribed by surgeon; avoid heavy work, such as gardening, mowing the lawn, or moving furniture • Avoid reading until allowed by surgeon, and then read in moderation during healing • Use measures to prevent constipation, such as adequate fiber and fluid intake, maintaining mobility as able, and possible use of stool softener • Wear sunglasses with side shields when outdoors (photophobia commonly occurs) • New corrective lenses (if needed) will not be prescribed until vision stabilizes, which may take several weeks; make and keep all recommended follow-up appointments with physician • Proper techniques for use of eye patch or shield and/or instillation of eye drops • Medication names, dose, schedule, side effects, purpose, and anticipated duration of use • Symptoms to report to physician: new, increased or severe eye pain or pressure, decreased vision, redness, cloudiness, drainage, floaters or light flashes, halos around brightly lit objects

VI. NURSING MANAGEMENT OF CLIENT HAVING EAR SURGERY

A. Preoperative period

1. Reduce anxiety through preoperative teaching about procedure and postoperative course and care

2. Complete a baseline assessment of client's hearing ability to use as a comparison postoperatively; establish a means of communication to be used after surgery; reassure client that decreased hearing acuity immediately after surgery is expected

3. Assess client's support systems and ability to care for self after surgery, including assessment of environmental safety (such as handrails, absence of throw rugs)

4. Teach that blowing of nose, coughing, and sneezing are restricted postoperatively to prevent pressure changes in middle ear and potential disruption of surgical site; if a cough or sneeze is necessary, keep mouth open to minimize pressure changes in middle ear

5. Complete shampoo or scrub around ear if ordered; complete usual preoperative activities and checklist; administer preanesthetic medications as ordered

B. Postoperative period

1. Perform baseline assessments as for all postoperative clients (vital signs, level of consciousness, bleeding or drainage from dressing, pain, recovery from anesthesia)

2. Implement standard interventions for care of postoperative client (pain control, mobility, prevention of postoperative complications)

3. Keep client on bedrest for 24 hours with head of bed either elevated or flat (depending on surgeon's order but usually elevated to decrease pressure in middle ear) and lying on nonoperative side (operative ear upward) for 12–24 hours

4. Change internal or external dressings if ordered; wipe away discharge from ear with dry sterile dressing material

5. Assess for nausea and vomiting; medicate with antiemetics prn to avoid vomiting, which can disrupt surgical site by increasing pressure in middle ear

6. Assess for dizziness and vertigo postoperatively; avoid unnecessary movements or turning in bed; provide antivertigo medications; and provide assistance when allowed to ambulate to reduce falls

7. Assess client's hearing postoperatively and compare to baseline; use alternate communication means as needed

8. Remind client that decreased hearing immediately after surgery may be due to edema and drainage at operative site; permanent hearing loss may be expected if cochlea is involved or no middle ear reconstruction is done

9. Teach client and family about postdischarge care (see Box 16-2)

Box 16-2	Include the following points in client and family discharge instructions after ear surgery:
Client Education Following Ear Surgery	• Keep the outer ear dressing clean and dry; change it as ordered if needed; do not remove inner ear dressing until allowed by surgeon; do not insert small objects to clean external ear canal
	• Whenever possible, avoid activities that increase middle ear pressure, such as blowing nose, sneezing, coughing, straining
	• If it is necessary, cough or sneeze with mouth open; blow nose one nostril at a time with mouth open; avoid drinking through a straw for 2–3 weeks; avoid air travel until allowed by surgeon
	• Use measures to prevent constipation, such as adequate fiber and fluid intake, maintaining mobility as able, and possible use of stool softener
	• Do not shower or shampoo hair until allowed by surgeon (usually restricted for 1 or more weeks)
	• Keep ear dry for 6 weeks with use of petrolatum-coated cotton ball placed in external auditory canal as ordered, if used change it daily; do not swim or dive until allowed by surgeon (when full healing occurs)
	• Reduce risk of infection by avoiding those with respiratory infections
	• Medication names, dose, schedule, side effects, purpose, and anticipated duration of use (antibiotics, antiemetics, antivertigo agents)
	• Symptoms to report to physician: persistent postoperative headache, increased drainage or bleeding from site, fever, new or increased ear pain or dizziness, decreasing hearing

VII. GLAUCOMA

A. Description

1. **Glaucoma** is an optic neuropathy with gradual loss of vision that usually involves an imbalance between aqueous humor production and drainage, leading to increased IOP; it affects 2% of those over age 40 and is a leading cause of blindness worldwide

2. Primary glaucoma can be of two types: open angle or angle closure (narrow angle, closed angle)

3. Secondary glaucoma is related to infection, inflammation, cataracts, tumors, hemorrhage, or trauma

B. Etiology and pathophysiology

1. Usually exists as a primary condition without identified precipitating cause; most frequent in adults over 60 years of age; may be a congenital condition in infants and children

2. Open-angle glaucoma: most frequent form with unknown cause although heredity suspected; the angle of the anterior chamber between iris and cornea is normal; flow of aqueous humor through trabecular network to Canal of Schlemm is obstructed; it is usually a bilateral process

3. Angle-closure (narrow-angle, closed-angle) glaucoma: less common form, is often unilateral, although the other eye can be affected at a later time
   a. Anterior chamber narrows due to corneal flattening or bulging of iris
   b. When iris thickens (pupil dilation) or lens thickens (during visual accommodation), angle can close completely, blocking outflow and causing sudden elevation of IOP
   c. Damage to neurons in retina and optic nerve can occur, rapidly lead to loss of vision if not treated quickly

C. Assessment

1. Open angle
   a. Loss of peripheral vision, mild headaches, difficulty adapting to the dark, seeing halos around lights, and difficulty focusing on near objects
   b. Symptoms may be vague with client unaware of them for a time; damage to optic disc causes a painless, progressive narrowing of visual fields; visual acuity deteriorates over time with rising IOP

2. Angle closure
   a. Triggered by pupil dilation, such as with high emotions and darkness, among others
   b. Symptoms include severe eye and face pain, nausea and vomiting, malaise, colored halos around lights, and episodes of sudden decline in vision; possible reddened eye, cloudy cornea from edema, and pupil fixed at midpoint
   c. Rapid and permanent loss of vision can occur if not treated promptly

3. Diagnosed by history; presenting symptoms; *tonometry*; ophthalmoscopy; **gonioscopy** (measurement of anterior chamber angle, differentiates open-angle from angle-closure glaucoma)

D. Priority nursing problems: reduced visual perception, potential for injury, pain, anxiety, inadequate knowledge

E. Planning and implementation

1. Acute glaucoma: medical emergency; vision loss can occur within 1–2 days if untreated; provide information to client and administer ordered therapies such as osmotic diuretics or carbonic anhydrase inhibitors to lower IOP (see Table 16-1); surgical intervention may be needed

2. Chronic glaucoma: interventions primarily consist of medication therapy and client education

3. Provide pre- and postoperative care as previously outlined in Section V A and B, if eye surgery is needed; surgical procedures to facilitate drainage of aqueous humor can include trabeculectomy, laser trabeculoplasty, iridectomy, or laser iridotomy

Practice to Pass

A client who has just been diagnosed with glaucoma states that she is not worried about the condition because she has no symptoms. How should you respond?

F. Medication therapy: prostaglandin analogs are treatment of choice due to once daily administration and low adverse effect rate, **miotic** drugs that constrict pupils, carbonic anhydrase inhibitors to decrease production of aqueous humor, and beta-adrenergic blockers to constrict pupils and reduce production of aqueous humor (refer again to Table 16-1)

G. Surgical treatments: indicated for clients with acute angle-closure glaucoma and those with chronic open-angle glaucoma that is not effectively controlled by medication

1. Noninvasive treatments
   a. Trabeculoplasty using a laser to create multiple burns around trabecular network; as the burns heal, the scars they create cause stretching and opening of network
   b. Laser iridotomy using a laser to create multiple small perforations in iris of eye which allows aqueous humor to drain
2. Trabeculectomy is an invasive surgery that involves general anesthesia; a permanent fistula is created to drain aqueous humor

H. Client education

1. Drug therapy is needed for life; noncompliance can lead to loss of vision that cannot be regained
2. Avoid mydriatic medications such as atropine that dilate pupils
3. Obtain MedicAlert card or bracelet specifying type of glaucoma
4. Use safety precautions at night (lighting, handrails) to compensate for reduced ability of pupils to dilate because of miotics, and remove obstacles in environment for safety
5. Follow general instructions following eye surgery (see Section V B)
6. Review specific drug information and procedures for self-administration

I. Evaluation: client verbalizes medication understanding and demonstrates use correctly, utilizes safety measures, identifies measures to prevent increases in IOP, has relief of eye pain, maintains existing vision, and complies with postoperative instructions

VIII. CATARACTS

A. Description

1. Progressive and gradual development of opacity in lens or lens capsule that results in loss of vision
2. Incidence increases with age (found to some extent in 50–70% of adults over 65 years of age), called "senile cataracts"

B. Etiology and pathophysiology

1. Other risk factors besides age include long-term exposure to ultraviolet light (UVB rays), cigarette smoking, heavy alcohol use, eye injury or inflammation, congenital defect, diabetes mellitus, and some medications (such as systemic corticosteroids, chlorpromazine [Thorazine], busulfan [Myleran])
2. Fibers and proteins of lens degenerate with age or following insult; opacity often begins at periphery of lens and moves to center
3. Partial opacity is termed "immature cataract"; opacity of entire lens is termed "mature cataract"
4. Opacity tends to occur bilaterally but is asymmetric in development, with one maturing faster than the other

C. Assessment

1. Decline in close and distance vision, blurred vision, changes in color vision (loss), glare, halos around lights, object distortion, white or cloudy gray pupil
2. Diagnosed by history and physical exam, results of visual acuity tests and slit-lamp exam; absence of red reflex with ophthalmoscopy

D. Priority nursing problems: reduced visual perception, potential for injury, potential for falls, inadequate knowledge

E. Planning and implementation

1. Provide emotional support since impaired vision is anxiety-producing for clients

2. Identify safety concerns in environment related to impaired vision and correct them
3. Surgical removal of lens is sole treatment option and is accompanied by lens implant or is treated with corrective lenses
4. Assist client in decision making about surgery, which is indicated when vision or activities of daily living are affected, or if causing secondary problems such as uveitis or glaucoma
5. Reinforce explanations about surgical extraction of lens
   a. Cryoextraction: forceps or supercooled probe used to extract lens after making small incision in cornea
   b. Phacoemulsification: ultrasound vibrations break lens into fragments that are aspirated (suctioned) from eye
   c. Intracapsular extraction: removal of entire lens and surrounding capsule (see Figure 16-2a)
   d. Extracapsular extraction: removal of lens nucleus and cortex, leaving posterior capsule intact to support lens implant; currently most popular method (see Figure 16-2b)

Figure 16-2

Cataract removal with lens implant. A. Intracapsular cataract extraction removes entire lens and capsule, with lens implantation in anterior chamber, B. Extracapsular cataract extraction removes lens and anterior capsule, with lens implantation within the intact posterior capsule.

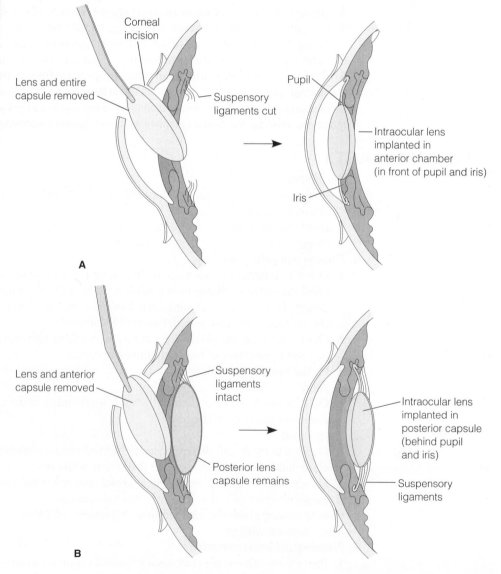

6. Surgery is done on one eye at a time, usually on an outpatient basis and using local anesthesia
7. Intraocular lens implant rapidly restores binocular vision and depth perception
8. If intraocular lens implant is not used, a thick convex corrective lens or contact lens is needed to provide light refraction and restore visual acuity to surgical eye
9. Provide preoperative and postoperative care as outlined in previous section

F. **Medication therapy**
1. Indicated for temporary use after surgery
2. Generally includes antibiotic and anti-inflammatory agents

G. **Client education**
1. Include adaptive strategies to compensate for changes in vision and depth perception if surgery not currently indicated or desired
2. Instruct postoperative client as outlined in previous section on eye surgery
3. Teach client to leave eye patch or shield in place until changed or removed by surgeon at postoperative visit, usually within 24-48 hours
4. Eye protection may include use of sunglasses during day in bright light and use of eye shield at night
5. Teach client information and procedures for medication use after surgery, such as acetaminophen for general discomfort, combination steroid (anti-inflammatory) and antibiotic eye drops, and others as needed by individual client (refer back to Table 16-1)
6. Teach client about insertion and care of postoperative contact lenses if prescribed
7. Teach client that when convex corrective lenses are worn postoperatively, visual field is narrowed by thick convex lens, so client must move head side to side (rather than just look side to side) to compensate; depth perception may also be affected, requiring attention to safety
8. Permanent eyeglasses will be prescribed several weeks after surgery when healing is complete and vision has stabilized

H. **Evaluation**: client exhibits behavior changes as needed to adapt to vision changes, remains free of injury, and demonstrates understanding of pre- and postoperative eye care

IX. DETACHED RETINA

A. **Description**
1. Separation of sensory layer of retina from choroid, the pigmented vascular layer
2. Retina may tear and fold back onto itself, or remain intact and be pulled away from choroid by shrinking of vitreous humor
3. Loss of contact between retina and choroid causes ischemia to neurons of retina

B. **Etiology and pathophysiology**
1. Most frequently occurs due to aging with shrinkage of vitreous humor, which pulls on retina at points of attachment, such as optic disk, macula, and periphery of eye
2. Can also be caused by trauma, inflammation, tumor, or complication of eye surgery (lens removal)
3. With a retinal break or tear, fluid enters defect, possibly leading to further rapid tearing and separation due to pressure
4. Incomplete area of detachment can progress slowly or can enlarge quickly and become complete
5. Will lead to permanent blindness if untreated, so is considered a medical emergency

C. **Assessment**
1. Initial: presence of floating spots (floaters) and/or flashing lights; eye appears normal to visual inspection

2. Progressive blurring of vision, visual field deficits corresponding to area of damage, sense of curtain or veil coming down, up or across field of vision, painless

3. Ophthalmic exam shows area of gray opaque retina, with possible accompanying tears, holes, or folds

D. **Priority nursing problems**: reduced visual perception, reduced retinal tissue perfusion, potential for injury, anxiety or fear, inadequate knowledge

E. **Planning and implementation**
   1. Preoperative care
      a. Protect eye from further damage: bed rest, cover both eyes with eye patches to limit movement and prevent eye stress, instruct client not to bend forward or make sudden or jerking head movements
      b. Position client with detached area dependent/inferior so gravity pushes detachment closer to choroid (for example, with left eye superior temporal detachment, keep client supine with head turned toward left)
      c. Protect client from injury keeping bed low, side rails up, call bell within reach; talk to client before approaching bed, assist with self-care
      d. Reinforce explanations about surgical repair
         1) Laser photocoagulation or cryotherapy (cold probe): creates a local inflammation that will locally adhere retina onto the choroid
         2) Scleral buckling: holds retina and choroid together with an implant or encircling strap or "buckle"
         3) Pneumatic retinopexy: injects air/gas into vitreous with adjustment of client's head position to push detached portion of retina back into contact with choroid
         4) Surgical instrument manipulation to move detached segment of torn retina into place, followed by laser therapy or injection of gas or silicone oil to create a bond
      e. Provide psychological support to alleviate anxiety associated with sudden loss of vision; reassure client most detachments are successfully treated (often on outpatient basis)
      f. Provide preoperative care as described in Section V A
   2. Postoperative care
      a. Provide standard postoperative care as described in Section V B
      b. Stress importance of maintaining prescribed position (affected eye inferior or dependent to maintain contact between retina and choroid)

F. **Medication therapy**: usually includes antibiotic, anti-inflammatory, and analgesic medications

G. **Client education**: as previously described in Box 16-1

H. **Evaluation**: client demonstrates understanding of pre- and postoperative eye care, exhibits behavior changes as needed to promote surgical healing, and remains free of injury

X. MACULAR DEGENERATION

A. **Description**
   1. Defined as degeneration of macular area (center area) of retina, which normally receives light from center of visual field and has greatest visual acuity
   2. Most common type is age-related macular degeneration (AMD), currently the leading cause of legal blindness in the United States for those over 65 years of age

B. **Etiology and pathophysiology**
   1. Causes of age-related macular degeneration are unknown, although heredity, smoking, injury, inflammation, and nutritional factors are suspected to play a role; females, whites and Hispanics are at higher risk
   2. Risk may be reduced with a diet high in omega-3 fatty acids, lutein, and zeoxanthin

---

Practice to Pass

A client tells you that "all of a sudden" it seems like a window shade is being pulled down over one eye. What are your immediate assessments and interventions?

3. In AMD, there is gradual failure of outer layer of retina (pigmented epithelium that attaches retina to choroid layer and removes cellular wastes); in this process, photoreceptor cells are lost, metabolic wastes accumulate in subretinal space, leading to cell death

4. There are 2 types of macular degeneration
   a. Atrophic ("dry") form: bilateral and gradual but progressive loss of vision occurs because of atrophy and degeneration of macula (90% of cases)
   b. Exudative ("wet") form: presence of new, weak blood vessels that are prone to leakage form; there is accumulation of serous fluid or blood in subretinal space, which leads to more rapid, severe loss of vision; scar tissue forms and leads to cell death and vision loss (10% of cases but responsible for 90% of legal blindness)

C. **Assessment**
   1. Clinical manifestations include loss of central vision while peripheral vision remains intact), appearance of pale yellow spots on macula called *drusen*, visual distortion of images (for example, straight lines may appear wavy) and difficulty with activities requiring focused and close central vision (for example, sewing, needlepoint, reading)
   2. Diagnostic tests: vision testing, fundoscopy (examination of fundus of eye); fluorescein angiography (for wet form only); and electroretinography (ERG) to measure retinal responses to light

D. **Priority nursing problems**: reduced visual perception, potential for injury, anxiety, inadequate knowledge

E. **Planning and implementation**
   1. Currently there is no treatment for dry macular generation but progress may be slowed with high-dose antioxidants and zinc; there is no curative therapy for either wet or dry macular degeneration
   2. Wet macular degeneration may be treated by
      a. Laser photocoagulation
      b. Photodynamic therapy, in which a light-activated drug is injected into vein and circulates to retinal blood vessels; a low-intensity laser light is shone on retina; this activates drug to eventually occlude blood vessel and stop leakage; note that it is possible for the process to recur in another area
   3. Nursing measures
      a. Standard nursing interventions to prevent falls and other injuries stemming from impaired vision
      b. Standard measures to assist those with impaired vision (see also Section XIV D, planning and implementation for legal blindness)
      c. Obtain home safety evaluation prior to discharge to minimize risk of injuries and falls in the home setting

F. **Medication therapy**: no medications are available to treat this condition

G. **Client education**
   1. Need for regular eye examinations to determine disease progression
   2. Use of Amsler grid for self-monitoring of central vision (available from eye care professionals or on the Internet)
   3. Measures to maintain safety at home and adapt to visual changes
      a. Obtain aids to enhance vision and promote safety (for example, magnification devices, enhanced lighting)
      b. Determine availability of large print books and newspapers and audio books
   4. Postprocedure self-care for photodynamic therapy includes use of dark glasses and protective clothing as well as avoiding bright indoor light for 5 days after treatment

H. **Evaluation**: client is free of injury; adapts to vision changes effectively; verbalizes an understanding of importance of continued monitoring of sight; and verbalizes adaptation to changing vision

XI. DIABETIC RETINOPATHY

A. Description and assessment findings
1. A vascular disorder affecting capillaries of retina
2. Capillaries become sclerotic and lose ability to transport sufficient oxygen and nutrients to retina

B. Etiology and pathophysiology
1. In the United States, is the leading cause of new blindness in people ages 20 to 74
2. Nearly half of Hispanic/Latino adults with diabetes mellitus (DM) have diabetic retinopathy
3. Risk is directly related to duration of the DM, degree of glycemic control, and presence of hypertension
4. Is seen in both type 1 and type 2 DM
5. Progresses from mild nonproliferative to proliferative retinopathy with leaking of venous capillaries of eye; new blood vessels form but are fine and fragile, resulting in being easily ruptured

C. Collaborative management
1. Yearly eye examination of all clients with DM by an ophthalmologist
2. Strict control of blood glucose levels and blood pressure
3. Laser photocoagulation of leaking vessels slows progression but does not cure disorder

XII. EYE INFECTIONS OR INFLAMMATIONS

A. Description and assessment findings
1. Blepharitis (inflammation of eyelid margin glands and lash follicles): red-rimmed eyes; irritation, burning, itching of eyelid margins; mucous discharge with crusting and scaling of lid margins
2. Hordoleum or sty (infection of sebaceous glands of eyelid): raised area of lid, pain, redness, tenderness, possible photophobia, tearing, and sensation of foreign body in eye
3. Chalazion (granulomatous eyelid cyst or nodule): hard swelling, painless, reddened local conjunctival tissue, possibly due to inadequately treated hordoleum
4. **Conjunctivitis** (infection of conjunctiva, or inflammation caused by allergen, toxin, other irritant): eye redness and itching; possible scratchy, burning, or gritty sensation; photophobia, tearing, discharge (watery, purulent, or mucoid); usually not painful; if severe, possible conjunctival edema, hemorrhage, or perforation
5. Corneal ulcer (local necrosis of cornea): caused by infection, trauma, or misuse of contact lenses; manifested by: photophobia, discomfort ranging from gritty sensations to severe pain, excessive tearing; possible discharge; decreased visual acuity, inability to open eye or spasm of eyelid, visible area of ulceration
6. Keratitis (inflammation of cornea): similar to conjunctivitis, can lead to ulceration and blindness
7. Uveitis (inflammation of uveal tract, e.g., vascular layer): pupillary constriction, erythema around limbus, severe eye pain, photophobia, blurred vision

B. Collaborative management
1. Medication therapy with topical or systemic antibiotics or antiviral agents, antihistamines, and corticosteroids
2. Promote infection control through diligent hand hygiene and proper care of contact lenses; teach client that conjunctivitis can be highly contagious
3. Reduce pain or discomfort with warm compresses, dark sunglasses, and analgesics (acetaminophen and/or codeine)
4. If corneal perforation is suspected, have client lie supine, close eye, and cover with dry, sterile dressing to avoid loss of eye contents until surgery is done

XIII. EYE INJURY

A. **Description and assessment findings**
1. Corneal abrasion (disruption of superficial cornea from drying, contact lenses, eyelashes, or foreign bodies such as dust, dirt, or fingernails): pain, photophobia, tearing
2. Burns (from chemicals, heat, radiation, explosion): eye pain, decreased vision, swollen eyelids, burns, reddened and edematous conjunctiva, possible corneal haziness or cloudiness, ulcerations
3. Blunt trauma (caused by sports injuries, motor vehicle crashes, falls, physical assault): includes lid ecchymosis (black eye), conjunctival hemorrhage (painless erythema), hyphema (bleeding into anterior chamber with eye pain, decreased vision, and seeing a reddish hue), and orbital fractures (diplopia/double vision, pain with upward eye movement, limited eye movements, sunken appearance to eye, and decreased sensation on affected cheek)

B. **Collaborative management**
1. If chemical burn present, irrigate eye with copious amounts of normal saline (preferred) or water (if necessary), until pH of eye is in range of 7.2–7.4; use topical anesthetic to make irrigation easier; then evaluate vision with and without any corrective eyeglasses; follow with antibiotic ointment
2. If no chemical burn injury is present, first evaluate vision with and without eyeglasses to provide data about extent of injury and for use as a baseline
3. Remove loose foreign bodies quickly using a sterile moistened cotton-tipped applicator or by irrigation to prevent corneal abrasion; follow with antibiotic ointment
4. Apply eye patches or sterile gauze dressings over both eyes if severe or penetrating eye injury occurs to reduce eye movements; stabilize any penetrating objects until surgery is done to help preserve vision; institute bed rest
5. Enucleation (surgical removal of eye) may be necessary because of trauma, infection, glaucoma, intractable pain, or malignancy; schedule placement of a temporary prosthesis within 1 week of surgery with permanent fitting 1–2 months after surgery
6. Care after blunt trauma includes bedrest in semi-Fowler's position with an eye shield to both eyes to decrease eye movement; may need medications to decrease intraocular pressure
7. Provide follow-up client education about purpose, effects, and use of medications, use of eye patch or shield, avoidance of activities that increase intraocular pressure during healing (lifting, bending, straining), and how to avoid future injury

XIV. LEGAL BLINDNESS

A. **Description**: visual acuity that is no better than 20/200 even with correction in better eye, or a visual field of less than 20 degrees (instead of 180 degrees)

B. **Etiology**
1. In United States, glaucoma and cataracts are 2 most common causes, followed by other retinal disorders (macular degeneration, diabetic retinopathy, congenital disorders)
2. Worldwide, the causes include cataracts, glaucoma, trauma, eye infections, and nutritional deficiencies; two-thirds of worldwide cases are preventable and result from lack of access to care, fear or ignorance about treatment or its need, poor sanitation, and poor nutrition

C. **Priority nursing problems**: reduced visual perception, decreased ability to perform activities of daily living, inadequate knowledge, reduced self-esteem, grief response, loss of hope, loss of power

D. **Planning and implementation**
1. Assist client to move through grieving process that accompanies vision loss, not only because of loss of sight, but because of its interference with mobility, self-sufficiency, and possibly financial status

Practice to Pass

You are admitting a client who is legally blind to the nursing unit. How would you orient this client to the bedside unit?

2. Support client who is experiencing changes in roles and relationships, communication patterns (through loss of ability to perceive nonverbal cues), and possibly sexual expression
3. Foster independence in hospital environment
   a. Verbally and physically orient client to room using bed as a reference point
   b. Keep room and hallway free of clutter
   c. Introduce yourself when entering client's room and state when you are leaving
   d. Use increased verbal communication: describe activities in environment and provide stimuli such as radio or television; ask client what assistance is needed
   e. Ensure that call bell and other needed articles are within easy reach of client and that client knows where they are located
   f. Describe location of food on plate using a clock face description (for a client who was previously sighted and knows what a clock face is)
   g. Assist with ambulation, walking slightly ahead and allowing client to hold your arm (not the reverse); describe the environment that lies ahead, such as turns or stairs

E. **Client education**: teach client and family measures to minimize risk of injury in home setting and adapt to performing ADLs with impaired vision
F. **Evaluation**: client exhibits adaptation to vision loss by moving purposefully within environment without injury, providing self-care for ADLs, and coping verbally and behaviorally with loss of vision

XV. EAR INFECTIONS

A. **Description and etiology**
   1. Otitis externa: infectious, inflammatory, or allergic response in external auditory canal or auricle; also called "swimmer's ear;" more frequent in warm, humid areas
   2. Otitis media: infection or inflammation of middle ear; often a consequence of upper respiratory infection when organisms travel from nose and throat via Eustachian tube; may be acute or chronic
   3. Mastoiditis: infection of the mastoid process (temporal bone adjacent to middle ear), usually a consequence of untreated or inadequately treated otitis media

B. **Assessment**
   1. Otitis externa: redness, swelling, and exudate in external auditory canal, earache, itching, sensation that ear is "plugged" or "blocked," hearing loss in affected ear; manipulating the auricle increases pain
   2. Otitis media
      a. Acute: severe earache or ear pain (classic), ear pressure, fever, malaise, diminished hearing, dizziness or vertigo, nausea and possible vomiting, possible tinnitus, presence of fluid behind a bulging or retracted tympanic membrane
      b. Chronic: slight fever, diminished hearing, chronic ear discharge
   3. Mastoiditis: fever, malaise, possible tinnitus and headache, persistent throbbing ear pain worsened by head movement, tenderness behind ear (over mastoid process), local cellulitis of skin, drainage from ear, diminished hearing in affected ear; manifestations usually develop 2–3 weeks after an episode of acute otitis media

C. **Priority nursing problems**: pain, alteration in auditory perception, potential for injury, potential for falls

D. **Planning and implementation**
   1. Apply local heat 3 times per day for 20 minutes at a time as prescribed
   2. Encourage bed rest as applicable to reduce head movements and pain
   3. Administer prescribed antibiotics (otic or systemic), decongestants, antihistamines, analgesics (acetaminophen or aspirin), and antivertigo agents

   4. Teach client to use caution while hearing is diminished
   5. Otitis externa
      a. Stay out of water until acute inflammatory process is completely resolved (7–10 days)
      b. Use precautions to keep ear canal dry while in water
      c. Immediately after swimming, dry ear canal by tilting head and jumping to shake out water; dry with a towel, then use a hair dryer on lowest setting to dry canal; do *not* insert cotton swabs or other objects into ear canal
      d. Use a drying agent such as 2% acetic acid solution in ear canal
      e. If impacted debris is present, irrigate ear with warm tap water
   6. Acute otitis media
      a. Teach that air travel, rapid changes in elevation, or diving may increase pain significantly and should be avoided
      b. Explain that abrupt relief of pain may indicate spontaneous perforation of tympanic membrane and should be reported immediately
   7. Provide care to clients undergoing ear surgery as per Section VI

E. Surgical procedures
   1. Myringotomy: surgical perforation of tympanic membrane to allow drainage of middle ear secretions and relieve pain and pressure (otitis media)
   2. Tympanocentesis: insertion of a 20-gauge spinal needle through inferior portion of tympanic membrane to drain secretions, possibly to obtain culture, and relieve pain and pressure (otitis media)
   3. Mastoidectomy: surgical removal of infected mastoid air cells, bone, and pus; radical mastoidectomy involves removal of middle ear structures such as incus and malleus as well as diseased tissue (conductive hearing loss then occurs unless reconstructive surgery is done as well)
   4. Tympanoplasty: surgical reconstruction of ossicles and tympanic membrane of the middle ear to help restore hearing

F. Evaluation: resolution of signs and symptoms of infection

> ▶ *Practice to Pass*
>
> A client is being discharged to home following myringotomy. What would you include in postoperative discharge teaching?

XVI. OTOSCLEROSIS

A. Description: hereditary disorder of labyrinthine capsule in which abnormal bone growth occurs around ossicles and causes fixation of stapes, leading to conductive hearing loss

B. Etiology and pathophysiology
   1. Is an autosomal dominant hereditary disorder most common in Caucasians and females; onset is in adolescence or early adulthood; pregnancy exacerbates condition
   2. Stapes do not vibrate as easily due to stiffening, thus reducing sound transmission to inner ear

C. Assessment
   1. Bilateral conductive hearing loss that is progressive and asymmetrical, tinnitus, possible retention of bone conduction (so client has difficulty in ordinary conversation but can use telephone adequately)
   2. Reddish or pinkish-orange tympanic membrane from increased vascularity (Schwartz's sign)
   3. Rinne test results: bone sound conduction equal to or longer than air conduction (abnormal finding) if hearing loss greater than 25 decibels (dB)
   4. Weber test results: lateralization to ear with greater conductive hearing loss

D. Priority nursing problems: pain, altered auditory perception, potential for injury or falls, possible interference with communication or socialization

E. Planning and implementation
   1. Encourage use of hearing aid(s) to augment sound

2. Administer sodium fluoride as ordered to slow bone resorption and overgrowth

3. Implement strategies to enhance communication with a hearing-impaired client
   a. Approach client from within client's line of vision or tap client lightly on shoulder to get attention before beginning to speak
   b. Reduce background noise, such as radio or TV, before beginning to speak
   c. Avoid covering mouth with hands or other objects while speaking
   d. Face client and speak slowly and clearly—pronounce words clearly without overarticulating them; speak using low pitch and normal loudness
   e. Use nonverbal cues and written messages to enhance communication
   f. Repeat sentences using different words if client has difficulty understanding
   g. Ask client to repeat directions or teaching that was done to ensure client's understanding
4. Surgical intervention
   a. Stapedectomy with fenestration: microsurgical removal of diseased stapes, with drill or laser, creation of a hole in footplate, followed by insertion of a steel or synthetic prosthesis to restore hearing
   b. Stapedotomy: insertion of a wire or platinum ribbon prosthesis into a small hole created in stapes footplate

F. **Client education**: referral to appropriate community agencies; postoperative care as outlined in Section VI

G. **Evaluation**: client uses alternate communication means as needed, indicates improved hearing postoperatively or with use of aids, does not suffer injury, and maintains social contacts

Practice to Pass

A client has just been given a diagnosis of otosclerosis. How would you explain the disorder? What communication strategies will you use?

XVII. MÉNIÈRE'S DISEASE

A. **Description**: **Ménière's disease** is an inner ear disorder with excessive accumulation of endolymphatic fluid in membranous labyrinth; also called idiopathic endolymphatic hydrops

B. **Etiology and pathophysiology**
   1. Unknown etiology, possibly heredity, viral influence, and immune dysfunction play a role; affects men and women equally; highest risk between ages 35–60 years
   2. Impaired reabsorption of endolymph leads to dilation of lymph channels, which causes symptoms

C. **Assessment and diagnostic findings**
   1. Recurrent severe attacks of vertigo accompanied by sense of fullness in ears, roaring or ringing tinnitus, nausea, headache, and gradual but progressive sensorineural hearing loss (often unilateral)
   2. Attacks may last minutes to hours with possible associated symptoms of hypotension, diaphoresis, and nystagmus
   3. Attacks may be triggered by increased sodium intake, vasoconstriction, premenstrual fluid retention, stress, or allergies, although sometimes no trigger is identified
   4. Diagnosis is by electronystagnography (including caloric testing), Rinne and Weber tests, x-ray, CT scan, evaluation of response to a test dose of an osmotic or loop diuretic

D. **Priority nursing problems**: potential for injury, alteration in sleep pattern, possible reduced auditory perception, anxiety

E. **Planning and implementation**
   1. Low-sodium diet and, if symptoms are severe, fluid restriction
   2. Avoid use of alcohol, caffeine, nicotine
   3. Bed rest to control vertigo; assist with ambulation for safety
   4. Medication therapy: atropine (to reduce parasympathetic response) or CNS depressant as an alternative to atropine, diuretics, antihistamines (if allergy present), antivertigo and antiemetic drugs

      5. Surgical procedures (postoperative care as per Section VI)

        a. Endolymphatic decompression: relieves pressure in labyrinth and creates shunt between membranous labyrinth and subarachnoid space for fluid drainage (preserves hearing in most cases, relieves vertigo in approximately 70% of cases, relieves tinnitus and sensations of ear fullness in 50% of cases)

        b. Vestibular neurectomy: severing of portion of eighth cranial nerve that controls balance and sensation of vertigo (relieves vertigo in up to 90% of cases)

        c. **Labyrinthectomy**: complete removal of labyrinth, destroying cochlear function, relieving vertigo but causing loss of any minimal remaining hearing as well ("last resort")

F. Client education

    1. Follow restrictions in sodium, fluid, nicotine, alcohol, and caffeine

    2. Take medications as prescribed

    3. Learn signs of an impending attack: fullness in affected ear, increasing tinnitus, headache; lie down in bed in a dark quiet room if at home when an attack begins, or pull off the road for safety if driving

    4. Avoid sudden movements or position changes; move head slowly, and do not get up unassisted during an attack

    5. Wear a MedicAlert bracelet or necklace to indicate the condition

    6. Learn stress reduction techniques of choice to help reduce severity of attacks

    7. If tinnitus persists between attacks, use white noise or ambient sound machine to mask tinnitus and promote sleep; consider use of medication most commonly effective—oral antidepressant nortriptyline (Pamelor) taken at bedtime

    8. Practice balance training exercises to help brain learn to compensate for damage to vestibular system; these consist of moving head up and down, side to side, and tilting head to the left and right; repeated 10 times each twice a day

G. Evaluation: client identifies how to prevent injury during an attack, complies with measures to reduce frequency of attacks, maintains normal sleep patterns and daily interactions with others

Case Study

A 65-year-old female client is scheduled for cataract surgery this morning. You are the nurse working in the ambulatory surgery center where the client's ophthalmic surgery will be performed.

1. What questions will you ask the client when she arrives prior to surgery?

2. What assessments will you make before the procedure begins?

3. What are the priorities of care for the client immediately after the procedure?

4. What discharge instructions will you give to the client?

5. When the client asks you about what to expect regarding vision changes after surgery, how would you respond?

For suggested responses, see page 626.

POSTTEST

1 The nurse is giving discharge instructions to a client who had a cataract removed a few hours earlier. Which instructions must the nurse include?

1. Report itching and redness.
2. Resume all preoperative activities.
3. Report visual changes immediately.
4. Creamy white discharge is a sign of infection.

2 A client is being admitted to the postanesthesia recovery area following cornea removal of the left eye following a chemical injury. Which intervention is appropriate during the immediate postoperative period?

1. Encourage deep breathing and coughing to prevent atelectasis.
2. Position client on the right side with the head of bed elevated 30 degrees.
3. Ask client to perform eye exercises to maintain eye mobility.
4. Position upright with the head and neck turned to the left.

3 A client who has developed impaired vision because of previously undiagnosed glaucoma asks the nurse if the lost vision will return. Which reply by the nurse is most accurate?

1. "Vision that is lost will not return, but adhering to therapy can help to maintain current vision."
2. "It will take at least 2 to 3 months for vision to return to baseline."
3. "It is difficult to answer that question with accuracy. Some clients experience return of vision, while others do not."
4. "Vision will return to normal within a week or so if intraocular pressure is reduced quickly."

4 A client is seen at the health care provider's office and diagnosed with a detached retina of the right eye. The nurse should place highest priority on doing which of the following?

1. Preparing for tonometry testing
2. Allowing client to get out of bed but keeping room darkened
3. Giving eye drops every hour and allowing bathroom privileges only
4. Positioning on the left side and patching both eyes

5 When planning care for a client who is legally blind, the nurse should take which action that is most important to ensure the client's safety?

1. Leave doors partially closed.
2. Orient client verbally and physically to the room.
3. Provide radio and television for stimulation.
4. Describe the weather and community events for client.

6 The nurse is caring for a 48-year-old client who has just been told that he is legally blind. Which of the following would be appropriate interventions for this client? Select all that apply.

1. Instructions regarding daytime driving only
2. Immobility to promote retinal repair
3. Home assessment prior to discharge
4. Psychological support
5. Provide referral to vocational rehabilitation

7 The nurse is providing instructions to a client who has been diagnosed with hearing impairment and has just received a hearing aid. The nurse would include which statement in discussion with the client?

1. "Immerse hearing aid daily in warm water for 15 minutes to clean it."
2. "Leave hearing aid on at all times to keep battery charged."
3. "Avoid use of aerosol sprays near the aid, because particles can clog the receiver."
4. "Adjust volume control to maximum setting for efficient use."

8 The nurse is caring for a client who had a myringotomy. Which activities that are safe should the nurse plan to teach the client after surgery?

1. Close mouth when coughing.
2. Change outer ear dressing as needed.
3. Turn or reposition self frequently.
4. Shampoo only unaffected side of head.

9 A 72-year-old client reports to the nurse during a health history that the healthcare provider previously diagnosed an age-related hearing loss. The nurse documents in the medical record that the client reports which disorder?

1. Otosclerosis
2. Méniére's disease
3. Presbycusis
4. Otalgia

10 The nurse would prioritize that which nursing diagnosis has highest priority for a client experiencing an attack of Méniére's disease?

1. Risk for Injury
2. Risk for Disturbed Sleep Pattern
3. Impaired Sensory Perception: Auditory
4. Risk for Ineffective Coping

➤ *See pages 562–564 for Answers and Rationales.*

ANSWERS & RATIONALES

Pretest

1 **Answer: 1** **Rationale:** Fluorescein is a dye that is used to visualize corneal damage from any type of trauma Tonometry measures the pressure in the eye to determine the presence of glaucoma. Gonioscopy and fundoscopy are also used for diagnosing glaucoma. **Cognitive Level:** Applying **Client Need:** Reduction of Risk Potential **Integrated Process:** Nursing Process: Assessment **Content Area:** Adult Health **Strategy:** Recognize that a diagnostic study that allows the practitioner to ascertain the type and amount of damage is indicated. **Reference:** LeMone, P., Burke, K. M., & Bauldoff, G. (2011). *Medical-surgical nursing: Critical thinking in patient care* (5th ed.). Upper Saddle River, NJ: Pearson Education, pp. 1587, 1593.

2 **Answer: 4** **Rationale:** Brimonidine is a direct-acting mydriatic eye drop. It works by dilating the pupil, reduce the production of aqueous humor, and increase its absorption, therefore lowering intraocular pressure. If the medication is absorbed, it can produce systemic side effects so pressure is placed on the inner canthus after administration to minimize systemic absorption. Immediately following instillation, the client can experience blurred vision for 1–2 hours. **Cognitive Level:** Applying **Client Need:** Pharmacological and Parenteral Therapies **Integrated Process:** Nursing Process: Planning **Content Area:** Adult Health **Strategy:** Recall information about the pathophysiology of glaucoma, the mechanism of action for medications used to treat glaucoma, and side effects in order to answer this question. In addition, visualize the correct

procedure for instilling eye drops. **Reference:** LeMone, P., Burke, K. M., & Bauldoff, G. (2011). *Medical-surgical nursing: Critical thinking in patient care* (5th ed.). Upper Saddle River, NJ: Pearson Education, pp. 1593–1595.

3 **Answer: 3** **Rationale:** It is important to share with the client that lifelong medication therapy is needed to preserve vision. Glaucoma involves a gradual loss of peripheral fields that the patient is often unaware of. Education on this visual field loss is important to help improve adherence to therapy. Increased intraocular pressure does not respond to a decrease in fluid intake. Glaucoma is typically diagnosed through a routine comprehensive vision examination. **Cognitive Level:** Analyzing **Client Need:** Health Promotion and Maintenance **Integrated Process:** Nursing Process: Implementation **Content Area:** Adult Health **Strategy:** To answer this question, you need to understand what glaucoma is and then eliminate any answer choice that is unrelated. **Reference:** LeMone, P., Burke, K. M., & Bauldoff, G. (2011). *Medical-surgical nursing: Critical thinking in patient care* (5th ed.). Upper Saddle River, NJ: Pearson Education, p. 1592.

4 **Answer: 2** **Rationale:** A cloudy-appearing lens is characteristic of cataract development. Early symptoms of cataract formation include blurred vision and a loss of ability to see colors. Seeing bright flashes of light across the field of vision characterizes detached retina. Night blindness, particularly from childhood, characterizes retinitis pigmentosa. Photophobia characterizes chalazion and inflammation of the sebaceous gland of the eye. **Cognitive Level:** Analyzing **Client Need:** Physiological Adaptation **Integrated Process:** Nursing Process: Assessment

Content Area: Adult Health **Strategy:** Between the age and description, the conclusion of a cataract should be evident. Then compare the distracters to the effects of cataracts on vision. **Reference:** LeMone, P., Burke, K. M., & Bauldoff, G. (2011). *Medical-surgical nursing: Critical thinking in patient care* (5th ed.). Upper Saddle River, NJ: Pearson Education, pp. 1585–1586, 1589, 1600–1602.

5 **Answer: 1** **Rationale:** The client has adequate central vision and objects directly in front of him can be seen adequately. Glaucoma causes loss of peripheral vision. Clients who see shadows are more inclined to benefit from direct light over an area. An unobstructed pathway is important for all clients to prevent injury but does not help specifically compensate for the client's visual changes. **Cognitive Level:** Applying **Client Need:** Safety and Infection Control **Integrated Process:** Nursing Process: Implementation **Content Area:** Adult Health **Strategy:** Each eye disorder affects vision in a different way. Understanding the type of vision loss seen in glaucoma enables the nurse to provide care that can compensate for the specific loss. **Reference:** LeMone, P., Burke, K. M., & Bauldoff, G. (2011). *Medical-surgical nursing: Critical thinking in patient care* (5th ed.). Upper Saddle River, NJ: Pearson Education, p. 1592.

6 **Answer: 4** **Rationale:** It is essential to determine that the tympanic membrane is intact before completing an otic irrigation. If a perforation is present sterile technique must be used. No more than 50 to 70 mL of solution should be drawn up at one time, and the fluid should be at body temperature. The client may be positioned wherever it is comfortable and needs only a receptacle to hold the drainage and a waterproof pad to protect clothing. **Cognitive Level:** Applying **Client Need:** Physiological Adaptation **Integrated Process:** Nursing Process: Implementation **Content Area:** Adult Health **Strategy:** Note the terms *otic* and *cerumen*. Recall normal ear anatomy to determine the correct procedure that will minimize damage to the ear. **Reference:** Berman, A. J., & Snyder, S. (2011). *Kozier and Erb's fundamentals of nursing: Concepts, process, and practice* (9th ed.). Upper Saddle River, NJ: Pearson Education, pp. 906–908.

7 **Answer: 3** **Rationale:** Ear pain is a primary or classic symptom associated with otitis media. Pus is usually located behind the tympanic membrane and drainage occurs if the membrane ruptures. Loss of balance occurs with Méniére's disease or inner ear disorders. Otitis media is a disorder of the middle ear. Tinnitus occurs with labyrinthitis and other inner ear disorders. **Cognitive Level:** Analyzing **Client Need:** Physiological Adaptation **Integrated Process:** Nursing Process: Evaluation **Content Area:** Adult Health **Strategy:** The core issue of the question is the ability to differentiate the symptoms of middle ear infections from inner or outer ear infections. Recall basic physiology and use the process of elimination to make a selection. **Reference:** LeMone, P., Burke, K. M., & Bauldoff, G. (2011). *Medical-surgical nursing: Critical thinking in patient care* (5th ed.). Upper Saddle River, NJ: Pearson Education, pp. 1606–1611.

8 **Answer: 2, 3, 5** **Rationale:** Clients should be taught to wash hands and use aseptic technique prior to administering eye drops to prevent transmission of organisms to the eye. Eye drops should be instilled into the lower conjunctiva where there is a capillary bed that can absorb the medication. Because pilocarpine contains epinephrine, pupillary constriction usually occurs rather than dilation. **Cognitive Level:** Applying **Client Need:** Pharmacological and Parenteral Therapies **Integrated Process:** Nursing Process: Implementation **Content Area:** Adult Health **Strategy:** Visualize the procedure for administering eye drops to make the correct selections, and recall that pupil dilation is contraindicated in glaucoma to help you choose correctly. **Reference:** Smith, S. F., Duell, D. J., & Martin, B. C. (2012). *Clinical nursing skills: Basic to advanced skills* (8th ed.). Upper Saddle River, NJ: Pearson Education, pp. 593–594.

9 **Answer: 4, 1, 3, 2, 5** **Rationale:** The client is first positioned in a manner that allows easy access and visualization of the ear. Starting with the ear to be treated upward decreases the amount of movement required by the client. After positioning the client, the nurse cleans the pinna and meatus of the ear. Cleaning prior to administering the medication decreases the risk of flushing an external infection or debris to the inside of the auditory canal. The pinna is then pulled up and back in order to straighten the ear canal. The medication is administered. Pressure is applied to the tragus to assist the flow of medication into the ear canal. **Cognitive Level:** Applying **Client Need:** Pharmacological and Parenteral Therapies **Integrated Process:** Nursing Process: Implementation **Content Area:** Adult Health **Strategy:** Picture the steps of the procedure. **Reference:** Berman, A. J., & Snyder, S. (2011). *Kozier and Erb's fundamentals of nursing: Concepts, process, and practice* (9th ed.). Upper Saddle River, NJ: Pearson Education, pp. 907–908.

10 **Answer: 4** **Rationale:** The client with Méniére's disease should limit intake of salty foods and possibly concentrated sugars that could cause an increase in endolymphatic fluid in the inner ear. The other foods listed pose no problem. **Cognitive Level:** Applying **Client Need:** Physiological Adaptation **Integrated Process:** Nursing Process: Evaluation **Content Area:** Adult Health **Strategy:** An understanding of the pathophysiology of Méniére's disease is needed to determine the correct response as well as an identification of high-sodium foods. **Reference:** LeMone, P., Burke, K. M., & Bauldoff, G. (2011). *Medical-surgical nursing: Critical thinking in patient care* (5th ed.). Upper Saddle River, NJ: Pearson Education, pp. 1611–1613.

Posttest

1 **Answer: 3** **Rationale:** Itching and redness are a normal response to cataract removal and will respond to mild analgesics or cool compresses. Any activities that increase intraocular pressure should be avoided. Visual changes could occur if there is bleeding into the eye and must be reported immediately. Creamy drainage is normal; yellow drainage represents an infection. **Cognitive Level:** Applying **Client Need:** Reduction of Risk Potential **Integrated Process:** Teaching and Learning **Content Area:** Adult Health **Strategy:** Eliminate options that are normal findings. Eliminate false statements. Select the option that indicates that there is a complication that could affect the client's vision. **Reference:** LeMone, P., Burke, K. M., & Bauldoff, G. (2011). *Medical-surgical nursing: Critical thinking in patient care* (5th ed., Vol. Single). Upper Saddle River, NJ: Pearson Education, pp. 1585, 1591.

2 **Answer: 2 Rationale:** Any activities that increase intraocular pressure must be avoided after eye surgery. Following eye surgery, the head of bed should be elevated 30 to 45 degrees and the client should lie on back or unaffected side to reduce intraocular pressure. The eye is covered following lens removal to minimize eye movement, and eye exercises are not ordered. **Cognitive Level:** Applying **Client Need:** Reduction of Risk Potential **Integrated Process:** Nursing Process: Implementation **Content Area:** Adult Health **Strategy:** The principle being tested is that clients with eye surgery must avoid activities that increase intraocular pressure. Select the answer choice that is consistent with this principle. **Reference:** LeMone, P., Burke, K. M., & Bauldoff, G. (2011). *Medical-surgical nursing: Critical thinking in patient care* (5th ed., Vol. Single). Upper Saddle River, NJ: Pearson Education, p. 1585.

3 **Answer: 1 Rationale:** Glaucoma is characterized by a gradual loss of vision that is irreversible because of the effects of increased intraocular pressure on the optic neurons. Compliance with medication therapy is important to preserve the current level of vision, although vision that is lost cannot be regained. **Cognitive Level:** Analyzing **Client Need:** Physiological Adaptation **Integrated Process:** Communication and Documentation **Content Area:** Adult Health **Strategy:** Recall glaucoma causes irreversible loss of vision. Select the answer choice that is consistent with this fact. **Reference:** LeMone, P., Burke, K. M., & Bauldoff, G. (2011). *Medical-surgical nursing: Critical thinking in patient care* (5th ed., Vol. Single). Upper Saddle River, NJ: Pearson Education, pp. 1591–1592.

4 **Answer: 4 Rationale:** The client with a detached retina should have activity restricted with eyes patched to reduce eye movement and prevent worsening of the detachment. Tonometry testing is done to measure the intraocular pressure of a client's eye, it is inappropriate for a client with a detached retina. Eye drops are not necessary. **Cognitive Level:** Analyzing **Client Need:** Physiological Adaptation **Integrated Process:** Nursing Process: Planning **Content Area:** Adult Health **Strategy:** The principle being tested is that eye movement can cause further damage to the eye. Select the answer choice that minimizes eye movement. **Reference:** LeMone, P., Burke, K. M., & Bauldoff, G. (2011). *Medical-surgical nursing: Critical thinking in patient care* (5th ed., Vol. Single). Upper Saddle River, NJ: Pearson Education, pp. 1600–1602.

5 **Answer: 2 Rationale:** The nurse should orient the client to the room for safety, using both words and a physical walking tour for best effect. Sensory input and conversation assists with orientation, not directly with safety. Leaving doors partially closed is hazardous because the client could inadvertently walk into the door during ambulation. Pathways should be free of obstacles. **Cognitive Level:** Analyzing **Client Need:** Safety and Infection Control **Integrated Process:** Nursing Process: Planning **Content Area:** Adult Health **Strategy:** The goal is to enable the client to remain independent despite being legally blind. Select the answer choice that is consistent with this goal and simultaneously prevents injury to the client. **Reference:** LeMone, P., Burke, K. M., & Bauldoff, G. (2011). *Medical-surgical nursing: Critical thinking in patient care* (5th ed., Vol. Single). Upper Saddle River, NJ: Pearson Education, pp. 1596–1597.

6 **Answer: 3, 4, 5 Rationale:** Legal blindness prohibits any driving. Immobility is appropriate for an acute retinal detachment. A client with legal blindness will not benefit from immobility. Clients who are legally blind are capable of living alone, but the home must be assessed and appropriate accommodations made to minimize injury. Newly diagnosed clients must be supported as they grieve for the loss of certain aspects of their life and adjust to the changes that will be required. People who are blind can receive mobility training, assistance with relearning self-care activities, education in the use of Braille to communicate, and vocational and other forms of rehabilitation **Cognitive Level:** Applying **Client Need:** Safety and Infection Control **Integrated Process:** Nursing Process: Implementation **Content Area:** Adult Health **Strategy:** Select the answer choices that would help the client to adapt to his diagnosis and still maintain his independence. **Reference:** LeMone, P., Burke, K. M., & Bauldoff, G. (2011). *Medical-surgical nursing: Critical thinking in patient care* (5th ed., Vol. Single). Upper Saddle River, NJ: Pearson Education, p. 1578.

7 **Answer: 3 Rationale:** The client should avoid the use of aerosol sprays, cosmetics, or other hair or facial products near the hearing aid. The aid should not get excessively wet. The hearing aid should be turned off when not in use and should be maintained on the lowest setting that is comfortable and effective. **Cognitive Level:** Applying **Client Need:** Health Promotion and Maintenance **Integrated Process:** Nursing Process: Implementation **Content Area:** Adult Health **Strategy:** This question asks for identification of the answer choice representing correct care of a hearing aid. Use information about this assistive device and the process of elimination to make a selection. **Reference:** Berman, A. J., & Snyder, S. (2011). *Kozier and Erb's fundamentals of nursing: Concepts, process, and practice* (9th ed.). Upper Saddle River, NJ: Pearson Education, pp. 793–795.

8 **Answer: 2 Rationale:** Following ear surgery, clients should avoid activities that could result in increased pressure in the middle ear. These include blowing the nose, sneezing, coughing, or doing any activities that involve holding the breath or bearing down. If it is necessary to cough, the client should keep the mouth open. The outer ear dressing can be changed as needed to keep clean and dry. The inner ear dressing should not be removed until advised to do so by the physician. Turning or repositioning should be minimized to avoid disruption to equilibrium. The client should avoid activities that might result in water in the ear canals. **Cognitive Level:** Applying **Client Need:** Reduction of Risk Potential **Integrated Process:** Nursing Process: Planning **Content Area:** Adult Health **Strategy:** Recall what a myringotomy is and how and why it is done to select the correct answer choice. Recall how important it is to avoid activities that could result in increased intracranial pressure that can be transmitted to the area behind the tympanic membrane. **Reference:** LeMone, P., Burke, K. M., & Bauldoff, G. (2011). *Medical-surgical nursing: Critical thinking in patient care* (5th ed., Vol. Single). Upper Saddle River, NJ: Pearson Education, pp. 1607–1609.

9 **Answer: 3 Rationale:** Presbycusis is an age-related decline in hearing. Otosclerosis is a familial disorder characterized by hearing loss. Méniére's disease is a disorder of the inner ear that results in vertigo. Otalgia is an earache. **Cognitive Level:** Applying **Client Need:** Physiological Adaptation **Integrated Process:** Nursing Process: Assessment **Content Area:** Adult Health **Strategy:** Recall general information about each of the disorders listed in the options. Select the one that is most likely related directly to advancing age. **Reference:** LeMone, P., Burke, K., & Bauldoff, G. (2011). *Medical-surgical nursing: Critical thinking in patient care* (5th ed.). Upper Saddle River, NJ: Pearson Education, pp. 1610–1611, 1614.

10 **Answer: 1 Rationale:** Méniére's disease is characterized by bouts of vertigo, which place the client at risk for falls and injury. The client may have manifestations of the other nursing diagnoses as well, but the highest priority is on preventing injury. **Cognitive Level:** Analyzing **Client Need:** Physiological Adaptation **Integrated Process:** Nursing Process: Planning **Content Area:** Adult Health **Strategy:** The correct answer choice directly relates to the primary disturbance of Méniére's. **Reference:** LeMone, P., Burke, K. M., & Bauldoff, G. (2011). *Medical-surgical nursing: Critical thinking in patient care*. Upper Saddle River, NJ: Pearson Education, pp. 1612–1613.

References

Berman, A., & Snyder, S. (2012). *Kozier & Erb's fundamentals of nursing: Concepts, process, and practice* (9th ed.). Upper Saddle River, NJ: Pearson Education.

D'Amico, D., & Barbarito, C. (2012). *Health & physical assessment in nursing* (2nd ed.). Upper Saddle River, NJ: Pearson Education, Inc.

Ignatavicius, D. D., & Workman, M. L. (2013). *Medical-surgical nursing: Critical thinking for collaborative care* (7th ed.). Philadelphia: W. B. Saunders Company.

Kee, J. L. (2010). *Laboratory and diagnostic tests* (8th ed.). Upper Saddle River, NJ: Pearson Education.

Lehne, R. (2010). *Pharmacology for nursing care* (7th ed.). St. Louis, MO: Saunders.

LeMone, P., Burke, K., & Bauldoff, G. (2011). *Medical-surgical nursing: Critical thinking in patient care* (5th ed.). Upper Saddle River, NJ: Pearson Education.

Lewis, S., Dirksen, S., Heitkemper, M., Bucher, L., & Camera, I. (2011). *Medical surgical nursing: Assessment and management of clinical problems* (8th ed.). St. Louis, MO: Elsevier.

McCance, K. L., & Huether, S. E. (2010). *Pathophysiology: The biologic basis for disease in adults and children* (6th ed.). St. Louis, MO: Mosby, Inc.

Osborn, K. S., Wraa, C. E., & Watson, A. (2010). *Medical surgical nursing: Preparation for practice* (Vol. Combined). Upper Saddle River, NJ: Pearson Education.

Smith, S. F., Duell, D. J., & Martin, B. C. (2012). *Clinical nursing skills: Basic to advanced skills* (8th ed.). Upper Saddle River, NJ: Pearson Education.

Common Problems Encountered in Emergency and Critical Care Nursing

17

Chapter Outline

Objectives

- ➤ Describe the pathophysiology and etiology of common problems seen in emergency and critical care settings.
- ➤ Discuss expected assessment data and diagnostic findings for common problems seen in emergency and critical care settings.
- ➤ Identify priority nursing problems commonly encountered in emergency and critical care settings.
- ➤ Discuss therapeutic management of common problems seen in emergency and critical care settings.
- ➤ Discuss nursing management of common problems seen in emergency and critical care settings.
- ➤ Identify expected outcomes for common problems seen in emergency and critical care settings.

NCLEX-RN® Test Prep

Use the accompanying online resource, NursingReviewsandRationales, to test yourself with hundreds of NCLEX®-style practice questions.

Review at a Glance

asphyxiation effects of decreased amount of oxygen and increased carbon dioxide in body tissues and blood

autotransfusion therapeutic method of transfusing client's own shed and filtered blood back to client

cardiac index (CI) a measurement of cardiac performance that considers client's body surface area; is equal to cardiac output divided by body surface area

defibrillation asynchronous external application of electrical charge to depolarize myocardial cells, terminating abnormal cardiac activity to reestablish a normal rhythm

dysrhythmia abnormal cardiac activity

emergent immediate care required; condition presents a threat to life or limb

Glascow Coma Scale assessment tool that evaluates client's level of consciousness through eye opening, best motor response, and best verbal response

morbidity illness

mortality death

non-urgent routine care is required; may delay care for a period of time

phlebostatic axis point where fourth intercostal space and midaxillary line meet; serves as reference point for right atrium

primary assessment assessment of airway, breathing, circulation, and brief neurological status

secondary assessment a head-to-toe assessment of client to identify all injuries

triage method of determination of priority of clients cared for in emergency care

PRETEST

1 The client has severe continuous bleeding from a self-inflicted wrist laceration. While applying direct pressure to the area with a dry, sterile dressing, what should be the nurse's next action?

1. Call for a psychiatric evaluation since this was a self-inflicted injury.
2. Apply ice to lower the body temperature to slow circulation.
3. Lower the extremity to below heart level.
4. Assess for signs of shock.

2 The nurse suspects that the client has developed a tension pneumothorax. Which of the following assessment findings would support this conclusion?

1. Decreased tidal volume and normal respiratory rate
2. Hypertension
3. Cough productive of frothy, pink mucus
4. Mediastinal shift toward uninjured side

3 A client is exhibiting signs of an allergic reaction to a bee sting. Which of the following symptoms would the nurse anticipate being present?

1. Pulsus paradoxus
2. Prolonged expiratory phase
3. Petechiae
4. Distant heart sounds

4 The nurse is preparing to suction a client on a ventilator who desaturates easily. In what sequence should the nurse perform the following actions? Place the choices in order from first to fifth.

1. Hyperoxygenate the client.
2. Monitor for adverse effects.
3. Assess lung sounds.
4. Insert suction catheter.
5. Apply suction.

5 Which clients should the nurse monitor closely for manifestations of multiple organ dysfunction syndrome (MODS)? Select all that apply.

1. Client with sepsis
2. Client with a gastrointestinal bleed
3. Client with acute respiratory failure
4. Client with diabetic ketoacidosis
5. Client with a basilar skull injury

6 A nurse caring for a client with a human bite to the hand anticipates that the health care provider will prescribe which of the following therapies?

1. Antibiotics to prevent infection from oral bacteria
2. Application of a tourniquet to prevent the spread of the microorganisms
3. Administration of antivenom
4. A pressure dressing to control swelling and pain

7 The client is being weaned from a ventilator. Arterial blood gases drawn prior to extubation reveal pH 7.32; PaO_2 90 mmHg; $PaCO_2$ 56 mmHg; HCO_3^- 26 mEq/L. What acid–base imbalance is reflected by these results?

1. Metabolic alkalosis
2. Respiratory alkalosis
3. Respiratory acidosis
4. Metabolic acidosis

8 A nurse in the triage area of the emergency unit would prioritize and assist in the treatment of which client first?

1. A client with unifocal premature ventricular contractions
2. A client who has developed pulseless ventricular tachycardia and is nonresponsive
3. A client with a severe frostbite injury to the foot
4. A client who has just undergone escharotomy to the arm

9 The nurse is walking past a client's room and hears a visitor calling for help. Upon entering the room, the client is noted to be choking. What should be the nurse's first action?

1. Call a code.
2. Ask him if he can speak.
3. Begin cardiopulmonary resuscitation (CPR).
4. Perform the Heimlich maneuver.

10 The health care provider performs a pericardiocentesis for a client diagnosed with acute pericardial tamponade. If the procedure is ineffective, the nurse should expect the return of which symptoms? Select all that apply.

1. Muffled heart sounds
2. Decrease in blood pressure
3. A sudden drop in heart rate
4. Inspiratory crackles
5. Jugular venous distention

➤ *See pages 607–608 for Answers and Rationales*

I. INTRODUCTION TO EMERGENCY NURSING

A. Emergency nursing

1. The practice of providing *episodic* (as needed), primary, critical, and acute nursing care to clients of all ages who experience physical, emotional, or psychological health alterations; care may be given in a variety of practice settings and ranges from minimal intervention to life support

2. The emergency nurse can become certified in emergency nursing (CEN) by passing a certification exams offered through Board of Certification for Emergency Nursing

3. Emergency nursing requires a broad knowledge of pathophysiology of diverse disease processes, disease and injury prevention, life-saving measures, cultural characteristics, legal and ethical issues, mental health issues, and age-specific health care requirements

B. Care of client presenting to an emergency department

1. **Triage**: classification of all clients for purpose of prioritizing treatment

   a. Is used to promptly identify clients requiring immediate, life-saving treatment and those who would receive more efficient and effective care in a less acute area (outpatient clinic or fast track area)

   b. Triaging is done using a set of guidelines prioritizing into level I to level IV based on client's medical need, mental health status, and psychosocial needs; priority is given to client with airway dysfunction unless there is a disaster requiring other priority

   c. Triage requires a brief, thorough interview and assessment of client's reason for presenting to emergency department (ED), determination of acuity, and initiation of care; also begins process of identifying emotional and psychosocial needs of client and family

   d. Triage rating systems frequently include 3 categories:

      1) **Emergent**: conditions requiring immediate care and intervention because of increased risk of **mortality** (death) or threat to life, limb, or vision; examples include major burns, cardiac arrest, chest pain, respiratory distress, major blunt or penetrating trauma, hemorrhage, or ectopic pregnancy

      2) *Urgent*: conditions that require care generally within 1 hour because condition may lead to deterioration of health if not treated as soon as possible; clients will have stable vital signs but have acute illness and must be treated to prevent increased **morbidity** (illness); examples include fever (including rectal temperature greater than 101°F in an infant less than 3 months old), abdominal pain, stable fractures, headache, lacerations with controlled bleeding, or dehydration

3) Non-urgent: conditions requiring routine care that can be delayed safely for more than 2 hours without client deterioration; clients with non-urgent conditions often use ED because they don't have a primary care provider; examples of non-urgent conditions include colds, sore throat, toothache, rashes, or abrasions

2. Disaster management plan: a community-wide, hospital-wide, or ED plan to handle mass casualty incidents that may occur at any time
   a. Involves coordinated planning of how each unit will respond to a disaster occurrence, care of victims following disaster, and recovery of victims and staff after incident
   b. Requires planning, mock drills, and refinement of plan for optimal preparedness

C. **Assessment of client presenting to ED**
   1. **Primary assessment**: rapid initial assessment of presenting symptoms to determine presence of life-threatening conditions while simultaneously intervening
      a. <u>A</u> = Airway with C-spine (cervical spine) immobilization
         1) Assess and maintain a patent airway; assessment includes determining ability to speak, checking for foreign body in airway, and evaluating chest expansion
         2) If airway appears compromised, observe for possible causes such as foreign body (tongue, teeth, dentures, food, vomitus), airway or facial trauma, edema of face, neck, or trachea, or smoke inhalation as appropriate
         3) Possible interventions to maintain a patent airway include chin lift or jaw thrust maneuvers, suctioning, oropharyngeal or nasotracheal intubation, cricothyrotomy or tracheostomy
         4) During this evaluation and all interventions, C-spine must remain in an anatomically neutral position and may be immobilized with cervical collar or manually stabilized to prevent morbidity due to possible spinal cord injury
      b. <u>B</u> = Breathing
         1) Assess effectiveness of breathing and ventilation ability
         2) Normal findings are spontaneous, unlabored respirations with full bilateral equal chest expansion and bilateral breath sounds
         3) Abnormal findings are apnea; weak, shallow, or labored respirations; diminished or absent breath sounds; unequal chest expansion; retractions or paroxysmal chest wall movement; tracheal deviation; distended neck veins; open chest wound or signs of chest trauma; and subcutaneous emphysema
         4) Possible interventions for ineffective breathing pattern include application of supplemental oxygen (O_2) by face mask or bag-valve-mask device (Ambu bag), assisting with intubation or chest tube insertion, covering of open chest wound with a 3-sided occlusive dressing, and use of a pressure dressing on a flail segment of ribs
      c. <u>C</u> = Circulation and controlled hemorrhage
         1) Assess for adequate circulation to maintain cellular tissue perfusion; signs of adequate perfusion include full, regular, and normal pulse rate; pink, warm, and dry skin with capillary refill less than 3 seconds; absent external uncontrolled bleeding; and ability to respond appropriately
         2) Indications of decreased circulation include bradycardia or tachycardia; hypotension; cool, pale and diaphoretic skin, obvious uncontrolled external bleeding; or decreased level of consciousness (LOC)
         3) Signs of hypovolemia, pericardial tamponade, or cardiac arrest indicate that an immediate life-threatening condition exists
         4) Possible interventions to enhance circulation include direct pressure to control external bleeding; insertion of large bore intravenous (IV) access device; fluid volume replacement with normal saline (NS), blood or blood products;

cardiopulmonary resuscitation (CPR), pericardiocentesis (aspiration of blood from pericardial sac); or **autotransfusion** (transfusion of one's own blood)

  d. <u>D</u> = Disability

  1) Complete a brief neurological assessment to determine baseline functioning, potential life-threatening complications, and LOC

  2) Glasgow Coma Scale assesses arousal component of responsiveness; it measures eye opening, best verbal response, and best motor response; minimum score is 3 and maximum score is 15

  3) Normal findings include client is alert and responding appropriately to questioning; pupils are equal and reactive to light; and appropriate motor and sensory functioning

  4) A client who is unresponsive, demonstrates decreased LOC, loss of sensory motor function, pupillary response abnormalities, or fixed pupils has possible neurological dysfunction; these findings require more extensive assessment during secondary assessment and require added attention to maintaining a patent airway

  e. <u>E</u> = Expose: remove all clothing to facilitate a thorough complete secondary assessment examination

2. Secondary assessment: a brief systematic head-to-toe assessment that identifies all injuries; maintain C-spine immobilization; assessment of hemodynamic and oxygenation status continues

  a. <u>F</u> = Fahrenheit: provide measures to prevent body heat loss through use of warmed IV fluids, warmed blankets, or heating lamps

  b. <u>G</u> = Get vital signs (VS): obtain a full set of VS (with rectal temperature if possible); use other assessment aids such as cardiac monitor, pulse oximeter, urinary catheter, and nasogastric (NG) tube; laboratory studies can be drawn (often include complete blood count [CBC], electrolytes, coagulation studies including fibrin degradation products [FDP], amylase, lactate, hepatic and renal studies, arterial blood gases [ABGs], urinalysis, blood type and cross-match, and occasionally toxicology studies)

  c. <u>H</u> = History and head-to-toe assessment: obtain from client, family, or pre-hospital care provider a thorough history of mechanism of injury, client presentation at time of injury, pre-hospital VS and treatment, and past medical history, allergies, and medications; then complete a detailed head-to-toe assessment to assess for all injuries

  1) Head and face: bleeding, deformities, ecchymosis, wounds, drainage from ears, eyes, or nose, and eyes for pupil size, reaction to light, accommodation, and extraocular movement; palpate head and face for bony deformities, tenderness, crepitus, or swelling

  2) Neck: if post injury and neck is immobilized carefully remove anterior portion of cervical collar while another team member maintains C-spine stabilization; inspect neck for wounds, bleeding, swelling, or tracheal deviation; palpate neck for pain, tenderness, and crepitus; auscultate carotid arteries for bruits

  3) Chest: breathing pattern, depth, chest symmetry, ecchymosis, wounds, paradoxical movement, or use of accessory muscles; palpate for tenderness, bony crepitus or deformities, or subcutaneous emphysema; auscultate breath and heart sounds

  4) Abdomen and flanks: wounds, bleeding, distention, ecchymosis, or scars; auscultate bowel sounds and vessels for bruits and pulses; palpate in all 4 quadrants and costovertebral angle (CVA) for tenderness, guarding, masses

  5) Pelvis and perineum: wounds, deformities, ecchymosis, blood at urinary meatus or perineum, or priapism (erection of penis that often accompanies spinal cord injury); palpate pelvis for tenderness, stability, or fractures; assess sphincter tone

6) Extremities: wounds, bleeding, deformities, and movement; palpate for pulses, temperature, sensation, tenderness, deformities, or bony crepitus

7) Posterior surfaces: while maintaining C-spine stabilization, logroll client to inspect back for wounds, bleeding, ecchymosis, or deformities; palpate for tenderness or deformities

II. COMMON PROBLEMS SEEN IN EMERGENCY SETTINGS

A. Airway obstruction

1. Description: partial or complete obstruction of airway

2. Etiology and pathophysiology

   a. Facial and neck trauma can cause foreign bodies such as teeth, tongue, or vomitus to block airway

   b. Mechanical obstruction can also occur from loss of structural support or narrowing of airway from accumulation of fluid or blood in airway tissues

   c. Allergic reactions, infection, exposure to chemical irritants, or burns can cause bronchospasm, laryngospasm, and laryngeal edema

   d. Medical and neurological conditions such as stroke, seizures, drug or alcohol intoxication, or mental retardation can predispose client to airway obstruction

3. Assessment

   a. Clinical manifestations depend on etiology of obstruction

   1) Airway obstruction: inability to speak, breathe, or cough

   2) Partial obstruction: stridor, wheezing, choking, gagging, or drooling

   3) Late manifestations: cyanosis, shortness of breath, altered mental status, bradycardia, hypotension, and cardiopulmonary arrest

   4) Diminished or absent breath sounds or adventitious breath sounds may be present as a result of decreased airflow into lungs

   b. Diagnostic and laboratory tests

   1) Neck x-rays: altered tissue densities or foreign body in airway

   2) ABGs: respiratory acidosis in later stages of airway obstruction; rarely used

4. Therapeutic management

   a. Allow conscious clients with partial airway obstruction to attempt to clear their own airway

   b. Clients may require suctioning assistance to remove foreign bodies such as blood or vomitus as a result of trauma; use care when suctioning with a hard suction catheter to avoid further airway obstruction or stimulating vomiting

   c. Unconscious clients with partial or complete airway obstruction must receive immediate life-saving measures; perform chin-lift or jaw-thrust maneuver; if airway remains obstructed, ET intubation, cricothyrotomy, or tracheostomy must be performed (remember to remove dentures)

5. Priority nursing problems: impairment of airway, alteration in respiratory pattern, fear

6. Planning and implementation

   a. Goal of care for client with ineffective airway clearance is to maintain airway patency

   b. Monitor respiratory pattern, rate, and detect signs of further airway obstruction (stridor, hoarseness, cough, increased edema or swelling); keep suction equipment available to remove blood, vomitus, or foreign bodies

   c. Maintain C-spine immobilization until x-rays rule out cervical fractures

   d. Provide emotional support and provide alternative communication methods if ET intubation is required

   e. Supplemental humidified O_2 will also be used

   f. Assist with treatment of underlying cause of airway obstruction

7. Medication therapy: possible antibiotics if edema is caused by bacterial infection; bronchodilators may reduce bronchospasm; possible sedatives and muscle relaxants for ET intubation and mechanical ventilation

8. Client education
   a. Ways to prevent specific cause of airway obstruction
   b. Treatment procedures (explain to client and family to allay anxiety)

9. Evaluation: client maintains a patent airway with adequate oxygenation and ventilation; O_2 saturation is greater than 90%; breathing pattern is regular and unlabored; ABGs and VS are appropriate for client

B. Tension pneumothorax

1. Description: occurs when air enters pleural space through a tear during inspiration and accumulates because it cannot escape during expiration

2. Etiology and pathophysiology
   a. Can be caused by blunt or penetrating trauma, fractured ribs that penetrate pleura, barotrauma, injury to tracheobronchial tree, infection, ruptured bleb or positive-pressure mechanical ventilation
   b. Increased intrathoracic pressure is caused by a "one-way valve effect" that leads to hyperinflation, lung collapse on injured side, increased mediastinal pressure and shift towards uninjured side
   c. Mediastinal shift causes compression of vena cava, decreased cardiac output (CO) and a potentially life-threatening condition due to circulatory failure if not corrected

3. Assessment
   a. Clinical manifestations: labored respirations, dyspnea, tachypnea, hypoxia, decreased or absent breath sounds on side of injury, tracheal deviation away from injured side, distended neck veins caused by impeded return of blood to heart, and decreased CO
   b. Diagnostic and laboratory findings: usually diagnosed by clinical manifestations and mechanism of injury; an upright posterior-anterior (PA) chest film will confirm diagnosis, but upright films should not be done unless spine is without injury

4. Therapeutic management: administer high-flow O_2 and prepare for a needle thoracostomy or chest tube placement; a needle thoracostomy involves insertion of a large bore (16- or 18-gauge) needle above third rib in mid-clavicular line to allow for release of pressure; a chest tube of appropriate size for client may also be placed using sterile technique and attached to water seal drainage

5. Priority nursing problems: alterations in respiratory pattern or gas exchange, reduced cardiac output, risk for hemodynamic instability

6. Planning and implementation
   a. Goals: respiratory rate (RR) is 12–20 breaths/min, ABGs are within normal parameters, and client remains hemodynamically stable
   b. Administer supplemental O_2, assist with chest tube insertion or needle thoracostomy, closely monitor for signs of hypoxia (restlessness, anxiety, and mental status changes), and monitor patency and functioning of closed chest-drainage system (especially monitor for signs of resolution of air leak)
   c. Encourage client to take deep breaths and to change position every 2 hours to promote full lung expansion and prevent atelectasis

7. Medication therapy: analgesics to promote comfort during chest tube insertion and during deep-breathing exercises

8. Client education: purpose of therapeutic interventions, how to perform deep-breathing exercises, and to report increasing shortness of breath

9. Evaluation: client maintains an effective breathing pattern and adequate gas exchange, remains hemodynamically stable, and pain is controlled to level acceptable to client

C. Flail chest

1. Description: force of impact to chest wall during injury causes fracture of 3 or more contiguous ribs in 2 or more places, resulting in a "floating" segment; usually results from blunt trauma to chest wall such as falls, when striking steering wheel, etc.

2. Etiology and pathophysiology

   a. Because rib cage is no longer intact, as intrathoracic pressure increases with normal inspiration, flail segment is drawn inward and conversely bulges outward with expiration

   b. Pain, pulmonary contusion (which frequently coexist), and increased work of breathing cause clinical manifestations

3. Assessment

   a. Clinical manifestations: dyspnea, poor air movement, chest wall pain, ecchymosis, splinting respirations, hypoxia, pain on inspiration, paradoxical chest wall movement, possible palpable subcutaneous emphysema

   b. Diagnostic and laboratory findings: chest x-rays confirm multiple rib fractures; ABGs may reveal extent of hypoxemia

4. Therapeutic management: initial stabilization with supplemental O_2, IV access, O_2 saturation monitoring, and ABGs; with severe hypoxia, client may require ET intubation to prevent respiratory failure; adequate pain management is essential; stabilize chest wall with elastoplast dressing

5. Priority nursing problems: alterations in respiratory pattern or gas exchange, pain, alteration in tissue integrity

6. Planning and implementation

   a. Goal: client has effective breathing pattern and perfusion with tolerable pain management

   b. Because of increased risk of concurrent pulmonary tissue damage, assess for pulmonary contusion and use measures to maintain airway, breathing, and circulation (ABCs)

   c. Administer supplemental O_2 to maintain O_2 saturation greater than 90%

   d. Maintain IV access and titrate fluids to avoid overhydration, which may exacerbate interstitial pulmonary edema if present from damage

   e. Pain management is necessary to avoid hypoventilation that may lead to atelectasis and pneumonia; positioning client on affected side (a form of splinting) may also assist with pain control

7. Medication therapy: pain management with opioid analgesics such as morphine sulfate, hydromorphone, fentanyl, or acetaminophen with oxycodone; intercostal nerve blocks, epidural or patient-controlled analgesia (PCA) may also be used, particularly for hospitalized client

8. Client education: how to use PCA if ordered, splinting techniques to control rib pain, treatment approaches used, and medication side effects

9. Evaluation: client achieves an effective breathing pattern; ABGs are within normal limits, pain management is effective

D. Uncontrolled hemorrhage

1. Description: uncontrolled bleeding

2. Etiology and pathophysiology

   a. Can result from blunt or penetrating trauma, gastrointestinal (GI) or genitourinary (GU) bleeding, or hemoptysis

   b. Clinical manifestations result from inadequate circulating volume that leads to decreased tissue perfusion

   c. Decreased tissue perfusion and metabolism results in hypoxia, vasoconstriction, and shunting of available circulating volume to vital organs (brain and heart)

Practice to Pass

A client involved in a motor vehicle crash (MVC) has experienced multiple contiguous fractured ribs. What are the goals for your nursing care?

          d. Sympathetic nervous system (SNS) stimulation, hormonal release of antidiuretic hormone (ADH) and angiotensin-renin mechanisms, and neural responses attempt to compensate for loss of circulating volume, but over time these mechanisms fail

          e. Eventually metabolic acidosis, multiple organ system failure, respiratory failure, and cardiac arrest occur

    3. Assessment

          a. Clinical manifestations: cool, clammy, pale skin and distal extremities, delayed capillary refill (greater than 3 seconds), weak, rapid pulses, decreased blood pressure (BP) with systolic BP less than 90 mmHg), rapid, shallow respirations greater than 28/min or RR less than 10/min, restless, anxious, or decreased LOC, cardiac **dysrhythmias** (abnormalities of cardiac rhythm), and decreased urine output (UO)

          b. Diagnostic and laboratory findings

              1) Evidence of bleeding from thoracostomy or a thoracostomy that indicates bleeding from chest area

              2) Abdominal or pelvic CT scan, abdominal ultrasound, or peritoneal lavage indicate intra-abdominal bleeding

              3) Endoscopy indicates upper or lower GI bleeding

              4) Angiography procedures diagnose severe vascular damage

              5) Extremity x-rays show presence of long bone fractures

              6) Hemoglobin and hematocrit from CBC are decreased due to blood loss

              7) Elevated serum lactate if bleeding continues and client becomes acidotic

              8) ABGs show metabolic acidosis as blood loss continues

              9) Baseline coagulation studies: initial PT, PTT, and platelet count will be normal but as coagulation factors become depleted, clotting times will increase and platelet count will decrease

              10) Other laboratory tests would include serum electrolytes to assess renal function and intravascular volume state; these values will vary based upon level of fluid loss and length of time of blood depletion

    4. Therapeutic management: note that medical interventions carried out by nurses are in collaboration with provider or part of protocol orders

          a. Perform initial stabilization of uncontrolled bleeding simultaneously with assuring an effective patent airway

          b. Maintain C-spine immobilization

          c. Use respiratory adjuncts to establish effective breathing pattern for O_2 delivery to circulating volume

          d. Stop obvious bleeding with direct pressure and find a hidden source of bleeding quickly; if bleeding cannot be stopped immediately, surgery may be needed

          e. Initiate IV fluid resuscitation with warmed balanced salt solutions such as Lactated Ringer's or NS solution

          f. Initiate blood replacement therapy as needed (with typed and cross-matched blood if time permits), however, type-specific packed red blood cells (PRBCs) or low titer, type O-negative RBCs may be used until type specific blood becomes available; transfuse platelets and coagulation factors as indicated by laboratory results; 1 unit of PRBCs is needed for each 3 liters of crystalloid solution to prevent hemodilution

          g. Monitor cardiac rhythm, VS, central venous pressure (CVP) if available, mental status, and UO to evaluate effectiveness of interventions

    5. Priority nursing problems: reduced tissue perfusion, fluid volume loss, reduced cardiac output, risk for hemodynamic instability

6. Planning and implementation
   a. Goals: reestablishment of adequate tissue perfusion and prevent tissue damage
   b. After establishing an adequate airway, breathing pattern, and applying supplemental O_2, give priority to interventions to control external bleeding, such as direct pressure to wound site, or assisting with surgical interventions
   c. Establish IV access with 2 large-bore (14-, 16-, or 18-gauge) catheters and begin fluid replacement with crystalloid solutions such as lactated Ringer's or NS at a rate of 3 mL crystalloid solution for every 1 mL estimated blood loss
   d. Draw blood specimens as ordered for evaluation of hemoglobin, hematocrit, electrolyte, oxygenation, and hydration status
   e. Insert an indwelling urinary catheter and NG tube to assist in accurate recording of fluid balance
   f. Perform and document continuous serial assessments of hemodynamic parameters such as VS, capillary refill, CVP, cardiac rhythm, LOC, UO and laboratory findings
   g. Keep client warm to prevent hypothermia
7. Medication therapy: crystalloids and blood products to maintain adequate circulating volume; sodium bicarbonate to correct acidosis; vasopressors such as dopamine if necessary (only after providing appropriate fluid resuscitation)
8. Client education: explain procedures to client and support family by explaining emergency measures and interventions
9. Evaluation: improved and adequate tissue perfusion is noted by improved LOC; VS and other hemodynamic parameters are within normal limits; UO is greater than 30 mL/hr; capillary refill less than 3 sec; bleeding is controlled; client is normothermic; ABGs are within normal limits; client has an adequate breathing pattern and tissue oxygenation

E. **Motor vehicle crashes (MVCs)**: blunt and multiple trauma
   1. Description: injuries sustained from MVC, including blunt injuries and multiple trauma; high incidence of morbidity and mortality in MVCs are due to blunt trauma
   2. Etiology and pathophysiology
      a. Three types of forces commonly occur with blunt MVC trauma
         1) Acceleration-deceleration forces occur when velocity of a moving object increases and then decreases, either from speed of vehicle, speed of occupant, or speed of internal organs
         2) Compression forces occur when organs or body parts are pressed against immovable objects; can result in explosive injury to air-filled organs (such as bowel) or crush injury to solid organs such as liver or spleen
         3) Shearing forces occur when there is a rotational force exerted around a fixed site
      b. Type of impact, speed at impact, point of impact, restraint systems used, organ systems involved, and client's preexisting conditions also affect results of these forces
      c. Blunt trauma injuries can involve fractures, lacerations, contusions, rupture or tearing of solid or hollow organs and major blood vessels
   3. Assessment
      a. Clinical manifestations: generally depend on organ system impacted and mechanism of injury
         1) Signs of hypovolemia (tachycardia, mental status change, pale, cool skin, hypotension, etc.), respiratory distress or inadequate breathing pattern may be due to bruising of lung tissue, pneumothorax, hemothorax, or loss of functional structure of thoracic cage as with flail chest or rib fractures

          2) Blunt trauma to head, neck or spine may result in decreased LOC, loss of sensation or decreased motor ability due to spinal fracture or damage to central nervous system (CNS); it may also cause impaired respiratory function from swelling or loss of integrity of upper airway

          3) Blunt abdominal trauma may result in signs of hypovolemia from bladder, liver, or spleen rupture as well as damage to GI tract

          4) Blunt trauma to extremities may cause fractures, pain, swelling, loss of function, and loss of large quantities of blood into surrounding cavities

      b. Diagnostic and laboratory findings: effects of blunt trauma are usually more difficult to diagnose because of their frequent lack of external signs of injury

          1) Based on physical assessment and mechanism of injury, x-rays, CT scans, ultrasounds, and MRIs may be used to assess injuries

          2) Diagnostic peritoneal lavage may help detect abdominal injury or intra-abdominal bleeding; abdomen can contain RBCs, white blood cells, bile, feces, or food products if rupture is in abdominal cavity or GI tract

          3) Electrocardiogram (ECG) will help determine myocardial damage

          4) Laboratory tests such as a CBC, electrolytes, urinalysis, serum amylase and lactate, liver enzymes, cardiac enzymes, type and cross or screen, clotting studies, ABGs, and toxicology studies will establish baseline or detect abnormal findings

    4. Therapeutic management

      a. Initially assess and stabilize ABCs while assuring C-spine immobilization; depending upon injury pattern, intubation may be necessary

      b. Provide supplemental O_2

      c. Place client in modified Trendelenburg position (legs elevated, thorax level) if shock symptoms are present; control obvious bleeding using direct pressure

      d. Insert 2 large-bore IV lines and infuse lactated ringers or NS as ordered; aggressively manage signs of shock while diagnostic procedures and preparation take place

      e. Complete NG and indwelling urinary catheter insertion, radiological procedures, and ECG to determine what injury management will be required

      f. Use positioning, splinting, ice, and elevation for closed fractures

      g. Prepare client for surgery if needed

    5. Priority nursing problems: impaired airway, alterations in respiratory pattern or gas exchange, dehydration, reduced cardiac output, reduced tissue perfusion, anxiety, pain

    6. Planning and implementation

      a. Goals: focused on adequate oxygenation, tissue perfusion, comfort, and supportive measures

      b. Maintain airway management with least invasive yet most effective method; nasopharyngeal, oropharyngeal, or ET intubation may be needed to maintain a patent airway, especially in clients with blunt trauma to face or neck

      c. Immobilize C-spine with a cervical collar and keep collar in place until C-spine has been cleared by radiography

      d. Continuously observe breathing pattern to ensure effective oxygenation and gas exchange for tissue perfusion; also check O_2 saturation levels

      e. Be prepared to assist with chest tube insertion and then continuously monitor quantity and character of drainage and presence of any air leak

      f. Assist with diagnostic procedures as ordered and continually monitor client's response

      g. Perform serial assessment of VS, LOC, characteristics and location of pain; initiate pain management as soon as possible

      h. Initiate measures to provide psychological support to client and family as soon as possible; advise client and family of plan of care and offer information about tests to be performed

  7. Medication therapy: immediate fluid resuscitation with NS or Ringer's lactate if shock is present; stable clients may receive tetanus immunization, antibiotics, analgesics, and vasopressors if needed to maintain adequate perfusion pressures after hydration has been completed

  8. Client education: explain all procedures to client; provide explanations of resuscitative procedures to families of clients with trauma

  9. Evaluation: client demonstrates a patent airway, effective breathing pattern, and hemodynamic stability; all injuries are identified and appropriate interventions are completed; pain is controlled to an acceptable level and client and family are aware of plan of care and extent of injury as appropriate

F. Penetrating injuries (stab wounds, gunshot wounds)

  1. Description: penetrating injuries are those caused by an object or missile set in motion that penetrates body

    a. Extent of penetration and damage depends on velocity of missile, energy created by missile, area of body penetrated, and missile characteristics

    b. Low-velocity missiles such as knives, pencils, or forks generally create tissue damage only along path of weapon because of low energy force of weapon

    c. Penetrating injuries from high-velocity, high-energy missiles such as from guns, rifles, or high-pressure injection devices such as paint guns, cause damage to tissue immediately in path of missile but also tissue damage caused by stress and strain to surrounding tissues and toxins of any chemicals injected

  2. Etiology and pathophysiology

    a. Low-velocity missiles or those weapons with low kinetic energy have little energy to be dissipated as they penetrate body

      1) Damage caused by these weapons can be calculated by many factors, including weapon used, structure of weapon (such as length and shape), position of victim when struck, and position of attacker

      2) Gender of attacker is also appropriate in estimating penetrating injury damage; men usually stab with an upward motion and women usually stab with a downward motion since this is how they generate most of their power

      3) Assessment of possible injuries must take into consideration possibility of more extensive internal injury than entrance wound indicates because of victim movement; a low-velocity weapon can be life threatening if it strikes a highly vascular or vital organ

    b. High-velocity, high-kinetic energy missiles cause a great deal more damage to tissues directly affected by missile and also those tissues affected by cavitation, shock wave, and heat of missile

      1) Severity of wound can be predicted by knowing caliber (diameter), type of missile (potential to fragment or deform, yaw [veer from a straight path], or tumble), distance from victim, and trajectory into body

      2) High-pressure injection missile injuries, such as from paint guns, usually appear as a minor puncture wound; however, major damage is caused by injection of toxic, foreign substances into surrounding tissues, which causes infection, pain, swelling, and potential compartment syndrome

  3. Assessment

    a. Clinical manifestations: an open wound is present; symptoms of shock exist, such as hypotension, tachycardia, dyspnea, pallor, cool and clammy skin, and changes in mental status

    b. Diagnostic and laboratory findings: generally the extent of wound and damage to surrounding tissues are diagnosed by direct assessment and radiographic studies (presence of blood, air or fluid in body compartments; location of missile, and integrity of organ systems); soft tissue damage is usually diagnosed by ultrasound; CBC, electrolytes, cardiac and hepatic enzymes, amylase, and ABG help determine extent of damage to various organ systems

4. Therapeutic management
   a. Determined by extent of tissue damage; initially stabilize ABCs
   b. Penetrating trauma to lungs may require chest tube placement to reinflate a lung
   c. Penetrating trauma to heart may require surgical exploration and repair; usually leads to traumatic full arrest and open cardiac massage
   d. Penetrating trauma to bowel or GI tract will require surgery (probable bowel resection or ostomy) to prevent development of peritonitis caused by leakage of GI contents into peritoneal cavity
   e. Bladder rupture or tears will also require surgical repair
   f. Management of penetrating trauma to head, neck, and face may also require surgery to determine extent of injury or repair it
   g. Penetrating trauma of high velocity to soft tissue such as in leg may be monitored for complications, whereas trauma to firm tissues such as bone may require surgery (including amputation) to prevent infection or further neurovascular damage

5. Priority nursing problems: impaired airway, alterations in respiratory pattern or gas exchange, dehydration, reduced cardiac output, reduced tissue perfusion, interrupted skin integrity, potential for infection, anxiety, pain, body image alteration

6. Planning and implementation
   a. Goals: adequate oxygenation and tissue perfusion, prevention of further alterations in body systems affected, comfort and supportive measures
   b. Provide airway management as needed if there is trauma to face or neck; use least invasive but effective management device; if an effective breathing pattern has been disrupted because of loss of lung or diaphragm integrity or because of pain, prepare to assist with ET intubation and mechanical ventilation if needed
   c. Initiate noninvasive methods of splinting area and coughing and deep breathing if chest has been site of trauma
   d. Assess for excessive blood loss, whether overt or covert, by initial and serial VS; administer prescribed fluids and blood products as quickly as possible to avoid inadequate tissue perfusion
   e. Disruption of skin integrity presents a risk for infection; provide sterile dressing changes; monitor puncture site for drainage, redness, and signs of healing; administer antibiotics as prescribed
   f. Provide pain management as necessary to encourage mobility and for psychological well-being
   g. Keep client and family informed of plan of care and prognosis as much as possible

7. Medication therapy: tetanus immunization, antibiotics for infection control, and analgesics for pain
8. Client education: provide explanations of all procedures done; families usually require emotional support and honest discussions about therapeutic interventions and plans
9. Evaluation: client maintains a clear airway, effective breathing pattern, and adequate tissue perfusion; client remains free of signs of infection; pain and anxiety are minimized; client and family are aware of plan of care and prognosis as appropriate

G. Hypothermia
1. Description: a condition where core body temperature is 36°C (96.8°F) or less
2. Etiology and pathophysiology

    a. Exposure to extreme cold causes a decrease in basal metabolic rate after a period of compensatory mechanism attempts to increase body temperature

    b. As body uses all its energy stores, decreased circulation and cellular perfusion cause a state of acidosis, which causes further metabolic cellular dysfunction and eventual death

3. Assessment

    a. Clinical manifestations

        1) Core body temperature of 36°C (96.8°F) or less

        2) In mild hypothermia (33–36°C or 91.4–96.8°F), client will appear lethargic, shivering, mildly confused, ataxic, and demonstrate diminished fine motor skills

        3) In moderate hypothermia (28–32°C or 82.4–91.3°F), shivering will cease, LOC will decrease to coma, bradycardia and bradypnea will be present, and pupils will be dilated; cardiac rhythm will show atrial and ventricular dysrhythmias

        4) With a core body temperature below 28°C (82.4°F), client will have severely depressed respiratory, cardiovascular, and neurological function and appear dead; client's ECG may show asystole, and there will be muscle rigidity; may defibrillate once but then must rewarm to 85°F before second attempt

    b. Diagnostic and laboratory findings: core temperature is decreased; ABGs show level of acidosis

4. Therapeutic management

    a. Initially stabilize airway and breathing with supplemental O_2; mechanical ventilation may be needed if there is absent or ineffective respiratory effort

    b. Observe cardiac monitor continuously for dysrhythmia development

    c. Faster rewarming is usually more effective than slow rewarming, particularly with a core body temperature less than 32°C; active rewarming involves use of heated humidified O_2 delivered at 40–44°C, heated IV solutions delivered at 40–42°C, heated gastric lavage if airway has been secured, heated peritoneal lavage at 40–45°C, and heated pleural irrigation through inserted chest tube at 40–42°C if no cardiac activity is present; cardiopulmonary bypass may also be used in severe hypothermia

    d. If CPR and **defibrillation** (application of asynchronous external electrical charge to depolarize myocardial cells) attempts were unsuccessful initially, they should be retried after rewarming; monitor ABGs and electrolytes for hyperkalemia caused by cellular damage and fluid shifts

5. Priority nursing problems: hypothermia, reduced cardiac output, alterations in respiratory pattern or gas exchange, impaired airway maintenance, reduced tissue perfusion

6. Planning and implementation

    a. Assist with establishing an effective airway and breathing

    b. Initiate cardiac monitoring and assess for development of dysrhythmias

    c. Assist with rewarming measures

    d. Monitor UO after indwelling urinary catheter insertion

    e. Frequently assess pulmonary status for development of pulmonary edema

    f. Monitor ABGs and electrolytes and assist in treatment of acidosis and electrolyte imbalances, which may contribute to cardiac dysrhythmias

    g. Keep client and family informed of plan of care and prognosis

7. Medication therapy: Dextrose 50% 50 mL IV to correct hypoglycemia, and amiodarone (Cordarone) 300 mg IV push; repeat 150 mg every 3 to 5 minutes as needed with maximum 2.2 grams IV over 24 hours to correct ventricular dysrhythmias, followed by IV drip at 15 mg/minute

8. Client education: provide emotional support to families of client in severe hypothermia; explain treatments and interventions; teach prevention techniques related to cold exposure when client is stable

9. Evaluation: body temperature is greater than 36°C; effective airway and breathing pattern is established with ABGs within normal limits; CO is adequate for perfusion, and dysrhythmias are absent; LOC is improved; UO is greater than 30 mL/hr; client and family verbalize understanding of plan of care

H. Frostbite

1. Description: injury caused by exposure to cold temperature
2. Etiology and pathophysiology
   a. Exposure to cold results in loss of body heat and vasoconstriction to preserve core body heat
   b. As vasoconstriction occurs at periphery, tissue ischemia occurs
   c. As tissue freezes, ice crystals form in extravascular space, causing edema and mechanical damage to cells
   d. Cellular damage causes clumping of platelets and RBCs when thawing is attempted with risk for progressive ischemic damage
3. Assessment
   a. Clinical manifestations: pain, loss of sensation and paresthesia of affected body parts; area may be edematous, red, blistered, white, hard and cold to touch, or necrotic depending upon extent of exposure and stage of frostbite; client may describe pain as stinging, burning, or aching
   b. Diagnostic and laboratory findings: diagnosis is based on clinical findings; in case of severe frostbite, baseline CBC, electrolytes, BUN, creatinine, and glucose determine organ system status; a urinalysis may reveal myoglobinuria (seen in muscle damage)
4. Therapeutic management
   a. Remove client from cold environment before thawing is attempted because refreezing after thawing can increase risk of permanent loss of affected extremity
   b. Immerse areas in warm water (100–106°F), gently circulating water around extremity
   c. Do not rub area but client may move affected extremity during warming process; mechanical friction can increase tissue damage
   d. Monitor client's core body temperature to prevent hypothermia caused by return of cold blood into central circulation
   e. After thawing, gently wrap extremity and elevate it to prevent edema formation
   f. Blisters may or may not be debrided based upon provider preference
   g. Amputation of affected extremities will not be considered until extent of permanent tissue damage is known, which may take several months
5. Priority nursing problems: reduced tissue perfusion, interrupted skin integrity, potential for infection, pain, inadequate knowledge
6. Planning and implementation
   a. Assist with thawing process; monitor for signs of further tissue ischemia
   b. Remind client not to rub areas but that gentle movement is appropriate
   c. Antibiotics and sterile bulky dressings will be used to prevent infection
   d. Newly thawed areas will be very painful and pain should be managed at a tolerable level
   e. Since client is expected to undergo an extended period of care, client and family should understand plan of care and expected outcomes
7. Medication therapy: aloe vera (topical) can be used because of its thromboxane-inhibiting effect, which inhibits platelet aggregation; possible tetanus prophylaxis based on immunization status; both topical and parenteral antibiotics may be prescribed to prevent infection; pain should be controlled with parenteral and oral analgesics

   8. Client education: pain management, signs of infection, importance of adhering to follow-up care, methods to prevent future cold-related injuries, and importance of avoiding nicotine to maintain circulatory integrity

   9. Evaluation: function and sensation are restored to affected area; pain and infection are minimized; client states understanding of follow-up care

I. Heat exhaustion

   1. Description: vasomotor collapse from prolonged exposure to heat

   2. Etiology and pathophysiology

   a. Dehydration occurs because of increased sweating through evaporation; this results in loss of salt and water; symptoms associated with heat exhaustion result from these losses

   b. Condition usually results from exercising vigorously in hot weather

   c. Predisposing factors include advanced age, use of diuretics, and a preexisting fluid disorder such as diarrhea

   3. Assessment

   a. Clinical manifestations

   1) Nausea, vomiting, headache, lightheadedness, malaise, or myalgia

   2) Pale, warm, and moist skin

   3) Core body temperature ranges from 39–41°C (103–105°F)

   4) Possible impaired judgment and mild confusion

   b. Diagnostic and laboratory findings

   1) Serum electrolytes show a decrease in potassium level

   2) Decrease in serum sodium (depletes in 2 hours with excessive perspiration)

   3) Increased hematocrit from hemoconcentration

   4. Therapeutic management: rest in cool, shaded area; sponge with tepid water and direct fans toward client; fluid and electrolyte replacement orally and IV, if needed

   5. Priority nursing problems: dehydration, fever, inadequate knowledge of measures to prevent heat exhaustion

   6. Planning and implementation

   a. Key measures include preventing further fluid and electrolyte loss and increasing body temperature

   b. Rehydrate using fluids with electrolytes and assist client to rest in a cool environment

   c. May sponge client with tepid water and allow evaporation to occur

   d. Attempt to prevent shivering, which may raise temperature

   7. Medication therapy: fluid and electrolyte solutions

   8. Client education: prevent future exposure to heat; drink fluids containing electrolytes before and after strenuous exercise; may also mix 1 teaspoon of salt in 500 mL of water and drink to maintain sodium level; watch for signs and symptoms of electrolyte abnormalities

   9. Evaluation: body temperature returns to normal; serum electrolytes are within normal limits and adequate hydration status is maintained; client and family verbalize understanding of preventive measures

J. Heat stroke (hyperthermia)

   1. Description: an extremely elevated core body temperature caused by a failure of hypothalamus' perspiration-regulating mechanism; carries 70% mortality rate

   2. Etiology and pathophysiology

   a. Most serious heat-related emergency; results in death if untreated

   b. Common predisposing factors include older adults, high humidity and temperature, preexisting illnesses such as diabetes, cardiovascular disease, previous stroke, obesity, medications such as phenothiazines, tricyclic antidepressants, diuretics, and beta blockers

c. Street drugs such as alcohol, amphetamines, and phencyclidine can also predispose to development of heat stroke

d. A person who is exposed to hot environments normally perspires, but with progressive fluid loss through evaporation, he or she eventually cannot produce enough perspiration to normalize body temperature

e. When sweating stops, core body temperature increases, leading to cardiac collapse

f. If heat stroke is left untreated, serious brain injury and nervous system damage results

3. Assessment

a. Clinical manifestations

1) Core body temperature greater than 42°C (105°F)

2) Ataxia, stupor, delirium, seizures, coma, tachycardia, tachypnea, hypotension, dysrhythmias, nausea, vomiting, and diarrhea

3) Dry, hot, flushed skin

b. Diagnostic and laboratory findings

1) CBC to rule out contributory factors causing high temperature, such as infection

2) Serum electrolytes reveal hypernatremia, hypokalemia, and hypoglycemia

3) Liver function tests may reveal liver failure and possible rhabdomyolysis

4) Prothrombin time (PT) or partial thromboplastin time (PTT) may indicate clotting abnormalities

5) ABGs indicate metabolic acidosis

4. Therapeutic management: institute aggressive cooling measures, including full body exposure and cooling by evaporation; prevent shivering (raises body temperature); use cardiac monitoring to assess for dysrhythmias; assist with ice water gastric and peritoneal lavage; continually monitor core temperature to prevent overcorrection and hypothermia

5. Priority nursing problems: hyperthermia, hemodynamic instability

6. Planning and implementation

a. Ensure establishment of stable airway and monitor breathing pattern

b. Maintain circulatory status with IV access and infusion of NS or D_5 ½ NS; do not use lactated Ringer's solution because liver is unable to metabolize lactate in acidosis

c. Insert urinary catheter to maintain accurate UO

d. Initiate cooling measures with cold solutions and cooling by evaporation; cold packs may be placed in areas of large blood volume such as groin, axilla, neck, and head

e. Continually monitor cardiac rhythm for dysrhythmias

f. Prevent shivering, acidosis, and cerebral edema

7. Medication therapy: chlorpromazine (Thorazine) 10–25 mg to prevent shivering (do not use aspirin or acetaminophen [Tylenol]; they are ineffective); benzodiazepines to prevent seizures; mannitol (Osmitrol) and methylprednisolone (Solu-Medrol) to decrease cerebral edema

8. Client education: how to prevent this type of injury; clients at risk (older adults, those receiving phenothiazines) should take extra precautions to avoid prolonged heat exposure

9. Evaluation: body temperature returns to normal; effective airway, breathing pattern, and gas exchange are maintained; cardiac dysrhythmias are recognized and treated; client and family verbalize understanding of treatment regime and preventive measures

K. Drowning and near drowning

1. Description: drowning is death caused by asphyxia and aspiration after submersion in water; near drowning is risk of death occurring within 24 hours after submersion in water

2. Etiology and pathophysiology
    a. **Asphyxiation** (suffocation) can be caused by laryngotracheal spasm from a small amount of water entering larynx or large amounts of water swallowed and then vomited and aspirated into lungs
    b. In most cases, water enters lungs from aspiration, which cause drowning or near-drowning symptoms
    c. Depending on type of fluid aspirated, water entering lungs displaces surfactant and increases alveolar surface tension, reducing O_2 perfusion
    d. Chlorinated swimming pool water will also cause a chemical pneumonitis because of chemical destruction of alveolar membrane
    e. Saltwater, because of its hypertonic state, will lead to pulmonary edema (causes a fluid shift from vascular space into alveolar space)
    f. As alveolar ventilation decreases, inflammation, obstruction, and collapse of smaller alveolar and capillary membranes cause pulmonary edema, decreased lung capacity, hypoventilation, O_2 desaturation, and eventually cardiac arrest
    g. Although victims of near-drowning events do not expire immediately, the severe hypoxia, alveoli membrane damage, possible aspiration of gastric secretions, and acidosis produce cardiac, renal, hepatic, metabolic, and neurological dysfunction
3. Assessment
    a. Clinical manifestations: hypoxia, dyspnea, wheezing, crackles, rhonchi, cough with pink, frothy sputum, tachycardia, cyanosis, mental confusion, seizures, cardiac or respiratory arrest
    b. Diagnostic and laboratory findings: ABGs reveal acidosis; CBC reveals hemodilution; serum sodium level may be elevated or decreased depending on fluid aspirated (in freshwater drowning, serum electrolytes will be reduced; in saltwater drowning, serum sodium and chloride will be elevated); serum osmolality is elevated in saltwater drowning; chest x-ray reveals bilateral infiltrate (best method to determine amount of fluid in lungs)
    c. Monitor LOC, even if client presents being conscious, sudden cerebral edema can occur
4. Therapeutic management
    a. Establish a patent airway and effective breathing pattern
    b. ET intubation and mechanical ventilation with PEEP may be needed for adequate ventilation with pulmonary edema and low lung compliance
    c. Use CVP monitoring, pulmonary capillary wedge pressure monitoring, and arterial line monitoring to monitor fluid resuscitation and fluid volume status
    d. Correct hypoxia and correct acidosis with sodium bicarbonate
    e. If near drowning occurred in cold water, undertake rewarming measures
    f. Initiate CPR and advanced cardiac life support (ACLS) measures until client's body temperature has returned to normal
    g. Manage developing pulmonary infections as a result of near-drowning incidents aggressively with appropriate antibiotics
5. Priority nursing problems: alterations in gas exchange or respiratory pattern, ineffective cough, reduced cardiac output, anxiety
6. Planning and implementation
    a. Ensure ABCs
    b. Provide frequent suctioning and supplemental O_2 to enhance ventilatory efforts
    c. Infuse lactated Ringer's IV for saltwater drowning and NS solutions IV for freshwater drowning to prevent hypervolemia or hypovolemia
    d. Use cardiac monitoring to diagnose and appropriately treat developing dysrhythmias
    e. Insert a urinary catheter to aid in maintaining accurate UO

      f. Assist with correction of acidosis and rewarming if immersion occurred in cold water

      g. Closely monitor and record cardiac, respiratory, and neurological status; report changes as they occur

      h. Assist client and family to understand prognosis and plan of care

  7. Medication therapy: epinephrine 1 mg IV push (IVP), lidocaine 1–1.5 mg/kg IVP, amiodarone 150 mg IVP, atropine 1 mg IVP per ACLS protocol for cardiac arrest; sodium bicarbonate to correct acidosis; steroids, bronchodilators, and isoproterenol to counteract effects of edema and bronchospasm; antibiotics for respiratory infections caused by aspiration

  8. Client education

      a. Strategies to prevent drowning: wear lifejackets or vests when engaging in water activities; learn to swim; never swim alone; keep gates locked in swimming pools to prevent accidental drowning of children; and never swim immediately after a meal

      b. Importance of knowing CPR; refer clients to agencies where they could be trained

  9. Evaluation: client exhibits effective breathing pattern with adequate gas exchange; acidosis is corrected; complications of respiratory, cardiac, and neurological systems are avoided; family and client verbalize understanding and agreement with plan of care

L. Bites (dog, cat, rodent, human, insect/bee, spider, tick, snake)

  1. Description: a break in continuity of skin caused by a bite from an animal, reptile, insect, or human

  2. Etiology and pathophysiology

      a. It is assumed that all bites that break skin surface will potentially inoculate area with bacteria or viruses

      b. Presence of bacteria is most common in human, dog, and cat bites

      c. Venom from poisonous spiders and snakes has substances capable of causing localized tissue damage because of enzyme effects and cardiotoxic, neurotoxic, and hematological effects

      d. Inoculation with toxins from bee stings and venomous bites can cause an anaphylactic reaction

  3. Assessment

      a. Clinical manifestations

         1) Initial presentation reveals a break in skin integrity caused by bite from animal, reptile, human, or insect

         2) Pain and tenderness are usually seen with fresh bites

         3) Further underlying damage such as bruising or swelling from crush injury to surrounding tissues, fractures of bone, tendon, or nerve damage may also be found, particularly with large animal or human bites

         4) If wound occurred several hours or days before seeking care, redness, swelling, or cellulitis symptoms may be observed

         5) Bites from insects, spiders, and snakes may have local reaction of itching, swelling, and local inflammation, but some spider and snake bites cause a systemic reaction as severe as nausea, vomiting, respiratory difficulty and seizures; assess nature of bite, time of injury, location of wound, and what interventions were completed before seeking treatment

      b. Diagnostic and laboratory findings: diagnosis is based on clinical findings; cultures of injury sites and baseline electrolyte and CBC may be done; white blood cell count will be elevated with an "old" bite indicating presence of infection

4. Therapeutic management
   a. For most human and animal wounds, the most important treatment is meticulous wound cleaning and follow-up care
   b. Thoroughly clean and irrigate wound with copious amounts of solution
   c. Debride macerated tissue and apply a topical antibiotic as prescribed
   d. Leave wound open and apply a bulky dressing
   e. For most human bites and severe, high-risk animal bites, IV antibiotics will be ordered
   f. Rabies prophylaxis is based upon type of animal bite and risk of animal carrying rabies
   g. All carnivores have potential for carrying rabies, so bites from bats, raccoons, and most wild animals should be considered contaminated unless proven otherwise
   h. Herbivores, such as mice and other rodents, usually do not carry rabies; in most communities, local public health department should be contacted for regional information about other diseases carried
   i. Venomous bites such as those from black widow spiders and poisonous snakes require antivenom treatment and methods such as a constricting band or ice to slow circulation and spread of venom throughout circulation (a good description of offending snake, spider or animal behavior helps determine which antivenom or treatment to administer)
   j. Allergic reactions and systemic allergic reactions are treated with epinephrine and diphenhydramine (Benadryl) quickly to avoid system-wide vascular collapse and histamine response
5. Priority nursing problems: interrupted skin integrity, potential for infection, inadequate knowledge, potential alteration in respiratory pattern, potential for reduced cardiac output
6. Planning and implementation
   a. Priority nursing care is to prevent further tissue damage
   b. General measures are to clean wound thoroughly, leave open, and apply topical antibiotic ointment
   c. Apply dry sterile dressing if prescribed and monitor for signs of infection or wound healing
   d. Provide rabies prophylaxis based upon information obtained from local public health department
   e. Administer antibiotics (IV or oral) as prescribed
   f. Spider bites, such as from a black widow spider, require symptomatic care; apply ice to bite area to decrease absorption while antivenom therapy is being administered; observe for signs of neurotoxicity and administer muscle relaxants as prescribed
   g. Maintain an effective airway and breathing pattern to prevent hypoxia
   h. Treat bites from poisonous snakes aggressively also and closely monitor for signs of systemic reaction such as syncope, paralysis, paresthesia, or seizures
   i. Because snake venom can also affect clotting factors, monitor for signs of hemorrhage such as excessive bleeding or hematuria
   j. Prevent further systemic spread of venom through use of a constricting band to extremity and ice while antivenom therapy is initiated
   k. Continuously monitor VS, cardiac rhythm, and neurological status
7. Medication therapy: tetanus prophylaxis based upon immunization history (most common); antibiotics based on type of bite and clinical signs; rabies prophylaxis as indicated; species-specific antivenom for poisonous snake and spider bites (may need to be obtained from local public health department)

8. Client education
   a. Methods to avoid reinjury if appropriate
   b. Need to notify animal control for animal bite and impound animal for 10 days to evaluate for rabies; notify police for human bites if occurred during an altercation
9. Evaluation: in all bite cases, further tissue damage is absent; there is reduced infection potential, and client understands plan of care; client is aware of need for strict follow-up if rabies and tetanus prophylaxis are started; clients exposed to venomous bites maintain effective cardiorespiratory and neurological function

M. Poisonings

1. Description: substances that are harmful to humans when inhaled, ingested (food, drug overdose), or acquired by contact (insecticides)
2. Etiology and pathophysiology
   a. Carbon monoxide inhalation signs and symptoms are caused by cellular toxicity and tissue hypoxia that result from formation of carboxyhemoglobin, which replaces O_2 on hemoglobin molecule; as a result, O_2 is not released to tissues and cellular destruction occurs; organ systems most critically affected are those that require most O_2 (cardiovascular and CNS); because of tissue hypoxia, lactic acid also builds up causing metabolic acidosis
   b. Food poisoning is most often caused by *Staphylococcus aureus*, *Salmonella*, *Escherichia coli*, *Clostridium perfringens*, or *Bacillus ceruns*; these bacteria release a toxin into body; symptoms are generally self-limiting and non–life-threatening except in debilitated clients
   c. Drug overdose: depends on type and amount of medication or drug ingested and speed of medical intervention; pathophysiological changes are usually caused by toxic effect of drug; some examples include the following:
      1) Salicylate overdose symptoms result from overstimulation of respiratory center and metabolic acidosis, which cause hyperventilation, hyperthermia, and hyperglycemia
      2) Narcotic or opioid overdoses generally cause CNS depression, hypotension, nausea and vomiting, and respiratory depression
      3) Excessive acetaminophen causes liver damage because of increased amounts of hepatotoxic metabolites
   d. Insecticide surface absorption: both organophosphates and carbamates are cholinesterase inhibitors and allow acetylcholine to accumulate and can cause a cholinergic crisis
3. Assessment
   a. Clinical manifestations
      1) Carbon monoxide inhalation: mild exposure—nausea, vomiting, mild throbbing headache, flulike symptoms; moderate exposure—dyspnea, dizziness, confusion, visual disturbance, increased severity of mild symptoms; severe or prolonged exposure—seizures, coma, respiratory arrest, hypotension, and dysrhythmias, there may be redness to face
      2) Food poisonings: nausea, vomiting, diarrhea, abdominal cramps, fever, chills, dehydration, headache
      3) Drug overdose: depends on substance ingested; symptoms may include nausea, vomiting, CNS depression or agitation, altered pupil response, tachypnea or bradypnea, alterations in temperature control, seizures, or cardiac arrest
      4) Surface absorption of insecticides (organophosphates or carbamates): nausea, vomiting, diarrhea, headache, dizziness, weakness or tremors, mild to severe respiratory distress, slurred speech, seizures, and cardiopulmonary arrest
   b. Diagnosis and laboratory findings: diagnosis is often based on history and clinical manifestations; serum and urine toxicology screens determine extent of absorption;

baseline blood work such as CBC, electrolytes, renal and hepatic studies help identify organ and tissue damage

4. Therapeutic management
   a. Generally, ABC interventions take priority
   b. Initiate IV access and infused prescribed fluids
   c. Give antagonists such as naloxone (Narcan) for respiratory depression caused by narcotic overdose and flumazenil (Romazicon) for benzodiazepine ingestions
   d. Initiate treatment of life-threatening dysrhythmias, seizures, or shock
   e. To prevent further absorption of drug ingested and to hasten elimination, vomiting may be induced, or charcoal and a cathartic can be administered either orally or by NG tube
   f. Gastric lavage (irrigation of stomach using large volumes of solution) is controversial in many cases
   g. Vomiting is contraindicated in cases of decreased LOC, absence of gag reflex, and ingestion of corrosive materials
   h. Administer antidotes if available, such as physostigmine for anticholinergic drugs such as antidepressants, tricyclics, or antihistamines or atropine for cholinergic crisis from insecticides

5. Priority nursing problems: potential for ineffective airway maintenance, potential for alteration in breathing pattern, potential reduced cardiac output, possible dehydration, reduced tissue perfusion, potential for injury, anxiety, risk for suicide, loss of hope

6. Planning and implementation
   a. Nursing interventions aim to decrease further damage to organ systems, assist with treatment of life-threatening conditions
   b. Assist with maintaining an effective airway, breathing pattern, and circulatory status
   c. Give treatment for life-threatening dysrhythmias and conditions as prescribed; continually monitor VS, cardiac rhythm, and neurological status
   d. Assist in hastening elimination of poison and decreasing absorption; administer antidotes as ordered
   e. Assist client and family in seeking appropriate referrals and provide client education to prevent further complications or incidence of overdose
   f. Ensure that client and family understand discharge instructions for follow-up care or reason for admission

7. Medication therapy: antidotes will vary with medication ingested; activated charcoal powder slurry orally or per NG tube; magnesium citrate for GI evacuation; other medications may be needed for supportive care

8. Client education: varies depending on nature of poisoning

9. Evaluation: client maintains effective O_2 and perfusion status as seen by regular RR and normal ABGs; no further organ system damage or injury occurs; absorption is minimized and toxic by-products are reduced; client and family verbalize measures to prevent further occurrences and need for follow-up care or admission

N. Electrocution
1. Description: injury sustained by electric current
2. Etiology and pathophysiology
   a. Electrical energy converts to heat energy as it passes through body
   b. Heat energy (which increases with amperage of current), causes extensive underlying tissue damage
   c. Entrance and exit wounds may be small, but current can cross blood vessels, nerves, and muscles as it passes through body
   d. Damage to myocardium and electrical conduction system of heart occurs from heat transfer, causing ventricular fibrillation

   e. Smaller body parts (such as fingers, hands, toes, and feet), because of smaller surface area and ability to dissipate heat, will suffer extensive damage if in path of current

 3. Assessment

  a. Clinical manifestations

   1) Are related to strength of electrical current encountered, type of current, path of current through body, and duration of contact

   2) Cardiac dysrhythmias may include sinus tachycardia, atrial tachycardias, premature ventricular contractions, ventricular fibrillation, or asystole

   3) Respiratory arrest may occur from inhibition of respiratory center, tetany of chest muscles or diaphragm, or paralysis of respiratory muscles

   4) Neurological symptoms may include altered LOC, amnesia, seizures, coma, and paresthesia

   5) Musculoskeletal injuries may include fractures, compartment syndrome, corneal burns, and thermal burns

  b. Diagnostic and laboratory findings: ECG shows conduction changes; creatinine phosphokinase (CK-MB) is elevated with myocardial tissue damage; hyperkalemia indicates cellular damage; metabolic acidosis occurs with extensive tissue and organ system damage; myoglobin in urine indicates significant muscle damage

 4. Therapeutic management

  a. Stabilize and ensure adequate ABCs

  b. Initiate spine immobilization due to possibility of a fall

  c. Begin fluid resuscitation to maintain UO of 1 mL/kg/hr because of third-spacing of fluids to injured muscles; an adequate UO also decreases complication of renal failure due to myoglobinuria

  d. Immobilize fractures of extremities to prevent further tissue damage until definitive care can be provided

  e. Provide wound care to external thermal burns, including cleansing, possible debridement, and dressing to prevent infection

  f. Administer tetanus prophylaxis based on client's immunization history

 5. Priority nursing problems: interrupted tissue integrity, reduced cardiac output, pain, potential for infection

 6. Planning and implementation

  a. Assist with measures to stabilize ABCs

  b. Initiate continuous cardiac monitor and administer antidysrhythmic drugs as ordered

  c. Continuously monitor VS, breath sounds for development of pulmonary edema, neurovascular status of extremities, and UO; all clients (regardless of visible damage) should have continuous cardiac monitoring for at least 24 hours to detect dysrhythmias

  d. Elevate affected limbs to decrease edema and monitor for signs of compartment syndrome, which may develop due to potential extensive internal muscle and tissue damage

  e. Provide support to family and client; answer questions as appropriate and advise regarding plan of care and procedures being completed

 7. Medication therapy: bicarbonate added to IV solutions maintains a urinary pH greater than 7.45 to increase myoglobin solubility in urine; mannitol increases UO; tetanus prophylaxis 0.5 mL IM is administered based on immunization status; antidysrhythmics such as lidocaine, amiodarone, and epinephrine are used for cardiac arrest

 8. Client education: focused on prevention of future injury

 9. Evaluation: client is hemodynamically stable with dysrhythmias appropriately treated; risk for infection or further tissue damage is minimized; client and family verbalize understanding of plan of care

III. COMMON PROBLEMS SEEN IN CRITICAL CARE SETTINGS

A. Critical care nursing

1. Description
   a. Critical care (CC) nurse is a licensed professional who provides care to meet individualized needs in response to potentially life-threatening conditions in an environment supportive of highly technological, collaborative, and holistic care; CC nurses may seek certification as a critical care nurse by exam offered through American Association of Critical Care Nursing
   b. CC nurse serves as a client advocate, provider of comprehensive care, and coordinator of interdisciplinary care aimed at achieving optimum outcomes to life-threatening conditions; care is given in collaboration with physicians and may use standard order sets

B. Problems encountered by client in a critical care setting

1. Anxiety
   a. Is related to fear of death and the unknown for both client and family
   b. Change in health status is frequently due to an unexpected and unfamiliar stressor; clients' usual coping mechanisms are often ineffective initially
   c. Anxiety may be increased because of unfamiliar surroundings, care providers, and technology to which they are exposed
   d. Overt and covert client symptoms can include verbalization of feelings of fear and excessive concern for family, restlessness, irritability, preoccupation with surroundings and asking many questions, rapid speech, physiologic symptoms of increased heart rate (HR), hyperventilation, nausea, vomiting, and palpitations
   e. Encourage client to discuss concerns about situation and anticipated outcomes
   f. Introduce all interdisciplinary care providers involved in client's care and thoroughly discuss plan of care with client and family to alleviate anxiety
   g. Allow family to participate in client care as appropriate; encourage use of touch, relaxation, and imagery therapies and manage physiological symptoms as prescribed

2. Impaired communication
   a. May occur because of physical barriers such as ET intubation, new tracheostomy, or as a sequelae of trauma
   b. Cultural and language differences may also make communication difficult and anxiety producing
   c. Preexisting conditions (such as inability to read or write or new sensory, motor, and neurological conditions such as hearing or visual impairment or new onset stroke), may also make it difficult for client and family to express needs and concerns
   d. First acknowledge client's communication concern
   e. Use reassurance and attempt to alleviate communication difficulties with such measures as translators, word cards, paper and pencil, picture cards, or facial or hand gestures
   f. Family may be an excellent source of information about client's usual communication methods
   g. Collaborate with client about method(s) to be used
   h. Communication among health care providers is also essential to successful client

3. Sleep deprivation
   a. Occurs because of alteration in usual sleeping pattern, lack of consistent periods of rapid eye movement (REM) and non-REM (NREM) sleep, care interventions and treatments, anxiety, and some medications
   b. Clinical signs of sleep deprivation may be restlessness, increased irritability or sensitivity to pain, confusion, hallucinations, decreased ability to concentrate or apparent excessive sleepiness

       c. Be aware of risk for or presence of this condition and make reasonable attempts to decrease causative factors

       d. Attempt to determine client's usual sleeping patterns such as body position, favorite bedtime routine, and sleeping pattern

       e. If possible, schedule nursing interventions, treatments, assessments, and family visits to allow for several 90-minute rest periods per day

       f. Make attempts to decrease stimulation by dimming lights, decreasing alarm limits within a safe range, providing soft music, providing ear plugs or eye covers

       g. Discourage staff from loud talking or activity in immediate vicinity of client's bed

       h. Provide pain relief as needed; nonpharmaceutical methods such as relaxation exercises, guided imagery and audiotapes may enhance rest

    4. ICU psychosis

       a. Is an acute confusional state that may develop in CC environment from many factors

       b. Commonly used drugs such as narcotics, anticholinergics, CNS stimulants and depressants, and steroids may cause a state of confusion

       c. Sleep deprivation, sensory overload, fluid and electrolyte imbalances, inadequate oxygenation, infection, head trauma, and underlying preexisting conditions such as confusion or chronic brain disorders also contribute

       d. Symptoms of loss of orientation, ability to reason, concentrate, or follow directions develop abruptly

       e. Client may attempt to remove all monitoring lines, catheters, and dressings while in a state of confusion

       f. Visual and auditory hallucinations may be observed

       g. Nursing management involves a multidisciplinary approach; collaboration with other health care providers to communicate with client is essential

       h. Treatment for physiological conditions should be aggressively pursued

       i. Frequently orient client to person, place, and time, provide reality orientation, and explain reason for presence in ICU, rationale and process of treatment

       j. Frequently explain noises and activities within environment

       k. Use measures to prevent or minimize sleep deprivation

       l. Provide medications as ordered and monitor for and report undesirable effects

  C. Common nursing procedures in critical care setting

    1. Hemodynamic monitoring

       a. Concepts important in hemodynamic monitoring

          1) *Cardiac output* (CO): volume of blood ejected from heart in 1 minute; it is determined by multiplying HR by stroke volume (mL of blood expelled per heartbeat); normal CO is 4–8 liters/minute

          2) *Preload*: amount of stretch in left ventricle just before ventricular contraction at end of diastole; is affected by volume of blood in left ventricle (which is influenced by venous return or amount of blood returned to ventricles); is measured by CVP on right side of heart and pulmonary artery wedge pressure (PAWP) on left side of heart

          3) *Afterload*: tension that ventricles must overcome to eject blood into arterial systems (pulmonary and aortic); is measured by systemic vascular resistance (SVR) on left side of heart and pulmonary vascular resistance (PVR) on right side of heart

          4) Cardiac index (CI): is CO divided by body surface area; is a better indicator of body's ability to perfuse tissues than CO; normal CI is 2.5–4.0 liters/minute/meters^2

       b. Types of hemodynamic monitoring

          1) Arterial lines

             a) Purpose: provide a direct, continuous intra-arterial measurement of BP (systolic, diastolic, and mean)

b) Methods and equipment: a 20-gauge arterial catheter is inserted into radial, brachial, or femoral artery and connected to high-pressure tubing leading to a pressure transducer and amplifier; transducer converts mechanical physiologic waves to electrical energy, which are displayed on a monitor screen as pressure waves and digitally read in mmHg; patency of arterial catheter is maintained by a saline flush infusion that may or may not be heparinized (flush is contained within a pressure bag at 300 mmHg; is connected to IV tubing and a 3-way stopcock); site is covered and maintained with a sterile dressing (see Figure 17-1)

c) Indications for use: clients requiring accurate perfusion pressures (low CO, excessive vasoconstriction, unstable conditions requiring vasopressor or vasodilator drug titration, or frequent ABG analysis)

d) Nursing management: level and calibrate or "zero" the system (normalize system to a built-in constant) at beginning of each shift to accurately trend readings; ensure no air is in transducer tubing; correlate arterial pressure readings with indirect sphygmomanometer pressures each shift; observe waveform at eye-level and assess for a sharp normal waveform frequently throughout shift; draw arterial blood samples through 3-way stopcock after aspirating approximately 5 mL blood and discarding specimen to prevent contamination by flush solution; flush line with valve flush device after completing blood collection; change sterile dressings and IV solution and tubing as needed or per hospital policy; usually IV solution is changed every 24 hours with tubing and dressing changes every 24–48 hours

e) Provider prescribes removal of arterial catheter; using sterile technique, remove catheter from artery with one smooth motion while applying direct pressure to site, use a dry sterile dressing and keep pressure on area for at least 5 minutes; then observe site for oozing or swelling and continue pressure if needed; after oozing stopped, apply a new dry sterile dressing and check site frequently for rebleeding; check distal pulses and motor and sensory function frequently for complications caused by thrombosis

!

Practice to Pass

Your client is to have an arterial line placed prior to surgery. What is the preferred site for placement?

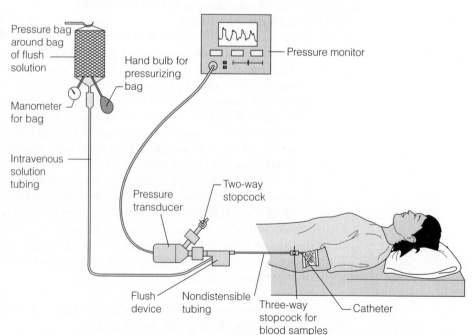

Figure 17-1

Components of a hemodynamic monitoring system

Pressure bag around bag of flush solution

Hand bulb for pressurizing bag

Pressure monitor

Manometer for bag

Intravenous solution tubing

Pressure transducer

Two-way stopcock

Flush device

Nondistensible tubing

Three-way stopcock for blood samples

Catheter

           f) Possible complications: bleeding from insertion site, hemorrhage, infection at insertion site or systemic, air embolus, thrombus formation; occlusion of circulation with loss of circulation distal to insertion site; perform Allen test (compress radial and ulnar arteries for 3–5 seconds, release pressure on ulnar artery and watch for brisk return of circulation to hand) before radial artery line insertion; frequently monitor distal pulses to decrease adverse effects

           g) Priority nursing problems: potential for reduced tissue perfusion, potential for infection, potential for reduced cardiac output

      2) Pulmonary artery (PA) or Swan-Ganz catheter

           a) Purpose: provide indirect measurement of left ventricular function to detect and treat cardiac and pulmonary changes

           b) Methods and equipment: a 5-lumen, balloon-tipped, flow-directed catheter connected to a pressure transducer and pressurized heparin flush system is inserted often through a subclavian or jugular vein and directed into right atrium; balloon tip is inflated in atrium to allow normal blood flow to carry catheter tip through tricuspid valve, right ventricle, pulmonary valve and into PA; once in PA, balloon is deflated and PA systolic, diastolic and mean pressures are recorded; balloon is again inflated until pulmonary capillary wedge pressure (PCWP) and waveform is obtained—may require up to 1.5 mL air; balloon is then completely deflated and locked to prevent accidental wedging and pulmonary infarction; perform ongoing cardiac monitoring because of risk for PVCs to develop from myocardial irritation during insertion; catheter is sutured in place and a dry sterile occlusive dressing is applied; a chest x-ray is done to check placement and ensure absence of pneumothorax

           c) Indications for use: when there is need to monitor PA pressure and/or PCWP that indirectly reflects left ventricular function; provide information about CO, tissue perfusion, and blood volume; obtain venous blood specimens; proximal ports can be used for continuous fluid or medication infusion

           d) Nursing assessment and management: level and secure transducer at **phlebostatic axis** (fourth intercostal space, mid-axillary line), which serves as reference point for right atrium; to ensure accurate readings ensure that system is free of air bubbles that will dampen waveform and digital measurement; zero and calibrate the system at least once a shift; maintain sterility with dressing and line changes; notify provider if waveforms dampen or evidence of a permanent wedge form develops; because line is present in heart, client is at risk for microshock and development of ventricular fibrillation

           e) Taking readings: record PA systolic and diastolic pressures (usually about 25/10 mmHg); to obtain a PCWP or left ventricular end-diastolic (LVEDP) reading, inflate catheter balloon slowly and watch for dampening of waveform that indicates wedging (normal 5–12 mmHg); after reading has been noted, allow balloon to fully deflate passively and lock it to prevent accidental wedging; take all readings at end of expiration

           f) Continue to monitor PA waveform, noting any inadvertent wedging; respond immediately to reposition catheter according to agency policy

           g) Potential complications: dysrhythmias, infection, air embolism, pneumothorax, catheter occlusion, or thrombus formation

           h) Priority nursing problems: potential for reduced tissue perfusion, potential for infection, potential for reduced cardiac output, potential for alterations in gas exchange, inadequate knowledge

2. Circulatory assist device (intra-aortic balloon pump, or IABP)
   a. Purpose: a counterpulsation device that augments CO to provide adequate tissue perfusion while allowing myocardium to rest and recover
   b. Methods and equipment: IABP is a mechanical circulatory support device consisting of a 30–40 mL balloon catheter and a console that mechanically inflates and deflates balloon; balloon is placed into descending aorta distal to subclavian artery via femoral artery and sutured in place; console is set to trigger balloon inflation during diastole and deflation during systole to decrease afterload and myocardial workload; initially, it is set to trigger with every client heartbeat (1:1) and, as myocardial strength improves, it can be decreased to 1:2, 1:4, or 1:8 intervals; inflation and deflation sequence is triggered by client's ECG pattern that is displayed on console
   c. Indications for use: cardiogenic shock, heart failure, support before heart transplantation, unstable angina and/or failure to wean from cardiopulmonary bypass after coronary artery bypass surgery
   d. Nursing management
      1) Assist with placement and maintain sterility with dressing changes
      2) Monitor and record effectiveness as indicated by increased CO, increased BP, increased UO, increased LOC, palpable peripheral pulses, improved ischemic ECG changes
      3) Monitor and record ECG rhythm, VS, heart and lung sounds, IABP settings, and waveforms
      4) Monitor neurovascular status in leg of insertion; keep affected leg straight at all times
      5) Client positioning; maintain stable position in bed; slight head of bed (HOB) elevation may minimize balloon migration while HOB greater than 30 degrees may decrease blood flow distal to catheter insertion site (causing lower extremity ischemia) or may crimp catheter itself; log roll client from side to side to reposition
      6) Because client will be receiving anticoagulants, monitor for signs of hematuria, excessive oozing from insertion or hemodynamic catheter sites, positive stool guaiac, bleeding gums or abnormal PT, PTT, or platelet counts
   e. Potential complications: air or foreign body embolus if balloon ruptures; thrombus formation at insertion site and loss of distal circulation; migration of catheter; dissection of aorta; sepsis; complications of immobility
   f. Priority nursing problems: potential for reduced tissue perfusion, potential for infection, potential for reduced cardiac output, interrupted skin integrity, inadequate knowledge
3. Airway maintenance adjuncts
   a. Endotracheal (ET) tube
      1) Purpose: to assist in maintaining a patent airway when client is unable to maintain an airway or requires mechanical ventilation
      2) Methods and equipment: a laryngoscope and blade are used to visualize vocal cords and trachea for insertion of ET; after insertion, ET cuff is inflated to ensure minimal occlusion and lungs are auscultated for bilateral breath sounds; ET position is marked at client's mouth and secured with twill or adhesive tape to prevent displacement; supplemental O_2 is delivered by t-piece or ventilator; ET placement is confirmed by chest x-ray
      3) Indications: inability to maintain an effective airway for oxygenation; presence of facial or neck trauma where swelling may cause potential airway obstruction; altered LOC; absence of gag or swallow reflex

4) Nursing management
  a) Gather equipment
  b) Check O_2 saturation, color, dysrhythmias, and hyperoxygenate using bag-valve-mask device prior to initiating 30-second attempt to place ET tube
  c) Assist with intubation by providing cricoid pressure during insertion of ET tube
  d) Evaluate bilateral lung sounds before inflating cuff to determine tube placement above carina (not in right mainstem bronchus)
  e) Monitor for cuff pressure, that tube placement remains as initially marked, and continued presence of bilateral breath sounds
  f) Provide oral and tracheal suctioning, mouth care (every 4 hours) and observe for development of pressure areas or ulceration around mouth
  g) Provide alternative communication means and emotional support
5) Potential complications: migration of tube causing airway obstruction; laryngeal damage due to prolonged intubation; accidental extubation; aspiration from inadequate cuff inflation
6) Priority nursing problems: possible reduced tissue perfusion, potential for infection or injury, potential for alterations in gas exchange, inadequate knowledge, anxiety, inability to verbally communicate

b. Tracheostomy
  1) Purpose: maintain an effective airway in clients who are unable do so or who require prolonged mechanical ventilation
  2) Method and equipment: tracheostomy placement requires surgical creation of a stoma into trachea; a sterile tracheal tube with obturator is inserted into incisional area and obturator is removed to allow for air passage; client is hyperoxygenated and suctioned using sterile technique; tracheostomy tube area is then cleansed and secured with twill tape or trach ties
  3) Indications: upper-airway trauma or obstruction; facial or neck trauma with risk for airway obstruction; head or neck surgery that may impair maintenance of an effective airway; or need for long-term mechanical ventilation
  4) Nursing management
    a) Explain procedure and rationale and assist with placement
    b) Keep the area clean with frequent dressing changes and suctioning to prevent infection after placement
    c) Maintain appropriate tracheal cuff inflation to prevent aspiration and prevent tracheal pressure necrosis
    d) Monitor respiratory status and monitor for signs of hemorrhage with new tracheostomy
    e) Perform routine cleansing of inner cannula and ostomy site
  5) Potential complications: accidental extubation; airway obstruction from dried secretions; hemorrhage from tracheostomy site; excessive secretions blocking tube; tracheal necrosis due to elevated cuff pressure
  6) Priority nursing problems: possible reduced cough, potential for reduced tissue perfusion, potential for infection, inadequate knowledge, anxiety

c. Mechanical ventilation
  1) Purpose: assist with breathing to provide for adequate gas exchange for tissue perfusion
  2) Method and equipment: ventilator that is connected to ET or tracheostomy tube
  3) Types of ventilators
    a) Positive-pressure volume-cycled, which exerts a positive pressure on airway delivering a predetermined volume of gas; this type allows for pressure and time limits to be set and is most common ventilator used

        b) Positive-pressure time-cycled ventilator, which exerts a positive pressure on airway, delivering a set volume of gas over a preset time

        c) Positive-pressure pressure-cycled ventilator, which exerts positive pressure on airway within pressure limits set to stop inspiration when that pressure is exceeded

        d) Positive-pressure jet ventilators, which exert a positive pressure on airway and deliver small volumes of gas at a very high rate

        e) Negative-pressure ventilators, which exert a negative pressure on external chest and do not require intubation (is rarely used today; an iron lung used for polio clients is an example)

4) Modes of ventilation

        a) Intermittent mandatory ventilation (IMV): delivers a preset tidal volume (V_T) at a preset rate despite client breathing spontaneously at his/her own rate and V_T

        b) Assist control ventilation (ACV): delivers a preset V_T for every breath set on machine as well as those initiated by client; allows for hyperventilation when needed

        c) Controlled mandatory ventilation (CMV): delivers a preset V_T at a preset rate and is most frequently used for clients with no ventilatory effort

        d) Synchronized intermittent mandatory ventilation (SIMV): delivers a preset, mandatory V_T that is synchronized to client's inspiratory effort; is the most common mode currently used

        e) Airway pressure release ventilation (APRV): a time-triggered pressure controlled mode that delivers a volume of gas to a preset inspiratory pressure and then allows exhalation to a second preset pressure at a preset time interval

5) Key ventilator settings

        a) Rate: number of breaths/minute delivered; is a number that is combined with mode frequently in clinical practice (for example, SIMV of 6/min)

        b) FiO_2: fraction of inspired O_2 or O_2 percent; is amount of O_2 in inhaled air via ventilator; is expressed as a decimal instead of a percentage for example, FiO_2 of 0.4 versus 40%)

        c) Tidal volume (V_T): amount of air delivered with each breath; often expressed in mL or liters (for example, 700 mL or 0.7 L)

        d) PEEP: abbreviation for *positive end expiratory pressure*; is the amount of positive pressure at end of exhalation; serves to keep alveoli open during exhalation to increase time for gas exchange to occur; is expressed as centimeters of pressure (for example, 5 cm)

6) Indications: ineffective breathing pattern or hypoxia (for example, dyspnea, cyanosis, altered mental status, absent breath sounds, tachycardia with no underlying cardiac disease); O_2 saturation levels of less than 80 mmHg, pH less than 7.35, $PaCO_2$ greater than 50 mmHg; tidal volumes less than 5 mL/kg, or minute volumes less than 10 L/min

7) Nursing management

        a) Position client for maximum alveolar ventilation and comfort; maintain soft restraints to avoid accidental extubation

        b) Monitor for any changes in respiratory status or effort

        c) Maintain ventilator settings as prescribed and troubleshoot ventilator alarms (high pressure frequently indicates need for suctioning or kinking or compression of ET; low pressure indicates leak or disconnection); manually ventilate client if alarms sound without apparent cause or problem cannot be fixed quickly; do not shut off alarms

        d) Monitor ABGs and maintain continuous O_2 saturation monitoring

        e) Complete a thorough physical assessment with emphasis on cardiac, neurological, and respiratory systems

        f) Administer antibiotics, neuromuscular blocking agents, and sedatives as ordered

        g) Maintain NG suction to prevent aspiration

        h) Supply nutritional support as ordered

        i) Perform frequent oral care and suctioning to maintain airway patency

        j) Provide emotional support to client and family and alternate communication method

    8) Potential complications: pneumothorax, GI stress ulcers, hypotension caused by decreased venous return from increased intrathoracic pressure, increased intracranial pressure, infection

    9) Priority nursing problems: alterations in gas exchange or respiratory pattern, ineffective cough, potential for infection, anxiety

D. Common complications seen in critical care setting

  1. Sepsis

    a. Description: a diffuse inflammatory systemic response to a chemical, mechanical, bacterial, or microbial assault; if untreated, can lead to shock

    b. Etiology and pathophysiology

      1) A bodily insult leads to an inflammatory response, which is intended to protect body from further injury and promote healing

      2) Vascular response consists of a massive release of histamine, prostaglandin, bradykinin, and other mediators, which cause vasodilation, increased capillary membrane permeability, and initiation of clotting cascade

      3) Maldistribution of circulating blood volume causes decreased cellular O_2 supply, impaired tissue perfusion and impaired cellular metabolism; impaired perfusion can be monitored by increasing saturation of central venous oxygenation ($ScvO_2$) and level less than 70% indicates significant problem with systemic O_2 delivery

      4) Severe sepsis, which is characterized by hypoperfusion, organ dysfunction, and hypotension, can lead to septic shock and death caused by multiple organ system failure

      5) In early sepsis (hyperdynamic phase), body attempts to compensate for decreasing oxygenation at cellular level; HR and RR increase and UO decreases because of shunting of blood to vital organs; body temperature increases as metabolic activity increases, and skin becomes warm and flushed because of vasodilation

      6) In late stage of sepsis, compensatory mechanisms begin to fail; SNS compensatory mechanisms cause extreme tachycardia but CO is low because of vasoconstriction and poor stroke volume; peripheral pulses become weak or absent and skin becomes cool, pale, and cyanotic (vasoconstriction); respirations become labored and decreased because of toxin accumulation and hypoxia in CNS; LOC decreases to coma because of severe hypoxia

    c. Assessment

      1) Clinical manifestations: early signs are fever greater than 38°C (100.4°F) or less than 36°C (96.8°F), tachypnea, hypocarbia, $ScvO_2$ less than 70%, tachycardia, restlessness, and hyperglycemia; late signs are diminished LOC, coma, respiratory failure, heart failure, and oliguria

      2) Diagnostic and laboratory findings

        a) WBCs increase initially because of inflammatory process and later decrease because of bone marrow exhaustion

      b) Glucose levels are high in early sepsis from glucogenesis and decrease in later sepsis because of hepatic failure

      c) Serum lactate levels are elevated because of cellular hypoxia, and renal, hepatic, and cardiac enzymes show abnormalities as organ systems begin to fail

      d) Blood cultures done early usually show causative agent and should direct antibiotic therapy regime

      e) ABGs demonstrate increasing metabolic acidosis and respiratory acidosis as respiratory failure occurs

      f) Clotting studies show increasing clotting times as clotting factors begin to be consumed beyond available reserves

      g) Chest x-ray and other radiographic studies may be used to determine site of underlying cause of infection

      h) Procalcitonin (PCT) level will be elevated, is often used in cases where there may be sepsis without real signs of infection, for example in client with severe burns

  d. Therapeutic management

    1) Directed at early recognition and resuscitation to resolve inadequate systemic O_2 delivery using $ScvO_2$ as measurement; goal of $ScvO_2$ should be at least 70% using these parameters and goals:

      a) Administer fluids to achieve a CVP of 8–12 mmHg

      b) Transfuse RBCs to achieve a hematocrit of at least 30%

      c) Use vasopressors such as dopamine (Intropin), norepinephrine (Levophed), or phenylephrine (Neosynephrine) to achieve a mean arterial pressure (MAP) of at least 60 mmHg

    2) Corticosteroids to treat relative adrenal insufficiency often accompanying severe sepsis

    3) Tight glycemic control to minimize glycation products and O_2-free radical formation

    4) Nutritional support to prevent tissue malnutrition

    5) Early antibiotic therapy with high-end dosing regimens considering pharmacokinetics

  e. Priority nursing problems: reduced tissue perfusion, reduced circulating volume, reduced cardiac output, hemodynamic instability, alterations in gas exchange, insufficient nutrients to meet bodily needs, fever, anxiety

  f. Planning and implementation

    1) Goal: provide collaborative supportive measures while antibacterial therapy is being administered

    2) Assist with establishing and managing ABCs; infuse IV solutions of NS or lactated Ringer's to maintain systolic BP above 100 mmHg and CVP of 5–10 mmHg

    3) Use continuous cardiac monitoring and 12-lead ECG to detect and manage dysrhythmias

    4) Use aseptic technique at all times to prevent further infectious processes and administer organism-specific antibiotics as ordered

    5) Keep client comfortable and begin attempts to reduce fever, such as use of antipyretics and hyperthermia measures

    6) Keep client and family informed of plan of care and procedures

  g. Medication therapy: antibiotics based on causative agent; antidysrhythmics to control cardiac dysrhythmias; positive inotropes such as dopamine and dobutamine, vasodilators such as nitroglycerine, and vasopressors such as epinephrine

      h. Evaluation: client is hemodynamically stable, normothermic, and free of dysrhythmias; antibiotic therapy is effective and no additional organ system injury has occurred; client and family state follow-up plan of care and preventive measures

  2. Multiple organ dysfunction syndrome (MODS), formerly called multiple system organ failure (MSOF)

      a. Description: failure of one or more body systems after a major insult to body, such as infection, trauma, or severe illness

      b. Etiology and pathophysiology

          1) Cause of MODS is some type of inflammatory response or infection, persistent hypotension, and hypoxia

          2) In general, as body responds to an uncontrolled inflammatory process, damage at organ system level results from hypoperfusion, hypoxia, and necrosis of tissue

          3) The 6 major organ systems affected most by MODS are pulmonary, renal, cardiovascular, hematological (coagulation), liver, and neurological

          4) Pulmonary dysfunction and development of acute respiratory distress syndrome (ARDS) result from pulmonary vascular endothelium and alveolar epithelial damage with resultant surfactant deficiency, mild pulmonary hypertension, and pulmonary edema and hypoxia

          5) Renal dysfunction results from prolonged hypovolemia, hypoperfusion, and acute tubular necrosis; nephrotoxic drugs used in resuscitation efforts intensify renal damage

          6) Cardiovascular dysfunction results from prolonged compensatory efforts to increase CO and vasoconstriction to enhance organ perfusion; during resuscitation efforts, cardiac function becomes vasopressor dependent and eventually becomes unresponsive even to vasopressor; another influence on myocardium is release of myocardial depressant factor (MDF) from pancreas

          7) Coagulation system failure is seen with disseminated intravascular coagulopathy (DIC), an uncontrolled excessive consumption of coagulation factors

          8) Liver bilirubin levels are affected and ability to synthesize substances is impaired, often leading to impaired clotting factor production, bilirubin clearance and low serum albumin level

          9) CNS change is seen as decreasing LOC, confusion and psychosis

      c. Assessment

          1) Clinical manifestations: general symptoms relate to organ system affected; all are a result of decreased O_2 supply, increased O_2 demands, and circulating toxins; there are 4 stages:

             a) Stage 1: Systemic inflammatory response syndrome (SIRS), with 2 or more of these: temp greater than $38°C$ or less than $36°C$, HR greater than 90. RR less than 20 breaths/min or $PaCO_2$ level less than 32 mmHg by ABG, WBC count greater than 12,000 cells/mcL or 10% bands

             b) Stage 2: Sepsis, includes SIRS, plus a documented positive culture

             c) Stage 3: Severe sepsis, includes Stage 2 plus organ impairment, hypotension or evidence of hypoperfusion

             d) Stage 4: Septic shock, includes Stage 3 changes with *both* hypotension and hypoperfusion; a Sequential Organ Failure Assessment (SOFA) score may be given to gauge severity

             e) GI: abdominal distention, paralytic ileus, diarrhea, and GI bleeding

             f) Pulmonary: tachypnea, pulmonary hypertension and ARDS

             g) Renal: worsening renal failure with oliguria, anuria, and rising BUN and creatinine levels

        h) Cardiovascular: early compensatory signs of tachycardia, increased CO and decreased SVR; in later stages there is increased SVR, decreased CO, and absent or weak peripheral pulses

        i) Decreasing LOC to coma

        j) Excessive bleeding and fibrinolysis

    2) Diagnostic and laboratory findings

        a) ABGs: severe acidosis with pH less than 7.35 and pCO_2 less than 32 mmHg

        b) WBC counts decreased and platelet counts less than $80,000/mm^3$

        c) Fibrinogen level decreased

        d) PT and PTT increase and hemoglobin and hematocrit show severe anemia

        e) Creatinine levels and BUN increase

        f) Cardiac and hepatic enzymes are elevated

        g) Serum potassium is severely elevated from cellular damage

        h) ECG findings show ST-segment changes indicating ischemia

        i) Chest x-ray show interstitial edema and hypoperfusion

  d. Therapeutic management

    1) Goals: support tissue oxygenation, reduce O_2 consumption, reduce organ system damage, control causative agent; specifically, client will receive supplemental O_2 and mechanical ventilation as symptoms of ARDS develop

    2) Give fluid resuscitation to maintain CVP of at least 8–10 mmHg

    3) Infuse blood and blood products including platelets and clotting factors to control bleeding and enhance O_2-carrying capacity

    4) Hemodialysis or hemofiltration filters waste products and excessive fluid volume

    5) Nutritional support enhances tissue regeneration and provides glucose stores

    6) Antibiotic therapy is used based upon causative agent

  e. Priority nursing problems: alterations in gas exchange, reduced tissue perfusion, risk for dehydration or fluid overload, insufficient nutrients to meet bodily needs, potential for infection, anxiety

  f. Planning and implementation

    1) Assess perfusion by monitoring LOC, VS, peripheral circulation and UO; titrate medications as ordered

    2) Provide hydration and nutritional support as prescribed with assessment of intestinal status, weight, and ability to tolerate supplemental feedings

    3) Carefully assess respiratory status, including adventitious breath sounds, effectiveness of supplemental O_2 and mechanical ventilation; provide meticulous oral care; suction as needed

    4) Continuously monitor cardiac rhythm and treat any dysrhythmias

    5) Monitor for signs of coagulation dysfunction; reduce bleeding potential by avoiding procedures that may interrupt skin integrity (such as IV starts, invasive procedures, or aggressive turning)

    6) Implement emotional and comfort measures (limit activities, provide a calm environment, reduce external stimuli as possible, and keep client and family informed of condition and plan of care)

  g. Evaluation: client is hemodynamically stable; respiratory status is improved without mechanical ventilation; signs of increased tissue perfusion and organ system healing are present; bleeding is controlled and UO is improving; client and family state understanding of follow-up care and preventive measures

3. Shock

  a. Description: a state of imbalance between O_2 supply and demand that leads to inadequate blood flow to organs, poor tissue perfusion, and possibly fatal cellular dysfunction

    b. Etiology and pathophysiology

        1) Etiology can be classified as due to loss of circulation volume (hypovolemic or hemorrhagic), decreased pump function (cardiogenic), or distributive (anaphylaxis, spinal cord injury [neurogenic], or overwhelming inflammatory response from infection [septic])

        2) All forms of shock cause reduction in oxygenation and tissue perfusion, which lead to cellular damage and eventual organ system failure because of hypoxia

        3) SNS and endocrine system attempt to compensate for loss of oxygenation capability

            a) A decrease in circulating volume in right atrium and near carotid artery and aortic baroreceptors stimulates massive release of norepinephrine, which stimulates SNS to increase HR and RR, increase glycolysis, decrease UO, shunt blood from less vital organs such as GI tract, liver and kidneys, and cause vasoconstriction

            b) Endocrine system attempts to increase circulating blood volume and O_2 carrying capacity by secreting high levels of ADH for water reabsorption; decreased renal blood flow also stimulates release of angiotensin II, which causes vasoconstriction and water reabsorption

            c) If initial compensatory responses do not restore homeostasis, further hypoperfusion and hypoxia lead to cellular death, which ultimately leads to multiple organ system failure and death

    c. Assessment

        1) Clinical manifestations will be varied

            a) In early stages of shock, body attempts to compensate for a decreased perfusion and oxygenation state

            b) Generally, early findings will reveal a normal BP, slightly increased pulse rate, normal or slightly decreased UO, slight restlessness, anxiety, and thirst

            c) During next stage (progressive shock state), classic shock symptoms are present: cool, clammy, and pale skin, decreased capillary refill, tachycardia, tachypnea, decreased BP, decreased CO, decreased temperature, decreased UO, decreasing LOC; metabolic acidosis will begin to develop

            d) During later stages of shock, signs of specific organ failure will be seen such as anuria, slow, thready pulse, ARDS, bleeding and coagulation dysfunction, and coma

        2) Diagnostic and laboratory findings

            a) Hemoglobin and hematocrit are decreased

            b) ABGs show an acidotic state

            c) Serum lactate and potassium levels are elevated

            d) Cardiac, hepatic, and GI enzymes are elevated

            e) Increased creatinine and BUN levels will indicate renal failure

            f) Serum glucose levels initially increase and then decrease as glucose stores are depleted

            g) Urine specific gravity is increased

            h) Clotting studies show depletion in fibrinogen, platelets, and other clotting factors; PT/PTT and fibrinogen split/degradation products (FSP/FDP) are elevated

            i) ECG shows ST ischemic changes

    d. Therapeutic management

        1) Goal is to restore O_2 delivery to tissues and decrease O_2 consumption

        2) First establish an effective airway and breathing pattern with supplemental O_2 and possible mechanical ventilation

        3) Next, establish, adequate circulating volume with IV infusion of NS, lactated Ringer's, or blood products if needed

               4) Use vasopressor, vasodilating, and positive inotropic medications to enhance CO and systemic perfusion

               5) Correct acidotic state and provide treatment of specific causative agent in the case of anaphylactic reaction or sepsis

       e. Priority nursing problems: alterations in gas exchange, reduced tissue perfusion, risk for dehydration or fluid overload (depending on cause), reduced cardiac output, potential for infection, anxiety

       f. Planning and implementations

               1) Assess perfusion by monitoring LOC, VS, peripheral circulation, and UO; titrate medications as ordered

               2) Complete careful respiratory assessment, including adventitious breath sounds, effectiveness of mechanical ventilation and supplemental O_2 administration methods; provide meticulous oral care and suctioning as needed

               3) Institute continuous cardiac monitoring to assess and treat cardiac dysrhythmias that may develop

               4) Monitor for signs of coagulation dysfunction; maintain strict intake and output records

               5) Document continual serial assessments of VS, LOC, hemodynamic status, and response to treatments and report changes to provider as needed

               6) Provide emotional and comfort measures such as limited activities, calm environment, reducing external stimuli, teaching about condition and plan of care

       g. Evaluation: adequate tissue perfusion as measured by hemodynamic stability, improved LOC and UO; bleeding is controlled; effective breathing pattern, resolved acidosis; client and family state understanding of plan of care and follow-up care needed

   4. Acute respiratory distress syndrome (ARDS)

       a. Description: a syndrome characterized by a noncardiac type of pulmonary edema and increasing hypoxemia despite treatment measures

       b. Etiology and pathophysiology (see Figure 17-2)

               1) Injury to alveolar and capillary membranes of lungs can be caused by aspiration of gastric contents or water, inhalation agents, embolism, endotoxins, or multiple trauma

               2) Fluid and protein then shift into alveoli and interstitial tissue

               3) With increase in edema, terminal bronchioles collapse and alveolar space fills with fluid

               4) Lung compliance and functional residual capacity decrease, dead space increases, and work of breathing begins to increase O_2 consumption while O_2 perfusion capability has decreased

       c. Assessment

               1) Clinical manifestations: labored respirations, restlessness, and dry, nonproductive cough are early symptoms of ARDS; cyanosis, pallor, adventitious breath sounds, use of accessory muscles and retraction are late findings

               2) Diagnostic and laboratory findings: chest x-ray will initially appear normal and then progress to complete "white out" with bilateral diffuse infiltrates; pulmonary function tests show decreased compliance, lung capacity and elevated peak inspiratory pressures; ABGs initially show respiratory alkalosis (hyperventilation) and then respiratory acidosis; elevated PA systolic and diastolic pressures with a normal PCWP/LVEDP

       d. Therapeutic management

               1) Provide O_2 therapy and mechanical ventilation in late stages

               2) Neuromuscular blocking agents and sedation may be needed to allow client to tolerate mechanical ventilation

Practice to Pass

Medical and nursing management of the client exhibiting signs of shock are directed toward what three concerns?

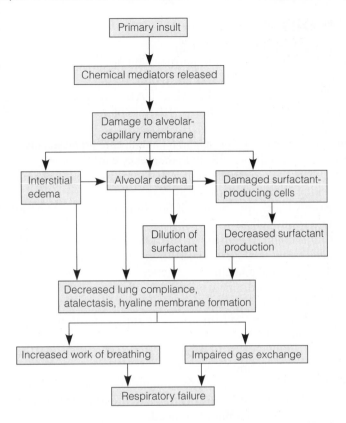

Figure 17-2

Cascade of pathophysiology events in ARDS

3) Fluid therapy: crystalloids and colloids to maintain intravascular volume

4) Use hemodynamic monitoring to assess pulmonary and cardiac function

5) Treat underlying cause of ARDS (use antibiotics if infection present)

6) Provide nutritional support with positive protein balance for healing

7) Administer prescribed corticosteroids to stabilize cellular membranes and decrease fluid shifts

8) Initiate support of other body systems to prevent further damage

e. Priority nursing problems: alterations in gas exchange, reduced tissue perfusion, inability to endure activity, potential for infection, insufficient nutrients to meet bodily needs

f. Planning and implementation

1) Assist and maintain mechanical ventilation

2) Monitor O_2 saturation; provide thorough suctioning, oral care, and sedation as needed to tolerate mechanical ventilation

3) Administer diuretic therapy and nutritional support as ordered

4) Monitor effectiveness of treatment plan through serial assessments of VS, heart, lung and bowel sounds, ECG rhythm, UO, and neurological status

5) Position client for comfort, turn frequently, and elevate head of bed to enhance respiratory effort

6) Schedule rest periods to conserve energy

7) Keep client and family informed of plan of care and prognosis

g. Evaluation: client demonstrates improved oxygenation and gas exchange; further organ system failure is decreased; family and client state understanding of prognosis and plan of care

IV. BASIC LIFE SUPPORT

A. Overview of basic life support (BLS)

1. Is a mechanical attempt to perfuse vital organs, especially brain; also known as cardiopulmonary resuscitation (CPR)
2. Follows a series of steps known as CAB (circulation, airway, and breathing), which is American Heart Association's 2010 revision to old ABC (airway, breathing, circulation) of resuscitation

B. Summary of adult basic life support for health care professionals

1. Recognize need for CPR and emergency cardiac care
   a. Determine unresponsiveness by tapping or gently shaking client's shoulder and asking loudly, "Are you okay?"
   b. Briefly check for absence of breathing or abnormal breathing while checking unresponsiveness
   c. Call for help or activate emergency medical system (EMS); dial 911 if outside a health care facility; use institutional policy for calling a code or in-house response team if inside a health care agency
   d. Retrieve an automatic external defibrillator (AED) if readily available or send someone else to do so
   e. Place client on flat firm surface in supine position
2. C = Circulation
   a. Place 2 or 3 fingers on Adam's apple and slide fingers into groove between Adam's apple and neck muscle
   b. Palpate for carotid pulse for minimum of 5 seconds but not more than 10 seconds
   c. If pulse is present, assess airway and breathing; provide rescue breathing at rate of 10–12 breaths per minute if needed
   d. If no pulse is present, begin external cardiac compressions
      1) Using hand closest to client's feet, place heel of hand at nipple line and place second hand on top of first
      2) Place middle finger on notch and index finger next to middle finger
      3) Place heel of opposite hand next to index finger (hand position is now on lower half of sternum); proper positioning is critical for success of CPR and to avoid injuring client
      4) Position own body directly over hands, with shoulders above hands, and elbows straight
      5) Provide compressions at rate of at least 100/minute and at depth of at least 2 inches; 2010 AHA guidelines state to "push hard, push fast," and allow chest to recoil after each compression (AHA, 2010, p. 5).
      6) Use a 30:2 compression to ventilation ratio for either 1- or 2-rescuer CPR; change positions for "switch" as needed after 5 cycles of 30:2
   e. Do not interrupt chest compressions for more than 10 seconds at a time except for defibrillation or intubation; interruptions for rescue breaths should take less than 10 seconds; "switches" during 2-person CPR should take less than 5 seconds
   f. When automated external defibrillator (AED) is available, continue CPR while AED pads are being placed on chest and stop CPR only when AED is analyzing cardiac rhythm
3. A = Airway
   a. Use gloves and barrier device if available
   b. Open airway using head tilt-chin lift method by lifting chin with 2 fingers while pushing down on forehead with other hand; kneel parallel to client's sternum
   c. If head or neck (cervical spine) injury is suspected or has occurred, use jaw thrust maneuver to open airway by lifting mandible on both sides with fingertips while positioning hands on sides of client's face; kneel at client's head

Practice to Pass

What assessment findings indicate a need for cardiopulmonary resuscitation?

4. B = Breathing
   a. Inadequate or absent breathing
   1) If client is not breathing adequately, maintain head tilt-chin lift and give 2 rescue breaths at rate of 1 second/breath; use breath sufficient to produce a rise in chest
   2) If chest does not rise with breath, reposition airway and try again (incorrect airway position is most common cause of obstructed rescuer ventilations)
   3) If chest still does not rise and fall, perform finger sweep of mouth to check for foreign body; clear airway and try again; remove dentures only if obstructing airway
   4) Provide one breath every 5–6 seconds or 10–12 breaths per minute; allow time to exhale between ventilations (rescue breathing)
   b. Breathing client
   1) If client is breathing adequately and has suspected or actual head or neck trauma, do not move client
   2) If client is breathing adequately and does not have suspected head or neck trauma, logroll client onto side as a unit (maintaining alignment of spine) and continue to monitor; this position is also called recovery position
   c. Improper ventilation technique could lead to ineffective ventilations or gastric distention
   d. Use mouth-to-nose ventilation if mouth cannot be sealed, has serious injuries, or cannot be opened for any reason
   e. Use mouth-to-stoma ventilation after temporary tracheostomy or laryngectomy; seal client's mouth and nose to ensure adequate ventilation
C. Summary of pediatric BLS for health care providers
   1. Overview
   a. Principles are same as for adult CPR; differences relate to smaller body size and needs of client
   b. Use child CPR if client is age 1 to 8
   c. Use infant CPR for clients less than 1 year old
   2. Circulation
   a. Check carotid or femoral pulse for child and brachial or femoral pulse for infant (health care providers only, not lay rescuers)
   b. Provide compressions at ratio of 30 compressions to 2 breaths for both child and infant CPR; when there are 2 health care provider rescuers, may use a 15:2 ratio
   c. Maintain rate of at least 100 compressions per minute for both child and infant CPR; same as for adult
   d. Use heel of 1 hand or 2 hands for compressions to child with compression depth of at least 1/3 of anterior-posterior (AP) diameter of chest (about 2 inches or 5 cm); use same hand placement as adult
   e. Use middle and ring fingers for compressions to infant at a depth of at least 1/3 AP diameter of chest (about 1.5 inches or 4 cm)
   f. Determine correct hand placement for infant by placing index finger of hand furthest from infant's head on sternum just below an imaginary line between nipples; lower middle and ring fingers onto sternum and then lift index finger; provide compressions with middle and ring fingers
   3. Airway: open airway using head tilt-chin lift method (infant and child)
   4. Breathing
   a. After checking breathing, if needed, provide 2 rescue breaths initially for both infant and child CPR with visible chest rise (same as for adult client); cover mouth and nose with infant breaths

        b. After initial 2 breaths, provide 2 breaths after each 30 compressions for both child and infant with single rescuer

        c. Deliver a breath every 3–5 seconds for a total ventilation rate of 12–20 breaths per minute

D. Foreign Body Airway Obstruction

  1. Adult or child who is choking

    a. Conscious

      1) Ask client, "Are you choking?" (will not be able to cough or speak with severe or complete airway obstruction; will also have increasing respiratory distress and developing cyanosis)

      2) Encourage client to cough if crowing noise is heard (partial obstruction)

      3) Use Heimlich maneuver (stand behind client; encircle client with arms; make fist with one hand above umbilicus and below xiphoid process; deliver upward and inward thrusts with fist until client becomes unconscious or blockage is relieved)

    b. Unconscious (health care provider directions)

      1) Place client on back

      2) Proceed to sequence for chest compressions

      3) Observe for breathing; if chest does not rise, return to compressions

      4) Repeat sequence until obstruction is cleared

  2. Infant who is choking

    a. Conscious

      1) Observe respiratory difficulty in infant

      2) Use series of 5 back blows and 5 chest thrusts on infant (positioned with head lower than trunk) until relieved

      3) Check mouth of infant for foreign object after each series, but avoid blind finger sweeps that could push obstruction further into airway

    b. Unconscious

      1) Assess unconsciousness of infant

      2) Institute sequence of chest compressions

      3) Assess breathing and observe for foreign object; remove if seen

      4) Attempt ventilation

      5) Repeat CAB sequence until successful or code team or EMS personnel arrive

  3. Pregnant or obese client who is choking

    a. Conscious

      1) Stand behind client and put own arms around client's chest

      2) Place fist on middle of sternum between nipples (be sure to avoid xiphoid process)

      3) Grasp fist with other hand and deliver firm backward thrusts until object is removed or victim becomes unconscious

    b. Unconscious

      1) Position victim lying on back; use a small pillow or wedge under right hip of pregnant client to shift uterus to left side of abdomen

      2) Institute chest compressions using ratio of 30 compressions to 2 ventilations

      3) Assess breathing and observe for obstruction; remove if seen

      4) Attempt to ventilate

      5) Repeat CAB sequence until successful or code team or EMS personnel arrive

E. Nursing role during a code

1. Call code: upon finding client and confirming need for assistance, initiate calling code team per hospital or agency protocol
2. Ensure appropriate CPR procedure is done
3. Once team and equipment has arrived, ensure placement of backboard under client and effective placement of cardiac monitor, defibrillator, medication and supply cart or "code cart"
4. Determine who is the team leader so that all will know who is responsible for code management
5. Assist as needed with airway management and IV access and provide for timely administration of medications, treatments, and transportation of labs as indicated
6. Assist with dysrhythmia recognition, defibrillation, and treatment as needed
7. Continue making serial assessments of client
8. Document in a thorough and concise manner all actions and responses during code process
9. Crowd control: all persons not actively participating in code should be excluded from the vicinity
10. Assist with psychosocial needs of family, roommates, and staff after a code

Practice to Pass

Your client's monitor is showing ventricular tachycardia. The client is unresponsive, and has no pulse or blood pressure. What would your immediate response be?

Case Study

A client presents to the emergency department reporting of "accidental overdose" of acetaminophen. You are working in the department.

1. What would the triage category be for this client?
2. What are the priorities in treating this client?
3. What methods could be utilized to decrease absorption of this medication?
4. What would be 3 priority nursing problems for this client?
5. What would be 3 evaluation criteria indicating successful treatment of this client?

For suggested responses, see pages 626–627.

POSTTEST

POSTTEST

❶ A client suddenly becomes unresponsive and pulse-less. The cardiac monitor shows this rhythm. What is the first action the nurse should take?

1. Administer sodium bicarbonate for developing acidosis.
2. Initiate cardiopulmonary resuscitation (CPR).
3. Immediately defibrillate the client.
4. Administer oxygen.

❷ The nurse is caring for a client who had a chest tube placed for treatment of an open pneumothorax caused by a stab wound. In what chamber of the chest drainage system will blood from the injury accumulate? Draw an "X" in the correct area on the image shown.

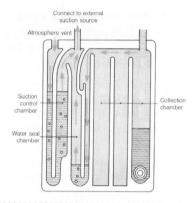

❸ The nurse prepares a client for insertion of a pulmonary artery catheter. Preprocedure teaching for this client will include which of the following statements?

1. "The catheter will assist in directly monitoring your systemic arterial pressure."
2. "The catheter will provide direct information about your cardiac output."
3. "The catheter will provide indirect information about your left ventricular function."
4. "The catheter will provide indirect information about your right ventricular function."

❹ The nurse suspects that the client is in cardiogenic shock based upon which of the following findings?

1. Decreased or muffled heart sounds
2. Cardiac index > 3.2 L/min/m^2
3. Bounding pulses
4. Cardiac output 5 L/min

❺ The nurse is caring for a client with a diagnosis of acute myocardial infarction (AMI). The client's cardiac alarm sounds, and the nurse assesses the client, who is unresponsive, pulseless, and not breathing. Which of the following rhythms is the client likely to be in when placed on a monitor? Select all that apply.

1. Supraventricular tachycardia
2. Atrial flutter
3. Ventricular fibrillation
4. Asystole
5. Pulseless electrical activity

❻ During the insertion of a pulmonary artery (Swan-Ganz) catheter, the client reports shortness of breath and the nurse notes labored respirations, decreased breath sounds on the side of the insertion, and asymmetrical chest movement. The nurse recognizes these manifestations as characteristic of which complication?

1. Pulmonary embolism
2. Myocardial infarction
3. Pneumothorax
4. Anxiety

❼ A client presents in acute respiratory distress after an automobile collision. The nurse observes that the client has facial trauma. The most urgent nursing diagnosis for this client would be which of the following?

1. Impaired Gas Exchange
2. Ineffective Airway Clearance
3. Decreased Cardiac Output
4. Anxiety

❽ A client presents with circumferential burns to the chest and shortness of breath following an electrical burn injury. The nurse identifies that the priority nursing diagnosis for *this* injury would be which of the following?

1. Deficient Fluid Volume
2. Risk for Injury
3. Ineffective Breathing Pattern
4. Decreased Cardiac Output

9 A client is brought to the emergency department after being found with a body temperature of 106°F. The client is unresponsive, hypotensive, and tachypneic. A medical diagnosis of heat stroke is made. What would be the nurse's priority nursing intervention in the care of this client?

1. Obtain a health history and assessment.
2. Obtain an oral temperature to monitor effectiveness of treatment.
3. Contact next of kin for any advance directives.
4. Remove all clothing, wrap in wet sheets, and cool with fans.

10 The nurse is preparing to assist with endotracheal intubation of a client. In what order will the following actions occur? Place the following choices in order from first to fifth.

1. Obtain chest x-ray.
2. Obtain informed consent.
3. Secure endotracheal tube.
4. Insertion of endotracheal tube.
5. Auscultate for bilateral breath sounds.

➤ *See pages 608–610 for Answers and Rationales.*

ANSWERS & RATIONALES

Pretest

1 **Answer: 4** **Rationale:** Excessive blood loss will result in the development of shock symptoms such as tachycardia, cool, clammy skin, and changes in mental status, because hypovolemia leads to vasoconstriction and shunting of blood to the central circulation. Applying ice to lower the body temperature would not be appropriate since the body temperature is usually decreased with hypovolemia. Measures to decrease circulation to the affected extremity, such as elevation of that extremity to heart level would be appropriate, although elevating it further could lead to ischemia. A psychiatric evaluation would be appropriate after the client has become hemodynamically stable. **Cognitive Level:** Applying **Client Need:** Physiological Adaptation **Integrated Process:** Nursing Process: Implementation **Content Area:** Adult Health **Strategy:** Consider the ABCs (airway, breathing, and circulation). After these have been addressed, additional interventions can be implemented safely. **Reference:** Wagner, K., Johnson, K., & Hardin-Pierce, M. (2010). *High acuity nursing* (5th ed.). Upper Saddle River, NJ: Pearson Education, p. 871.

2 **Answer: 4** **Rationale:** In a tension pneumothorax air enters the pleural space but is unable to escape. Tracheal and mediastinal shifting will occur to the uninjured side because of increased intrathoracic pressure on the side of the injury. The client will exhibit hypotension caused by the decreased cardiac output (related to pressure on the heart and great vessels). As tidal volume decreases there will be a decrease in gas exchange. The hypoxemia will cause an increase in the respiratory rate. Frothy pink mucous is a characteristic of pulmonary edema, not of a pneumothorax. Mediastinal shift is always a late sign and requires immediate treatment to relieve the buildup of trapped air to prevent death. **Cognitive Level:** Analyzing **Client Need:** Physiological Adaptation **Integrated Process:** Nursing Process: Assessment **Content Area:** Adult Health **Strategy:** This question requires an understanding of the

pathophysiology of a tension pneumothorax. Apply this pathophysiology to each distracter to determine the correct response. **Reference:** Wagner, K., Johnson, K., & Hardin-Pierce, M. (2010). *High acuity nursing* (5th ed.). Upper Saddle River, NJ: Pearson Education, pp. 284–285.

3 **Answer: 2** **Rationale:** The expiratory phase of respiration is prolonged, caused by the air trapping and alveoli distention that occurs as a result of the anaphylactic response. Pulsus paradoxus (an exaggerated decrease of the systolic blood pressure during inspiration) is seen with obstructive shock due to cardiac tamponade. Petechiae are seen with thrombocytopenia. Distant heart sounds are associated with cardiogenic shock states and cardiac tamponade. **Cognitive Level:** Analyzing **Client Need:** Physiological Adaptation **Integrated Process:** Nursing Process: Assessment **Content Area:** Adult Health **Strategy:** Selecting the correct response requires an understanding of what happens to the airway during an allergic response. Use nursing knowledge and the process of elimination to make a selection. **Reference:** Wagner, K., Johnson, K., & Hardin-Pierce, M. (2010). *High acuity nursing* (5th ed.). Upper Saddle River, NJ: Pearson Education, p. 484.

4 **Answer: 3, 1, 4, 5, 2** **Rationale:** First assess the client's lung sounds. If adventitious lung sounds are not present, suctioning may not be necessary. If suctioning is necessary hyperoxygenate before suctioning to avoid dangerous drops in oxygen saturation. Insert the catheter without suction. Then apply suction intermittently as the catheter is withdrawn. Monitor for adverse effects of suctioning after the procedure is completed. **Cognitive Level:** Applying **Client Need:** Basic Care and Comfort **Integrated Process:** Nursing Process: Implementation **Content Area:** Adult Health **Strategy:** Picture the steps of the procedure and choose the order in which they would be completed. **Reference:** Wagner, K., Johnson, K., & Hardin-Pierce, M. (2010). *High acuity nursing* (5th ed.). Upper Saddle River, NJ: Pearson Education, p. 322.

5 **Answer: 1, 2, 3** **Rationale:** Infection (such as sepsis) is the most common cause of multiple organ dysfunction syndrome (MODS). Hemorrhage and respiratory failure are other causes. Primary MODS is believed to be the result of inadequate oxygen delivery to cells and a failure of the microcirculation to remove metabolic end products as seen with hypoxemia or hemorrhage. Head trauma and diabetic ketoacidosis do not place a client at risk for MODS. **Cognitive Level:** Analyzing **Client Need:** Physiological Adaptation **Integrated Process:** Nursing Process: Assessment **Content Area:** Adult Health **Strategy:** Recall that multiple organ dysfunction syndrome (MODS) is most commonly the result of infection, hemorrhage, or hypoxemia. Identify disorders that fit these categories. **Reference:** Wagner, K., Johnson, K., & Hardin-Pierce, M. (2010). *High acuity nursing* (5th ed.). Upper Saddle River, NJ: Pearson Education, pp. 497–500.

6 **Answer: 1** **Rationale:** Human bites are considered highly contaminated wounds because of the bacteria present in the oral cavity. Antibiotics are ordered prophylactically and are usually begun by the IV route prior to discharge. A pressure dressing may be applied to the site after cleaning and application of triple antibiotic ointment. Neither administration of antivenom nor application of a tourniquet is an appropriate intervention for a human bite. **Cognitive Level:** Analyzing **Client Need:** Physiological Adaptation **Integrated Process:** Nursing Process: Planning **Content Area:** Adult Health **Strategy:** The oral cavity has multiple organisms endemic to the area. Eradication of the risks associated with these organisms is the immediate priority. **Reference:** Ball, J. W., Bindler, R. M. W., & Cowen, K. (2010). *Child health nursing: Partnering with children and families* (2nd ed.). Upper Saddle River, NJ: Pearson Education, pp. 1541–1542.

7 **Answer: 3** **Rationale:** Evaluate the pH first to determine acidosis or alkalosis. Then evaluate $PaCO_2$ as the respiratory component and HCO_3^- as the metabolic component. The client's pH < 7.35 and $PaCO_2$ > 45 mmHg indicate a state of respiratory acidosis and indicate that the client is not tolerating the weaning process. Metabolic alkalosis would be indicated by a pH > 7.45 and a HCO_3^- >26 mEq/L. Respiratory alkalosis would be seen in a client with a pH > 7.45 with a $PaCO_2$ < 35 mmHg. Metabolic acidosis would be indicated in a client with a pH < 7.35 with a HCO_3^- < 21 mEq/L. **Cognitive Level:** Analyzing **Client Need:** Reduction of Risk Potential **Integrated Process:** Nursing Process: Assessment **Content Area:** Adult Health **Strategy:** Determine if the results are acidic or basic then eliminate distracters that do not reflect this. Then use the PCO_2 and HCO_3 to determine if it is a respiratory or metabolic problem. **Reference:** Berman, A. J., & Snyder, S. (2011). *Kozier and Erb's fundamentals of nursing: Concepts, process, and practice* (9th ed.). Upper Saddle River, NJ: Prentice Hall, pp. 1457–1458, 1467–1469.

8 **Answer: 2** **Rationale:** A client in pulseless ventricular tachycardia has a life-threatening dysrhythmia that will cause irreversible brain injury within minutes because of a lack of effective circulation. Immediate defibrillation and CPR should be completed. Premature ventricular contractions are of greater concern if they are multifocal rather than unifocal. A client with frostbite injury needs attention rapidly, but this would not precede the need for resuscitation in a cardiac arrest. An escharotomy releases pressure within a compartment and restores circulation to the hand. This is a helpful treatment. **Cognitive Level:** Analyzing **Client Need:** Management of Care **Integrated Process:** Nursing Process: Planning **Content Area:** Adult Health **Strategy:** Consider life-threatening options first. These often involve airway, breathing, or circulation. Consider which client best meets these criteria. **Reference:** Wagner, K., Johnson, K., & Hardin-Pierce, M. (2010). *High acuity nursing* (5th ed.). Upper Saddle River, NJ: Pearson Education, pp. 401–402.

9 **Answer: 2** **Rationale:** Asking the client if he can speak establishes that the client has something in his airway and does not have a patent airway. The ability to speak or cough strongly indicates that the airway is clear or only partially obstructed. Calling a code, beginning CPR, or performing the Heimlich maneuver would not be appropriate initial interventions until the status of the airway is assessed. **Cognitive Level:** Applying **Client Need:** Physiological Adaptation **Integrated Process:** Nursing Process: Assessment **Content Area:** Adult Health **Strategy:** Review the ABCs (airway, breathing, and circulation) and the procedures involved with the Heimlich maneuver or CPR. Use the process of elimination, recalling that it is important not to interfere with a client who has a functional airway, so this must be assessed first. **Reference:** Berman, A. J., & Snyder, S. (2011). *Kozier and Erb's fundamentals of nursing: Concepts, process, and practice* (9th ed.). Upper Saddle River, NJ: Pearson Education, p. 735.

10 **Answer: 1, 2, 5** **Rationale:** A pericardiocentesis is not always a definitive treatment. After a pericardiocentesis is performed, the nurse must assess for the recurrence of the cardiac tamponade. This could be evidenced by muffled heart sounds, decreased blood pressure, and jugular venous distention. A sudden drop in heart rate and inspiratory crackles are not part of this clinical picture. **Cognitive Level:** Applying **Client Need:** Reduction of Risk Potential **Integrated Process:** Nursing Process: Assessment **Content Area:** Adult Health **Strategy:** Review the clinical presentation of pericardial tamponade and the effectiveness of a pericardiocentesis. **Reference:** Wagner, K., Johnson, K., & Hardin-Pierce, M. (2010). *High acuity nursing* (5th ed.). Upper Saddle River, NJ: Pearson Education, p. 459.

Posttest

1 **Answer: 3** **Rationale:** The dysrhythmia shown is ventricular fibrillation, the most common cause of sudden death. Defibrillation is the definitive treatment for this life-threatening arrhythmia when a defibrillator is immediately accessible. CPR would be used if defibrillation is not successful in converting this arrhythmia. Oxygen should be administered but does not take priority over defibrillation; sodium bicarbonate is used to treat acidosis that may develop with prolonged CPR but also does not take priority. **Cognitive Level:** Analyzing **Client Need:** Physiological Adaptation **Integrated Process:** Nursing Process: Implementation **Content Area:** Adult Health **Strategy:** The correct answer choice is the definitive treatment for this dysrhythmia. Use specific nursing knowledge to make your selection. **Reference:** Wagner, K., Johnson, K., & Hardin-Pierce, M. (2010). *High acuity nursing* (5th ed.). Upper Saddle River, NJ: Pearson Education, pp. 401–402.

2 **Answer:**

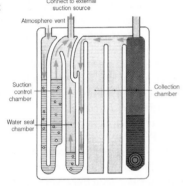

Rationale: The largest chamber of the chest drainage system is connected to the chest tube and collects drainage, including blood, from the chest tube. **Cognitive Level:** Applying **Client Need:** Physiological Adaptation **Integrated Process:** Nursing Process: Evaluation **Content Area:** Adult Health **Strategy:** All chest drainage systems have a collection chamber, a water seal chamber, and a suction control chamber. Of these, the collection chamber will be the largest. **Reference:** Wagner, K., Johnson, K., & Hardin-Pierce, M. (2010). *High acuity nursing* (5th ed.). Upper Saddle River, NJ: Pearson Education, pp. 288, 878.

3 **Answer: 3** **Rationale:** A pulmonary artery catheter will provide information about the function of the left ventricle when the balloon is wedged and is the most global response. It does provide direct information (not indirect information) about right ventricular function because it can measure central venous pressure. The pulmonary artery catheter does not directly determine the cardiac output or cardiac index. An arterial line is used to directly monitor the client's arterial pressure. **Cognitive Level:** Applying **Client Need:** Reduction of Risk Potential **Integrated Process:** Nursing Process: Implementation **Content Area:** Adult Health **Strategy:** Eliminate answer choices that are inconsistent with the direct actions of a pulmonary artery catheter and choose a global answer. **Reference:** Wagner, K., Johnson, K., & Hardin-Pierce, M. (2010). *High acuity nursing* (5th ed.). Upper Saddle River, NJ: Pearson Education, p. 352.

4 **Answer: 1** **Rationale:** Cardiogenic shock is caused by a decrease in pumping ability of the myocardium. The decrease can be caused by a weakened myocardium or

restriction of the myocardium by fluid or blood. Decreased or muffled heart sounds would be indicative of a fluid restriction in the pericardial sac, causing restriction of the heart's ability to pump effectively. Decreased pumping ability would cause a decrease in the cardiac index (normal 2.5–4.0 L/min/m^2), thready, weak pulses, and decreased cardiac output (normal 4 to 8 liters/minute). **Cognitive Level:** Analyzing **Client Need:** Physiological Adaptation **Integrated Process:** Nursing Process: Assessment **Content Area:** Adult Health **Strategy:** The correct answer choice is related to one of the mechanical causes of cardiogenic shock. Eliminate answer choices that are inconsistent with the shock state. **Reference:** Wagner, K., Johnson, K., & Hardin-Pierce, M. (2010). *High acuity nursing* (5th ed.). Upper Saddle River, NJ: Pearson Education, pp. 335, 479–480.

5 **Answer: 3, 4, 5** **Rationale:** In ventricular fibrillation, asystole, or pulseless electrical activity there is no effective electrical activity in either the atria or ventricles. As a result, the client is unresponsive, pulseless, and not breathing. The other rhythms demonstrate possible or actual effective ventricular contraction. **Cognitive Level:** Analyzing **Client Need:** Reduction of Risk Potential **Integrated Process:** Nursing Process: Assessment **Content Area:** Adult Health **Strategy:** Consider the rhythms that are likely to occur when a client presents in cardiac arrest. The wording of the question indicates that more than one option is correct. **Reference:** Wagner, K., Johnson, K., & Hardin-Pierce, M. (2010). *High acuity nursing* (5th ed.). Upper Saddle River, NJ: Pearson Education, pp. 401–402.

6 **Answer: 3** **Rationale:** The anatomical proximity of the apex of the lung and the subclavian vein increases the possibility of the development of a pneumothorax caused by accidental puncture of the lung. The client was demonstrating classic signs of pneumothorax. Pulmonary embolism, myocardial infarction, and anxiety do not cause asymmetrical chest movement. **Cognitive Level:** Analyzing **Client Need:** Reduction of Risk Potential **Integrated Process:** Nursing Process: Assessment **Content Area:** Adult Health **Strategy:** The principle being tested is that with any insertion of a central venous catheter there is a risk of collapsing the lung from a puncture during insertion. Select the answer option that is consistent with this complication. **Reference:** Wagner, K., Johnson, K., & Hardin-Pierce, M. (2010). *High acuity nursing* (5th ed.). Upper Saddle River, NJ: Pearson Education, pp. 285–286.

7 **Answer: 1** **Rationale:** Facial trauma can prevent the client from having a patent airway and lead to subsequent respiratory distress. Impaired gas exchange will occur as a result of the client's inability to maintain a patent airway. Decreased cardiac output can be a result of tissue hypoxia. Anxiety may be an appropriate diagnosis for this client, but is not the most life threatening. **Cognitive Level:** Analyzing **Client Need:** Physiological Adaptation **Integrated Process:** Nursing Process: Diagnosis **Content Area:** Adult Health **Strategy:** In any emergency situation always institute the ABCs to stabilize the client. This is especially true with injuries around the head and neck. **Reference:** Wagner, K., Johnson, K., & Hardin-Pierce, M. (2010). *High acuity nursing* (5th ed.). Upper Saddle River, NJ: Pearson Education, p. 802.

8 **Answer: 3** **Rationale:** Electrical burns cause massive soft tissue and muscle injury from the inside out. Circumferential burns to the chest wall will decrease chest expansion and ventilation and will compromise breathing. An ineffective breathing pattern is evident as a result of this injury. There is potential for further tissue damage, decreased cardiac output, and fluid volume deficit caused by hypoxia and edema formation for burn with third-spacing of fluids. However, breathing and airway are priorities in this case. **Cognitive Level:** Analyzing **Client Need:** Management of Care **Integrated Process:** Nursing Process: Diagnosis **Content Area:** Adult Health **Strategy:** This item is testing knowledge of the mechanism of injury for an electrical burn and the implications for the client. Select the answer option that reflects the extent of injury and associated risk. **Reference:** Wagner, K., Johnson, K., & Hardin-Pierce, M. (2010). *High acuity nursing* (5th ed.). Upper Saddle River, NJ: Pearson Education, p. 838.

9 **Answer: 4** **Rationale:** Heat stroke is a life-threatening situation, and interventions to cool the body must be accomplished quickly. Removing the clothing and cooling by evaporation is the most effective intervention to accomplish cooling quickly. A health assessment and communication are important, but only after the cooling

process has begun. Core body temperatures (not oral) will be utilized to monitor effectiveness of treatment. **Cognitive Level:** Applying **Client Need:** Physiological Adaptation **Integrated Process:** Nursing Process: Implementation **Content Area:** Adult Health **Strategy:** The immediate priority is to begin cooling the client so long-term damage or death is avoided. Select the distracter that indicates that this is the priority. **Reference:** Murray, R. B., Zentner, J. P., & Yakimo, R. (2009). *Health promotions strategies through the life span* (8th ed.). Upper Saddle River, NJ: Pearson Education, pp. 650–651.

10 **Answer: 2, 4, 5, 3, 1** **Rationale:** Informed consent must be obtained before initiation of the procedure. The endotracheal tube is inserted after consent is obtained. Auscultation for equal breath sounds is done immediately after insertion to insure that the endotracheal tube is not positioned in the esophagus or in the right bronchus. The tube is not secured until initial placement is confirmed through auscultation of lung sounds. The chest x-ray is obtained after initial placement is confirmed by auscultation of lung sounds and the tube is secured. **Cognitive Level:** Analyzing **Client Need:** Reduction of Risk Potential **Integrated Process:** Nursing Process: Implementation **Content Area:** Adult Health **Strategy:** Consider requirements for procedures and actions that must be taken to prevent or identify complications. **Reference:** Wagner, K., Johnson, K., & Hardin-Pierce, M. (2010). *High acuity nursing* (5th ed.). Upper Saddle River, NJ: Pearson Education, pp. 219, 300–304.

References

American Heart Association (2010). *Highlights of the 2010 American Heart Association Guidelines for Cardiopulmonary Resuscitation and Emergency Cardiac Care.* Retrieved February 9, 2011, from http://www.heart.org/idc/groups/heart-public/@wcm/@ecc/documents/downloadable/ucm_317350.pdf.

Berman, A., Snyder, S., Kozier, B., & Erb, G. (2011). *Fundamentals of nursing: Concepts, process, and practice* (9th ed.). Upper Saddle River, NJ: Pearson Education.

Kee, J. F. (2010). *Laboratory and diagnostic tests with nursing implications* (8th ed.). Upper Saddle River, NJ: Prentice Hall.

D'Amico, D., & Barbarito, C. (2012). *Health & physical assessment in nursing.* Upper Saddle River, NJ: Pearson Education.

Lehne, R. (2010). *Pharmacology for nursing care* (7th ed.). St. Louis, MO: Saunders.

LeMone, P., & Burke, K. M., & Bauldoff, G. (2011). *Medical-surgical nursing: Critical thinking in patient care* (5th ed., Vol. Single). Upper Saddle River, NJ: Pearson Education.

Huether, S. E., & McCance, K. L., (2012). *Understanding pathophysiology:* (5th ed.). St. Louis, MO: Mosby.

Wagner, K., Johnson, K., & Kidd, P. (2010). *High acuity nursing* (5th ed.). Upper Saddle River, NJ: Pearson Education.

Appendix

➤ *Practice to Pass Suggested Answers*

Chapter 1

Page 8: *Suggested Answer*—To increase the ability to obtain an accurate health history, the nurse should do the following:

1. Determine if the client uses any sensory aids such as a hearing aid, reads lips, utilizes sign language, communicates in writing, or uses a companion for communication purposes; and utilize those methods as much as possible.
2. Convey presence in the room by approaching from the front or by a gentle touch to the shoulders.
3. Face the client at all times and speak in a normal tone and amplitude of voice. Increased volume and exaggerated articulation can cause distortion and misinterpretation of information.
4. Validate all information.

Page 11: *Suggested Answer*—The questions should be directed to obtain the following information:

- When did the nausea begin (i.e., time, setting)?
- What were you doing at the time and what had you recently eaten?
- Is pain associated with the nausea and, if so, where is the pain located?
- If there is pain, does it radiate anywhere?
- Are there foods, medications, and activities that aggravate or alleviate the nausea?
- How disruptive is the nausea to your normal activities?

Page 12: *Suggested Answer*—In general, the physical examination should proceed as usual with the following exceptions. Inspection of the abdomen will include an assessment of the status of the incisional area (drainage, redness, approximation, etc.). Auscultation should be completed next since palpation and percussion can cause activation of bowel activity and distort assessment findings. Percussion and palpation should be done in all quadrants as usual; however, it is advisable to assess the area of an incisional wound or an area of discomfort at the end of the exam to prevent an extended period of discomfort.

Page 24: *Suggested Answer*—Coumadin is an oral anticoagulant that serves as an antagonist of vitamin K. Because it increases clotting time, it is essential that the PT be measured frequently. Usually clotting times with Coumadin are controlled at 1.5–2.0 times the normal clotting time of 10–13 seconds. It is important to remind the client to advise the provider of any changes in other medications and the use of any herbal remedies that may affect the client's clotting times. The client must also be advised to report any signs of bleeding to the provider immediately.

Page 26: *Suggested Answer*—The RPR test is a screening test for syphilis. A positive finding can be the result of syphilis; however, certain chronic diseases or exposure to many other diseases can also cause reactivity. Diseases such as TB, mononucleosis, chickenpox, smallpox, recent vaccinations, systemic lupus erythematosus, and pneumonia can cause reactivity of the test. Review with the client possible sexual history exposures and a history of any of the other identified diseases. The client should also be informed that the positive results can be verified with additional testing to eliminate false-positive results.

Chapter 2

Page 52: *Suggested Answer*—Ventilation and perfusion are gravity dependent, so when the client is lying on one side, gravity accounts for greater ventilation and perfusion to the dependent lung. Since pneumonia produces excess secretions and possible obstructed airways, ventilation and perfusion will be optimized when the client is placed in a position with the good lung in a dependent position.

Page 53: *Suggested Answer*—Carbon dioxide (CO_2) level in the blood is a major stimulus for breathing. Clients with COPD retain CO_2 and typically have higher than normal blood levels of CO_2 and develop a hypoxic drive. Administration of high concentration of oxygen O_2 lowers or removes this stimulus for breathing. Initial O_2 supplementation for clients with suspected or known COPD should be low concentration, 1–2 L/min via nasal cannula to avoid respiratory depression or arrest.

Page 54: *Suggested Answer*—The priority for the client with a tracheostomy is maintenance of a patent airway. Equipment for suctioning, tracheostomy cannula, supplemental O_2, and a call signal should be available at the client's bedside at all times. Additionally, a note should be placed near the call light console in the nurses' station indicating that the client cannot speak, and that calls must be answered in person.

Page 57: *Suggested Answer*—The main nursing measure to prevent recurrence of pneumothorax is to maintain water seal of the chest tube. This means that the chest tube should not be clamped. The provider should be notified immediately of a suspected obstruction of a chest tube such as might occur from a blood clot. Chest tubes should not be milked except by specific order for a specific reason, since this can cause tissue damage inside the chest.

Page 58: *Suggested Answer*—In the postoperative pneumonectomy client, positioning includes lying on the back and turning toward the operative side. The client may be turned temporarily slightly toward the nonoperative side, but should not remain in this position. Turning the client with the operative side in the dependent position promotes desired consolidation of fluid in the pleural space previously occupied by the removed lung and prevents the heart and remaining lung from shifting into the operative side. The client should not be positioned in a completely lateral position on the operative side, however, to avoid shifting of mediastinal contents.

Page 59: *Suggested Answer*—Emphysema is a chronic disease with progressive destruction of alveoli and loss of alveolar area available for gas exchange. Paralysis of respiratory muscles, airway obstructions, and pleural effusion would diminish ventilatory capacity that could ultimately lead to decreased oxygen supply.

Page 60: *Suggested Answer*—The primary cause of chronic bronchitis is cigarette smoking, so smoking cessation is the priority lifestyle change to enhance wellness. Clients who utilize multiple approaches to smoking cessation, such as nicotine withdrawal medications and social support, are usually more successful at achieving and maintaining smoking cessation than those without a support system.

Page 64: *Suggested Answer*—Chylothorax is the abnormal accumulation of lymph fluid within the pleural cavity. Chylothorax can be caused inadvertently during a surgical procedure by disruption of lymph vessels. Disease or traumatic processes that erode into lymph vessels can also produce chylothorax. Clients with chylothorax are unable to absorb lipids from the intestinal tract, so they may need intravenous administration of lipids to prevent fatty acid deficiency until the chylothorax is resolved.

Page 66: *Suggested Answer*—Tension pneumothorax is the accumulation of free air within the pleural cavity. When there is no mechanism for this air to escape into the atmosphere, the pressure caused by this air continues to increase. Increasing pressure on the great vessels within the chest can progress until the vessels actually collapse and interrupt blood supply to the heart and lungs, thereby causing the clinical condition known as cardiovascular collapse. This condition is life-threatening within a few seconds to a few minutes.

Page 67: *Suggested Answer*—The primary cause of atelectasis is diminished breathing activity such as occurs with anes-

thesia or immobility. The easiest maneuver to prevent atelectasis is to encourage, teach, and assist the client to cough and deep breathe frequently (every hour). Enhancing mobility as soon as feasible is also beneficial in preventing atelectasis.

Page 68: *Suggested Answer*—

	Bacterial	**Viral**
Temp	High	Normal or low-grade
Cough	Productive	Nonproductive
Chest x-ray	Diffuse infiltrates	Often normal
Clinical course	More severe	Less severe

Page 70: *Suggested Answer*—Antibiotic prophylaxis for individuals exposed to clients with active disease includes isoniazid as the drug of choice for 6 months if there is no clinical evidence of disease. Among clients with an abnormal chest x-ray, or high-risk population such as clients with HIV or drug-induced immunosuppression, isoniazid is the drug of choice for 12 months.

Page 72: *Suggested Answer*—The primary cause of pulmonary emboli is immobility. Therefore, optimizing mobility as soon as feasible is beneficial. Among clients who are immobilized due to severe illness, the use of passive range of motion, anti-embolism devices, and anticoagulation may be indicated to prevent pulmonary emboli.

Chapter 3

Page 96: *Suggested Answer*—A priority for a client with new atrial fibrillation is the prevention of thrombus formation due to blood pooling in the atria. The client should report calf tenderness or pain and should avoid calf massage. If warfarin (Coumadin) is prescribed, instruct the client about the importance of getting blood tests for prothrombin time (PT) and INR at regular intervals, and to maintain a steady amount of vitamin K–rich foods in the diet (green leafy vegetables), because vitamin K decreases the effectiveness of warfarin (Coumadin). Maintaining steady intake helps keep INR levels more consistent.

Page 101: *Suggested Answer*—The nurse assessing a client for signs of MI should make frequent assessments of the level and type of client's pain, continuous ECG monitoring for dysrhythmias or ST elevations, blood pressure and pulse, O_2 saturation, and cardiac enzymes levels.

Page 103: *Suggested Answer*—The nurse should explain that although frequent urination poses difficulties, diuretic therapy is essential in preventing fluid overload on the heart and preventing acute episodes of heart failure. The nurse should work with the client to determine a diuretic schedule for the client that maintains the prescribed dosage at a time of the day that allows optimal activity.

Page 103: *Suggested Answer*—The nurse should explain that once a client has SBE, he or she has increased risk for repeat infections. In order to prevent future episodes, the client needs to be taught symptoms to report to the provider, and always remember to obtain a prescription for prophylactic antibiotics prior to invasive procedures including all dental work.

Page 105: *Suggested Answer*—The client who is taking warfarin (Coumadin) for valve repair should receive an explanation that this therapy will be a lifelong treatment. The nurse should explain the routine management of warfarin (Coumadin) therapy including blood tests for PT and INR. Dietary teaching regarding the high vitamin K content of green, leafy vegetables should be included. Inconsistent intake of these foods reduces the effect of warfarin and can alter the effectiveness of the anticoagulant therapy.

Page 106: *Suggested Answer*—Restrictive cardiomyopathy is associated with right-sided failure, and the nurse would expect to see peripheral edema and possible abdominal tenderness or ascites.

Page 107: *Suggested Answer*—Cardiac tamponade is a serious complication of pericarditis. The nurse would expect to see jugular venous distention (JVD) with clear lungs, high CVP, narrowing pulse pressure, decreased BP or urine output (signs of decreased cardiac output), and muffled heart sounds.

Chapter 4

Page 124: *Suggested Answer*—The DASH (Dietary Approaches to Stop Hypertension) diet is based on findings of several research studies that demonstrated lowered blood pressure through dietary modification. The diet is rich in fruits and vegetables and low in saturated and total fat. The DASH eating plan is based on a 2,000-calorie diet, although it can be modified if weight loss is also required. The client must be reminded to center the meal around carbohydrates, such as pasta, rice, beans, or vegetables. Meat is part of the meal, not the focus. The DASH diet should be used in combination with foods lower in salt, keeping a healthy weight, being physically active, and engaging in smoking cessation and stress reduction behaviors.

Page 126: *Suggested Answer*—Explain to the client that angiography allows for visualization of arteries to determine if there is occlusion or an aneurysm present. A local anesthetic will be used, so minimal discomfort will be felt. A catheter will be inserted, usually into the femoral artery, although a sub-clavian, axillary, brachial, or translumbar approach may be used. Contrast dye will be injected and then serial x-rays will be taken. After the catheter is removed, direct pressure is placed on the site. Nursing implications include:

- Assess for bleeding.
- Bed rest for several hours postprocedure
- Assess puncture site frequently and remind client to report any wetness, warmth or pressure at the site.

- Conduct neurovascular checks q 1–2 h on the extremities.
- Assess for embolism.
- Neurovascular checks of both extremities q 1–2 h. Have client report any feelings of pain, numbness, coolness, or tingling of the feet immediately.
- Administer anticoagulants as ordered.
- Assess for pseudoaneurysm.
- Observe puncture site for pulsatile mass.
- Neurovascular checks of lower extremities q 1–2 h

Page 128: *Suggested Answer*—Arterial thrombosis is usually due to arterial obstruction from a blood clot that formed *within* an artery damaged by atherosclerosis. An embolus is a clot that has traveled—the wall of the artery may be healthy and the thrombus most likely originated from the heart. Most of these emboli lodge in the legs with a small percentage lodging in the arms.

Surgical management of arterial thrombosis usually involves revascularization of the extremity by bypass grafting. Arterial emboli may be removed by an embolectomy. Emboli and thrombi may be treated medically with thrombolytic agents if ischemia is not present.

Page 130: *Suggested Answer*—Monitor graft site and report any signs of possible leakage evidenced by:

- Decreased CVP, pulmonary artery pressure or pulmonary artery wedge pressure
- Oliguria (output less than 30 mL/hr)
- Ecchymoses of the scrotum or perineum
- New or enlargement of incision site hematoma
- Increasing abdominal girth
- Diminishing/absent peripheral pulses
- Decreasing blood pressure and increasing pulse
- Sudden pain in the abdomen, back, or groin

Prevent hemorrhagic or hypovolemic shock by:

- Administering IV fluids as ordered
- Recording accurate intake and output
- Assessing blood pressure, pulse, and level of consciousness
- Monitoring incision site and assessing for graft leakage
- Monitoring lab values

Page 131: *Suggested Answer*—Your client is most likely experiencing a pulmonary embolism. Most pulmonary emboli arise from clots in the legs. Symptoms include dyspnea, tachpnea, tachycardia, cough, chest pain, fever, and hypoxia.

Nursing interventions include:

- Apply O_2 immediately.
- Assess pulse oximetry to determine oxygen saturation.
- Call provider and report findings.
- Establish an IV line if not present.
- Maintain bed rest.
- Encourage cough and deep-breathing exercises to prevent atelectasis.
- Prepare client for a lung scan.
- Provide preoperative teaching for an embolectomy if pulmonary artery obstruction is greater than 50 percent.

Page 135: *Suggested Answer*—The pain of varicose veins is due to prolonged interruption of blood flow back to the heart and pooling of blood in the lower extremity. This poor blood flow and pooling deprives the tissues of oxygen and nutrients, which results in pain. Over time, tissue necrosis and ulceration may occur.

Chapter 5

Page 151: *Suggested Answer*—Acute confusion and chronic confusion differ in a number of ways:

- Onset: acute confusion begins abruptly over hours to days, while chronic confusion develops slowly over a number of years.
- Memory: acute confusion results in limited immediate and recent memory, while chronic confusion can affect recent and remote memory.
- Timing: in acute confusion, alertness can fluctuate during the day and often occurs at night; in chronic confusion, there is no cycling that coincides with the time of day or night.
- Awareness: acute confusion presents with decreased alertness and awareness that is interspersed with lucid intervals; in chronic confusion there is no change in level of consciousness.
- Attention: acute confusion limits the client's attention, while chronic confusion does not.
- Language: acute confusion often leads to incoherent speech because of disorganized thinking, while chronic confusion often leads to aphasia.
- Perception: acute confusion can be marked by hallucinations, dreams, and vivid but frightening misperceptions, while chronic confusion is not marked by hallucinations until late in the disease process.
- Sleep cycle: acute confusion disturbs and may even reverse a client's sleep–wake cycle, while in chronic confusion, sleep may be interrupted but is not characterized by reversal in the day/night cycle.

Page 159: *Suggested Answer*—Signs of meningitis include the following:

- Restlessness, agitation, and irritability
- Abdominal and back pain
- Nausea and vomiting
- Severe headaches
- Signs of meningeal irritation, nuchal rigidity (stiff neck), Brudzinski's sign (pain, resistance and hip and knee flexion occur with flexion of the neck to the chest in the supine position), Kernig's sign (pain and/or resistance occurs with flexion of the knee and hip and straightening of the knee in the supine position), and photophobia
- Chills and high fever
- Confusion, altered LOC
- Seizures
- Signs and symptoms of increasing ICP

Page 162: *Suggested Answer*—While supportive nursing care is similar for clients who have had a stroke or CVA, the differences can be attributed to the pathophysiology of the stroke. In hemorrhagic CVA, bleeding into the ventricles or brain tissue has occurred, resulting in a subarachnoid hemorrhage or an intracerebral bleed. In these clients, it is important to ensure that rebleeding does not occur, making it important to institute subarachnoid or aneurysm precautions, which limit environmental and physiological stimuli. It is also important to recognize or prevent blood vessel spasm in the area of the bleed, which can trigger a rebleed. In contrast, a client with an ischemic stroke has suffered either thrombus formation or embolus. In these cases, the client may be treated with a thrombolytic agent to dissolve the clot, or may at least be given heparin, an anticoagulant, to prevent propagation of existing thrombus. These clients need the typical precautions used with any client receiving anticoagulant therapy.

Page 164: *Suggested Answer*—The client is likely to have need for physical therapy, occupational therapy, a medical social worker, nursing staff, and possibly a psychologist and a vocational counselor.

Page 167: *Suggested Answer*—

- This medication may cause drowsiness or dizziness, so tasks requiring alertness should be avoided until medication response is known.
- Carry medical identification stating disorder and the name of anticonvulsant used.
- Take exactly as prescribed; call prescriber if doses are missed for 2 consecutive days; if one dose is missed, take within 4 hours if multiple doses are taken each day, or when remembered when once daily dosing is done (time of regular administration may need to be changed).
- Avoid using OTC products or alcohol while taking phenytoin.
- See dentist regularly for cleanings to prevent gingival hyperplasia, gum tenderness, or bleeding.
- Do not switch brands of medication; bioavailability may be different.
- Phenytoin may change the color of urine to pink, red, or reddish brown, but this is insignificant.
- Do not take medication within 3 hours of antacids or 2 hours of antidiarrheals for best absorption.
- Use an additional nonhormonal contraceptive method (females) while taking phenytoin; notify prescriber if pregnant or plan to become pregnant.

Chapter 6

Page 197: *Suggested Answer*—The client may be having urinary retention with overflow. Since urine stasis becomes a good medium for bacterial growth, the client is at risk for developing urinary tract infection. In addition, decreased urinary output may also indicate other medical conditions such as dehydration. The client should be advised that an evaluation by a health care practitioner is necessary.

Page 199: *Suggested Answer*—The involuntary flow of urine from the bladder is incontinence. This client describes stress incontinence, an incontinence characterized by incompetence of the bladder outlet allowing for urine to escape involuntarily. The involuntary escape of urine is caused by increased intra-abdominal pressure, which occurs with laughing, sneezing, coughing, lifting, or Valsalva maneuver. This client should be advised to see a urologist because pharmacologic and surgical intervention, such as a vesicourethropexy, have successfully improved the lives of clients with stress incontinence.

Page 199: *Suggested Answer*—Anatomical differences between females and males predispose females to urinary tract infections (UTIs). The female has a shorter urethra and lacks prostatic fluid that can protect her from UTIs. In addition, the anatomical proximity of the urethra to the vagina and rectum predisposes the female to migration of bacteria from those orifices. Since *Escherichia coli* is the most frequent source of UTI infection, it underscores the necessity for good hygiene practices. Tissue trauma during sexual intercourse may also predispose the female to higher incidence of UTIs.

Page 202: *Suggested Answer*—Many medical conditions and diseases can cause hematuria or blood in the urine. What the client describes in this case is gross hematuria. Blood may also be present in the urine without the individual noticing it and may be observed with microscopic analysis. Any client with hematuria should seek evaluation from a health care provider. Since hematuria is the most frequent sign of renal cancer and tumors of the urinary tract, early diagnosis and intervention is vital.

Page 206: *Suggested Answer*—Since fluid retention is common in glomerulonephritis, sodium restriction should be included in the teaching plan. The client should learn to check labels on food products to ascertain the amount of sodium in them. A low-protein diet is also instituted particularly when there is elevation of BUN and creatinine levels. A high-carbohydrate, high-calorie diet is necessary to prevent utilization and breakdown of protein stores. Collaboration with the dietician for detailed meal planning should also be sought.

Chapter 7

Page 225: *Suggested Answer*—The client should keep the temperature of the room air cool (68–70°F) with the humidity maintained at 30–40%. Itching may be relieved by taking a cool or tepid bath containing colloidal substances such as oatmeal, cornstarch, or soybean powder. Emollient lotions should be used rather than lotions containing alcohol, which can dry the skin.

Page 225: *Suggested Answer*—There are several types of viral hepatitis. Transmission for hepatitis A is through the fecal–oral route. For example, people who have hepatitis A may

transmit it to others if they do not wash their hands well after using the toilet and then handle food. Hepatitis A is also transmitted in seafood harvested from contaminated water or food eaten raw that has been washed in contaminated water. It may be transmitted sexually by oral contact with the rectum of a contaminated individual. Hepatitis B, C, and D are transmitted through contact with blood and blood products of individuals with the disease. It is also transmitted sexually, and the hepatitis B virus has been found in saliva, semen, urine, feces, and other body fluids. Hepatitis C is found in blood and semen, but most people with hepatitis C have no known risk factors.

Page 233: *Suggested Answer*—The purpose of lactulose is ultimately to reduce the ammonia level. It is a disaccharide laxative that is not absorbed by the GI tract and pulls water into the bowel, causing diarrhea and preventing the absorption of ammonia.

Page 235: *Suggested Answer*—The client's vital signs are taken every 15 minutes for an hour, every 30 minutes for an hour, every hour for 2 hours, every 4 hours four times and then every 6 hours thereafter. The nurse should observe the dressing for oozing when checking vital signs. Direct pressure should be applied to the biopsy site directly after the procedure, and the client is positioned on the right side. The client is usually kept on bedrest for 24 hours and can resume fluids 2 hours after the procedure. Anything that increases intra-abdominal pressure should be avoided for 1–2 weeks (coughing, lifting, straining).

Page 237: *Suggested Answer*—The client with cholelithiasis should be instructed to eat small, frequent, low-fat meals. The obese client should be encouraged to lose weight, but very rapid weight loss with an extreme calorie restriction should be avoided since this increases the risk for developing gallstones.

Page 238: *Suggested Answer*—The client should be assessed for pain, and pain should be treated before it becomes too intense. Vital signs should be taken at least every 4 hours and the client should be monitored for signs of peritonitis. The incision should be kept clean and dry and monitored for bleeding and drainage. To prevent pulmonary infection the client should be encouraged to use the incentive spirometer every hour and cough and deep breathe at least every 2 hours.

Chapter 8

Page 256: *Suggested Answer*—Because there is radiation involved in this diagnostic test, all women of childbearing age should be asked if they are or could be pregnant. During the procedure, the client is placed in the CAT scan machine, which is just slightly larger than the body; therefore, anyone with claustrophobia may have difficulty completing this test. All clients should be asked if they have claustrophobia before the test. Some CAT scans are performed using a contrast medium containing iodine so the client should be questioned about allergy to shellfish or iodine.

Page 258: *Suggested Answer*—Each step of the procedure should be explained to the client so that the level of anxiety can be minimized. The client is placed in a high-Fowler's position. The tube is measured from the tip of the nose to the ear and down to the xyphoid process and marked at this place. The tube is inserted through the nose with the client's head bent slightly forward, which helps to close the epiglottis and promotes movement of the tube into the esophagus rather than the trachea. The client is asked to swallow or sip water during insertion for this reason as well. Once the predetermined mark is reached, the tube is taped to the nose. Placement is checked by instilling 10–20 mL of air into the tube and auscultating for the flow of air "burp" in the left upper quadrant.

Page 260: *Suggested Answer*—Initial assessment of the postoperative colostomy client includes vital signs, lung sounds, bowel sounds, intake and output, level of consciousness, level of pain, and drainage from any tubes and drains. The incision should be assessed for drainage, wound approximation, and signs of infection. Of particular importance is a thorough assessment of the stoma. The stoma should be red or pinkish red and shiny. A stoma that appears dark, purplish red or blue may be ischemic and should be reported to the surgeon immediately. Drainage from the stoma is typically bloody and scant immediately postop. The drainage will increase as the client begins to take fluids, but should not contain blood.

Page 267: *Suggested Answer*—Barrett's epithelium is the body's way of compensating for chronic exposure of the esophagus to gastric juice. The normal squamous epithelium in the distal portion of the esophagus is replaced with columnar epithelium, also called Barrett's epithelium. This columnar epithelium is more resistant to gastric acid and actually supports healing of the chronic inflammation. The one disadvantage is that this type of cell is a premalignant tissue and the client with Barrett's epithelium has an increased risk of developing cancer of the esophagus, and therefore, needs periodic follow-up and testing.

Page 269: *Suggested Answer*—Peptic ulcer is a generic term for ulceration of tissue in the GI tract that comes in contact with gastric juice. The most common locations are the stomach and duodenum. Gastric ulcers are not necessarily caused by increased gastric acid secretion as are duodenal ulcers, but rather, are caused from a disruption of the normal gastric mucosal protective barrier, which prevents the diffusion of acid back across the membrane. Gastric ulcers also involve an area of gastritis surrounding the ulcer crater, and duodenal ulcers do not have this feature. Prostaglandins produced in the gastric mucosa increase the resistance of the mucosa to the effects of acid. Drugs that inhibit prostaglandins, such as aspirin and NSAIDs, contribute to gastric ulcer formation.

Chapter 9

Page 286: *Suggested Answer*—The client should be told that he will be in a cylinder-like tube and that he will need to be still during the procedure. There is a possibility that a contrast medium might be used. If so, the provider will inform him and will ask him about allergies.

Page 287: *Suggested Answer*—MRI is contraindicated in any client who has a metal implant of any type such as a pacemaker, prosthetic, or surgical clip. Clients with a history of claustrophobia might have difficulty in some MRI machines that enclose them in the diagnostic imaging machine. Clients who are unstable, or who require intravenous pumps, are not good candidates for an MRI procedure.

Page 295: *Suggested Answer*—The risk factors associated with osteoporosis that are appropriate to include in teaching this client are inadequate dietary intake of calcium, sedentary lifestyle, smoking, and excessive alcohol intake. All these factors involve lifestyle modifications that can prevent the disease.

Page 301: *Suggested Answer*—Priority interventions include:

1. Immobilize the fracture by the application of a splint.
2. Assess neurovascular status. Check for the pulse distal to the injury. Evaluate for the presence of paresthesia, inability to move the toes, coolness of the distal extremity, or delayed capillary refill. The tibial artery and/or the peroneal nerve may have been damaged by the injury and can cause neurovascular deficits.
3. Cover the skin opening with a sterile dressing.
4. Assess for signs of hemorrhage and shock.

Page 305: *Suggested Answer*—Gout is characterized by elevated serum uric acid level. When serum uric acid levels increase, monosodium urate crystals form in tissues of the body. This initiates the inflammatory response that causes the pain of gout. Probenecid (Benemid) is a uricosuric drug. This drug acts by blocking the tubular reabsorption of urate and promotes elimination of uric acid through the kidneys.

Chapter 10

Page 322: *Suggested Answer*—Methods used to prevent spreading impetigo include good hand hygiene, keeping hands away from lesions, not sharing drinks or straws, and no kissing or allowing anyone to touch lesions. Inform contacts about the infection and encourage use of good preventive measures from contacting impetigo.

Page 323: *Suggested Answer*—Discuss with client that herpes virus remains in the body for life. The virus may lay dormant for long periods of time. The fact that she has not had any lesions for several years does not mean that the virus has disappeared. She still has the virus and the lesion she has today could possibly be a genital herpes lesion. The virus can be reactivated at any time and then present with active lesions. Things that cause reactivation of the virus include illness and stress. However, she needs to have the lesion evaluated today.

Page 324: *Suggested Answer*—Warts are caused by a virus that remains in the body for life, and the virus can be reactivated at any time. Even removal of the wart with treatments such as over-the-counter products and cryotherapy is not a guarantee that the wart will not reappear at a later date. Recommend to the client that there are options for removal, such as cryotherapy; however the wart may still reappear at a later time or place. Even if no treatment is applied to the wart, the likelihood of the wart resolving on its own within 6–12 months is likely.

Page 332: *Suggested Answer*—Evaluation of the mole should include the ABCDE (Asymmetry, Border, Color, Diameter, Elevation or evolving) method of evaluation. Encourage monthly evaluation of the skin, especially new moles that may be changing. If concerned about any changes in moles, the client should consult the healthcare provider for further evaluation.

Page 333: *Suggested Answer*—Encourage skin protection with the use of sunscreen with an SPF 15 or greater when outdoors. Using clothing for skin protection along with a hat is recommended. Also avoid peak sun hours when the rays are strongest between the hours of 10:00 a.m. and 2:00 p.m. Encourage clients to monitor the skin monthly with skin checks, using the ABCD method to evaluate any moles or skin lesions.

Chapter 11

Page 359: *Suggested Answer*—It is important to assess and monitor the client for a potential allergic reaction (Type 1 hypersensitivity). The basic concepts of ABC (airway, breathing, and circulation) are of critical importance. It is also important to determine whether the client has a history of having this type of reaction before, other allergic reactions associated with food and medication, and any other pertinent medical conditions that might affect the individual. If there is a positive client history, the client may already have an Epi-Pen in his or her possession and may have to utilize the device as directed by the prescribing provider. Removal of the offending agent is required and the client should not be allowed to eat further strawberries even if the breathing pattern returns to normal.

Page 360: *Suggested Answer*—The concept of autoimmune disease involves a chronic condition with acute exacerbations and remissions. Autoimmunity involves the body's inability to maintain normal lines of defense and reaction by not recognizing one's "self." This can lead to an overactive immune response where the body develops autoantibodies that can lead to organ and system damage.

Page 370: *Suggested Answer*—The vast number of medications used to control this disease can certainly cause one to feel like "there is no way to comply," but each prescribed medication provides a specific function. The medications are aimed at working together to provide the best therapeutic response in the hopes of decreasing symptoms, decreasing viral load, and promoting the immune response.

Page 371: *Suggested Answer*—Megace is being prescribed for its effect to be an appetite stimulant and to promote weight gain. Even though it is considered a female hormone, it does provide this effect and is used in many disease states where weight loss and decreased appetite has become a problem.

Page 374: *Suggested Answer*—An ANC of 500 indicates that the client is severely immunosuppressed and neutropenic precautions should be instituted. The client should be placed on reverse isolation and the ANC level should be monitored to see if immune system function returns. Medication therapy such as colony-stimulating factors may be used to boost the immune response. A neutropenic diet should be instituted for the client. Client, staff, and family members must be made aware of and educated regarding these precautions and they should be maintained until the ANC count raises to an acceptable level as determined by the provider.

Chapter 12

Page 392: *Suggested Answer*—First, recognize that cancer causes fear and anxiety in the client and psychosocial support should be ongoing. Acknowledge the client's fears and concerns and encourage expression of concerns. He may be responding to misconceptions told to him by others ("My mother had radiation and no one could get closer than 6 feet to her."). Teach the client about external radiation, and tell him that there is no risk of harm or exposure to radiation to his son or others coming in contact with him.

Page 395: *Suggested Answer*—Recall that the client with a decreased platelet count (thrombocytopenia) is at risk for bleeding. Precautions to prevent bleeding include avoiding intramuscular injections and monitoring intravenous site at least every 2 hours. Other interventions include monitoring stool, urine, and vomitus for blood, posting a bleeding precaution sign on the door to the client's room, and teaching client measures to prevent bleeding. The decreased leukocyte count places the client at high risk for infection. Interventions include placing client in private room, instituting protective isolation, maintaining strict aseptic technique, screening visitors for infection, avoiding raw fruits and vegetables, and teaching the client measures to prevent infection.

Page 396: *Suggested Answer*—The client is experiencing stomatitis, a common side effect of chemotherapy and radiation. Interventions include teaching client proper oral care, using a soft toothbrush, avoiding mouthwashes, and rinsing mouth with water or saline frequently. Because the ulcerations are painful and interfering with nutritional intake, the client may benefit from viscous lidocaine to rinse mouth with; teach client not to swallow xylocaine. To manage nausea, round-the-clock antiemetics may be necessary. Teach client dietary habits to help reduce diarrhea. Encourage client to eat small, frequent meals, as these may be tolerated easier. Since the client is at risk for inadequate nutrition, suggest maintaining a food diary to record daily intake of food and fluid.

Page 397: *Suggested Answer*—Severe pain at the infusion site can indicate infiltration. Discontinue the infusion immediately. If the chemotherapeutic agent is a vesicant, proceed with the protocol for infiltration of that agent and inform the oncologist for specific actions to be taken. Assess the intravenous site, document the infiltration, actions taken, appearance of the site, and provide written and oral instructions to client.

Page 400: *Suggested Answer*—Early symptoms of spinal cord compression include progressive back and leg pain and numbness. Because of the potential for irreversible paraplegia, spinal cord compression is considered an oncological emergency. Assessment includes a thorough investigation of all complaints of back pain and neurological changes. The health care provider should be notified immediately if spinal cord compression is suspected.

Chapter 13

Page 415: *Suggested Answer*—The treatment goal in a client with SIADH is to restore normal fluid volume and serum osmolality. The client should be taught that excess ADH causes volume expansion and dilutional hyponatremia. Ingestion of too much fluid will therefore aggravate the serum hypo-osmolality and hyponatremia. Limiting fluids to 1,000 mL per day will aid in normalizing serum sodium. The client can be taught to decrease thirst by using of ice chips and hard candy to blunt the thirst sensation.

Page 420: *Suggested Answer*—Treatment of Graves' disease does not reverse the changes associated with exophthalmos. Thus the client needs to know how to protect the eyes from injury, prevent infection and promote comfort and visual acuity.

Page 422: *Suggested Answer*—Low levels of thyroid hormone associated with hypothyroidism cause altered lipid metabolism, leading to elevated serum triglyceride and cholesterol levels, and thereby increasing the risk for atherosclerosis and cardiovascular disease. In hypothyroidism constipation results from decreased gastrointestinal motility, peristalsis, and the reduced physical activity associated with low thyroid hormone induced fatigue.

Page 426: *Suggested Answer*—The body needs a therapeutic level of glucocorticoids to maintain fluid and electrolyte balance. If the medication is going to be stopped or dose decreased it need to be done gradually. A sudden dose decrease or termination of the medication does not allow the adrenal gland to begin functioning to produce glucocorticoid. When people take additional glucocorticoid medication to treat a condition, the adrenal gland slows down or may stop its own production of the glucocorticoid as a negative feedback mechanism.

Page 433: *Suggested Answer*—Insulin availability at the beginning of exercise affects the body's response. During exercise the muscles get energy from the breakdown of muscle glycogen and liver production of glucose. During prolonged exercise fatty acids are broken down for energy. If there is an insufficient amount of insulin during exercise, the glucose produced by the body cannot be used by the muscles. The glucose accumulates in the body, causing hyperglycemia, and forces the muscles to use fatty acids for energy, causing ketosis. Hypoglycemia can occur 6 to 15 hours up to 24 hours after sustained high intensity exercise. Hyperglycemia can occur and last for several hours following exercise. Regular moderate exercise improves glucose control for the patient with diabetes, improves glucose clearance, lowers insulin requirements, and promotes weight loss. Prior to exercise the client should check his fasting blood glucose level, and if it is greater than 250 mg/dL, he should check his urine for ketones. Ketones in the urine are a contraindication for exercise indicating that fatty acids are currently broken down for energy and there is insufficient insulin present.

Chapter 14

Page 451: *Suggested Answer*—The nurse should make sure that a signed consent has been completed. The nurse explains to the client about the procedure. Instructions should be given about not moving during the procedure. After the bone marrow biopsy has been completed, the nurse should apply a sterile pressure dressing on the puncture site. Direct pressure should be applied for at least 5 minutes and may be longer in cases where the client has thrombocytopenia. Periodic checks to monitor for evidence of bleeding should be continued up to 4 hours after the procedure.

Page 453: *Suggested Answer*—If an immediate IV access cannot be established within 20 minutes, then the unit of blood should be returned to the blood bank. Unused blood may not be refrigerated in other areas except in the blood bank.

Page 453: *Suggested Answer*—Chills may be a sign of a transfusion reaction and therefore the nurse has to implement the specific protocol of the agency or setting in which this occurred. The blood transfusion should be discontinued immediately. The blood product and the IV tubing are disconnected from the IV access site. New IV tubing and normal saline will be initiated to keep the IV line open. The client will be assessed for other signs of reactions and to evaluate vital signs. The provider and the blood bank will be notified of this reaction and established protocol will be followed. Throughout this process the nurse establishes intensive monitoring of the client, and emergency interventions are provided as they arise.

Page 460: *Suggested Answer* — Folic acid anemia is most likely to occur in individuals who are undernourished. This group includes the elderly, alcoholics, and those with substance abuse. Alcoholics usually develop this type of anemia because alcohol interferes with the metabolism of folic acid. In addition to this group, other individuals who might be susceptible to folic acid deficiency anemia are those with high metabolic requirements, including those who are pregnant, infants, and teenagers. Additional factors to the development of this anemia are certain medications, hemodialysis, and total parenteral nutrition supplementation.

Page 463: *Suggested Answer* — An individual with sickle cell trait is heterozygous, with one-fourth of the hemoglobin in the S form. Sickle cell anemia is an autosomal recessive genetic disorder that results from the inheritance of the sickle cell hemoglobin gene. If an individual who has sickle cell trait has a child with another with the trait, there is 25% likelihood that a child may inherit 2 abnormal genes and thus will develop the disease.

Chapter 15

Page 493: *Suggested Answer* — The client receiving continuous bladder irrigation (CBI) who develops bladder spasms should be assessed to determine the cause. One of the most common causes of spasms is urinary drainage tubing that is kinked or blocked (by the client's leg, position, etc.), and this should be checked first. Another cause is the size of the balloon at the tip of the catheter. The pressure exerted by the balloon on the bladder and the straining to attempt to void "against" the catheter causes the spasms. In addition, blood clots and bleeding can cause the spasms. If the discomfort is due to the pressure of the balloon and straining, then pain medication, including antispasmodics, should be given as prescribed. The client should also be instructed to avoid straining. If the spasms are caused by blood clot formation and urinary catheter obstruction, then increasing the instillation flow of the CBI or manual irrigations of the bladder should be performed.

Page 499: *Suggested Answer* — The client should be instructed to use condoms in the future and to avoid sexual intercourse until all sexual partners have been examined and treated. Sexually transmitted disease is the most common factor in causing the disorder in younger men. In older men, the most common etiology is urinary tract infection or prostatitis.

Page 500: *Suggested Answer* — Males between the ages of 15 and 40 are more likely to develop a varicocele. The major complication in this disorder is that varicocele could cause testicular atrophy, resulting in infertility, or it could cause diminished sperm count (the major complication).

Page 502: *Suggested Answer* — Testicular torsion or twisting of the testes and spermatic cord is a potential medical emergency because compromised blood flow may lead to testicular ischemia and necrosis. Detorsion of the testicle and fixation to the scrotum is performed immediately to prevent the necrosis from occurring.

Page 506: *Suggested Answer* — The classic symptoms of an enlarged prostate gland include difficulty starting and stopping urinary stream, overflow dribbling, and urinary frequency. Narrowing of the prostatic urethra causes all these symptoms.

Page 510: *Suggested Answer* — Client education is very important in treating clients with syphilis to prevent recurrence of the disease and to prevent infection of the client's sexual partner. Sexually transmitted diseases, including syphilis, are common in individuals who lack motivation for seeking early treatment, which underscores the importance of education to help in arresting the spread of the disease.

Page 511: *Suggested Answer* — The client should be informed that there is no cure for herpes. This disease has a latency period however, which is characterized by the virus remaining dormant in nerve fibers until its recurrence. During this stage, there may be no symptoms but is not an indication that the condition has been cured.

Page 514: *Suggested Answer* — Chlamydia, which is the most common sexually transmitted disease in the United States, is difficult to diagnose based on physical examination alone because most clients are asymptomatic. Female clients seek consultation when the infection has invaded the uterus and uterine tubes causing acute symptoms. Nearly a third of men with the infection remain asymptomatic.

Chapter 16

Page 549: *Suggested Answer* — There are no symptoms in the early stages of glaucoma. This disorder is characterized by a loss of peripheral vision that is so gradual it is virtually unnoticeable to the person affected. The vision that is lost, however, cannot be regained. The condition can lead eventually to blindness unless eye medications are taken daily for life, and periodic eye exams are done to monitor intraocular pressure and disease progression.

Page 552: *Suggested Answer* — The client's reported symptom is a classic finding with detached retina. The nurse should question the client about other manifestations, such as the presence of floating spots (floaters), flashing lights, blurring of vision, visual field deficits, and presence of pain (detached retina is painless). Immediate interventions are to:

- Protect the eye from further damage (bed rest, cover both eyes with eye patches).
- Instruct the client not to bend forward or make sudden or jerking head movements.

- Position the client with detached area dependent/inferior as ordered.
- Protect the client from injury by keeping the bed low, side rails up, call bell within reach, and assisting with care.
- Reinforce explanations about surgical repair.
- Provide psychological support to alleviate anxiety.

Page 555: *Suggested Answer*—Use the bed as a reference point to orient the client to the room and the bedside area. Using the face of a clock as an analogy, describe the location of different parts of the room in terms of where they are located on the clock face, such as "When you are lying in bed, the bathroom is at 3 o'clock in reference to you." Point out and demonstrate the use of the call bell for the client, and have the client practice to ensure it can be used when needed. Also point out controls for radio and TV to provide diversion. Encourage the client to call for assistance before getting out of bed to prevent injury, and check on the client often.

Page 557: *Suggested Answer*—Instruct the client to:

- Keep the outer ear dressing clean and dry.
- Avoid activities that increase middle ear pressure, such as blowing nose, sneezing, coughing, straining; if necessary, cough or sneeze with mouth open; blow nose one nostril at a time with mouth open.
- Avoid drinking through a straw for 2 to 3 weeks and avoid air travel until allowed by surgeon.
- Prevent constipation by increasing fluids and fiber and maintain mobility.
- Do not shower or shampoo hair until allowed by surgeon, and no swimming or diving until fully healed.
- Take medications as ordered and report persistent postoperative headache, increased drainage or bleeding from site, fever, new or increased ear pain or dizziness, or decreasing hearing to the surgeon.

Page 558: *Suggested Answer*—Otosclerosis leads to conductive hearing loss. It is a hereditary disorder of the labyrinthine capsule, in which abnormal bone growth occurs around the ossicles and causes stiffening or fixation of the stapes bone. Surgical correction may be needed. To enhance communication, the following should be done:

- Approach the client from within the client's line of vision or tap the client lightly on the shoulder to get attention before beginning to speak.
- Reduce background noise, such as radio or TV, before beginning to speak.
- Avoid covering mouth with hands or other objects while speaking.
- Face the client and speak slowly and clearly—pronounce words clearly without overarticulating them; speak using low pitch and normal loudness.
- Use nonverbal cues and written messages to enhance communication.
- Repeat sentences using different words if client has difficulty understanding.
- Ask client to repeat directions or teaching that was done to ensure the client understands.

Chapter 17

Page 572: *Suggested Answer*—The goals for the care of the client with multiple contiguous fractured ribs would be to:

1. Ensure ABCs.
2. Maintain an effective breathing pattern; mechanical ventilation may be necessary.
3. Achieve pain control.
4. Maintain hemodynamic stability.

Page 590: *Suggested Answer*—The preferred placement for an arterial line would be the radial artery. Other sites that can be used would be the femoral and brachial arteries.

Page 600: *Suggested Answer*—The primary areas of concern for shock are maintenance of adequate oxygenation, adequate cardiac output and tissue perfusion, and resolution of underlying cause.

Page 602: *Suggested Answer*—No spontaneous respirations and/or no palpable pulse are indications for cardiopulmonary circulation.

Page 605: *Suggested Answer*—Immediate, definitive care would be defibrillation (for a total of 3 shocks if needed). If no defibrillator is available, call for assistance and begin CPR until a defibrillator is available.

➤ Case Study Suggested Answers

Chapter 1

1. The questions should be directed to obtain the following information:
   - When did the abdominal pain, nausea, and vomiting start (time, setting)?
   - What were you doing at the time? What had you been eating or drinking?
   - Is there pain associated with the nausea or does it occur without nausea at times?
   - If there is pain, where is the pain located and does it radiate anywhere?
   - Are there any foods, medications, or activities that aggravate or alleviate the pain, nausea, or vomiting?
   - How disruptive is this to your normal activities?
2. Tests would likely include:
   - Serum amylase: indicates pancreatic tissue damage
   - Serum lipase: usually elevated with acute pancreatitis
   - Serum glucose: may be elevated because of pancreatic cell damage
   - WBC: indicates inflammation or infection
3. Diagnostic procedures may include the following:
   - Ultrasound to assess for the presence of gallstones or pancreatic mass
   - CT of the abdomen to assess for pancreatic size, fluid, or necrosis
   - Abdominal x-ray to assess for the presence of stones or fluid accumulation in the area of the pancreas

4. Client teaching related to these procedures would include the following:
   * The client will require no special preparation for the abdominal x-rays, however, ultrasound and CT procedures require special preparation.
   * Ultrasound of the abdomen will require that the client have a relatively clean bowel and be NPO for a period of time prior to procedure. Stool, gas, and air can alter the transmission of the sound waves and cause altered recorded images.
   * The CT of the abdomen will require that the client drink approximately 42 ounces of contrast media prior to the test. The client will also need to have IV access for administration of additional contrast material as needed.
5. Three possible nursing diagnoses that would be appropriate for this client are Pain, Risk for Imbalanced Nutrition: Less than Body Requirements, and Risk for Deficient Fluid Volume. Other possible nursing diagnoses based upon the particular client assessment may include Ineffective Breathing Pattern related to pulmonary effusion or pain, Risk for Activity Intolerance, Ineffective Health Maintenance related to knowledge deficit of disease process, Sleep Pattern Disturbance related to pain.

Chapter 2

1. Impaired Gas Exchange. Maintaining adequate gas exchange is the physiological priority for the client with acute exacerbation of COPD and acute lung infection of pneumonia. Activity Intolerance and Self-Care Deficit are also reasonable nursing diagnoses for this client who has been hospitalized.
2. Debris produced by dead bacteria accounts for purulent secretions in the client with a bacterial origin of pneumonia. This finding is a classic sign that helps to distinguish bacterial pneumonia from other etiologies of pneumonia. With viral pneumonia, the client typically has a nonproductive cough.
3. Clients with COPD are often underweight because of the fatigue associated with eating. This client has acutely increased energy needs because of the hypermetabolism associated with acute infection of pneumonia. Providing small quantities of calorie-dense foods will help to achieve needed calorie and protein intake while perhaps avoiding increased fatigue associated with eating.
4. Ventilation and perfusion are gravity-dependent, so when the client is lying on his or her side, gravity accounts for greater ventilation and perfusion to that dependent lung. Since pneumonia produces excess secretions and possible obstructed airways, ventilation and perfusion will be optimized when the client is placed in a position with the good lung in a dependent position.
5. Carbon dioxide (CO_2) level in the blood is a major stimulus for breathing. Clients with COPD retain CO_2 and typically have higher than normal blood levels of CO_2 and develop a hypoxic respiratory drive. Lowering CO_2 levels by administering high concentration of O_2 lowers or removes this stimulus for breathing. Initial O_2 supplementation for clients with suspected or known COPD should be low concentration, 1–2 L/min via nasal cannula to avoid respiratory depression or arrest.

Chapter 3

1. Instruct client in routine preoperative teaching, turning, and deep breathing (vigorous coughing is discouraged because it may increase intrathoracic pressure and cause instability in the sternal area), incentive spirometry to prevent respiratory complications, and leg exercises to prevent emboli formation. Explain expected client status immediately postoperatively including respiratory support on a ventilator with an endotracheal tube; suctioning; surgical incisions, chest tubes, multiple intravenous lines, tubes, drains, and monitors with alarms and noises; pain management, communication techniques, visiting policies, and expected length of hospitalization and recovery period. Include family members in preoperative teaching and explanations. Ensure that all consents are signed. Evaluate the client's understanding of the preoperative teaching. Ensure that all preoperative orders are complete.
2. In the preoperative phase, the nurse monitors the hemodynamic status of the client, and carefully monitors for signs of ischemia or decreased cardiac output. This includes continuous ECG monitoring, vital signs, and careful assessment and monitoring of any chest pain or dyspnea.
3. Nursing diagnoses that are appropriate for a client in the postoperative period are Pain, Ineffective Breathing Pattern, Risk for Decreased Cardiac Output, Risk for Dysrhythmia, Risk for Infection, Anxiety, Fear.
4. In the period after critical care, the nurse monitors the client for potential complications. These include decreased cardiac output, ineffective breathing and fluid accumulation in lungs, infection in surgical wounds, activity intolerance, or dysrhythmias.
5. When the client is ready to go home after surgery, the nurse will instruct client about new medication regime, symptoms to report to provider upon discharge including chest pain, shortness of breath, decrease in activity tolerance, fever, redness, swelling or drainage from surgical incisions, activity plan for home, cardiac rehabilitation, and resumption of sexual activity. The client may resume sexual activity when he or she can walk up two full flights of stairs without shortness of breath or chest pain. The client should be rested when resuming sexual activity. Sexual activity should be avoided after a heavy meal or after the intake of alcohol. Instruct client that clinical depression occurs in about 20% of clients up to 6 months after cardiac surgery, and client should notify provider because antidepressants are very effective. Include family in teaching and planning for discharge.

Chapter 4

1. The most likely cause of Mr. B.'s foot ulcer is venous insufficiency. Venous ulcers usually develop around the ankles, especially in the area of the medial malleoli.

2. Venous insufficiency may present with edema of the lower extremities, ulcerations that are moist around the ankles, complaints of aching or heaviness in the calf or thigh, cyanosis of the extremity when dependent, and a leathery or brawny appearance to the skin of the lower extremities. Pulses and normal hair distribution are usually present and the skin is warm to touch.

3. Nursing diagnoses include Impaired Skin Integrity, Risk for Infection related to decreased peripheral circulation and skin ulcers; Impaired Tissue Perfusion; Ineffective Health Maintenance related to lack of knowledge of venous insufficiency

4. Primary nursing interventions include:
   Education on improving venous return
   - Keep legs elevated above heart level as much as possible.
   - Avoid prolonged standing/sitting or flexing legs.
   - Wear support hose when ambulatory.
   - Do not wear tight or restrictive clothing or shoes.
   - Avoid injury or trauma to legs and feet.
   Treating venous stasis ulcer
   - Open sores treated with hydrocolloid or wet dressings of boric acid, Burrow's solution, or normal saline QID
   - Unna boot may be applied and changed every 1 to 2 weeks.
   - Teach client proper hand washing and infection control measures.
   - Assess for infection.
     Education on high-protein, low-sodium diet and proper weight control.

5. Outcomes of nursing care include:
   - No infection and healing of venous ulcers
   - Decreased peripheral edema
   - Verbalization of knowledge of wound care, improved venous return, and diet

Chapter 5

1. The focal neurological assessment should include the client's level of consciousness, Glasgow Coma Scale score, mental status assessment, motor and sensory evaluation, and possibly cranial nerve testing. It is important to assess pupil reaction to light, hand grasps, and foot pushes for strength and equality. A full neurological exam can proceed when the client is stabilized.

2. Intracranial hemorrhage can be diagnosed by CT scan or MRI.

3. Increased ICP is indicated by a deteriorating level of consciousness, focal neurological deficits, and by the classic signs of increasing systolic blood pressure, widening pulse pressure, and bradycardia.

4. A quiet peaceful environment that minimizes environmental stimuli will help prevent rises in intracranial pressure. Keep lights low, provide physical care to client, maintain bedrest, minimize stimulants such as radio, TV, newspaper, and others. Ingested stimulants should also be avoided, including coffee, tea, cola drinks, cigarette smoke, and others.

5. No specific medication is indicated to treat hematomas; medication such as anticonvulsants and steroids could be used as indicated to treat seizures and increased ICP if they occur as complications.

Chapter 6

1. Aminoglycoside antibiotics are known to be nephrotoxic and should be used with extreme care for clients with decreased renal function.

2. The client's blood glucose level should decrease as waste products are removed from his blood. Monitor his glucose levels and observe for signs of hypoglycemia.

3. The client's lungs are already compromised by pneumonia. Missing his dialysis treatment may lead to fluid overload, which places him at risk for congestive heart failure and pulmonary edema.

4. Metabolic acidosis may lead to a fruity odor on the breath. Other signs of metabolic acidosis include general malaise, headache, nausea and vomiting, and abdominal pain.

5. A trophy of the sweat glands and metabolic wastes not eliminated by the kidneys can lead to dry, itching skin. To help with the client's pruritus, avoid harsh soaps; instead use mild soap or a cleansing cream and bath oils. If soap is used, rinse well. Use a humidifier to add moisture to the air. Apply unscented lotion when the skin is slightly damp after bathing. Teach him that it isn't necessary to bathe every day.

Chapter 7

1. Lab values will reflect liver injury and decreased liver function and include elevated ALT and AST, low serum albumin, prolonged prothrombin time, elevated total bilirubin, hyponatremia, possible elevated serum ammonia level, anemia, thrombocytopenia, and leukopenia.

2. Since the liver is such a vascular organ, the priority of care is to monitor for bleeding. Vital signs are taken q 15 min × 4, q 30 min × 2, q 1 hr × 2, q 4 hr × 4, then every 6 hours. The dressing should be monitored for bleeding and the client should be positioned on the right side, which helps apply pressure to the biopsy site. The client is usually maintained on bedrest for 24 hours to reduce the risk of bleeding.

3. Complications of hepatitis B include the development of chronic hepatitis, which destroys the liver and leads to cirrhosis and liver failure. The complications of cirrhosis are portal hypertension leading to esophageal varices, right-sided heart failure, and varicose veins. Ascites,

hepatic encephalopathy, and hepatorenal syndrome are also complications of cirrhosis.

4. The client with cirrhosis is usually on a protein, sodium, and fluid-restricted diet. Foods to avoid would be canned and processed foods (high in sodium), chicken, meat, eggs, and dairy products (high in protein), and fluids are usually limited.

5. The long-term outcome of cirrhosis is death. If the complications of cirrhosis can be controlled, the prognosis is better. Liver transplant is an effective treatment for end-stage liver disease for those individuals who meet certain criteria.

Chapter 8

1. An upper-GI series will probably be ordered and can show lower esophageal sphincter (LES) function as well as ulceration. An esophagogastroduodenoscopy can be more diagnostic because it is a direct visualization of the tissue of the esophagus and can show inflammation. The gastric and duodenal mucosa are also visualized directly and ulcerations are evident. The advantage of endoscopy over an upper-GI series is that tissue samples can be obtained for determining the presence of cancer, Barrett's epithelium, or *H. pylori*. Gastric analysis may also be used to determine the pH and acid output of the stomach.

2. An upper-GI series usually involves the ingestion of barium, which is constipating. The client should be encouraged to drink fluids and ambulate. Aspiration of barium during the procedure is a possibility, so the nurse should assess lung sounds and monitor for signs of aspiration such as fever, cough, and dyspnea. For the client after esophagogastroduodenoscopy, it is extremely important to assess for the return of swallowing and the gag reflex since the throat is anesthetized for the procedure. The client is sedated for the procedure, therefore general safety measures should be instituted (side rails up, bed in low position).

3. Lifestyle and diet modifications are key to controlling GERD. The client should be instructed to avoid eating within 2 hours of bedtime and should remain in an upright position after eating. Tight clothing (belts, tight waistbands), straining (weight lifting, bending over, lifting heavy objects), and vigorous physical activity increase intra-abdominal pressure aggravate GERD and should be avoided. A reduction in dietary fat and an increase in complex carbohydrates encourage more rapid gastric emptying and reduction in symptoms of GERD. The client should be instructed to avoid substances that decrease LES tone such as caffeinated beverages, chocolate, peppermint, spearmint, smoking, and fried foods. The client should be encouraged to elevate the head of the bed about 12 inches to prevent reflux at night.

4. The complications of GERD are limited to the development of Barrett's epithelium, cancer, and esophageal stricture. Symptoms include dysphagia, pain, and more systemic symptoms such as fatigue, dyspnea, and activity intolerance. Complications of PUD are perforation, hemorrhage, gastric cancer (gastric ulcer), and pyloric obstruction. The client should be instructed to report any of the following symptoms: vomiting, hematemesis, black tarry stools, pain, rapid heart rate, abdominal rigidity, and fever as they may indicate a complication.

5. Clients with GERD may develop Barrett's epithelium and be at a greater risk for cancer if GERD remains untreated, so it is important that the client follow the treatment regimen. If the client has a duodenal ulcer, the risk for developing cancer as a result is minimal; however, there is an increased incidence of gastric cancer in people with gastric ulcers. Continued follow-up is therefore important in this population.

Chapter 9

1. The nurse should perform a neurovascular assessment, which includes assessing the right lower extremity for pulses, capillary refill, temperature, movement, and paresthesias. The dressing should also be inspected for bleeding. The respiratory status should be assessed since the client is on a PCA pump for the management of pain. The client's level of pain should also be assessed to evaluate the effectiveness of the PCA dosing.

2. The client should be turned alternately on the back or the nonoperative side. Avoid positioning the client on the operative side. When the client is turned, abduction pillows or abduction splints should be used between the knees. The nurse can also support the client's right ankle and right thigh to maintain abduction of the hip during turning. Sandbags can also be used to prevent external rotation of the hip. When the head of the bed is raised, remember that the hip should not be flexed beyond 90 degrees.

3. The pillow (or an abduction splint) prevents external rotation, supports the legs and prevents adduction. Adduction of the right leg past the midline can cause the right hip to dislocate.

4. Any activity that forces the hip into more than 90 degrees of flexion puts this client at risk for hip dislocation. These activities include using a low chair or a low commode, stooping, and bending. Any activity that causes the leg on the operated side to cross the midline, such as leg crossing, can cause dislocation of the affected hip.

5. It is important that activities are normalized as early as possible to lessen the complications of bed rest. Specifically, complications such as skin pressure ulcers, venous thrombosis, atelectasis, pneumonia, and contractures are prevented with early mobility.

Chapter 10

1. Questions to ask the client regarding the rash include:
   - Is there a family history of psoriasis?
   - Are you on any current or new medications?
   - Has here been any local trauma or irritation to the skin recently?
   - Have you had any recent infections?
   - Have you ever been tested or diagnosed with HIV?
   - When did the rash begin?
   - Ask the client to describe the course of the rash.
   - Does the rash itch or is it painful?
   - Have you used any new soaps, detergents, or lotions?
   - Have you had any exposure to any toxic substances?
   - Have you ever noticed what time of year you usually experience the rash?
2. Psoriasis is a chronic skin condition that affects approximately 3% of the population. It usually peaks during adolescence and young adulthood, and then reoccurs in the later adult years. The cause of the skin disorder is unknown. Some evidence indicates the condition can be familial and can be exacerbated by stress and cold climates. The plaques are thought to be produced from an overactive production of the skin cells, along with inflammation of the dermis and epidermis.
3. Psoriasis is a chronic skin condition that may require long-term treatment. The goal of treatment for psoriasis is to control the skin condition. To maintain control of the disorder and/or to prevent psoriasis the client will need to be compliant with recommended therapies.
4. Over-the-counter products that are useful for controlling psoriasis include emollients such as Eucerin™ cream, Lubriderm Moisture Plus™, or Moisturel™. For scalp involvement, the coal tar shampoos are recommended. Encourage daily use of these products and stress the importance of daily routines.
5. Outdoor environments are safe as long as the client wears sunscreen with a sun protection factor (SPF) of 15 or greater to protect the skin from burning. Sunlight exposure may help this chronic skin condition. However, a few clients will react differently to the sun, and it may even cause the psoriasis to worsen. Therefore, initial exposure to the sun should be limited to determine how the skin will react to the sunlight exposure.

Chapter 11

1. Background information that would demonstrate how the client is "reacting" to the diagnosis would include identification of social support systems, religious and cultural beliefs, and discussion of coping strategies that the client has utilized in the past to deal with life's dynamic changes.
2. A multisystem disease is one that eventually can affect every body organ. The progression of a multisystem disease can lead to changes in how each of the body's organ systems handles everyday immune responses.

3. Diagnostic tests that would serve to provide a baseline include antinuclear antibody (ANA), complement assay, ESR, CBC, and urinalysis. Depending on client's status at time of diagnosis, specific symptom complaints and results from baseline labs may require further testing to determine organ involvement.
4. Discharge planning should include measures aimed at minimizing stress, and establishing rest periods. Symptom management may require the use of medications such as NSAIDs to provide relief from arthritis manifestations. Skin protection along with proper skin care should be promoted to prevent possible exacerbation of disease. Client should be instructed to avoid potential infection exposure as this can cause exacerbation of problems in a client who already has an altered immune response. Adequate nutrition should be stressed to help the client remain well hydrated and maintain ideal body weight. Since the client is of childbearing age, birth control selection should be discussed since certain methods may be contraindicated for clients with this disease. While pregnancy is not contraindicated, discussion can be directed towards the concept of a "planned" pregnancy at a time when the disease has been in a stable state. Additionally, since the effects of this disease are multisystemic in nature, the client may have to deal with concepts of altered body image and altered coping. Counseling and available support systems should be in place to help the client and family members live with this disease process.

Chapter 12

1. The client with cancer may experience anxiety, for example, as a response to the specific disease, fear of the unknown, and fear of pain, disfigurement, or death. Nursing interventions include allowing the client to express feelings, establishing a therapeutic relationship with client, and assessing the client's level of anxiety. Additionally, informing the client about the disease, expected treatments and outcomes will allow the client a sense of control. Provide the client with resources to assist with coping, such as the American Cancer Society's "I Can Cope" program, which provides counseling, education, and support for clients with cancer.
2. Begin by asking her what information has been provided to her. Even though clients have been provided information, they may not have understood the specific details. Knowing what the client has been told and her level of understanding will assist you in explaining or clarifying information to her. From this point, you will teach her about chemotherapy, radiation, and other treatments that are included in the treatment plan.
3. You will provide the client with information regarding the chemotherapeutic agent, which includes expected side effects, signs of reaction or infiltration, and interventions before chemotherapy, such as taking antiemetics. Side effects should be specific, for example,

nausea, alopecia, xerostomia, bone marrow suppression. To reduce potential complications, you should continually evaluate the client's understanding of the teaching you provide.

4. You should administer an anti-emetic before beginning the chemotherapy. Suggest that the client consume small, frequent meals and drink cool liquids. Provide an atmosphere that is calm and quiet and free from odors. The client may require anti-emetics around the clock to reduce the nausea and vomiting.

5. The client with hair loss may experience a body image disturbance. Interventions should include allowing the client to express feelings and concerns about the change in body appearance. Also, encourage active participation in the management of hair loss, such as purchasing a hairpiece or wig, hats, or scarves. Suggest support programs such as "Look Good … Feel Better." Instruct the client that hair will begin to grow back after the chemotherapy is completed, though the texture and color may be different.

Chapter 13

1. Oral tracheal suction supplies, emergency tracheostomy tray with tracheostomy kit, two sand bags, thermometer, sphygmomanometer, ice collar, and a pole for the IV infusion should be placed in the client's room.

2. Respiratory distress and hemorrhage are most likely to occur during the first 24 hours postsurgery.

3. The client should keep the head neutral while lying in semi-Fowler's position with an ice collar over the incision area when in bed. The client should support her head and neck with her hands behind the neck when turning in bed. The client should turn to her side, then move to sitting at the bedside, and then walk to the bedside chair.

4. You should monitor the dressing for amount and frequency of drainage and degree of tightness around the neck. Assess the lower neck, back of neck, and below the dressing for bleeding. Auscultate the neck for stridor and stertor. Assess the client for numbness or tingling of extremities, lips, or mouth, and for Trousseau's and Chvostek's signs. Assess vital signs, breathing effort, skin color and ask the client about a sensation of tightness around the neck. Assess the client's voice for weakness and tone indicating laryngeal nerve damage.

5. The medication should be taken daily for life, in the morning 1 hour before food or 2 hours after food. The client should not change the brand without consulting the physician.

Chapter 14

1. The predisposition to develop disseminated intravascular coagulopathy in this client may be due to septic shock. Both septicemia and shock are conditions that predispose an individual to the development of DIC. Endotoxins from gram-negative bacteria activate several steps in the coagulation cascade and therefore increase the likelihood of the development of DIC.

2. The nurse has to perform a thorough assessment of the client for other signs and symptoms of this syndrome to be able to do appropriate planning and intervention. In DIC, there are both thrombotic and bleeding manifestations. The assessment finding relating to the left lower extremity points to the possibility that this client has a thrombotic phenomenon occurring in that area. Other areas should be explored to assess the extent of this thrombotic possibility. In addition, measures to assess and control bleeding should be instituted, particularly in areas where direct pressure could be applied. The provider should be notified of these observations so that appropriate interventions could be instituted.

3. Clients who have DIC will have screening tests which includes prothrombin time (PT), partial thromboplastin time (PTT), thrombin time, fibrinogen, platelets, fibrin split products, antithrombin III, and D-dimers. These laboratory tests attempt to evaluate the degree of fibrinolysis that is occurring. In DIC, the normal coagulation mechanisms are enhanced initially. However, excessive clotting activates the fibrinolytic system eventually, which in turn lysis the newly formed clots. This process increases the fibrin split products, which inhibit normal clotting because of their anticoagulant properties. These mechanisms can be deduced by examining the results of these laboratory tests.

4. The typical DIC presentation will show the following laboratory results: prothrombin time—prolonged; PTT—prolonged; thrombin time—prolonged; fibrinogen—reduced; platelets—reduced; fibrin split products—elevated; antithrombin III—reduced, and D-dimers—elevated.

5. Ineffective Tissue Perfusion, Decreased Cardiac Output, Acute Pain

Chapter 15

1. The procedure is usually done under local anesthesia. A piece of tissue will be surgically removed from the breast, using a small incision. The section of removed tissue will be sent to the laboratory for histologic examination.

2. The client who undergoes a breast biopsy and is later informed that she has a malignancy will have the following possible nursing diagnoses included in her care plan: Anxiety, Decisional Conflict, Anticipatory Grieving, Risk for Disturbed Body Image.

3. A mastectomy causes changes in the client's body image. The client and her husband may have anxiety and fear about the diagnosis and the resulting body changes that may occur with treatment and interventions.

4. The nurse should provide up-to-date written material and assist the client understand the options she has for treatment. The nurse should answer all questions posed by the

client. For those questions she is unable to answer, the nurse should assist the client in writing them down so that the provider may clarify them. Attentive listening and therapeutic communication techniques should be employed throughout the discussion with the client. The nurse should also share information about the American Cancer Society's programs for the woman with breast cancer, making a referral as soon as the diagnosis is made.

5. Modified radical mastectomy is the removal of breast tissue and lymph nodes under the arm, leaving the chest wall muscles intact.

Chapter 16

1. This procedure is typically done on an outpatient basis and generally requires less intensive nursing care than with some other types of surgery. Questions to ask this client include the questions typically asked of a preoperative client as well as a few particular to this procedure:
   - The time of the last intake of food or fluids (includes smoking and gum chewing)?
   - What medications, if any, were taken on the morning of surgery?
   - Are there any remaining questions about the procedure?
   - Who is available to drive the client home after surgery?
   - Does the client have someone to help at home as needed after the procedure?
   - Does the client have dark glasses available to use following surgery?

2. Assessments typically done in the preoperative period: baseline vital signs, general physical assessment, and results of preoperative laboratory or diagnostic tests.

3. Postoperative care includes the following:
   - Baseline assessments as for all postoperative clients: vital signs, level of consciousness, status of dressing
   - Maintain eye patch or eye shield in place to prevent injury to eye, and instruct client not to rub or touch the area.
   - Elevate head to 30–45 degrees and have client lie on back or unaffected side (to reduce intraocular pressure); use small pillows at sides of head to immobilize head when lying on back.
   - Instruct and assist the client to avoid activities that increase IOP, such as coughing or sneezing. If these are necessary, client should do so with mouth open.
   - Maintain client safety: orient to environment, keep articles and call bell on unaffected side, use side rails with stretcher/bed/chair in low position, and assist with ambulation.
   - Give antibiotic, anti-inflammatory, and other prescribed topical (eye) or systemic medications.
   - Give analgesics as ordered, avoiding or using caution with opioids to prevent postoperative nausea, vomiting, and constipation; discomfort may be described as achy or scratching; avoid morphine, which can cause miosis.

- Assess for possible surgical complications that should be reported immediately to preserve sight: sudden sharp eye pain (possibly indicating hemorrhage, sudden rise in IOP or other ocular emergency), hemorrhage, retinal detachment (client sensations of flashes of light, floaters, or a curtain being drawn over the eye), corneal edema—noted by a cloudy appearance to cornea (may not be visible if dressing in place).

4. The following points are included in discharge teaching:
   - Leave eye shield in place until the surgeon's office visit; then use eye shield at night during sleep for eye protection.
   - Avoid rubbing, scratching, touching, squeezing, or putting pressure on surgical eye.
   - Avoid activities that increase intraocular pressure (sneezing, coughing, vomiting, straining, moving rapidly, bending, or lifting more than 5 pounds).
   - Maintain sedentary lifestyle for approximately 2 weeks or as prescribed by surgeon.
   - Avoid reading until allowed by surgeon, and then read in moderation during healing.
   - Use measures to prevent constipation (adequate fiber and fluid intake, maintain mobility, use stool softener prn).
   - Wear sunglasses with side shields when outdoors (photophobia).
   - Proper techniques for use of eye patch or shield and/or instillation of eye drops
   - Medication names, dose, schedule, side effects, purpose, and anticipated duration of use
   - Symptoms to report to provider: new, increased or severe eye pain or pressure, decreased vision, redness, cloudiness, drainage, floaters or light flashes, halos around brightly lit objects

5. The client's vision may take several weeks to stabilize as healing occurs. A final prescription for corrective lenses will be given once vision has stabilized. In the meantime, it is very important to keep all follow-up appointments.

Chapter 17

1. The triage category would be "emergent" based upon potential for extensive organ system damage.

2. The priorities in treating this client are:
   - Stabilization of ABCs
   - Supplemental oxygen
   - IV access
   - Determination of medication serum level at present and serial levels
   - Prevention of further absorption and enhanced elimination of medication
   - If acetylcysteine (Mucomyst) is used, do not give charcoal to prevent binding of the antidote to the drug.

3. The methods that could be utilized to decrease absorption of this medication are:
   - Gastric lavage
   - Administration of activated charcoal

- Enhanced elimination may be of some use for medications primarily absorbed in the lower GI tract
- Hemoperfusion
- Remember that an alteration in mental status may preclude the use of any or all of these methods unless the airway has been protected by endotracheal intubation.

4. Suggestions for the three priority nursing diagnoses for this client would be:
   - Fluid Volume Deficit related to detoxification and elimination treatments
   - Risk for Impaired Tissue Perfusion
   - Risk for Injury

5. Three evaluation criteria indicating successful treatment of this client could include any of the following:
   - Absorption is minimized and toxic by-products are reduced.
   - Tissue integrity is maintained.
   - Fluid volume deficit is corrected.
   - Tissue and organ perfusion is adequate.
   - No further organ damage occurs.

Index

Page numbers followed by b indicate box; those followed by f indicate figure; those followed by t indicate table.